BASIC SKILLS

IN

# INTERPRETING
# LABORATORY DATA

ILLUSTRATED WITH CASE STUDIES

SECOND EDITION

SCOTT L. TRAUB, EDITOR

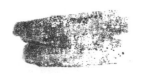

Correspondence to the authors should be sent in care of the publisher, American Society of Health-System Pharmacists, 7272 Wisconsin Avenue, Bethesda, MD 20814.

The information presented herein reflects the opinions of the authors and reviewers. It should not be interpreted as official policy of ASHP or as an endorsement of any product(s).

The authors and ASHP have made every effort to ensure the accuracy and completeness of the information presented in this book. However, the reader is advised that the publisher, authors, contributors, editors, and reviewers cannot be responsible for the continued currency of the information, for any errors or omissions, and for any consequences arising therefrom. Both internal and external reviewers have scrutinized the information presented. However, tests are continually subject to improvements, new applications, changes in reference ranges, and the discovery of interferences. Final determination of the information's suitability remains the sole responsibility of the practitioner.

Produced by the American Society of Health-System Pharmacists' Special Projects Division.
Page design: Hector L. Coronado.

ISBN: 1-879907-62-3

# Contents

## Chapters

## Appendices

*This book is dedicated to*

*my mother (in memoriam),* whose memories inspired me to persevere;

*my father,* for his example in pursuing and accomplishing difficult goals;

*my wife,* for her encouragement, understanding, sacrifice, and devotion to our family;

*my children,* for making this and everything worthwhile.

# Introduction

This book aims to familiarize allied health care providers with the fundamentals of interpreting clinical laboratory test results. Most of the tests discussed are performed in the clinical laboratory and involve biochemistry. Pulmonary function tests, some cardiac tests (e.g., electrocardiogram), and arterial blood gases are exceptions. They are included because of their importance in diagnosis and in the selection and monitoring of drug therapy. The scope of this book is limited to tests that are routinely available at most laboratories and hospitals. With few exceptions, investigational or research assays are not included.

This book is geared primarily to the entry to midcareer, general practitioner who has had only limited experience working with laboratory test results but who wants to develop skills in this area. A glossary of *contextual* definitions is included (Appendix C) to help readers who do not have an extensive medical vocabulary. The allied health student (who does not need to study the analytical and procedural aspects of tests) also may find this book useful as a primary text in a clinical laboratory data course or as a reference for a therapeutics or diagnostics course.

Chapters and discussions are organized primarily by disease or organ system; however, some sections use a "test" perspective (e.g., Chapters 14, 16, and 17). Consequently, some tests are described in more than one chapter. To minimize redundancy, each chapter covers only pertinent aspects of such tests but interchapter referrals are given. In addition, comprehensive indexing allows the reader to locate various clinical applications and interpretations of these tests easily.

Readers must have a basic knowledge of anatomy and physiology, at least as they relate to the mechanisms behind the changes in test results. Therefore, chapters on tests related to specific organ systems or diseases (Chapters 6–17) are prefaced with pertinent anatomy and physiology.

As its title implies, this book emphasizes the *interpretation* of laboratory test results as opposed to the (1)

chemical or procedural aspects of assays or (2) decisions regarding appropriate test selection. All chapters begin with learning objectives. Chapters 1–3 cover fundamental definitions, concepts, and technologies relating to laboratory testing and should facilitate comprehension of subsequent chapters. Chapters 4 and 5 deal with drugs and are written from a test viewpoint. Chapters 6–17 cover common laboratory tests to assess functional status of and gain information on various body systems.

All material from the first edition has been updated and expanded. Unlike the first edition, *all* chapters (except Chapter 2) include case studies and real-life practical examples of interpreting test results. Although this book is not a "therapeutics" text, the authors have been encouraged to use drug-therapy-related examples to reinforce important points or concepts concerning interpretation of a laboratory test. This emphasis is based on the assumption that many readers already have a sound knowledge base in the drug area and will be able to integrate the new knowledge more easily in this context.

New to this edition are QuickView charts for pertinent tests. These charts provide a "snapshot" of important clinical information, including reference ranges for adults and pediatrics, "critical" values, major tissue or organ locations of natural substances and whether the substances have inherent physiological activity, major causes and mechanisms of "true" abnormal (high, positive, or low) results, time course (after insult) of positive or high tests (i.e., time to onset, peak, and normalization of result), signs and symptoms associated with high (or positive) and low values, diseases and drugs monitored with the test, and significant in vitro drug interferences.

The index entries now include codes for readers to quickly identify whether the information is part of a table (t), figure (f), minicase (mc), or glossary (g).

Scott L. Traub, *Editor*

# Authors

Arasb Ateshkadi, Pharm.D.
Assistant Professor
College of Pharmacy
University of Utah
Salt Lake City, UT

Barry L. Carter, Pharm.D., FCCP
Professor and Chairman
Department of Pharmacy Practice
School of Pharmacy
University of Colorado Health Sciences Center
Denver, CO

Paul Farkas, M.D., FACP
Western Massachusetts Gastrointestinal Associates
Springfield, MA
Assistant Clinical Professor of Medicine
Tufts University School of Medicine
Boston, MA

Douglas R. Geraets, Pharm.D.
Clinical Specialist
Pharmacy Service
Veterans Affairs Medical Center
Iowa City, IA

James B. Groce III, Pharm.D.
Assistant Professor of Pharmacy
Campbell University School of Pharmacy
Buies Creek, NC
Clinical Pharmacist II
Moses Cone Health System
Greensboro, NC
Clinical Instructor of Medicine
University of North Carolina School of Medicine
Chapel Hill, NC

Thomas Hall, Pharm.D., BCPS
Manager, Barnes Inpatient Services
Department of Pharmacy
Barnes and Jewish Hospitals
St. Louis, MO
Associate Professor of Pharmacy Practice
St. Louis College of Pharmacy
St. Louis, MO

Gregory N. Hayner, Pharm.D.
Chief Pharmacist
Haight-Ashbury Free Medical Clinic
San Francisco, CA

Douglas Hyde, M.D.
Western Massachusetts Gastrointestinal Associates
Springfield, MA
Clinical Instructor
Tufts University School of Medicine
Boston, MA

Nancy S. Jordan, Pharm.D., BCPS
Director, Drug Information Services
Holyoke Hospital
Holyoke, MA

Robert J. Kandrotas, Pharm.D.
Director, Critical Care Pharmacology
Miami Childrens Hospital
Miami, FL

Dwight A. Marble, Pharm.D.
Clinical Coordinator
Pharmacy Department
The Genesee Hospital
Greater Rochester Health System
Rochester, NY

Steven J. Melnick, Ph.D., M.D., FCAP
Director, Clinical Pathology
Miami Childrens Hospital
Miami, FL

Gary Milavetz, Pharm.D.
Assistant Professor of Pharmacy
Division of Clinical and Administrative Pharmacy
College of Pharmacy
University of Iowa
Iowa City, IA

Mitchell A. Pelter, Pharm.D., FCSHP
Drug Education Coordinator
Kaiser Permanente
Woodland Hills, CA

Scott L. Traub, Pharm.D.
Director of Clinical Research
Mercy Hospital
Springfield, MA
Adjunct Associate Professor of Clinical Pharmacy
Massachusetts College of Pharmacy
Boston, MA

# Nonreviewer Contributors

Roger S. Manahan

Mary Sheehan

Edmund Terwilliger

Alison Viturale

# Reviewers

Bruce H. Ackerman, Pharm.D.

William M. Bennett, M.D.

Rosemary R. Berardi, Pharm.D.

Paul M. Beringer, Pharm.D.

Marianne Billeter, Pharm.D., BCPS

James F. Buchanan, Pharm.D.

Henry L. Bussey, Pharm.D., FCCP

R. Keith Campbell, R.Ph., FASHP

Mary H. Chandler, Pharm.D., FASHP, FCCP

Judy W. M. Cheng, Pharm.D.

Elaine Chiquette, Pharm.D.

Larry A. Cohen, Ph.D.

Thomas J. Comstock, Pharm.D.

Betty L. Dong, Pharm.D.

David Dunlop, M.P.A., Pharm.D.

Douglas Fish, Pharm.D.

John F. Flaherty, Jr., Pharm.D., BCPS

Richard Gannon, Pharm.D.

Mary B. Gross, Pharm.D., FASCP

Robert L. Hagan, Ph.D.

Philip Hansten, Pharm.D.

Anthony Hill, M.S., S.M., ASCP

Cary E. Johnson, Pharm.D.

Marshal Jordan, M.D.

Hugh F. Kabat, Ph.D.

George E. Karras, M.D.

William D. Kiss, M.D.

Rachel L. Kleiman-Wexler, Pharm.D., M.S.

Karen E. Koch, Pharm.D., BCPS

Wayne A. Kradjan, Pharm.D.

Dustin G. LaBreche, Pharm.D., BCPS

Thomas Lachapelle, Pharm.D.

Dorothy Lakoma, M.T., M.S.T., ASCP

Neal Lakritz, M.D.

Victor Lampasona, Pharm.D.

Lewis Leffer, M.D.

Joanne Levin, M.D.

Maryann Liebel, M.T., S.C., ASCP

Thomas Lonergan, Pharm.D.

Joy Longley, Pharm.D.

David Lutomski, M.S.

Hilary D. Mandler, Pharm.D.

Howard E. McKinney, Jr., Pharm.D., DABAT

Michael Montagne, Ph.D.

Bruce A. Mueller, Pharm.D., BCPS

Sid Nelson, Ph.D.

David P. Nicolau, Pharm.D.

David J. Osterberger, Pharm.D.

I. Desmond Padhi, Pharm.D.

Kohar M. Pelter, R.N., M.N.

Roy A. Pleasants, Pharm.D.

Joan M. Poutre, M.T., ASCP

David M. Poppel, M.D.

Frank Pucino, Pharm.D.

Carol B. Pugh, Pharm.D.

Beth H. Resman-Targoff, Pharm.D.

William L. Rock, Jr., Pharm.D.

Arthur A. Schuna, M.S., FASHP

Kulvinder K. Singh, Pharm.D.

Julie A. Sjolander, Pharm.D.

James V. Snider, Ph.D.

Christine A. Sorkness, Pharm.D.

Sarah A. Spinler, Pharm.D.

James E. Tisdale, Pharm.D.

Wynn W. Waite, Pharm.D.

Robert T. Weibert, Pharm.D.

Laurie A. Wesolowicz, Pharm.D.

John R. White, Jr., Pharm.D.

David A. Williams, Ph.D.

Michael E. Winter, Pharm.D.

Ann K. Wittkowsky, Pharm.D.

Lloyd Y. Young, Pharm.D.

# Chapter 1

# Definitions and Concepts

*Scott L. Traub*

Like many fields, laboratory medicine has its own special jargon. This chapter aims to familiarize the reader with the common terms and concepts used. It also covers the underlying rationale and principles governing test selection and interpretation of results. Comprehension of the material in subsequent chapters can be facilitated by first understanding the discussion here.

The major definitions and concepts to be covered include quantitative and qualitative tests, normal or reference range, sensitivity and specificity, and predictive value. Without a working knowledge of this material, the practitioner cannot accurately interpret clinical laboratory test results. The basic discussion is supplemented by practical examples and case studies.

## OBJECTIVES

Upon completion of this chapter, the reader should be able to

1. Distinguish quantitative from qualitative laboratory tests.
2. Define and give an example of normal or reference range.
3. List factors that may alter the usual normal range and discuss how they impact the interpretation of laboratory results.
4. Differentiate between assay accuracy and precision.
5. Differentiate between assay specificity and sensitivity and calculate these parameters in a case study.
6. Discuss factors that affect a test's predictive value and calculate the positive and negative values of a test in a case study.
7. Compare and contrast various types of laboratory errors.
8. Identify the common units used in reporting test results and discuss the status of the movement toward the International System (SI).
9. Discuss the considerations and rationale for ordering laboratory tests.
10. Describe a rational approach to interpreting laboratory results.

## QUANTITATIVE AND QUALITATIVE TESTS

Depending on the way that results are reported, laboratory tests are called quantitative or qualitative. Tests, such as serum potassium, where normal values are reported in ranges (e.g., 3.5–5.0 mEq/L) are termed quantitative. Conversely, tests with only positive or negative outcomes are termed qualitative. A urine or serum pregnancy test is qualitative since a woman is either pregnant or not. Tests that are reported with varying degrees of positivity but that do not furnish an exact measurement are termed semiquantitative (e.g., urine glucose result of 1+, 2+, or 3+).

Results of some semiquantitative and qualitative tests are actually measured as a quantity, either automatically within the assay procedure or manually by the technologist. However, the practitioner does not usually see them. Predetermined cutoff points are used to categorize the results as either positive or negative or as small, moderate, or large for semiquantitative tests.

For example, pregnancy tests are based on the fact that concentrations of human chorionic gonadotropin (HCG) gradually rise during early pregnancy. HCG can be measured in the urine. Most assays can detect HCG as low as 25 IU/L, the concentration seen 1 week after conception. Other assays can only measure HCG as low as 500–800 IU/L, which occurs about 3 weeks after conception. By using the more sensitive assay, the technologist would read an HCG concentration of 25 IU/L or greater and would report this result as positive. If the less sensitive assay were used and the HCG concentration were even 50 or 100 IU/L, the result would be reported as negative. In home pregnancy test kits, a (+) sign or color change usually appears. This example illustrates that knowing the predetermined breakpoint may be important for accurate interpretation. (This concept is explored in more detail in the Sensitivity, Specificity, and Predictive Value section.)

In contrast to qualitative tests, the *numerical* result of a quantitative test is compared with its normal range.

## NORMAL OR REFERENCE RANGE

The normal range of a laboratory test is usually determined by applying statistical methods to results from a representative sample of the general population. The normal range represents the range of values where a large percentage (95%) of normal people (i.e., without the illness in question) fall. The mean, or average value, plus or minus two standard deviations is usually taken as the normal range.

Figure 1 shows a normal distribution curve for serum potassium concentrations found in a "healthy" population. The curve's height at each point reflects the number of patients with the corresponding serum concentration on the *x*-axis. The normal range (3.5–5.0 mEq/L) is derived by including the population mean (4.25 mEq/L) and values that fall within two standard deviations (0.75 mEq/L) on each side of the mean. This range encompasses 95% of all concentrations found in people tested.

With this distribution, five asymptomatic people in 100 probably would have a serum potassium lower than 3.5 mEq/L or greater than 5.0 mEq/L. Moreover, one person out of 100 probably would have a serum potassium concentration less than 3.1 mEq/L or greater than 5.4 mEq/L, with no related symptoms. The normal range for potassium, an intracellular cation, is narrow (1.5 mEq/L) compared with sodium (10 mEq/L), an extracellular cation. This difference is predictable since the specimen measured is an extracellular body fluid (i.e., serum).

Some clinical laboratory scientists want to replace the term normal range with reference range or reference interval. These scientists argue that the word "normal" is misleading because a test result may not imply normalcy, even when it falls within the predetermined range.[1] Moreover, the limits of the range are not absolute but, rather, are points beyond which the probability of diagnostic, prognostic, or therapeutic significance begins to increase. In fact, chances are that one in 20 normal individuals has a value outside that range.

Conversely, results within the normal range do not necessarily mean that the clinical picture is normal. For example, a patient with a serum calcium concentration of 10.5 mg/dL (reference range: 8.5–10.8 mg/dL) may exhibit hypercalcemic signs or symptoms (Chapter 6).

Because reference ranges are determined statistically, the practitioner must remember the laws of probability when interpreting them. With automated analyzers, 12 or more assays may be run quickly on a single specimen with no more effort and scarcely more cost than performing a single test. In fact, this procedure is done routinely on admission in some hospitals. If one test is run, a 5% chance exists that the result will be outside the normal range despite the absence of related disease. If 12 tests are run, a 46% chance $[1-(0.95)^{12}]$ exists that one test will have a false-positive result; if 20 tests are performed, a 64% chance exists. Although the result may be abnormal, it is meaningless clinically. The astute clinician should not take any action without the presence of related signs or symptoms unless the result is so far beyond the reference range that signs and symptoms are imminent.

Some laboratories use the term *critical value* for a result that is far enough outside the normal range that it portends impending morbidity (e.g., potassium <2.5 mEq/L). Because laboratory personnel are not in a position to consider mitigating circumstances, they would call a responsible primary care provider immediately (based solely on the numbers). Theoretically, values outside the predetermined breakpoints usually warrant immediate action, no matter what the mitigating factors. "Critical" values may not always be so critical, however, because the normal range may vary for many reasons.

## FACTORS AFFECTING NORMAL RANGE

Factors that may change the usual interpretation of the normal range, reported by the laboratory, appear in Table 1. Examples of some factors are discussed below. All of them are discussed more fully in later chapters. Because of the increasing geriatric population, the effect of old age on the normal range is covered in more detail than the other factors. Most potential pitfalls can be avoided by referring to the reference range printed on the lab report as opposed to comparing the patient's result to some generic range committed to memory.

### Specimen Analyzed

Specimens commonly analyzed for laboratory tests are se-

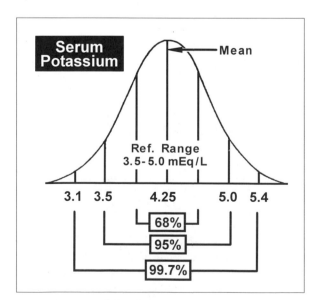

**FIGURE 1.** Normal distribution curve for serum potassium.

**TABLE 1.** Factors Affecting the Normal Range

| | |
|---|---|
| **Specimen analyzed** | **Assay used and form of analyte** |
| Serum | Free |
| Blood (venous or arterial) | Bound |
| Cerebrospinal fluid | **Nutritional status** |
| Urine | **Food and temporal relationships** |
| **Population studied** | Time of day |
| **Demographics** | Time of last dose |
| Age | Time of last meal |
| Sex | **Drugs** |
| Height | **Unit of measurement used** |
| Weight | |
| Body surface area | |

rum (or plasma), blood (venous or arterial), cerebrospinal fluid (CSF), and urine. The normal range for a substance in one body fluid may be quite different from that in another. For example, when diabetes is diagnosed or monitored, glucose is commonly measured in the serum where its reference range (depending on the laboratory) is 70–120 mg/dL if drawn during fasting. In contrast, the reference range for glucose in the CSF—a less frequently ordered test for the diagnosis of meningitis—is lower (50–75 mg/dL) and dynamic. A CSF glucose concentration that is less than 50% of a simultaneous serum concentration is consistent with bacterial meningitis.

Identifying the specimen type can be confusing because clinicians misuse terminology. For example, "serum glucose" is inappropriately referred to as "blood glucose" even though the use of whole blood for this assay is essentially obsolete. Therefore, a patient's value should be compared with the normal range used by the laboratory performing the assay, and the type of specimen analyzed (e.g., urine, plasma, serum, blood, CSF, and joint fluid) should be noted. The definitions for most specimen types can be found in the Glossary.

## Population Studied

Even if the same assay and equipment are used, reference ranges may differ among laboratories. This difference occurs because some laboratories determine their own normal ranges from local populations. The variability, however, is usually not significant. For example, one lab's range for sodium may be 136–145 mEq/L while another's range may be 134–143 mEq/L. Occasionally, however, local population differences can significantly affect a laboratory's reference ranges for some tests. For example, if iodine deficiency is endemic due to regional dietary factors, reference ranges for certain thyroid tests may be quite different compared with those from other areas.

## Demographics

In addition to population characteristics, the normal range of a given test may vary depending on a patient's demographics (e.g., age, sex, height, weight, and body surface

area). With respect to gender, a woman's normal creatinine clearance (CrCl) is typically less than a man's at any age (Chapter 7). Normal values for clearance or filtration rates (e.g., glomerular filtration rate or GFR) are often standardized to a body surface area of 1.73 $m^2$, where surface area is derived from the patient's height and weight.

Age is probably the most clinically important demographic factor. For example, a vast difference sometimes exists between the normal range in adults and that in newborns, infants, and children. In the adult age group alone, accepted "normal" cholesterol concentration increases with age. Until recently, research has been scarce on whether reference ranges should be adjusted for healthy persons over 65–70 years of age. Older studies looked at mean values in this population but often did not exclude patients with related diseases or abnormalities.

In an excellent review, Coodley and Coodley reached conclusions based primarily on studies that attempted to exclude elderly subjects with any trace of disease.[2] With these disease limitations, their conclusions were sometimes different from other authors. Table 2 combines their analysis with that of other recent reviews[3–6] where the four categories relate to healthy elderly persons. Relative to the usual normal range, tests results in this group are expected to change, and changes are clinically significant; expected to change, but changes are not clinically significant; expected not to change, yet results should be interpreted differently; or expected not to change, and values can be interpreted as they are in younger populations.

Unfortunately, with the exception of cholesterol, few clinical laboratories use age to adjust their reference ranges. The following discussion offers additional detail.

### *Electrolytes*

Serum electrolytes (e.g., sodium, potassium, chloride, carbon dioxide, magnesium, calcium, and phosphorus) do not move out of the usual normal range as one ages. The normal range for serum creatinine (SCr) is also stationary, but "normal" results must be interpreted differently in the elderly. CrCl, however, is a better assessor of renal function and the classic parameter that declines with age. In fact, age-adjusted normal values are widely accepted (Chapter 7). Calcium concentrations increase slightly in postmenopausal women, while men experience a slight decrease with age. Despite these changes, most authorities agree that separate calcium ranges are not needed for geriatric patients.

### *Glucose and Lipids*

Glucose tolerance decreases with age; 1-hr postprandial glucose concentrations rise by 10 mg/dL/decade after age 30. Although glucose tolerance diminishes, fasting blood glucose does not rise significantly (1–2 mg/dL/decade).

**TABLE 2.** Effects of Old Age and Its Clinical Significance on Laboratory Test Results[a]

| | Expected Test Results in Healthy Elderly Persons Compared to Young Adults | |
| Significance | Changed | Not Changed |
| --- | --- | --- |
| Clinically significant | Arterial oxygen pressure ($P_aO_2$) [↓][b]<br>1-hr postprandial glucose [↑]<br>Serum cholesterol [↑/↓]<br>CrCl [↓] | Serum creatinine (SCr)<br>Blood urea nitrogen (BUN) |
| Minimally or not clinically significant | Erythrocyte sedimentation rate (ESR) [↑]<br>Serum albumin [↓]<br>Serum uric acid [↓]<br>Fasting serum glucose [↑]<br>Creatine kinase (CK) [↓]<br>Serum iron [↓]<br>Alkaline phosphatase (ALP) [↑]<br>Triglycerides [↑] | Hemoglobin (Hgb), hematocrit (Hct), red blood cell (RBC) indices<br>White blood cells (WBCs) and differential<br>Platelets<br>Sodium, potassium, chloride, carbon dioxide, magnesium, calcium, phosphorus<br>Coagulation tests<br>Liver enzymes and bilirubin<br>Thyroid function tests<br>Uric acid |

[a]Compiled from References 2–6.
[b]Bracketed values [↑/↓] indicate the usual direction of the change in the elderly.

Chapter 12 offers further information on glucose.

Serum cholesterol concentrations increase with age from 20 to 65 years and then level off or decline slightly. This late decline may be a by-product of a survival phenomenon (i.e., individuals who had high cholesterol earlier in life have already died[2]). Triglyceride concentrations also increase between the 3rd and 8th decades, but the rise is only 30–50% and does not exceed 250 mg/dL. Therefore, only elderly patients with concentrations greater than 250 mg/dL (fasting) require further evaluation. No immediate morbidity is associated with hypertriglyceridemia until concentrations surpass 600 mg/dL. At this point, the risk of acute pancreatitis increases (Chapter 13).

### Enzymes

Enzymes, such as creatine kinase (CK), have been shown to decrease after 60–70 years of age in most groups. The mean values in men and women over 70 are 21 and 14.5% below the reference population, respectively.[7] Although these differences may be statistically significant, they are probably not clinically significant enough to establish a separate normal range or modify interpretation for elderly patients. The magnitude of increase in CK needed before disease [acute myocardial infarction (AMI), stroke, and muscle damage] is considered is great.

Serum concentrations of the pancreatic enzymes, amylase and lipase, do not change in the elderly. Most enzymes associated with the liver [SGOT or aspartate aminotransferase (AST) and SGPT or alanine aminotransferase (ALT)] and bilirubin change minimally in geriatric populations. One exception may be alkaline phosphatase (ALP), which increases by 20% between the 3rd and 8th decades. This increase may be due to age-related changes in bone metabolism. In the elderly, a significant increase (>20% above the upper limit of the reference range) is more likely to come from bone than liver.

### Hematological Tests

The normal ranges of most hematological tests [e.g., hemoglobin (Hgb), hematocrit (Hct), red blood cell (RBC) count, platelet count, mean cell hemoglobin (MCH) or other RBC indices, and white blood cell (WBC) count] do not change with age in the absence of disease (Figure 2). Even though mean serum iron concentrations drop in elderly patients, the decrease is within the usual reference range (50–150 µg/dL). In general, coagulation tests, such as prothrombin time and partial thromboplastin time (PTT) but excluding fibrinogen, do not change with age.

### Albumin

Some studies show decreased serum albumin in the elderly, but this change may be related to dietary intake (a factor that could have been controlled in studies).

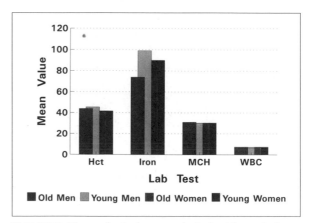

**FIGURE 2.** Hematological test results in healthy ambulatory adults. (Compiled from data in Reference 8.)

## *Erythrocyte Sedimentation Rate (ESR)*

Although the ESR (Westergren method) is listed in Table 2 as changing (clinically insignificant), there are conflicting opinions. A typical normal range is 1–15 mm/hr in men and 1–20 mm/hr in women. Some references use the following age-adjusted upper limits of "normal":[9]

> ➤ Men: $\dfrac{\text{age}}{2}$

> ➤ Women: $\dfrac{\text{age} + 10}{2}$

Although the percent increase in the mean ESR was substantial in one major study,[10] it was within the usual normal range. Some studies found the ESR to rise much higher in subjects older than 80; others found no difference.[8]

Some authors feel that age, per se, does not impact on the ESR and that a subclinical disease causes the gradual increase seen in geriatric populations (Figure 3). Increased plasma fibrinogen and decreased albumin (relative to globulins) in the elderly may be the cause of the rise.

Since in most clinical settings a workup is pursued only if the ESR is greater than 40 mm/hr, the ESR is in the clinically insignificant category in Table 2. ESRs of greater than 80 mm/hr are almost always associated with infection, rheumatic disease, or cancer. (Chapters 14 and 17 offer more information on the ESR.)

## *Thyroid Tests*

The usual normal range for serum thyroxine ($T_4$) remains applicable throughout life. Both production and degradation of $T_4$ decrease with age, so concentrations stay constant. Serum concentrations of the other major thyroid hormone, triiodothyronine ($T_3$), decline 10–15% in the elderly.

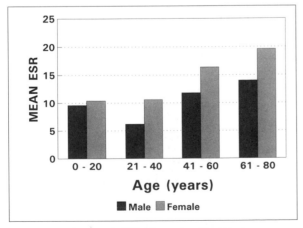

**FIGURE 3.** Changes in ESR (determined by Westergren method) with age and sex. Normal ranges are 1–15 mm/hr for males and 1–20 mm/hr for females. (Compiled from data in Reference 10.)

## Assay Used and Form of Analyte

A normal range may differ significantly with various methods of measurement. For example, the therapeutic range for quinidine varies, depending on the assay used. With a high-performance liquid chromatography assay, the normal range is 1–3 or 1–4 mg/mL; with the enzyme-multiplied immunoassay technique (EMIT, Syva), the normal range is 2–5 mg/mL; and with the single-extraction photofluorometric procedure, the normal range is 2–8 mg/mL.[11] These differences may not seem significant. However, small variations in a drug with a narrow therapeutic margin can mean the difference among nonefficacy, efficacy, and toxicity.

An analyte is the substance measured by the assay. The form of analyte (complexes with biological protein and salts) also influences the normal range. Some analytes, such as calcium and certain drugs, are bound extensively to proteins such as albumin. Only the unbound fraction elicits the physiological or pharmacological activity; bound substances are inert. Most assays measure the total—combination of bound and unbound—substance. Normal ranges for free (unbound) analytes may be quite different. For example, the normal range for *total* serum calcium is 8.5–11 mg/dL; for unbound or *free* (also called ionized) calcium, it is 4.6–5.2 mg/dL. (Chapter 6 and the following Nutritional Status section discuss other factors, such as albumin concentration, that may confound interpretation of serum calcium.)

Other analytes are divided into types, called fractions and subforms. Biological substances, such as bilirubin, are conjugated to form more water-soluble salt forms for easier excretion. For differential diagnosis purposes, clinicians often order bilirubin fractions or subtypes (Chapter 11). For example, the reference range for total bilirubin is 0.3–1 mg/dL. For the conjugated subform, it is 0.1–0.3 mg/dL; for the unconjugated fraction, it is 0.2–0.7 mg/dL. Similarly, total cholesterol can be separated into fractions such as low-density lipoproteins (LDL) and high-density lipoproteins (HDL). Subforms of enzymes [e.g., lactate dehydrogenase (LDH)] are called isoenzymes.

## Nutritional Status

Malnutrition is usually associated with hypoalbuminemia. As alluded to previously, low albumin concentrations lead to increased concentrations of unbound or ionized calcium ($Ca^{++}$), the physiologically active form. By way of a negative feedback loop, total serum calcium concentrations fall to maintain normal physiological concentrations of the unbound form. Teleologically, the normal range of (total) serum calcium is shifted lower in patients with hypoalbuminemia, a setting common in patients on parenteral nutrition. Low serum albumin concentrations can also affect the interpretation of concentrations of highly protein-bound drugs such as phenytoin and carbamazepine. (This subject is discussed in Chapter 5.)

## Food and Temporal Relationships

The impact of food and temporal relationships, or timing, on the normal range is illustrated best with tests that measure glucose and with drugs or cortisol. Timing refers to how the time of day or the time of blood draw relative to administration of an exogenous substance (e.g., food or drugs) affects expected test results. A fasting glucose concentration may appear abnormally high if a patient eats just before the blood sample is drawn. However, if the nonfasting status is known, the clinician would not misinterpret the concentration. The normal range as it relates to drug concentrations is called the *therapeutic range*. Interpretation of the drug level changes dramatically, depending on when the blood was drawn relative to when the patient received the last dose (Chapter 5).

Serum concentrations of many biological substances ebb and flow throughout the day. However, with the exception of just a few substances (e.g., cortisol and growth hormones), most laboratories and clinicians ignore these circadian rhythms. In a person who works during the day and sleeps at night, a normal 8 a.m. cortisol is 5–25 µg/dL. At 4 p.m., it is 2–9 µg/dL.

Research in chronobiology—the study of the timing of biological events—has intensified over the past 5–10 years. In one recent study of healthy adults in Spain, investigators looked for circadian rhythms of serum concentrations of CK [total creatine phosphokinase (CPK) and creatine kinase isoenzyme MB (CK-MB)], ALT or SGPT, AST or SGOT, γ-glutamyl transpeptidase (GGTP), ALP, cholinesterase, LDH and $LDH_1$, 5′-nucleotide, amylase (pancreatic), and lipase.[12] Except for amylase and lipase, a statistically significant rhythm was detected. Most enzyme concentrations were lower in the morning and peaked around 4 p.m.[12]

These investigators found a maximum daily rhythmic variation of about 10%.[12] Most enzymes that varied during the day had relatively wide references ranges. Furthermore, when clinicians interpret these enzymes in general practice, concentrations as high as 1.5–2 times the upper limit of normal do not raise concern unless (1) they have prior suspicion that something is wrong or (2) other test results assessing the same organ are also high. Therefore, these findings[12] are probably clinically insignificant.

## ACCURACY AND PRECISION

The quality of a quantitative assay is usually measured in terms of *analytical performance*, which includes accuracy and precision. Accuracy is defined as the extent to which the mean measurement is close to the true value. A sample spiked with a known quantity of an analyte is measured many times, and the mean measurement is calculated. An assay with high accuracy produces a mean value that is equal to or very close to the known quantity.

Accuracy of a qualitative assay is illustrated mathematically as

$$accuracy = \frac{TP + TN}{number\ of\ samples\ tested} \times 100\%$$

where TP is the number of diseased persons detected by the test (true positive), and TN is the number of nondiseased persons negative to the test (true negative).

Precision refers to the reproducibility of the assay (i.e., the agreement of results when the specimen is assayed many times). Measurements of accuracy and precision are among the many quality controls that are routinely done by laboratories. Analytical performance is often determined by an outside agency that provides samples to laboratories for testing. The laboratory sends the test results to the agency, which knows the true values, and performance results are then returned to the laboratory.

Practitioners usually assume that modern assays coupled with stringent quality-assurance measures, provided by clinical laboratories, lead to almost perfect analytical performance. This perception is confirmed in practice. Proper interpretation of results from these assays, however, also requires assessment of clinical performance.

## SENSITIVITY, SPECIFICITY, AND PREDICTIVE VALUE

The clinical usefulness or *clinical performance* of a test varies with its sensitivity, specificity, and predictive value. These variables, especially predictive value, depend on the prevalence of the disease in the population tested.[13,14] These concepts (Table 3) are easier to comprehend in the context of qualitative tests.

### Sensitivity

The sensitivity of a test refers to its ability to show positive results in patients who actually have the disease. Some practitioners use the mnemonic PID for "positivity in disease." It is also useful to remember the "n" versus "p" rule. Since sensitivity has no "p" (as in specificity), the clinician needs to remember that the missing letter deals with the opposite type of result. In other words, sensitivity deals with **p**ositive results and specificity deals with **n**egative results.

A test has 100% sensitivity if it is positive in every patient with the disease. For example, the test for phenylketonuria (a genetic error of metabolism) is 100% sensitive because a positive result is seen in all patients with the disease. However, one acquired immunodeficiency syndrome (AIDS) detection test on donated blood is 95% sensitive because it may be negative (in 5%) even though the donor is carrying the AIDS virus. If so, the result is a false negative. The lower the sensitivity, the higher is the chance of encountering a false-negative result and vice versa. Highly sensitive tests are best for ruling out a diag-

**TABLE 3.** Calculation of Sensitivity, Specificity, and Disease Prevalence[a]

| Screening Test Result | Diagnosis[b] | | Total |
| --- | --- | --- | --- |
| | **Diseased** | **Not Diseased** | **Total** |
| Positive | TP | FP | TP + FP |
| Negative | FN | TN | FN + TN |
| Total | TP + FN | FP + TN | TP + FN + FP + TN |
| | Sensitivity $= \dfrac{TP}{TP + FN} \times 100\%$ | | Specificity $= \dfrac{TN}{FP + TN} \times 100\%$ |

[a]*Sensitivity, specificity, and predictive value measure clinical performance, while accuracy measures analytical performance. Disease prevalence has a major impact on predictive value.*
[b]*TP = diseased persons detected by test (true positives); FP = nondiseased persons positive to test (false positives); FN = diseased persons not detected by test (false negatives); TN = nondiseased persons negative to test (true negatives).*

nosis. Since they are more likely to detect all patients with the disease, they are preferable when the clinician does not want to miss the disease in question because it can lead to serious, permanent consequences.

An example of a very sensitive test is the ESR. A normal ESR in patients with suspected temporal arteritis virtually rules out that disease since just about every patient with active disease has an abnormally high result. If not treated with steroids, this disease leads to blindness. Although the test is very sensitive, it is not very specific.

When applied to quantitative assays, sensitivity refers to the range over which the assay can accurately measure an analyte. If a quantitative assay is not very sensitive, it is not able to measure low levels of a substance accurately. For example, a digoxin assay with low sensitivity can accurately measure levels as low as 0.7 ng/mL. However, if the assay produces a reading of less than 0.7 (e.g., 0.4), the result would be reported as "less than 0.7 ng/mL."

At first glance, this result may appear to be clinically useful in all situations since the therapeutic range is 0.9–2 ng/mL. However, if the clinician is trying to determine whether a patient has been taking the prescribed medication, this result may not be useful. For example, the patient could have a level of 0.5 or just 0 ng/mL. The former level implies that the patient has been at least taking the digoxin, although the dose may be too low. However, if the patient's serum concentration is 0 ng/mL, noncompliance (or malabsorption) probably exists.

## Specificity

Specificity refers to the percentage of negative results among people who do not have the disease in question. A useful mnemonic is NIH for "negative in health"; the "p" versus "n" rule is also a memory tool. Since 99.9% of normal persons have negative results when tested for phenylketonuria, the test is 99.9% specific for the disease. The lower the specificity, the higher is the chance of generating a false positive. Tests with high specificity are best for confirming a diagnosis. They are rarely positive

in the absence of the disease in question.

As mentioned previously, an example of a test with low specificity is the ESR. The ESR can become elevated (prolonged) from practically any cause of inflammation, including trauma to the upper respiratory tract from sneezing too hard. The degree of specificity (and sensitivity) of a qualitative assay is determined by the manufacturer's breakpoints for positivity. There is usually a tradeoff between optimizing sensitivity and specificity. This concept of sensitivity was also illustrated previously using pregnancy tests.

When dealing with specificity of quantitative assays, many clinicians are concerned with cross-reactivity. For example, quinine may cross-react with or be measured as quinidine in some assays, thereby decreasing the test's specificity. In this case, the assay is not totally specific for quinidine. A similar interference is vitamin C being detected as glucose in some urine tests (e.g., Clinitest). (Drug interferences with laboratory tests are discussed in detail in Chapters 3 and 5.)

## Predictive Value

The predictive value of a positive result is the percentage of positive results that are actual (true) positives. In other words, it is the probability of disease given a positive test result. The predictive value of a negative result is the probability of no disease given a negative result. Predictive value depends on sensitivity, specificity, and the prevalence of the disease (in question) in the population tested. This concept is illustrated in Table 4.

For a test with equal sensitivity and specificity, the higher the prevalence of a disease in a population, the higher is the predictive value of a positive result. For example, a borderline abnormal SCr level has a higher predictive value for kidney disease in patients in a nephrology unit than in patients in a general medical unit. To reinforce this concept, refer to Minicase 1.

If recent onset of chest pain was not a prerequisite to enrollment in the minicase study, the predictive value would drop significantly. The existence of chest pain al-

**TABLE 4.** Relationship of Sensitivity, Specificity, Disease Prevalence, and Predictive Value of Positive Test

| Sensitivity and Specificity (%) | Prevalence (%) | Predictive Value of Positive Test (%) |
|---|---|---|
| 95 | 0.1 | 1.9 |
|  | 1.0 | 16.1 |
|  | 2.0 | 27.9 |
|  | 5.0 | 50.0 |
|  | 50.0 | 95.0 |
| 99 | 0.1 | 9.0 |
|  | 1.0 | 50.0 |
|  | 2.0 | 66.9 |
|  | 5.0 | 83.9 |
|  | 50.0 | 99.0 |

$$\text{Predictive value of positive test} = \frac{TP}{TP + FP} \times 100\%$$

$$\text{Predictive value of negative test} = \frac{TN}{TN + FN} \times 100\%$$

$$\text{Disease prevalence} = \frac{TP + FN}{\text{number of patients tested}}$$

ready preselects patients who are likely to have an AMI. The lower the prevalence of disease in the population tested, the greater is the chance that a positive test result is an error. This phenomenon is understood intuitively by most clinicians. Therefore, they expect the result to be consistent with the suspected diagnosis based on the patient's signs and symptoms. If the result is not consistent, they assume that the laboratory has made an error.[13]

## LABORATORY ERRORS

A laboratory error occurs when a test's reported result is not the true result. An error usually involves improper handling or timing of specimen collection, faulty reagents, inaccurate transcription, technical performance problems, or interfering substances. Lab errors may be suspected when one of the following situations occurs:

1. An unusual intrapatient trend develops.
2. The error's magnitude is great.
3. The result is not in agreement with a confirmatory test result.

---

### ✎ Minicase 1

A new derivative test for the early diagnosis of AMI, the $LDH_1:LDH_{total}$ ratio, was studied in 2000 patients with chest pain severe and persistent enough to bring them into the emergency room. Investigators argued that a ratio of at least 0.4 (≥40%) was "diagnostic" of an AMI in this setting. A typical reference range for $LDH_{total}$ is 100–250 IU/L; for $LDH_1$, it is 25–85 IU/L. Therefore, an $LDH_{total}$ of 200 with an $LDH_1$ of 80 (ratio = 0.4) would be consistent with an AMI, even though neither test alone is outside the normal range. An $LDH_{total}$ of 350 with an $LDH_1$ of 160 (ratio = 0.46), along with chest pain, would be diagnostic of an AMI. An $LDH_1:LDH_{total}$ ratio of at least 0.4 was considered a positive ratio.

*After reviewing the following results, what conclusions can be made about the clinical performance of this test?*

◆ 12–24 hr after the onset of chest pain:
   TP = 1200 patients with a positive ratio were ultimately diagnosed with an AMI.
   FP = 75 patients with a positive ratio were ultimately diagnosed not to have had an AMI.
   TN = 600 patients with a negative ratio were ultimately diagnosed not to have had an AMI.
   FN = 125 patients with a negative ratio were ultimately diagnosed with an AMI.
◆ 24 hr–5 days after the onset of chest pain:
   TP = 1350 patients with a positive ratio were ultimately diagnosed with an AMI.
   FP = 35 patients with a positive ratio were ultimately diagnosed not to have had an AMI.
   TN = 550 patients with a negative ratio were ultimately diagnosed not to have had an AMI.
   FN = 65 patients with a negative ratio were ultimately diagnosed with an AMI.

**Discussion:** To begin, the various measures of clinical performance must be calculated.

◆ 12–24 hr:
   Specificity = TN/(FP + TN) × 100%
     = 600/(75 + 600) × 100% = 88.9%
   Sensitivity = TP/(TP + FN) × 100%
     = 1200/(1200 + 125) × 100% = 90.6%
   Predictive value of (+) test = TP/(TP + FP) × 100%
     = 1200/(1200 + 75) × 100% = 94%
   Predictive value of (–) test = TN/(TN + FN) × 100%
     = 600/(600 + 125) × 100% = 82.8%
◆ 24 hr–5 days:
   Specificity = TN/(FP + TN) × 100%
     = 550/(35 + 550) × 100% = 94%
   Sensitivity = TP/(TP + FN) × 100%
     = 1350/(1350 + 65) × 100% = 95.4%
   Predictive value of (+) test = TP/(TP + FP) × 100%
     = 1350/(1350 + 35) × 100% = 97.5%
   Predictive value of (–) test = TN/(TN + FN) × 100%
     = 550/(550 + 65) × 100% = 89.4%

In general, this test has excellent clinical performance in diagnosing an AMI 12–24 hr after the onset of chest pain. The clinical performance is even better in patients tested 24 hr–5 days after their chest pain began, since the numbers of false positives and false negatives decline. This test may become as useful as the current gold standard, CK-MB, for the diagnosis of AMI within the first 1–3 days after the insult. It will be particularly useful 3–5 days after symptoms when the total CK and CK-MB have already returned to normal (Chapter 10).

4. The result is inconsistent with clinical information.

Some clinicians use the term lab error only if it leads to an inaccurate or false result—in other words, if a mistake occurs during performance of the assay. Other clinicians include any result (even if accurate) that, if interpreted as usual, would lead to inappropriate action. Laboratory error, in its broadest sense, may not be the fault of laboratory personnel or machinery as is the case in improper collection of a specimen. In these instances, "laboratory error" is a misnomer.

### Inaccurate Results

One type of lab error occurs when the assay does not render true results. This situation occurs if the reagents used have deteriorated or if the technologist misreads or miscalibrates an instrument or improperly prepares the sample. False results are also generated if an interfering substance (e.g., drug or cleaning reagent) is within the specimen to be analyzed or the assay machinery. If an error is suspected, the sample (if available) should be reassayed or the test should be repeated on another sample (Chapter 3).

### Accurate Results with Risk of Misinterpretation

Assays may give true readings, but sometimes the results are still not valid and should not be interpreted as usual or used at all. In this case, the analyte is measured correctly by the assay, but the quantity measured is not always what actually was in the serum (or other specimen) at the time of the draw. For example, improper handling (e.g., lack of refrigeration) could lead to spoiled specimens and falsely low concentrations, especially with enzymes. Incomplete collection of urine for measurement of CrCl or urea nitrogen (used to estimate nitrogen balance in patients receiving parenteral nutrition; Chapter 7) also leads to the reporting of falsely low numbers.

Conversely, excessive delays in running the assay or traumatic blood drawing may cause falsely high concentrations of certain intracellular electrolytes (e.g., potassium and phosphorus) due to hemolysis. With hemolysis, analytes that are in high concentrations within RBCs leak out into the serum (the substance being measured).

As mentioned previously, timing is important in interpreting drug and glucose concentrations. If the specimen is collected too early or too late, accurate but potentially misleading results may be reported. Finally, if patients become so dehydrated that their intravascular volume contracts, certain results will be high until the patient is rehydrated. The high concentration is accurately measured, but it does not reflect what the concentration would have been if fluids had not been depleted from the bloodstream. In this case, however, high concentrations

of some analytes (e.g., potassium) should be interpreted as usual because their physiological activity is still proportional to the measured concentration. If the elevation is from hemoconcentration, the concentrations will return to baseline when fluids are replaced.

## UNITS USED IN REPORTING LABORATORY DATA

As already mentioned, one cause of normal range variation among laboratories is the use of different assay methods. Another cause is the reporting of results with different units. For example, one laboratory may report magnesium concentration in mg/dL, and another may use mEq/L. Some laboratories describe the same units in different ways. The units mg/dL, mg/100 mL, and mg % are equivalent as are μg/mL and mg/L. Enzyme activity is usually reported in some type of unit, but the magnitude varies widely and depends on the method used. Clearance is most commonly measured in mL/min or L/hr, but coagulation test results are reported in seconds or minutes. This lack of standardization can cause confusion and misinterpretation.

During the last 15 years, the American National Metric Council has attempted to standardize units to the International System (SI). Most countries have already adopted this system for clinical chemistry. For example, in SI, the unit of concentration is the amount of substance (moles or millimoles) when the atomic composition is known per liter. Concentrations of substances whose atomic composition may vary (atomic weight is not fixed), such as vancomycin, are reported in traditional units. Most drugs measured in body fluids are expressed as mol/L, μmol/L, or mmol/L. In SI, enzyme activity is reported in moles transformed per second, and measurement of pH remains in its traditional form.[15]

SI was supposed to be used throughout the United States by 1987. In 1988, the *Journal of the American Medical Association* and other specialty journals began reporting SI units only, without conventional units in parentheses. Many other major journals followed. Then, in July 1992, the *New England Journal of Medicine* reversed its approach. Because of reader complaints and the reluctance of U.S. clinical laboratories to report results in the new system, the editors decided to return to conventional units (with corresponding SI units in parentheses).[16] This decision sparked an avalanche of letters published in the April 8, 1993 issue. Writers from the United States supported the retreat, while those from countries that had already adopted the new system were adamantly opposed to it.

The SI Convention, as well as some researchers and clinicians, has advised the pharmaceutical industry to measure and label drugs in moles so that the dosage given can be more closely related to the blood concentration of the drug (in SI units). The industry has not complied, nor does it have any plans to do so at this time. This reluctance probably stems from fears of decreased usage by practitioners who might be concerned about the increased risk of prescribing errors. However, administration of moles of drugs seems logical because each molecule—not each milligram—of drug elicits the pharmacological response when it attaches to its receptor.

Until the industry complies, practitioners should become familiar with moles and, thus, molecular weights of substances to make the conversion from milligrams. A list of commonly used laboratory tests with their usual reference ranges in the traditional and SI units appears in Appendices A and B. In addition, the SI unit equivalents of laboratory values are provided whenever possible throughout this book.

## RATIONALE FOR ORDERING LABORATORY TESTS

Laboratory tests are performed with the expectation that results will aid the practitioner or patient in the following:

1. Discovering occult disease.
2. Confirming suspected diagnosis after signs and symptoms appear.
3. Differentially diagnosing possible diseases.
4. Determining the stage or activity level of a disease.
5. Detecting the recurrence of a disease.
6. Measuring the effectiveness of therapy and guiding its course.

Tests can be categorized as either *discretionary* or *screening*. Some practitioners refer to discretionary tests as diagnostic or definitive. Discretionary investigations could include items 2–6 in the list above. As the name implies, these tests are performed at the discretion of the prescriber, based on a provisional diagnosis or proposal for treatment. Discretionary tests are usually requested after a history is taken and a physical examination is performed.

Screening tests, on the other hand, are performed without a clinical indication either on hospitalized patients (e.g., routine urinalysis or electrolytes) or on healthy outpatients as a preventive or early diagnostic measure (e.g., Pap smear, test for occult blood in stool, serum cholesterol, and tuberculosis skin test).[17] If a result is positive in preventive or early diagnostic tests (usually sensitive but not specific), more definitive or specific tests may be done to confirm the finding.

Screening tests are most valuable when the disease is common, silent, and treatable. Therefore, these tests are most cost effective when applied to the proper segments of the population. For example, colorectal cancer screening tests to detect occult blood in the stool have been shown to provide earlier diagnoses in asymptomatic individuals. As a result, survival rates have dramatically improved. The predictive value and, therefore, the cost effectiveness of this test should improve when screening is done primarily on persons over age 50. The incidence of the disease begins to increase at that age.[18]

Many laboratories group a series of related screening (and diagnostic) tests into one ordering block called a profile, although current trends discourage this practice. A six-test profile often includes the electrolytes (sodium, potassium, chloride, and carbon dioxide), blood urea nitrogen (BUN), and glucose. A 12-test battery may include electrolytes, calcium, glucose, BUN, uric acid, total protein, albumin, cholesterol, AST (formerly SGOT), LDH, and ALP. Depending on the type of information desired, the prescriber can request one or more of the profiles listed. Figure 4 shows a typical requisition or order form.

These profile requisitions are used primarily for the convenience of the requester, although some automated multitest analyzers can process only all or none of the individual tests. Also, the laboratory may spend less to process the entire profile than to perform only those tests that are truly desired. Some clinicians argue that the value of screening profiles is in their ability to provide baseline measurements for future reference. Others argue that the profiles lessen the chance of litigation.

The proponents of screening profiles rely on weak arguments, not actual research. In one study, investigators found that physicians tended to pay little attention to abnormal results from screens.[19] If such a result truly reflects an existing treatable disease, the physician's inaction could be labeled as negligent malpractice. Conversely, if further diagnostic investigation is ordered and no confirmatory results are found, time and money could be wasted. The efficiency of screens and profiles is a controversial subject.[20] In addition to the previously mentioned study, other investigators also suggested that these screening profiles may be wasteful.[13,21–23]

Many prescribers do not select laboratory tests with care or use them optimally.[24] In this era of diagnosis related groups (DRGs), health care reform legislation, and other cost-containment pressures (e.g., managed care programs), physicians, other clinicians, and laboratorians must choose, use, and perform tests cost effectively. A test should not be done if it will be directly or clinically redundant. In other words, the clinician should ask the following questions:

➤ Was the test run recently enough that the result probably has not changed significantly?
➤ Were other tests that provide the same information already done?
➤ Can the needed information be estimated with adequate reliability from existing data?

| CHEMISTRY PROFILE | | Date Ordered | Laboratory Request and Report |
|---|---|---|---|
| Glucose | | | |
| BUN | | | |
| Creatinine | | | |
| Protein, total | | | |
| Albumin | | Doctor | |
| Calcium | | | |
| Bilirubin | | | |
| SGOT—AST | | | |
| Uric acid | | | |
| Cholesterol | | | |
| ELECTROLYTE PROFILE | | Nurse | |
| Sodium | | | |
| Potassium | | | |
| Chloride | | | |
| Carbon dioxide | | | |
| HEART PROFILE | | | |
| CPK—CK | | | |
| CK-MB | | | |
| LDH | | | |
| $LDH_1$: $LDH_{total}$ ratio | | | |
| KIDNEY PROFILE | | | Imprint Patient's Card |
| BUN | | | |
| Creatinine | | | |
| Uric acid | | | |
| Osmolality | | | |
| LIVER PROFILE | | | |
| Bilirubin | | | |
| ALP | | | |
| SGOT—AST | | | |
| SGPT—ALT | | | |
| LDH | | | |
| Total protein | | | |
| Protein electrophoresis | | | |
| Prothrombin time | | | |
| THYROID PROFILE | | | |
| $T_3R$ Uptake | | | |
| $TT_4$ | | | |
| TSH | | | |
| Free $T_4$ | | | |

Date Ordered header box: Routine / Pre-op / Today / Other

Working Diagnosis

**FIGURE 4.** Typical laboratory test requisition form that includes selection by profile.

For example, serum osmolality can be estimated from electrolytes and glucose and CrCl can be estimated from age, weight, and SCr. Moreover, a clinician should ask, "What will I do if results are positive or negative (or abnormal or normal)?" If both answers are the same, the test should not be done.[25] In essence, if the results of a test will not change the diagnosis, prognosis, or therapy, the patient's benefits from this information are not worth the cost.

# RATIONALE FOR INTERPRETING LABORATORY TESTS

To understand the rationale for interpreting specific tests, a practitioner should learn the important characteristics of the substance being tested. Specific questions should be asked to clarify the rationale for requesting a test and for interpreting its result. (Most examples given below are explored in detail in later chapters.)

## Guidelines for Interpretation of Results

For most major tests discussed in this book, a QuickView chart answers the following questions and summarizes information helpful in interpreting results. For each test, only pertinent fields are shown and only concise descriptions are given. Figure 5 depicts the format and content of a typical QuickView chart.

### Does Measured or Isolated Entity Exist Naturally or Normally in Body (Compartment)? If So, Where?

Certain substances or contagium (e.g., bacteria) exist normally in the body, and some are at known concentrations. For example, urine is normally sterile; therefore, no bacteria should grow when it is cultured. Similarly, glucose exists naturally in the blood but not in the urine. If glucose is consistently found in the urine or found in excessive amounts in the blood, or both, diabetes mellitus is likely.

### How Might Entity Get into Body Fluid or Tissue Being Tested? What Is Its Usual Destiny?

Knowing how the substance or contagium gets into the body fluid or specimen being tested should make the rationale for test selection apparent and the interpretation logical. The processes closely resemble pharmacokinetics and may be dubbed "physiokinetics" for nondrug substances. The entity may normally exist outside of the body and enter via ingestion (oral drugs, glucose, and cholesterol), injection (hepatitis, human immunodeficiency virus, and drugs), inhalation (oxygen, carbon monoxide, and tetrahydrocannabinol from marijuana), and topical penetration (bacteria via skin abrasion and cocaine via absorption through nasal mucosa).

Analytes such as vanillylmandelic acid and conjugated bilirubin are metabolites. Their concentrations in body fluids depend on the production of precursors, the supply of enzymes (e.g., monoamine oxidase for vanillylmandelic acid) needed to catalyze their synthesis, their rate of degradation, and their ability to reach the specimen site.

Other substances, such as creatinine, are excreted into the specimen site (e.g., urine). Creatinine is a waste product of muscle metabolism. Because its clearance closely parallels the GFR, creatinine is used to estimate renal function.

Other analytes (usually hormones) are also secreted into the specimen site. For example, the adenohypophysis (anterior pituitary gland) secretes thyrotropin (TSH), growth hormone (somatotropin), corticotropin, follicle-stimulating hormone, and other substances into the bloodstream. Serum concentrations of all these hormones might decrease if the anterior pituitary is damaged.

### Is Entity Preferentially Stored or Concentrated in Any Body Compartments or Organs?

The entity may distribute to or naturally occur in higher concentrations in various parts of the body. With some blood tests, a clinician may assume that a substance has leaked or distributed from damaged tissue to the blood. This assumption is true with liver damage, where high concentrations of enzymes (e.g., AST, LDH, and ALP) leak into surrounding tissue and then into the circulation.

Another example involves bilirubin. Because bile is stored in the gallbladder, elevated serum concentrations of bilirubin are consistent with pathophysiology related to that organ. Likewise, because amylase is produced and stored only in the pancreas and parotid gland, elevated serum concentrations imply problems in one of these areas. In contrast, drugs such as benzodiazepines distribute to the central nervous system (CNS), but their concentration in the blood does not reliably reflect concentrations in the CNS or correspond with pharmacological activity.

### Does Entity Have Normal Function (Physiological Effect) in Body? If So, What Is It?

Hormonal secretion is usually controlled by a negative feedback loop. For example, when $T_4$ concentrations fall below a preset point, the hypothalamus secretes thyrotropin-releasing factor (TRF); TRF causes the anterior pituitary to secrete TSH. TSH then causes the thyroid gland to secrete $T_4$, which increases the basal metabolic rate. When $T_4$ concentrations increase beyond a preset point, inhibition of secretion of TRF occurs, closing the loop. Damage to any gland in the loop leads to decreased $T_4$ concentrations in the serum. All three hormones (and possibly others) should be measured to determine where the fault has occurred in the cycle (Chapter 12).

| Parameter | Description | Comments |
|---|---|---|
| **Common reference ranges** | | |
|    **Adults** | Normal range in adults | Variability and factors affecting range |
|    **Pediatrics** | Normal range in children | Variability, factors affecting range, age grouping |
| **Critical value** | Value beyond which immediate action usually needs to be taken | Disease-dependent factors; relative to reference range; value is a number or multiple of upper normal limit |
| **Natural substance?** | Does susbtance exist naturally in the body? | Is it formed only under abnormal circumstances? |
| **Inherent activity?** | Does substance have any physiological activity? | Description of activity and factors affecting activity |
| **Location** | | |
|    **Production** | Is substance produced? If so, where? | Factors affecting production |
|    **Storage** | Is substance stored? If so, where? | Factors affecting storage |
|    **Secretion/excretion** | Is substance secreted or excreted? If so, where/how? | Factors affecting secretion or excretion |
| **Major causes of . . .** | | |
|    **High (or positive) results** | Major causes | Modification of circumstances/other related causes |
|      **Associated signs and symptoms** | Major signs and symptoms with high or positive result | Modification of circumstances/other related signs and symptoms |
|    **Low results** | Major causes | Modification of circumstances/other related causes |
|      **Associated signs and symptoms** | Signs and symptoms associated with low result | Modification of circumstances/other related signs and symptoms |
| **After insult, time to . . .** | | |
|    **Initial elevation or positive result** | Minutes, hours, days, weeks | Assumes acute insult/modification of circumstances |
|    **Peak values** | Minutes, hours, days, weeks | Assumes insult not removed/modification of circumstances |
|    **Normalization** | Minutes, hours, days, weeks | Assumes insult removed and nonpermanent damage/modification of circumstances |
| **Drugs often monitored with test** | List of typical drugs | Suggested monitoring frequency/other (less typical) drugs |
| **Causes of spurious results** | List of common causes | Modification of circumstances/assay specific? |

**FIGURE 5.** Contents of a typical QuickView chart.

### *Does Assayed Entity Reflect (Patho)Physiology in Question Directly or Indirectly?*

Sometimes it is not possible or convenient to measure the substance desired. Instead, a closely related substance may be tested. For example, total (bound and unbound) serum calcium is an indirect measurement of free, ionized calcium. Similarly, measurement of vanillylmandelic acid, the predominant catecholamine metabolite in the urine, is sometimes used to evaluate patients for pheochromocytoma. Parent catecholamines (e.g., epinephrine and norepinephrine) could be measured directly, but the assay is more complex and not always readily available.

Therefore, vanillylmandelic acid may be used instead as an initial screen. Clinicians should know in which situations the ordered test is a surrogate and, thus, what limitations exist.

## Mechanisms of Abnormal Results

The specific mechanisms of truly abnormal results of quantitative tests are as diverse as the types of pathophysiology the mechanisms reflect. At the risk of oversimplification, the practitioner can separate the general causes into the following mnemonic arrangement:

   1.   Excessive or insufficient intake, production, re-

lease, or secretion *into* a body fluid of the substance being measured.

2.  Excessive or insufficient outflow *from* the body or metabolism within the body of the substance being measured.

3.  Dilution or concentration of the substance being measured, secondary to an increase or decrease in the usual amount of fluid in the compartment from which the specimen is taken.

Excessive intake, production, release, and secretion leads to abnormally high concentrations of the measured substance (e.g., potassium, creatinine, LDH, and $T_4$, respectively), whereas insufficient intake, production, secretion, or release could cause low readings. Excessive outflow also tends to cause concentrations below the normal range. For example, albumin leakage in glomerulonephritis, Hgb loss in hemorrhage, or chloride loss with nasogastric suction leads to low concentrations in the blood. In contrast, insufficient metabolism (e.g., ammonia in liver disease or drugs) causes accumulation and high or toxic concentrations.

The most pertinent example of dilution or concentration involves fluid status. If a patient becomes dehydrated, the amount of fluid in his or her bloodstream decreases, and certain constituents (e.g., sodium, glucose, Hgb, and BUN) become more concentrated. This effect is called "hemoconcentration." The absolute amount of the substance in the body may not have changed. However, because the amount of fluid in which it is dissolved has decreased, the concentration may become abnormally high. Relativity must be applied, or false impressions may arise (as in Minicase 2).

## Tips for Interpretation and Utilization

Clinicians should remember the following checklist when interpreting test results. The common theme is that laboratory test results should not be considered in isolation.

### Test Results versus Signs and Symptoms

Clinicians should consider a test result as only one piece of useful information for making diagnostic or drug therapy decisions. When planning subsequent action, the clinician should usually give more weight to the presence or absence of signs and symptoms associated with the medical problem rather than to a laboratory report. For example, a patient with a potassium level of 3 mEq/L (normal range: 3.5–5.0 mEq/L) who is asymptomatic should not cause as much concern as a patient who has a level of 3.3 mEq/L but is symptomatic. Tests that screen for occult diseases (e.g., colon cancer) are exceptions to this logic because, by definition, the persons being tested are asymptomatic.

---

### ✎ Minicase 2

Norma S., a 78-year-old female nursing home patient, suffered a minor stroke about 5 weeks ago. Her neurological deficits improved to only residual weakness on her left side. She returned from an acute care hospital 12 days ago. Since that time, Norma S. has not been eating much and has been drinking even less. She has a history of chronic iron and folate deficiency anemia with her usual Hgbs around 10 g/dL (normal range: 12–16 g/dL), Hcts around 30% (normal range: 37–47%), iron concentrations around 35 µg/dL (normal range: 40–160 µg/dL), and folates less than 1–3 ng/mL (normal range: 4–15 ng/mL).

Norma S. takes daily iron and folate supplements as well as many other drugs. Her blood pressure has remained stable, but her heart rate has increased (from 70s to 90s) over the past 5–7 days. Her mucous membranes became dry, her skin turgor diminished, and her urine output decreased over that same time. A complete blood count is ordered. Tests indicate that she is no longer anemic with a Hgb of 13 and a Hct of 40. Her BUN is 40 mg/dL (normal range: 8–20 mg/dL), and sodium is 145 mEq/L (normal range: 136–145 mEq/L).

*Has the patient's anemia resolved? What is happening here?*

**Discussion:** An astute clinician should realize that the Hgb, Hct, BUN, and possibly sodium concentrations have become temporarily hemoconcentrated because the patient is dehydrated. Thirst mechanisms sometimes are disrupted after a stroke. Her dry mucous membranes, decreased skin turgor and urine output, and increased heart rate are all consistent with dehydration. As the patient is rehydrated, the Hgb and Hct values should fall below the normal range to her usual baseline.

If the patient is overhydrated, the opposite scenario can occur. Of course, assay interference by drugs, metabolites, and other foreign substances (as well as laboratory error) should always be kept in mind. If hemoconcentration had not been so apparent, laboratory error and interferences might be considered. In that case, the tests should be repeated. (Test interference is discussed in detail in Chapter 3.)

---

### Isolated Results versus Trends

An isolated test result often is difficult to interpret. However, two or more results from the same test done at two different times allow the clinician to establish a more useful trend or pattern. For example, a glucose concentration of 300 mg/dL may cause some concern unless the patient was admitted yesterday for diabetes out of control with a concentration of 500 mg/dL. A series of results adds some perspective to an interpretation. Unfortunately, a series of tests may also increase overall costs.

### Baseline Studies

To establish relativity, some clinicians order baseline studies. Such studies are especially informative when normal ranges are wide or when normal values vary significantly among patients. An example of a test with a wide range is CK (normal range: 35–200 IU/L depending on assay and lab). Because of the potential for certain drugs (e.g., the newer hypolipidemics such as lovastatin) to cause increases in CK and "liver" enzyme concentrations with associated pathology, some practitioners request that this test be done before and intermittently during therapy. If no baseline value exists, it would be difficult to interpret a CK concentration of 200 IU/L (using the above reference range) after 1 month of therapy. Likewise, a baseline value may be important when PTT is used to adjust heparin therapy, since some practitioners use a PTT of 1.5–2.5 times the baseline (as opposed to mean control value) as their therapeutic goal.

### *Rate of Change*

The rate of change of a laboratory value is often related to the risk of presenting with associated signs and symptoms. A patient whose RBC count falls from 5 to 3.5 million/mm³ over several days is more likely to become symptomatic than if the decline took place over several months. Hence, practitioners must remember that temporal relationships are important when interpreting test results.

## SUMMARY

Clinical laboratory tests are convenient, usually noninvasive methods to investigate potential problems with a patient's anatomy or physiology. Without the ability to interpret laboratory test results accurately, knowledge of pathophysiology and therapeutics alone is insufficient to provide high-quality clinical consultations.

This chapter should help the clinician appreciate general causes and mechanisms of abnormal test results. However, results within the normal range are not always associated with lack of signs and symptoms. Many factors, including units used in reporting, can change the normal range. Additionally, knowing the sensitivity, specificity, and predictive value is important in selecting an assay and interpreting its results. An understanding of the definitions, concepts, and strategies discussed should also facilitate mastering information in the following chapters.

## REFERENCES

1. Killingsworth LM. What do the numbers say? *Clin Chem.* 1988; 35:996.
2. Coodley EL, Coodley GO. Laboratory changes associated with aging. *Hosp Physician.* 1993; Jan:12–8, 25–31.
3. Melillo KD. Interpretation of laboratory values in older adults. *Nurse Pract.* 1993; 18(7):59–67.
4. Duthie EH Jr, Abbasi AA. Laboratory testing: current recommendations for older adults. *Geriatrics.* 1991; 46:41–50.
5. Kelso T. Laboratory values in the elderly: are they different? *Emerg Med Clin North Am.* 1990; 8:241–54.
6. Fraser CG. Age-related changes in laboratory test results: clinical implication. *Drugs Aging.* 1993; 3:246–57.
7. Tietz NW, Wekstein DR, Shuey DF, et al. A two-year longitudinal reference range study for selected serum enzymes in a population more than 60 years of age. *J Am Geriatr Soc.* 1984; 32:563–70.
8. Zauber NP, Zauber AG. Hematologic data of healthy very old people. *JAMA.* 1987; 257:2181–4.
9. Wallach J. Interpretation of diagnostic tests: a synopsis of laboratory medicine, 5th ed. Boston, MA: Little, Brown; 1992.
10. Shearn MA, Kang IY. Effect of age and sex on the erythrocyte sedimentation rate. *J Rheumatol.* 1986; 13:297–8.
11. Wooding-Scott RA, Darling IM, Slaughter RL. Comparison of assay procedures used to measure total and unbound concentrations of quinidine. *Drug Intell Clin Pharm.* 1989; 23:999–1004.
12. Rivera-Coll A, Fuentes-Arderiu X, Diez-Noguera A. Circadian rhythms of serum concentrations of 12 enzymes of clinical interest. *Chronobiol Int.* 1993; 10:190–200.
13. Krieg AF, Gambino R, Galen RS. Why are clinical laboratory tests performed? When are they valid? *JAMA.* 1975; 233:76–8.
14. Kraemer HC. Evaluating medical tests. Newbury Park, CA: Sage Publications; 1992.
15. Council on Scientific Affairs, American Medical Association. SI units for clinical laboratory data. *JAMA.* 1985; 253:2553–4.
16. Campion EW. A retreat from SI units. *N Engl J Med.* 1992; 327:49.
17. Holland WW, Whitehead TP. Value of new laboratory tests in diagnosis and treatment. *Lancet.* 1974; 2:391–4.
18. Messner RL, Gardner SS, Webb DD. Early detection the priority in colorectal cancer. *Cancer Nurs.* 1986; 9:8–14.
19. Schneiderman LJ, DeSalvo L, Baylor S, et al. The abnormal screening laboratory result. *Arch Intern Med.* 1972; 129:88–90.
20. Lehmann C, Lekena A. The impact of technology on laboratory ordering strategies. *NY State J Med.* 1985; 85:690–3.
21. Kaplan EB, Sheiner LB, Boeckmann AJ, et al. The usefulness of preoperative laboratory screening. *JAMA.* 1985; 253:3576–81.
22. Durbridge TC, Edwards F, Edwards RG, et al. Evaluation of benefits of screening tests done immediately on admission to hospital. *Clin Chem.* 1976; 22:968–71.
23. Korvin CC, Pearce RH, Stanley J. Admissions screening: clinical benefits. *Ann Intern Med.* 1975; 83:197–203.
24. Kassirer JP. Our stubborn quest for diagnostic certainty: a cause of excessive testing. *N Engl J Med.* 1989; 320:1489–91.
25. Carter PM, Davison AJ, Wickings HI, et al. Quality and quantity in chemical pathology. *Lancet.* 1974; 2:1555–7.

## BIBLIOGRAPHY

Bakerman S, Bakerman P, Strausbauch P. ABC's of interpretive laboratory data, 3rd ed. Myrtle Beach, SC: Interpretive Laboratory Data; 1994.

Berwick DM. Screening in health fairs: a critical review of benefits, risks and costs. *JAMA.* 1985; 254:1492–8.

Fischbach F. A manual of laboratory & diagnostic tests, 4th ed. Philadelphia, PA: J. B. Lippincott; 1992.

Olsen DM, Kane RL, Proctor PH. A controlled trial of multiphasic screening. *N Engl J Med.* 1976; 294:925–30.

Sacher RA, McPherson RA. Widman's clinical interpretation of laboratory tests, 10th ed. Philadelphia, PA: F. A. Davis; 1991.

Speicher CE. The right test: a physician's guide to laboratory medicine. Philadelphia, PA: W. B. Saunders; 1990.

Wallach J. Interpretation of diagnostic tests, 5th ed. Boston, MA: Little, Brown; 1992.

Chapter 2

# Introduction to Common Laboratory Assays and Technology

*Robert J. Kandrotas and Steven J. Melnick*

Clinical laboratory data are used in the diagnosis and treatment of disease. The performance of laboratory tests involves clinical chemistry methodologies to identify and/or quantify clinically important endogenous or exogenous substances. Other laboratory methods—in the areas of hematology, microbiology, and molecular pathology—are used to evaluate a wide range of biological parameters. Although clinicians do not usually perform laboratory tests, they still need an introduction to and a basic understanding of the common methods and techniques. This chapter provides an introduction to these techniques.

Early methods for identification and separation of analytes included flame photometry and paper chromatography. Although recent technological advances have increased the sophistication and complexity of laboratory methodologies, many procedures still rely on the basic principles of those two tests: (1) changes in color or light absorbance and (2) various solubility and polarity characteristics. Even new developments in molecular biology and immunobiology utilize these principles in some test steps.

This chapter reviews the methodologies of some common laboratory tests as well as their principles, their advantages, and their disadvantages.

## OBJECTIVES

Upon completion of this chapter, the reader should be able to

1. List the primary analytes of ion-selective electrodes (ISE).
2. Explain the principles behind turbidimetry and nephelometry.
3. List the basic components of a spectrophotometer and describe the purpose of each.
4. Describe the basis for paper and thin layer chromatography.

5. Compare gas and high performance (or pressure) liquid chromatography (HPLC) with respect to equipment and methodology.
6. Explain the methodologic basis of immunoassays.
7. List common tests done using agglutination.
8. Compare and contrast radioimmunoassay (RIA), enzyme-linked immunosorbent assay (ELISA), enzyme-multiplied immunoassay technique (EMIT), and fluorescent polarization immunoassay (FPIA) with respect to methods and tests performed.
9. Describe the purpose of polymerase chain reaction (PCR).

## FLAME PHOTOMETRY

Although flame photometry is not used often in clinical laboratories today, it is discussed here as an historical framework for the tests currently in use. Concentrations of elements such as sodium, potassium, and lithium were classically determined by flame photometry. It is based on the elementary quantum principle that electrons in an atom are excited to a higher energy level by heat. The electrons, being unstable in this state, then return to a lower energy state; in doing so, the excess energy is liberated as photons in the visible light range.

Usually, multiple energy levels are involved and the resulting spectral patterns are characteristic of each element. When conditions are held constant, the concentration of each ion is proportional to the light intensity at its characteristic wavelength.

## ION-SELECTIVE ELECTRODES

The ISE method, having comparable or better sensitivity than flame photometry, has become the principal test for

**TABLE 1.** Routine Tests Performed by Common Laboratory Assays

| Assay | Analysis Time (min) | Common Tests | Use |
|---|---|---|---|
| ISE | 6–18 | Electrolytes (sodium, potassium, chloride, calcium, lithium, total carbon dioxide) | Primary testing method |
| GC | 30 | Toxicologic screens, organic acids, drugs [e.g., benzodiazepines and tricyclic antidepressants (TCAs)] | Primary testing method |
| HPLC | 30 | Toxicologic screens, vanilmandelic acid, hydroxyvanilmandelic acid, amino acids, drugs (e.g., indomethacin, steroids, cyclosporin) | Primary and secondary or confirmatory testing methods |
| RIA | 15 | Endocrinology (e.g., thyroid) and drugs (e.g., digoxin) | Secondary or confirmatory testing method |
| ELISA | 0.1–0.3 | Serologic tests (e.g., antinuclear antibody, rheumatoid factor, hepatitis B, cytomegalovirus, and human immunodeficiency virus antigens) | Primary testing method |
| EMIT | 0.1–0.3 | General chemistries [e.g., albumin, blood urea nitrogen (BUN), creatinine, glucose, cholesterol, bilirubin, total protein] and enzymes (e.g., acid and alkaline phosphatase, amylase, creatine kinase) Coagulation (e.g., antithrombin III, fibrinogen, fibrinogen degradation products, heparin, plasminogen) Therapeutic drug monitoring (e.g., aminoglycosides, vancomycin, digoxin, antiepileptics, antiarrhythmics, theophylline) Toxicology (acetaminophen, salicylate, barbiturates, TCAs, amphetamines, cocaine, opiates) | Primary testing method |
| FPIA | 0.1–0.2 | Therapeutic drug monitoring (e.g., aminoglycosides, vancomycin, antiepileptics, antiarrhythmics, theophylline, methotrexate, digoxin, cyclosporine) General chemistries (e.g., thyroxine, triiodothyronine, cortisol, amylase, BUN, lactate dehydrogenase, creatinine, glucose, cholesterol, iron) | Primary testing method |
| PCR | 0.1–0.2 | Microbiologic and virologic markers of organisms and genetic markers | Primary testing method |

determining urine and serum electrolytes in the clinical laboratory (Chapters 6 and 7). Typically, ion concentrations such as sodium and potassium are measured using this method (Table 1).

The principle of ISE involves the generation of a small electrical current when a particular ion comes in contact with an electrode. The electrode selectively binds the ion to be measured. To measure the concentration, the circuit must be completed with a reference electrode. The three types of electrodes are

➢ Ion-selective glass membranes.
➢ Solid-state electrodes.
➢ Liquid ion-exchange membranes.

As shown in Figure 1, ion-selective glass membranes preferentially allow hydrogen ($H^+$), sodium ($Na^+$), and ammonium ($NH_4^+$) ions to cross a hydrated outer layer of glass. An electrical potential is created when these ions diffuse across the membrane.

Solid-state electrodes consist of halide-containing

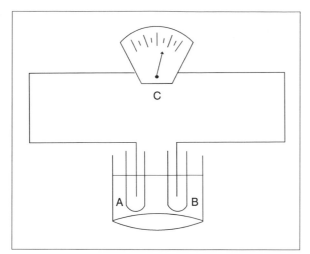

**FIGURE 1.** The pH meter is an example of a test that uses ISE to measure the concentration of hydrogen ions. An electric current is generated when hydrogen ions come in contact with the ISE (A). The circuit is completed through the use of a reference electrode (B) submerged in the same liquid as the ISE (also known as the liquid junction). The concentration can then be read on a potentiometer (C).

crystals for measuring specific ions. An example is the silver–silver chloride electrode for measuring chloride.[1]

Liquid ion-exchange membranes contain a water-insoluble, inert solvent that can dissolve an ion-selective carrier. Ions outside the membrane produce a concentration-related potential with the ions bound to the carrier inside the membrane.[1]

The electrodes are separated from the sample by a liquid junction or salt bridge. Since the liquid junction generates its own voltage at the sample interface, it is a source of error. This error is overcome by adjusting the composition of the liquid junction.[2] Another source of error is the selectivity of the electrode; therefore, careful electrode selection is important. Overall, this method is simple to use and more accurate than flame photometry for samples having a low plasma water due to conditions such as hyperlipoproteinemia.[3]

## TURBIDIMETRY AND NEPHELOMETRY

When light passes through a solution in a cuvet, it can be either absorbed or scattered. Turbidimetry is a simple technique for measuring the percent transmittance of light due to particles such as immune complexes. Nephelometry also is commonly used in immunoglobulin assays (Chapter 17).

The major advantage of turbidimetry is that measurements can be made with common laboratory instruments such as a spectrophotometer. Errors associated with this method center around sample and reagent preparation. Since the amount of light blocked depends on both the concentration and size of each particle, differences in particle size between the sample and the standard result

in error. The length of time between sample preparation and measurement should be consistent since particles settle to varying degrees, allowing more or less light to pass. Large concentrations are necessary because this test measures small differences in large numbers.

Nephelometry is similar to turbidimetry. The main differences are that (1) the light source is usually a laser and (2) the detector to measure scattered light is at a right angle to the incident light. The scattered light is a function of the size and number of particles in the beam. Nephelometric measurements are more precise than turbidimetric ones since the smaller signal generated for low analyte concentrations is more easily detected against a very low background.[4] Because antigen–antibody complexes are easily detected by this method, it is commonly employed in combination with the enzyme immunoassay (EIA) (discussed later).

## SPECTROPHOTOMETRY

Spectrophotometry is used to identify and/or quantify a given substance by measuring the light absorbed at a characteristic spectral region excited by a specific narrow wavelength of light. Because of its rapidity, ease of use, and relatively high specificity, spectrophotometry is commonly employed in conjunction with other methodologies such as nephelometry and EIA (e.g., the spectrophotometer is used to quantitate the reaction produced by an immunoassay). The high specificity typically achieved with spectrophotometry is obtained by reacting the analyte with various substances that produce a colorimetric reaction. This specificity can be further enhanced by first isolating the analyte.

The basic components of the two types of spectrophotometers (single and double beam) are depicted in Figure 2. Light from a source (I) (e.g., a tungsten bulb or

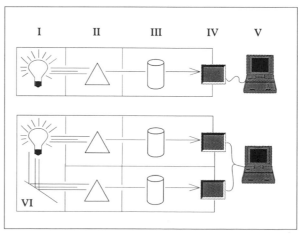

**FIGURE 2.** Schematic of single-beam (upper portion) and double-beam (lower portion) spectrophotometers. I = radiant light source; II = monochromator; III = analytical cuvet; IV = photomultiplier; V = recording device; VI = mirror.

laser) passes through an entrance slit which minimizes stray light. Specific wavelengths of light are isolated by a monochromator (II). The selected wavelength then passes through the exit slit and illuminates the analytical cell (cuvet) holding the test solution (III).

After passing through the test solution, the light strikes a detector—usually a photomultiplier tube (IV).[1] This tube amplifies the electronic signal, which is then sent to a recording device (V). The result is compared with a standard curve to yield a specific concentration.

The double-beam instrument is designed to compensate for changes in absorbance of the reagent blank and light source intensity. It utilizes a mirror (VI) to split the light from a single source into two beams, one passing through the test solution and one through the reagent blank. By doing so, it automatically corrects optical errors as the wavelength changes.

Most measurements are made in the visible range of the spectrum, with some made in the ultraviolet and still fewer in the infrared ranges. To achieve the greatest sensitivity, the selected wavelength of light is usually in the range of maximum absorption. If substances are known to interfere at this wavelength, however, measurements may be made at a different one. This procedure allows detection of the analyte of interest with minimal interference from other endogenous or exogenous substances.

# CHROMATOGRAPHY

Chromatography is used primarily for separation and identification of various compounds. Three types of chromatography are routinely used in the clinical laboratory: thin layer chromatography, gas chromatography (GC), and high performance (or pressure) liquid chromatography (HPLC). Although paper chromatography was used at one time, it is seldom employed today.

Because chromatographic assays require more time for specimen preparation and performance, they are usually performed only when another assay type is not available or when interferences are suspected with an immunoassay (discussed later). Chromatographic assays do not require premanufactured antibodies and, therefore, afford better flexibility than an immunoassay.

## Paper Chromatography

The principle behind paper chromatography is simple and applies in all forms of chromatography. However, quantification of a substance is not possible with this method.

A drop of the sample is placed at the bottom of a piece of chromatography paper and allowed to dry. The paper is then hung in a chromatography jar so that the bottom edge contacts a solvent. Each component, having a different solubility and polarity, migrates toward the top of the paper as the solvent moves by capillary action. After separation is complete (12–24 hr), the paper is sprayed with a developing solution. Various fractions can be identified by how far they migrated on the paper.

## Thin Layer Chromatography

Thin layer chromatography is used for drug screening (Chapter 4) and analysis of clinically important substances such as oligosaccharides and glycosaminoglycans (e.g., dermatan sulfate, heparan sulfate, and chondroitin sulfate). The principles of thin layer chromatography are identical to those of paper chromatography, except that a thin layer of gel applied to glass or plastic is used in place of paper. The gel may be composed of silica, alumina, polyacrylamide, or starch.

Thin layer chromatography is used for both

> Identification and separation of multiple components of a sample in a single step.
> Initial component separation prior to analysis by another technique.

Unlike with paper chromatography, quantification of various substances is possible because each spot can be scraped off and analyzed individually.[1]

While thin layer chromatography is a useful screening technique, it has lower sensitivity and resolution than either gas or high pressure chromatography. Another disadvantage, as with gas and high pressure chromatography, is that someone with skill and expertise must interpret the results.

## Gas Chromatography

GC is used to identify and quantify volatile substances such as alcohols, steroids, and drugs in the picogram range (Table 1). This technique is based on the principles of paper and thin layer chromatography but has better sensitivity. Instead of a solvent, GC uses an inert gas (e.g., nitrogen or helium) as a carrier for the volatile substance. A column packed with inert material, coated with a thin layer of a liquid phase, is substituted for paper or gel.

The sample is injected into the column (contained in a heated compartment) where it is immediately volatilized and picked up by the carrier gas. Heating at precise temperature gradients is essential for good separation of the analytes. The gas carries the sample through the column where it contacts the liquid phase (which has a high boiling point). Analytes with lower boiling points migrate faster than those with higher boiling points, thus fractionating the sample components.

When the sample leaves the column, it is exposed to a detector. The most common detector consists of a hydrogen flame with a platinum loop mounted above it. When the sample is exposed to the flame, ions collect on the platinum loop and generate a small current. This current is amplified by an electrometer, and the signal is sent on to an integrator or recorder.

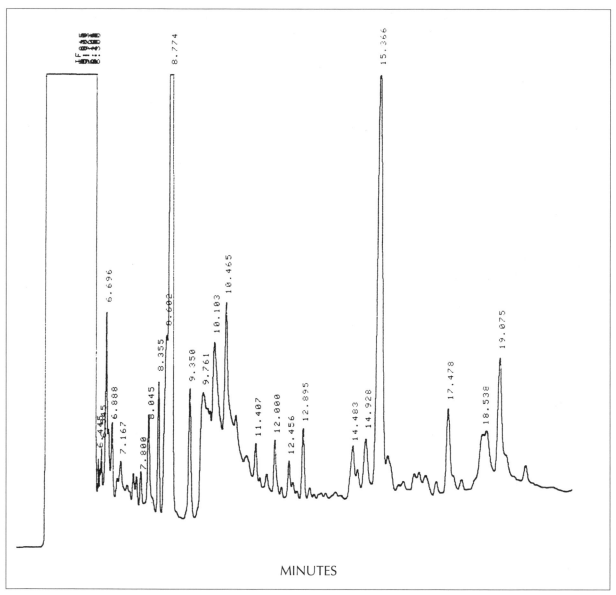

**FIGURE 3.** Gas chromatogram. Area under the curve or peak height of an analyte (e.g., drug or toxin) is compared to the area under the curve or peak height of an internal standard, and then the ratio is calculated. This ratio is compared to a standard curve of peak area ratios to give the concentration of the analyte.

The recorder produces a chromatogram, with various peaks being recorded at different times. Because each sample component is retained for a different length of time, the peak produced at a particular retention time is characteristic for a specific component (Figure 3). The amount of each component present is determined by the area of the characteristic peak or as the ratio of the peak heights calibrated against a standard curve.

This technique has many advantages, including high sensitivity and specificity. However, it requires sophisticated and expensive equipment. In addition, substances may produce interfering peaks with the same retention time as the analyte of interest. If such interference is suspected, the temperature and/or composition of the liquid phase can be adjusted for better peak resolution.

## High Pressure Liquid Chromatography

HPLC has been used for toxicologic screening and to measure various drugs (Table 1) (Chapter 5). Its basic principles are similar to those of GC, but it is useful for nonvolatile or heat-sensitive substances. Instead of gas, HPLC utilizes a liquid solvent (mobile phase) and a column packed with a stationary phase, usually with a porous silica base. The mobile phase is pumped through the column under high pressure to decrease the assay time.

The sample is injected onto the column at one end and migrates to the other end in the mobile phase. Various components move at different rates, depending on their solubility characteristics and how much time is spent in the solid versus liquid phases. As the mobile phase leaves the column, it passes through a detector that produces a peak proportional to the concentration of each sample component. The detector is usually a spectrophotometer with variable wavelength capability in the ultraviolet and visible ranges.

A signal from the detector is sent to a recorder or integrator, which plots peaks for each component as it elutes from the column (Figure 4). Once again, each component has its own characteristic retention time so each peak represents a specific component. As with GC, interferences may occur with compounds of similar structure or solubility characteristics; the peaks may fall on top of each other. Better resolution can be obtained by using a column packing with different characteristics or by changing the composition and/or pH of the mobile phase.

Compounds are identified by their retention times and quantified either by computing the area of the peak or by comparing the peak height or area to an internal standard to obtain a peak height or peak area ratio. This ratio is then used to calculate a concentration by comparison to a predetermined standard curve.

Although HPLC offers both high sensitivity and specificity, it requires specialized equipment and personnel. Furthermore, since the substance being determined usually is in a body fluid (e.g., urine or serum), one or more extraction steps are needed to isolate it. Another concern is that since many assays require a mobile phase composed of volatile and possibly toxic solvents, federal

guidelines (Occupational Safety and Health Administration) must be followed. In addition, initial assay development may be costly since modifications to published methods are almost always required.

## IMMUNOASSAYS

Immunoassays are all based on the reaction between an antigenic determinant or hapten (e.g., drug) and a labeled antibody. The label may consist of a radioisotope, an enzyme or enzyme substrate, a fluorophore, or a chromophore. The reaction may be measured by several detection methods including liquid scintillation, ultraviolet absorbance, fluorescence, fluorescent polarization, and turbidimetry or nephelometry. Serum drug concentrations are usually measured using immunoassays.

Immunoassays can be divided into two general categories: heterogeneous and homogeneous. In heterogeneous assays, the free and bound portions of the determinant must be separated before either or both portions can be assayed. This separation can be accomplished by various methods including protein precipitation, double antibody technique, adsorption of free drug, and removal by immobilized antibody on a solid phase.

Homogeneous assays do not require a separation step and, therefore, can be easily automated. The binding of the labeled hapten to the antibody alters its signal in a way (color change or reduction in enzyme activity) that

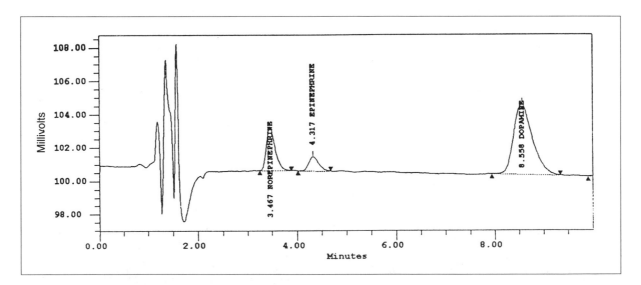

| Drug | Peak Results | | |
| | Retention Time (min) | Area (mV sec) | Height (mV) |
| --- | --- | --- | --- |
| Norepinephrine | 3.467 | 31,479 | 2612 |
| Epinephrine | 4.317 | 11,761 | 847 |
| Dopamine | 8.558 | 112,271 | 4249 |

**FIGURE 4.** HPLC chromatogram. Appearance of this chromatogram is similar to the gas chromatogram, and area or peak height ratio is used to quantify the analyte in a sample.

can then be used to measure the analyte concentration. Homogeneous assays are also suited to "stat" tests due to their rapid turnaround time.

Early immunoassays used polyclonal antibodies, generated as a result of an animal's natural immune response. Typically, an antigen is injected into an animal. The animal's immune system then recognizes the material as foreign and produces antibodies against it. These antibodies are then isolated from the blood.

Many different antibodies may be generated in response to a single antigen. The number as well as the specificities of the antibodies depend on the size and number of antigenic sites on the antigen. In general, the larger and more complex the antigen (e.g., cell or protein), the more antigenic sites it has and the more different antibodies formed.

Although polyclonal antibodies have been used successfully, both specificity and response may vary greatly because of their heterogeneous nature. The result is a high degree of cross-reactivity with similar substances. To address this problem, monoclonal antibodies have been developed.

Prior to 1975, the only monoclonal antibodies available were from patients with malignant plasma cells. In 1975, however, a technique was developed to make monoclonal antibodies in the laboratory.[5] The technique is based on the fusion of

> Genetic material from plasma cells that produce antibody but cannot reproduce.
> Myeloma cells that do not produce antibody but can reproduce.

The plasma cells and myeloma cells are cultured together, resulting in a mixture of both parent cells and a hybrid cell. This hybrid cell produces the specific antibody and reproduces.

The mixture is incubated in a special medium, which kills the parent cells and leaves only the hybrid antibody-producing cells alive. The hybrid cells can then be grown using conventional cell culture techniques, resulting in large amounts of the monoclonal antibody. The development of monoclonal antibodies has allowed for high sensitivity and specificity in immunoassay technology.

## Radioimmunoassay

As with flame photometry, RIA is rarely used in the modern clinical laboratory and is discussed largely from a historical perspective. RIA, a heterogeneous immunoassay, was developed in the late 1950s[6] and has been used primarily in endocrinology (Table 1). This technique takes advantage of the fact that certain atoms can be either incorporated directly into the analyte's structure or attached by antibodies. The primary atoms used in the clinical laboratory fall into two classes: gamma emitters and beta emitters.

Gamma emitters ($^{125}I$ and $^{57}Co$) are generally incorporated into compounds such as thyroid hormone and cyanocobalamin (vitamin $B_{12}$).[4] These isotopes can be counted directly with standard gamma counters that utilize a sodium iodide–thallium crystal. When the gamma ray hits the crystal, it gives off a flash of light. This light, in turn, stimulates a photomultiplier tube to amplify the signal.

Beta emitters ($^{14}C$ and $^{3}H$) are used primarily to measure steroid concentrations.[4] Beta rays cannot be counted directly since endogenous substances tend to absorb the radiation. Therefore, this technique requires a scintillation cocktail with an organic compound capable of absorbing the beta radiation and reemitting it as a flash of light. This light is then amplified by a photomultiplier tube and counted.

RIA is extremely sensitive and has been made more specific with the introduction of monoclonal antibodies. Unfortunately, this technique also has several significant disadvantages:[4]

> A short shelf-life for labeled reagents.
> Lead shielding, making the instrument heavy and bulky.
> Strict recordkeeping.
> Monitoring of personnel.
> Special licensing.
> Waste disposal issues.

Since EIAs have none of these problems, the clinical use of RIA has decreased in recent years.

## Agglutination

The simplest immunoassay is agglutination. Typical tests that can be performed using this assay include human chorionic gonadotropin, rheumatoid factor, antigens from infectious agents such as bacteria and fungi, and antinuclear antibodies (ANA). The agglutination reaction, used to detect either antigens or antibodies, results when multivalent antibodies bind to antigens with more than one binding site.

The reaction occurs through the formation of cross-linkages between antigen and antibody particles. When enough complexes form, clumping results and a visible mass is formed (Figure 5, next page). Since the reaction depends on the number of binding sites on the antibody, the greater the number, the better is the reaction. For example, immunoglobulin M (Chapter 17) produces better agglutination than immunoglobulin G because it has more binding sites.

The agglutination reaction is also affected by other factors:[6]

> Avidity and affinity of antibody.
> Number of binding sites on antigen as well as antibody.

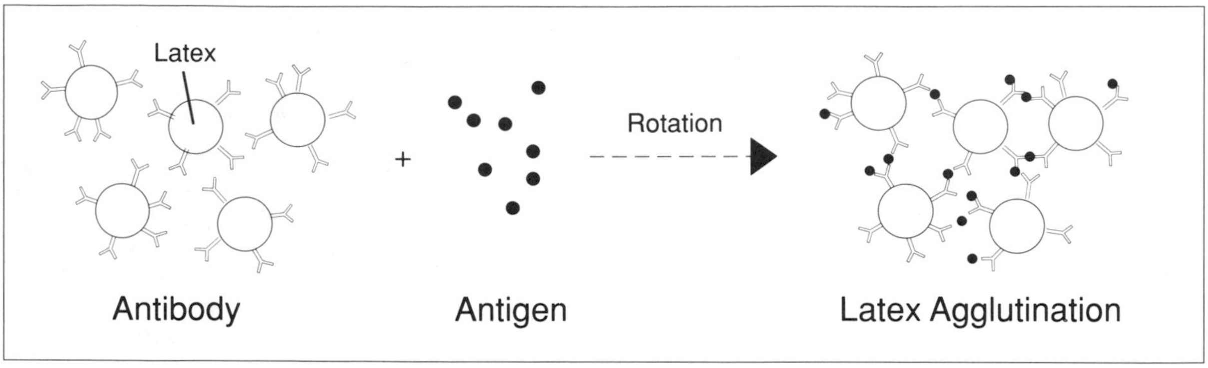

**FIGURE 5.** Schematic of latex agglutination immunoassay. The specimen (cerebrospinal fluid, serum, etc.) contains the analyte (in this case antigens to bacteria) that causes the latex particles (with corresponding antibody attached) to agglutinate. Interaction of the three components causes an easily readable reaction. (Adapted, with permission, from Power DA, McCuen PJ, eds. Manual of BBI products and laboratory procedures. Cockeysville, MD: Becton Dickinson Microbiology Systems; 1998:77.)

> ➤ Relative concentrations of antigen and antibody.
> ➤ $\zeta$-Potential (electrostatic interaction that causes particles in solution to repel each other).
> ➤ Viscosity of medium.

The two types of agglutination reactions are (1) direct and (2) indirect. Direct agglutination occurs when the antigen and antibody are mixed together, resulting in visible clumping. An example of this reaction is the test for *Salmonella typhi* antibody.

Indirect agglutination (also known as passive or particle agglutination) uses a carrier for either the antibody or antigen. Originally, erythrocytes were selected as the carrier, as described in hemolytic anemia tests (Chapter 14). Latex-coated particles are now commonly used, however, and this latex agglutination method is simpler and less expensive than the erythrocyte immunoassay. In addition, latex particles allow titration of the amount of antibody bound to the latex particle, thus reducing variability. Other advantages include a rapid performance time with no separation step, allowing full automation. Disadvantages include expensive equipment and lower sensitivity than either RIA or EIA. The use of an automated particle counter increases the sensitivity of the test 10–1000 times.[7]

### Enzyme Immunoassays

EIA employs enzymes as labels for specific analytes. When antibodies bind to the antigen–enzyme complex, a defined reaction occurs (e.g., color change, fluorescence, radioactivity, or altered activity). This altered enzyme activity is used to quantitate the analyte.

The advantages of EIA include commercial availability at a relatively low cost, long shelf life, good sensitivity, automation, and none of the specific requirements mentioned for RIA.

#### Enzyme-Linked Immunosorbent Assay

ELISA is a heterogeneous EIA. This assay employs the same basic principles as RIA, except that enzyme activity rather than radioactivity is measured. This assay is commonly used to determine antibodies directed against a wide range of antigens such as rheumatoid factor (Chapter 17), hepatitis B antigen (Chapter 11), and bacterial and viral antigens in the serum (Chapter 16) (Table 1).

In a competitive ELISA assay, the specific antibody is adsorbed to a solid phase. Enzyme-labeled antigen is incubated together with the sample and the antibodies attached to the solid phase. After a specified time, an equilibrium is reached and the solid phase is washed with buffer. The reaction then is stopped, and the reaction product is measured with a spectrophotometer or fluorometer.

#### Enzyme-Multiplied Immunoassay

EMIT is a homogeneous EIA; enzyme is used as a label for a specific analyte (e.g., a drug). Many drugs commonly assayed using EMIT are also measured by FPIA (e.g., digoxin, quinidine, procainamide, *N*-acetyl procainamide, and aminoglycoside antibiotics) (Chapter 5) as are substances like blood urea nitrogen (BUN) and creatinine (Chapter 7) (Table 1).

With the EMIT assay, the enzyme retains its activity after attaching to the analyte. For example, to determine a drug concentration, an enzyme is conjugated to the drug and incubated with antidrug antibody. As shown in Figure 6, the test drug (D) is covalently bound to an enzyme that retains its activity and acts as a label. When this complex is combined with antidrug antibody, the enzyme is inactivated. If the antibody and enzyme-bound drug are combined with serum that contains unbound drug, competition occurs. Since the amount of antidrug antibody is limited, the free drug in the sample and the enzyme-linked drug compete for binding to the antibody. When the antibody binds to the enzyme-linked drug, enzyme activity is inhibited. The result is that the serum drug concentration is proportional to the amount of active en-

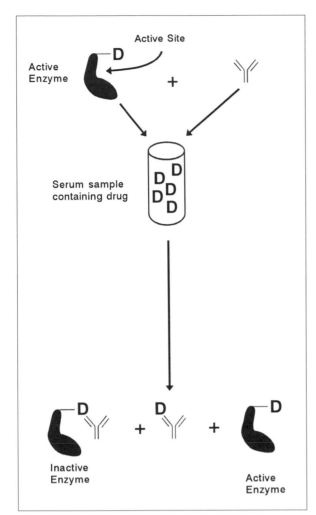

**FIGURE 6.** EMIT. This assay is used in quantifying the drug concentration in a serum sample, as described in the text.

zyme remaining. Since no separation step is required, this assay can be automated.

### Fluorescent Polarization Immunoassay

FPIA, the most common form of immunoassay, is used to measure concentrations of many clinical chemistries such as BUN and creatinine. It also is commonly employed for determining serum drug concentrations of aminoglycoside antibiotics, vancomycin, and theophylline (Table 1).

Molecules having a ring structure and large number of double bonds, such as some aromatic compounds, can fluoresce when excited by a specific wavelength of light. These molecules must have a particular orientation with respect to the light source for electrons to be raised to an excited state. When the electrons return to their original lower energy state, some light is reemitted as a flash with a longer wavelength than the exciting light. Fluorescent immunoassays take advantage of this property by conjugating an antibody or analyte to a fluorescent molecule.

The concentration can be determined by measuring either the degree of fluorescence or, more commonly, the decrease in the amount of fluorescence present.[4,7]

In FPIA, a polarizing filter is placed between the light source and the sample and between the sample and the detector. The first filter assures that the light exciting the molecules is in a particular orientation; the second filter assures that only fluorescent light of the appropriate orientation reaches the detector.

The fluorescent polarization of a small molecule is low because it rotates rapidly and is not in the proper orientation long enough to give off an easily detected signal. To decrease this molecular motion, the molecule is complexed with an antibody. Since this larger complex rotates at a slower rate, it stays in the proper orientation to be excited by the incident light.

When unlabeled analyte is mixed with a fixed amount of antibody and fluorescent-labeled analyte, a competitive binding reaction occurs between the labeled and unlabeled analytes. The result is a decrease in fluorescence. Thus, the concentration of unlabeled analyte is inversely proportional to the amount of fluorescence.[7]

Because of their simplicity, automation, and low cost, assays have been developed with relatively high sensitivity for many drugs (e.g., antiepileptics, antiarrhythmics, and antibiotics). The primary difficulty is interference from endogenous substances (lipids and bilirubin) or metabolites of the drugs.

## POLYMERASE CHAIN REACTION

PCR is used principally for detecting microbiologic organisms and genetic diseases (Table 1). Microorganisms identified by this process include chlamydia, cytomegalovirus (CMV), Epstein–Barr virus, human immunodeficiency virus (HIV), mycobacteria, and herpes simplex virus (Chapter 16). Although the number of organisms that can be identified is limited at present, this list is growing. Furthermore, PCR can often identify organisms with greater rapidity and sensitivity than conventional methods.

Genetic diseases diagnosed using PCR include α-1-antitrypsin deficiency, cystic fibrosis, sickle cell anemia, fragile X syndrome, Tay-Sachs disease, drug-induced hemolytic anemia, and von Willebrand's disease. In addition, cancer research has benefitted from PCR through the diagnosis of various cancers (e.g., chronic myeloid leukemia and pancreatic and colon cancers) as well as the detection of residual disease after treatment.[8] This technique is used to amplify specific DNA and RNA sequences enzymatically.

PCR takes advantage of the normal DNA replication process. *In vivo*, DNA replicates when the double helix unwinds and the two strands separate. A new strand forms on each separate strand through the coupling of

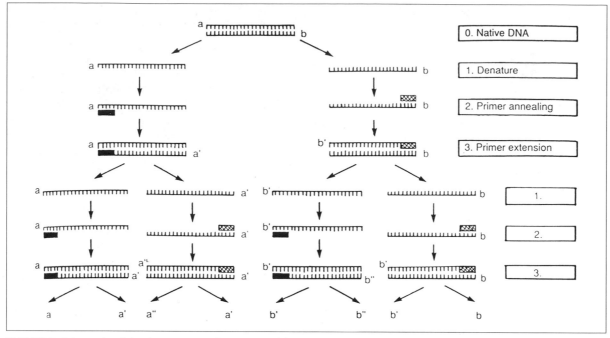

**FIGURE 7.** Schematic of the three steps in the PCR amplification of a specific DNA sequence, as described in the text. (Adapted from Reference 9.)

specific base pairs (e.g., adenosine with thymidine and cytosine with guanosine). The PCR cycle is similar and consists of three separate steps[7] (Figure 7):

1. Denaturation—the two strands of DNA are thermally separated.
2. Primer annealing—sequence-specific primers are allowed to hybridize to opposite strands flanking the region of interest by decreasing the temperature.
3. Primer extension—DNA polymerase then extends the hybridized primers, generating a copy of the original DNA template.

The efficiency of the extension step can be increased by raising the temperature. Typical temperatures for the three steps are 201.2 °F (94 °C) for denaturation, 122–149 °F (50–65 °C) for annealing, and 161.6 °F (72 °C) for extension. Since the entire cycle is completed in only about 3 min,[9] many cycles can occur within a short time, resulting in the exponential production of millions of copies of the target sequence.

The genetic material is then identified by agarose gel electrophoresis. While not truly a chromatographic technique, gel electrophoresis utilizes principles similar to thin layer chromatography in that the migration of bands is similar to the migration of spots. An electric current is applied to facilitate DNA migration, and the gene is identified by the distance it migrates through the gel.

One potential disadvantage of this method is contamination of the amplification reaction with products of a previous PCR (carryover), exogenous DNA, or other cellular material. Contamination can be reduced by pre-aliquoting reagents, using dedicated positive-displacement pipets, and physically separating the reaction preparation from the area where the product is analyzed. In addition, multiple negative controls are necessary to monitor for contamination.

## SUMMARY

This chapter presents a brief overview of the more common laboratory assay methodologies, including their potential advantages and problems. A number of these methodologies such as flame photometry, paper chromatography, and RIA are discussed primarily to provide an historical basis and description of the simple principles on which the more complex methods are based.

Due to its simplicity and improved sensitivity, ISE has replaced flame photometry as the principal method for measuring serum and urine electrolytes. Some methods such as turbidimetry, nephelometry, and spectrophotometry are used in conjunction with other tests such as the immunoassay. With these methods, concentrations of substances such as immune complexes can be determined.

Chromatography is one of the mainstays of the laboratory for drug detection. The two principal forms of chromatography are liquid and gas. Both types are similar in that they depend on differences in either solubilities or boiling points, respectively, to separate different analytes in a sample. Another group of important tests are the immunoassays: EIA, EMIT, ELISA, and FPIA. All of these methods depend on an immunologically mediated reaction that increases sensitivity and specificity. These assays are commonly used to determine routine clinical chemistries and drug concentrations. Finally, PCR—a relatively new technology—is used to amplify specific DNA and RNA sequences, primarily in the areas of microbiology and detection of genetic diseases.

A dramatic increase in the dependence on the clinical laboratory has occurred in the last 30–40 years. This increased use parallels an increase in the sophistication of the tests, improved sensitivities and specificities, and decreased turnaround time for obtaining the results. Because of the increasing complexity of test methodologies, today's clinician must have a basic understanding of the more common tests in order to select the most appropriate one in each case and to know how interferences occur. All of these developments have translated directly into improved patient care.

## REFERENCES

1. Evenson MA. Principles of instrumentation. In: Henry JB, ed. Clinical diagnosis and management, 18th ed. Philadelphia, PA: W. B. Saunders; 1991:27–48.
2. Burnett RW, Lee-Lewandrowski E, Lewandrowski K. Electrolytes and acid base balance. In: McClatchey KD, ed. Clinical laboratory medicine, 1st ed. Baltimore, MD: Williams & Wilkins; 1994:331–54.
3. Ladenson JH, Apple FS, Koch DD. Misleading hyponatremia due to hyperlipemia: a method-dependent error. *Ann Intern Med*. 1981; 95:707.
4. Moore RE. Immunochemical methods. In: McClatchey KD, ed. Clinical laboratory medicine, 1st ed. Baltimore, MD: Williams & Wilkins; 1994:213–38.
5. Kohler G, Milstein C. Continuous cultures of fused cells secreting antibody of predefined specificity. *Nature*. 1975; 256:445–97.
6. Berson SA, Yalow RS, Bauman A, et al. Insulin I131 metabolism in human subjects: demonstration of insulin binding globulin in the circulation of insulin treated subjects. *J Clin Invest*. 1956; 35:170.
7. Nakamura RM, Tucker ES, Carlson IH. Immunoassays in the clinical laboratory. In: Henry JB, ed. Clinical diagnosis and management, 18th ed. Philadelphia, PA: W. B. Saunders; 1991:848–84.
8. Erlich HA, Gelfand D, Sninsky JJ. Recent advances in the polymerase chain reaction. *Science*. 1991; 252:1643–51.
9. Remick DG. Clinical applications of molecular biology. In: McClatchey KD, ed. Clinical laboratory medicine, 1st ed. Baltimore, MD: Williams & Wilkins; 1994:165–74.

# Chapter 3

# Evaluating Potential Drug Interferences with Test Results

*Scott L. Traub*

If drug interferences with laboratory tests are not recognized, inappropriate changes in therapy or followup diagnostic evaluation can be made. Therefore, clinicians should consider such interferences when interpreting laboratory data.

The first section of this chapter covers the types of drug influences on test results, particularly in vitro perturbations. The actual chemistry of the assays is not discussed unless an understanding of the mechanism of interference is important. The effects of food, disease, exercise, and improper storage or collection of samples also are not included.

Later sections deal with the clinical events that should raise suspicions of a drug–test interference and present an approach to investigation. A case study (minicase) covers most of the principles and concepts discussed, and many practical examples are offered.

## OBJECTIVES

Upon completion of this chapter, the reader should be able to

1. Compare and contrast in vivo and in vitro drug interferences with clinical laboratory tests.
2. Compare the relative incidence of the two major types of drug effects on laboratory tests.
3. Predict a drug's potential for interference on an assay, given the drug's pharmacokinetic, chemical, and physical properties as well as the chemical basis for the assay.
4. Investigate a suspected drug–laboratory test interference in a logical, systematic manner, given an assay and a clinical situation.
5. Discuss the clinical relevance of analytical drug–laboratory test interferences and list the most commonly involved drugs or drug classes.
6. List various available resources on drug–laboratory test interferences.

## IN VIVO AND IN VITRO DRUG EFFECTS ON LABORATORY TESTS

Mechanisms of drug effects on clinical laboratory tests can be classified as either *in vivo* or *in vitro*. In vivo drug effects also can be called biological and be subclassified as pharmacological or toxicological. Likewise, the term "in vitro" is sometimes used synonymously with "analytical" or "methodological." The major differences are discussed here.

### In Vivo Effects

Although in vivo effects account for most influences by substances on laboratory tests, they are discussed here only briefly. An in vivo interference is an actual change in the analyte concentration or activity *prior* to collection and analysis. The assay measurement is true and accurate. The change usually occurs in the living organism, where an exogenous or endogenous substance accumulates enough to influence the analyte being measured.

Exogenous substances include drugs, toxins, and food. Ammonia, blood urea nitrogen (BUN), and keto-acids are examples of endogenous substances. Infrequently, an abnormal decrease in an endogenous substance can affect a test result in vivo. For example, because of physiological influences, as serum albumin decreases so does total calcium. When an in vivo effect is at work, usually the test result accurately reflects the degree of physiological or anatomical normality (or abnormality) with which it correlates. In this case, the test can be interpreted as usual. However, in the case of albumin and calcium, the results cannot be interpreted as usual. The physiologically active form of calcium remains in the normal range (Chapter 6).

Several examples of in vivo drug effects should be helpful:

> *Pharmacologically,* the loop diuretic bumetanide

usually increases potassium excretion and may cause hypokalemia. The test result of low serum potassium concentration is true and expected. Therefore, although the assay value may be outside the normal range, the measurement is accurate.

➤ True in vivo hyperglycemia can be caused by more than 50 drugs (Chapter 12). Those drugs seen most commonly in practice include thiazide and loop diuretics, corticosteroids, and oral contraceptives.

➤ An overdose of acetaminophen, causing liver damage and a rise in hepatic transaminases (Chapter 11), is an in vivo *toxicological* drug effect.

## In Vitro Effects

Endogenous biochemicals (e.g., lipids and bilirubin) and other substances (e.g., drugs and metabolites) in a subject's body fluid or tissue can interfere with a clinical laboratory test *during* the in vitro analytical process. In addition, substances that are prepackaged in or added to the in vitro system before or after sample collection can interfere in vitro. For example, test tubes sometimes contain heparin or fluoride; heparin can interfere with aminoglycoside assays, and fluoride can cause false increases in BUN when measured by an Ekatchem assay. Although unlikely, interferences from detergents or antiseptics also can occur if equipment is not thoroughly washed and rinsed.

The concentration of *endogenous* substances usually must be well above normal levels before it significantly influences an assay. A common example is a jaundiced patient with a bilirubin of 10 mg/dL (170 μmol/L) (normal range: 0.3–1.0 mg/dL). Icteric samples cause many immunologically based drug concentration assays (Chapters 2 and 5) to generate spurious results. In contrast, interference by *exogenous* substances (e.g., drugs) may occur at concentrations resulting from just usual doses.

Unlike in vivo effects, analytical effects occur because of interference with a chemical step in an assay, causing erroneous results that *cannot* be interpreted as usual or expected. Interferences occurring in the collection tube are labeled in vitro but are not always *analytical* since the result reflects what is in the specimen at the time of measurement. For example, glucose concentrations are falsely lowered within the collection tube secondary to metabolism by red and white blood cells if the tube used for collection does not contain any inhibitors such as fluoride and is stored for prolonged periods.

### Mechanisms of In Vitro Interferences

To predict and identify analytical drug interferences, a clinician must know the various mechanisms. Basically, effects are related to the chemical (e.g., influence on pH

or reaction with reagents) or physical (e.g., color or fluorescence) properties of the interfering substance. Interference mechanisms can be classified as follows:

1. Drug reacts with reagent to form a chromophore (e.g., cefoxitin or cephalothin with Jaffe-based creatinine assay).
2. Drug or metabolite reacts, because of structural similarity, with immunoassay's antibody that is intended to be specific for the analyte. Examples of drugs interfering by this mechanism include caffeine for theophylline, digitoxin for digoxin, netilmicin for gentamicin, and cyclosporine metabolites for cyclosporine.
3. Drug alters the specimen pH (usually urine) so that reagent reactions are inhibited or enhanced (e.g., acetazolamide or bicarbonate causing false-positive proteinuria with reagent dip strips).
4. Drug has chemical properties similar to the analyte (e.g., acetaminophen with uric acid assays based on reducing activity of uric acid—both drugs act as reducing agents).
5. Drug chelates an enzyme activator or a cofactor [e.g., cysteine (as metabolite of *N*-acetylcysteine) chelation of magnesium ions, causing decreased alkaline phosphatase (ALP) activity].
6. Drug directly inhibits an enzyme (e.g., theophylline inhibition of ALP activity).
7. Drug directly activates an enzyme (e.g., cysteine's effect on creatine phosphokinase).
8. Drug absorbs at the same wavelength as the analyte (e.g., methotrexate with methods using an absorbance range of 340–410 nm).

### Inactive Ingredients in Drug Products

Rarely, components of pharmaceutical dosage forms themselves influence an assay. Examples include

➤ Excipients such as lactose and starch.
➤ Preservatives such as antioxidants and reducing agents (e.g., ascorbic acid, sodium sulfite, and dihydroguaiaretic acid).
➤ Microbicides such as phenol and various parabenzoates.
➤ Metallic compounds such as zinc oxide and titanium oxide.
➤ Colorants and flavorings.

Now that company disclosure of inactive ingredients is becoming common, practitioners should consider them as possible interferents. Unfortunately, little research has been performed in this area.

To investigate their possible interference, the *amount* of each inactive ingredient should be determined. Although a drug's chemical reactivity must be considered, the amount of chemical that might contact the test reagents is more important. The more interferent present, the higher is the probability for interference. Solid dosage forms often contain more excipient than drug (by weight) but much less colorant and preservative. These substances should be considered only if they enter the fluid or tissue to be analyzed.

However, all "inert" ingredients must be accounted for when a commercial drug product is used during in vitro research (e.g., adding an oral or injectable dosage form to serum and determining whether it interferes with specific tests). Prior extraction of the active drug may not separate additives from it. Therefore, unless additives are to be considered, samples should be spiked with pure drug alone.

An interesting example of inactive ingredients confounding test interpretation involves cimetidine and Hemoccult. This interaction is clinically relevant because cimetidine is often used in patients at risk for gastrointestinal (GI) bleeding; Hemoccult is a test for blood in the stool.

Initially, investigators found that gastric aspirates from patients taking cimetidine tablets produced a false-positive Hemoccult reaction.[1] Although a second researcher was unable to reproduce these findings using pure cimetidine in blank nasogastric aspirate, he could reproduce them using a dissolved tablet.[2] He postulated that the blue dye in the commercial product caused the problem (even though the dye constituted only 0.004% of the tablet's weight and should not impart much color or activity on the Hemoccult).

Later, other researchers in an in vitro experiment showed that the interference depended on concentration (>1.25 mg/mL) and was due to the cimetidine itself. These researchers made this conclusion after finding false positives with injectable, tablet, and liquid forms of cimetidine as well as the pure chemical.[3]

## Simultaneous In Vitro and In Vivo Effects

Some substances can affect an analyte both in vivo and in vitro. In these rare situations, interpretation is extremely difficult because the degree of impact in each environment cannot be easily determined. The prototypic example involves reaction of aminoglycosides with penicillins, which leads to a loss of antibacterial activity in vivo and can decrease measured aminoglycoside concentrations and antibacterial activity in vitro.[4,5] Although this inactivation mechanism is unclear, it seems to involve the formation of an adduct between the aminoglycoside and beta-lactam ring of the penicillins. Although only this interaction is discussed here, the concepts can be extrapolated to other drugs.

### In Vitro Effects

In vitro, of the penicillins, carbenicillin is the most potent inactivator of aminoglycosides; of the aminoglycosides, tobramycin is the most susceptible. Amikacin and netilmicin are degraded the least. Refrigeration does not significantly slow the reaction, but centrifugation with freezing does. Unreasonably low aminoglycoside concentrations in patients receiving concomitant high-dose penicillins should alert the practitioner to this in vitro interaction.

### In Vivo Effects

In vivo, inactivation of aminoglycosides by penicillins is a problem primarily in patients with renal failure; with normal renal function, these antibiotics are excreted at a rate faster than their interaction rate. In one study, the in vivo inactivation rate constant (Ki) of gentamicin in patients with renal failure receiving carbenicillin was 0.025 hr$^{-1}$. The inactivation rate constant was defined as the difference between the elimination rate constant (Ke) for gentamicin alone and that for its combination with carbenicillin. Thus, in renal failure patients, carbenicillin apparently "eliminates" gentamicin at the same rate as do the kidneys. The change corresponded to a shortening of the gentamicin half-life (t½) from 61.6 to 19.6 hr after carbenicillin was added.[6] Fortunately, carbenicillin is rarely used today.

### Minimizing Interactions

The effect of penicillins on aminoglycosides can be minimized in several ways:

1. To eliminate in vitro problems, the sample can be centrifuged and frozen soon after it is drawn.
2. Antibiotics with a lesser interaction (amikacin and piperacillin or a cephalosporin) can be used.
3. Administration times can be separated or blood can be drawn just before the next scheduled penicillin dose to decrease the penicillin concentration in the specimen tube, the concentration–exposure time (in vivo), and, therefore, the degradation time.

This last maneuver would be less fruitful in renal failure patients, especially if the penicillin dose were not adjusted. However, decreasing the daily penicillin dose according to renal function and required serum concentration would make testing more accurate even for these patients.[7] For example, some clinicians suggest carbenicillin 5 g every 24 hr if creatinine clearance is less than 10 mL/min. What impact penicillin and aminoglycoside interference has on outcome has not been studied.

## INCIDENCE OF DRUG INTERFERENCE WITH LABORATORY TESTS

The effects of drugs on laboratory tests can significantly increase health care costs if they lead to prolonged hospitalization, extra office visits, and unnecessary tests. In vitro interferences account for approximately 10–20% of af-

**TABLE 1.** Comparison of Reports of Drugs and Substance Effects on Laboratory Test Results—1975 versus 1990[a]

| Test | Physiological | | | | Analytical | | | | Total |
|---|---|---|---|---|---|---|---|---|---|
| | No effect | Increase | Decrease | Subtotal[b] | No effect | Increase | Decrease | Subtotal[b] | |
| Serum bilirubin (total) | | | | | | | | | |
| 1975 | 1 | 104 | 12 | 116 | 21 | 25 | 5 | 30 | 168 |
| 1990 | 77 | 349 | 19 | 368 | 181 | 34 | 12 | 46 | 672 |
| Serum creatinine | | | | | | | | | |
| 1975 | 2 | 52 | 1 | 53 | 28 | 22 | 0 | 22 | 105 |
| 1990 | 33 | 107 | 3 | 110 | 227 | 44 | 10 | 54 | 424 |

[a]Compiled from References 8 and 9. These data do not include influences other than drugs and chemicals (effects of storage, exercise, etc., are not included. Data from the 1991 supplement by the same author do not change the statistics substantially.
[b]Subtotal of tests where results were increased or decreased by drugs.

fected tests, based on an analysis of about 800 tests in 1975 and 1400 tests in 1990 as compiled by Young et al.[8,9]

For example, in the 1975 database, 146 substances reportedly influenced serum bilirubin; of these, 30 (almost 20%) involved an in vitro interference (Table 1). For some tests, such as serum creatinine (SCr), about one-third of the interferences were analytical. In the 1990 database, 46 of 414 (11%) bilirubin alterations and 54 of 164 (33%) SCr alterations were of the in vitro type.

In addition to new assays and drugs, Young's 1990 edition included all of the tests and drugs in the 1975 publication, although many were no longer used. Therefore, it is difficult to determine the true incidence of drug effects on assays in common use today. One can speculate that the relative incidence of in vitro interferences should decline over the years because some less specific assays either are no longer used or have been improved. Regardless of the real incidence, most drug effects on laboratory tests encountered in clinical practice reflect true physiological changes caused by pharmacological actions.

## PREDICTING A DRUG'S EFFECT ON ASSAYS

Clinicians should be able to anticipate the likelihood of assay interference by knowing a drug's pharmacological, chemical, and pharmacokinetic properties as well as clinical data. Moreover, it should be easier to identify or predict an interference accurately when a patient takes just a few drugs.

In addition to a drug's chemical properties, the chemical basis of the *assay* needs to be understood. As mentioned previously, a drug may be a chromophore and confuse colorimetric measurements. When the drug's color is close to the color of the substance being measured, interference occurs. Structural similarity of the drug or metabolite to the intended analyte also may cause erroneous results. This consideration is most important with immunoassays because antibodies rely on chemical structure for identification.

Assay methods that depend on a certain pH range may be altered by drugs that can affect the pH of the specimen or reagents. Likewise, drugs that act as reducing or oxidizing agents can interfere with assays that also rely on such properties. Finally, problems can occur if the drug affects enzymes used in the assay reactions.

Although *pharmacokinetic* and *pharmacological* information may be useful for making predictions, this information is more valuable when confirming suspicions by reproducing the occurrence in a controlled environment. Often helpful are serum peak and trough concentrations of the drug or metabolites achievable with usual clinical doses and overdoses. Levels achievable in other body fluids or tissue are sometimes needed, and occasionally the route of administration must be considered. If the interference is concentration dependent, the time to peak also is important. Finally, the protein- and tissue-binding characteristics of a drug may have to be considered to estimate tissue penetration (Chapter 5).

## WHEN TO SUSPECT DRUG–LABORATORY TEST INTERFERENCES

The clinician should suspect a drug–laboratory test interference when an inconsistency appears among related test results or between test results and the clinical picture. Specifically, clinicians should become suspicious whenever

1. Test results do not correlate with the patient's signs and symptoms.
2. Results of different tests—assessing the same anatomy, physiology, or pharmacology—conflict with each other.
3. Results from a series of the same test vary greatly over a short period.
4. Results from a series of the same test change in the wrong direction.
5. A single result is *extremely* high or low compared with the normal range or expected value.

Examples of each "interference-trapping" scenario are

discussed here. When confronted with these apparent inconsistencies, clinicians should consider causes other than laboratory error and, in particular, analytical interference by a drug.

## Test Results Do Not Correlate with Patient's Signs and Symptoms

As emphasized elsewhere in this book, when test results do not correlate with signs and symptoms, the signs and symptoms should be considered more strongly than the test results. This rule is especially true when test results are (1) being used to confirm suspicions raised by the signs and symptoms in the first place or (2) only surrogate or indirect indicators of underlying pathology.

For example, SCr is a close approximation of the glomerular filtration rate, which is used to approximate the kidneys' ability to make urine. Nevertheless, actual urine output is a more direct (and visible) marker of overall renal function. If a patient's urine output has not changed but a repeat SCr (normal range: 0.7–1.5 mg/dL or 62–133 µmol/L) 3 days later increases by 1–2 mg/dL (88–177 µmol/L), more credence should be given to the urine output when formulating a diagnosis or therapy plan. In other words, a false elevation is possible.

Another example of discordant findings is when a patient's total bilirubin is 6 mg/dL (102 µmol/L) or higher (normal range: 0.3–1.0 mg/dL or 5–17 µmol/L), but he or she is not jaundiced; scleral icterus is often apparent at 4 mg/dL (68 µmol/L). If these signs of hyperbilirubinemia are absent, bilirubin test results may be incorrect. One should be especially suspicious if other tests of liver-related disease [e.g., ALP, lactate dehydrogenase, alanine aminotransferase (ALT), and aspartate aminotransferase] are normal.

Still another example of this principle is a free serum thyroxine concentration of 4 ng/dL (51.5 pmol/L) (normal range: 0.8–2.7 ng/dL or 10–35 pmol/L) in a patient without signs or symptoms of hyperthyroidism (Chapter 12).

Finally, even a test result within the normal range may be suspect. If a patient arrives in the emergency department with fulminant acute pancreatitis and signs of severe hypocalcemia (hyperactive reflexes and tetany) but has a calcium concentration of 10 mg/dL (2.5 mmol/L) (normal range: 8.5–10.8 mg/dL or 2.1–2.7 mmol/L) and an albumin within normal limits (Chapter 6), the serum calcium result should be held suspect.

## Results of Different Tests Conflict with Each Other

Occasionally, results of two tests that assess the same anatomy, physiology, or pharmacology conflict with each other. For example, a presurgical test screen shows a SCr of 4.2 mg/dL (371 µmol/L) (normal range: 0.7–1.5 mg/

dL or 62–133 µmol/L) in an otherwise healthy 20-year-old patient with a BUN of 8 mg/dL (2.9 mmol/L) (normal range: 8–20 mg/dL or 2.9–7.1 mmol/L). Usually BUN is elevated in the presence of elevated SCr.

Further investigation reveals that the patient received a prophylactic dose of cefoxitin shortly before blood was drawn. Cefoxitin can falsely elevate creatinine concentrations (Chapter 7). Because of the predictive value concept (Chapter 1), even without a normal BUN, it is not likely that the elevated creatinine is from renal failure because the test was done in an asymptomatic patient as part of a routine screen. The conclusion would be different for a long-term diabetic patient with uncontrolled diabetes and a urinary tract infection who has a reason for diminished renal function.

## Results from Series Vary Greatly over Short Period

The same patient also would fall into this category if the SCr had been 1 mg/dL on the day before surgery. SCr rarely climbs that fast (Chapter 7). Likewise, some laboratory "error" should be considered in the following case.

An activated partial thromboplastin time (aPTT) of 25 sec is reported in a patient being treated for deep venous thrombosis (Chapter 15). Over the last few days, however, the aPTT was between 65 and 75 sec. There has been no change in the daily heparin dose or interruption of the constant infusion, and warfarin has neither been started nor stopped. Similarly, suspicion should arise if (1) hemoglobin (Hgb) drastically increases [e.g., from 11 g/dL (6.8 mmol/L) to 14 g/dL (8.7 mmol/L) over 2–3 days] in a normally hydrated patient who has not received any blood or (2) digoxin concentration (valley) suddenly increases [e.g., from 1.1 ng/mL (1.4 nmol/L) to 3.5 ng/mL (4.5 nmol/L) in 24 hr] in a patient without any change in dose (with or without a change in renal function).

With experience, a practitioner develops a feeling for how quickly a value can increase or decrease from day to day, even under the most drastic pathophysiological changes. Such knowledge is helpful in interpreting laboratory data and in identifying interferences. This information is provided in many of the QuickView charts in this book.

## Results from Series Change in Wrong Direction

This situation is best described using drug concentrations. For example, an elderly female is admitted with a digoxin concentration of 4.5 ng/mL (5.8 nmol/L) (normal range: 0.9–2 ng/mL or 1.2–2.8 nmol/L). Her digoxin is discontinued, and concentrations decline over the next 2 days to 3.8 and 3.1 ng/mL. On the 4th day, however, her concentration is 3.9 ng/mL. Lab error or interference must be suspected because concentrations should decrease—

not increase—when digoxin is not being given.

## Single Result Is Extremely Higher or Lower than Normal or Expected

Examples of this situation are

- ➤ An unusually high glucose of 800 mg/dL (45 mmol/L) in a 75-year-old, asymptomatic, nondiabetic nursing home patient.
- ➤ A peak gentamicin concentration lower than the trough within the same dosing interval.
- ➤ A theophylline concentration of 1 μg/mL (therapeutic range: 10–20 mg/L) drawn soon after administration of a usual loading dose.

(These last two examples also are discussed in Chapter 5.)

## INVESTIGATING SUSPECTED DRUG– LABORATORY TEST INTERFERENCE

When confronted with one of the preceding scenarios, the clinician must find the cause of the suspected interference. To investigate such an occurrence systematically, the reader can refer to the algorithm shown in Figure 1. No algorithm designed to assist with medical decisions or problem solving can include all possible paths. Nevertheless, this algorithm addresses the more common encounters and provides branches to practical options in the clinical setting. An explanation by major segments (A–D) of this algorithm follows.

For an integrated perspective, a single clinical case study (minicase) is used with this algorithm. An understanding of the relationship among phenacetin, sulfhemo-

globinemia, and methemoglobinemia and of the performance of a bromide level is not needed to comprehend the teaching points. This case actually occurred and was investigated using this algorithm.

### Algorithm Segment A

Brian R.'s bromide concentrations are suspicious for three reasons:

1. A concentration of 12 mg/dL is much too low to cause the signs and symptoms of bromism. (Rarely, bromide is used to treat refractory seizures; the therapeutic concentration is around 100 mg/dL.)
2. No drugs containing bromide were taken before admission.
3. The bromide concentration on day 7 should not have been higher than the concentration on day 1 since the patient ingested no bromide while hospitalized.

Because this case falls into the first, fourth, and fifth interference-trapping scenarios (page 32 of this chapter), the investigator should continue down the algorithm's "No" pathway.

Checking with the laboratory for a transcription error is the next step, and the technologist responsible for the assay is consulted rather than the receptionist. A transcription error can occur between the specialty area (e.g., immunology laboratory) and the data-entry person or receptionist. If there is no transcription error, the test should be repeated.

When the assay is repeated, the original specimen should be used. Brian R.'s original samples were retested

---

### ✎ Minicase

Brian R., an 83-year-old male, was admitted to the hospital with dyspnea, confusion, and ankle edema. His history included congestive heart failure, chronic obstructive pulmonary disease, hearing impairment, and several admissions for bleeding duodenal ulcer over the past few years.

Brian R. was now profoundly cyanotic (mucous membranes and periphery), but his partial pressure of oxygen ($pO_2$) was 83 mm Hg on room air (within normal range). Oxygen saturation was decreased (80%), but both Hgb and hematocrit were normal. Therefore, cyanosis was not due to polycythemia but may have resulted from a low percentage of oxygenated Hgb—findings consistent with methemoglobinemia. Over the next 3–4 days, Brian R. became increasingly confused and disoriented despite adequate arterial blood gas results.

Sulfhemoglobinemia, methemoglobinemia (secondary to phenacetin), and bromism (Brian R. had some old Bromo-Seltzer containing bromine and phenacetin at

home) were suspected; bromism is associated with confusion and disorientation. Methemoglobin was less than 3% (normal). A bromide concentration was 12 mg/dL (normal without ingesting drug: <5 mg/dL; therapeutic: 100 mg/dL) on day 1 and 42 mg/dL on day 7, despite no known bromide intake during that period. The values reported were verified by the technologist performing the assay. She repeated the test each time with essentially the same results.

Further questioning of the patient's wife revealed that it was unlikely that Brian R. took any drugs containing bromide prior to admission. He had been taking usual doses of furosemide, theophylline, lorazepam, digoxin, and potassium iodide (as an expectorant). His drugs were not changed in the hospital, except that multivitamins were added and his expectorant dose was increased.

*Why was Brian R.'s bromide concentration elevated? Was the elevation real? How might one investigate whether a drug–lab test interference was occurring?*

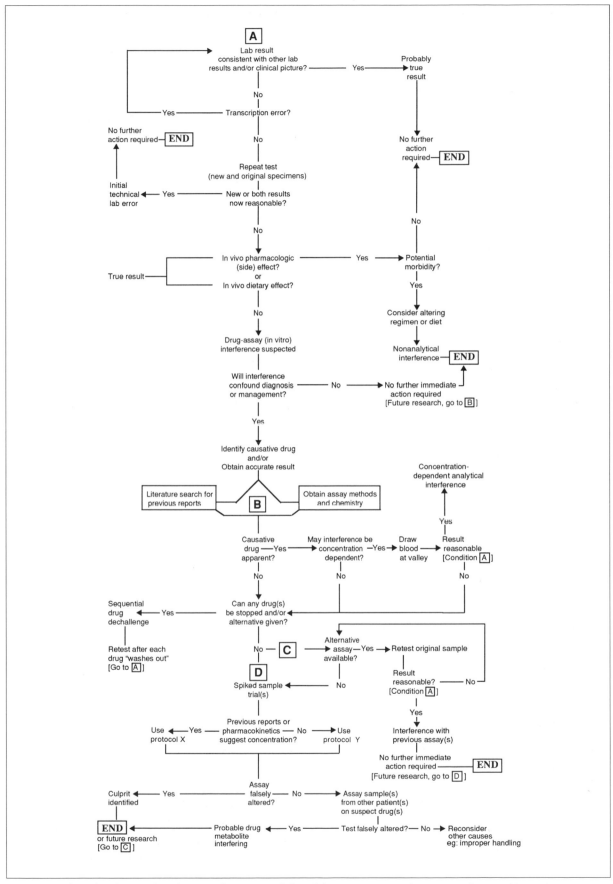

**FIGURE 1.** Algorithm for initial evaluation of a suspected drug–laboratory test interference (as discussed in text).

and yielded essentially the same numbers. In some cases, a second specimen should be tested; however, interpretation may be different because of the time differential. If the original specimen is no longer available, a second specimen is the only option. If results from the retested original and new specimens are both reasonable, some initial technical laboratory error probably occurred (e.g., one-time assay performance error). If the result from the retested original specimen does not change significantly but the result from the new specimen is reasonable, the original specimen may contain an interferent. Possible interferents include

> - A drug or metabolite whose concentration was higher during the first draw.
> - Residual detergent in the glassware.
> - The wrong type of collection tube (containing an interfering preservative).

In any case, if neither of the new results meets the criteria in A (as with Brian R.), the clinician should follow the algorithm down the "No" path for further investigation.

At this point, one should consider whether an in vivo pharmacological or dietary effect may be involved. The possibility of surreptitious or occult ingestion of substances containing bromide was ruled out by Brian R.'s wife and nurses.

In another example outside of this case, a practitioner may be unaware that platelet counts have been reported to increase substantially in some patients taking cefuroxime axetil. After further research, the practitioner finds that no morbidity is associated with the high count and that the count usually normalizes when the drug is discontinued. Further immediate exploration is unnecessary. If there were associated morbidity or if the pharmacological effect confounded diagnosis or therapy, the clinician would have to consider altering the regimen. The discovery would be an in vivo pharmacological effect.

Once an in vivo effect is ruled out, the clinician should redirect efforts toward in vitro, particularly drug–assay interferences. Again, action need not be taken at this time unless the interference confounds diagnosis or management. The goal is to identify the causative agent and/or obtain an accurate result. Segment B deals with this stage.

## Algorithm Segment B

The next step is to search the literature for related reports. Although reports of the same interference may not exist, those involving similar drugs or assays may furnish needed evidence. The clinician cannot assume that a drug does not interfere with a particular test just because it is not listed in the assay circular, or vice versa. Manufacturers of laboratory assays are not obliged to perform comprehensive analyses. A pharmaceutical company is most likely to study tests that

> - Are frequently performed in the general population.
> - Evaluate drug effectiveness or toxicity.
> - May be analytically affected based on the structure or chemical or physical properties of the drug or major metabolites.

An assay developer is most likely to study drugs and metabolites that

> - Are frequently prescribed in the general population.
> - Are prescribed for diseases monitored by the test.
> - May interfere analytically with the test based on the structure or chemical or physical properties of the drug or major metabolites.

These priorities are often also followed by outside researchers after the marketing of a new drug or assay.

Conversely, identification of a similar anecdotal report does not guarantee that the same problem is occurring in the present patient. As with drug–drug interactions, hundreds of reports are made every year. Unfortunately, many anecdotal reports do not give the dose, elimination capabilities of patients, drug concentration, time since last dose, other drugs, special diets, and assay methodology—information needed for a complete analysis. Also, drug effects may vary when multiple drugs are taken together. Few studies, however, have looked at laboratory test effects of combinations of drugs or drugs plus their metabolites.

In general, older literature tends not to be pertinent to today's practice. For example, a current assay used in an automated analyzer instrument may not be susceptible to the same drugs as its predecessor was. Often the methodology differs, or the assay has been altered to become more specific. Improved specificity is the case for immunoassays for drugs—more and more monoclonal antibodies are being used to increase specificity. These assays can even distinguish between drugs with very similar structures.

For the minicase, a search of the literature reveals that bromide and iodide can interfere with many chloride assays. However, iodide (which Brian R. was taking in the form of potassium iodide) had not been reported to interfere with bromide assays. Because of the patient's clinical history and the chemical similarity of iodide to other halides, the clinician should have strong suspicions of iodide interference. The assay chemistry, as obtained from the laboratory, is based on the anionic exchange of chlorine with bromine as gold salts:

$$AuCl_3 + 3Br^- \rightarrow AuBr_3 + 3Cl^-$$

**TABLE 2.** Protocol X—Spiking Body Fluid Samples Using Pharmacokinetic or NCCLS[a] Data

1. From general literature or NCCLS data,[10] estimate drug concentration range in body fluid based on dose, absorption, distribution, and excretion characteristics

2. For serum, spike "clean" serum samples at expected mean, valley, peak, and eight times peak concentrations. For urine, estimate amount of drug excreted in 24 hr and test four, two, and one times this quantity per liter of "clean" urine

3. If pure drug is unavailable, use pharmaceutical dosage form with least amount of nonactive ingredients, preferably injectable (if only solid form is available, extraction may be necessary)

4. Perform assay on specimens using blank fluid as control

5. If "spiked" sample results are above assay limits, retest serial dilutions

[a]NCCLS = National Committee for Clinical Laboratory Standards.

Gold bromide, which is yellow-brown, is then quantified colorimetrically. The suspected interference reaction assumes that iodide takes the place of bromide. A literature search reveals that gold iodide also is yellow-brown. Based on an increased bromide concentration with an increased potassium iodide dose, the interference is postulated to be concentration dependent. The apparent causative agent is discontinued. Since Brian R. is then discharged, however, no followup bromide or iodide levels are obtained. If Brian R. had not been discharged, another bromide level would have been taken after an iodide washout period.

When the causative drug is not apparent, a sequential discontinuation of drugs should be pursued, with bromide levels obtained after each. If the clinician cannot withdraw the suspect agents or replace them with a therapeutic equivalent and then remeasure bromide concentrations, paths C and D have to be considered.

## Algorithm Segment C

In this segment, the clinician confirms the existence of a drug–assay interference without necessarily identifying the specific interferent. At the time of the minicase, no alternative assay was available. Since then, assays that can distinguish bromide from iodide (ion-specific electrodes, ion chromatography, and gas chromatography as discussed in Chapter 2) have been introduced. If these assays had been available, Brian R.'s samples would have been retested.

An alternative assay with a different chemical or physical basis is preferred because it is less prone to the same interferences. Results should be more reasonable (in this case, bromide in the normal range) with the new testing method. To identify the interfering drug, spiked sample trials must be performed (segment D).

## Algorithm Segment D

Here the clinician attempts to identify the interferent and to characterize the interaction using samples spiked with known quantities of drug. If the literature provides information on concentrations to use in the trials, the investigator should follow protocol X (Table 2). This protocol also should be followed if enough pharmacokinetic data are available for estimating probable specimen concentrations for a given dose. On the other hand, protocol Y (Table 3) should be used if pharmacokinetic data are inadequate.

To avoid missing an interaction because of underestimation, both protocols start with higher than expected specimen drug concentrations. If an interference is seen only at the highest concentration of a particular drug, and this concentration is very unlikely for a particular patient, the drug should not be indicted.

For patient-specific investigations, the researcher should try to match the characteristics of the test sample specimens (and blank) with those of the patient. In other words, not adjusting for an unusually high or low blood or urine pH may prevent the interference from being reproduced, even though the interferent is being tested. Any effect caused by the unusual characteristics of a specimen—and not by a drug—would be apparent after a positive finding with a blank. In in vitro testing for an interference, the spiked sample may not interact—even though the "drug" is the cause—if a metabolite of the drug is affecting the assay. Extraction of active drug from dosage forms, preparation of test solutions, and statistical applications to data are beyond the scope of this book. The reader is referred to the National Committee for Clinical Laboratory Standards guidelines.[10]

**TABLE 3.** Protocol Y—Spiking Samples If Pharmacokinetic or NCCLS Data Are Not Available[a]

1. Serum: Use concentration equal to eight, four, two, and one times daily dose diluted in 5 L of "clean" serum if drug is unlikely to distribute much beyond bloodstream (i.e., hydrophilic or charged molecules); if drug probably distributes into extracellular fluid, dilute in 15 L; if unsure, use both diluent volumes

2. Urine: Use eight, four, two, and one times daily dose diluted in "clean" urine in volume close to that of patient's urinary output if known or 2 L if unknown

3. Gastric fluid: Estimate maximum concentration based on dose and gastric fluid volume (50–100 mL) and test four, two, one, and half times this concentration; oral forms may be ideal for GI specimens, so "inert" ingredients also may be added (if unlikely to be absorbed at time of interference)

4. Perform assay on specimens using blank fluid as control

5. If "spiked" sample results are above or at assay limits, retest serial dilutions

[a]Adapted from Reference 11.

For the minicase, a modification of protocol Y is used. Both 50- and 25-mg/dL dilutions of potassium iodide in blank serum are prepared. When the 50-mg/dL sample is assayed for bromide, the result is "above upper limit of assay." The 25-mg/dL sample is reported as bromide 47 mg/dL.

## CLINICALLY IMPORTANT ANALYTICAL DRUG–LABORATORY INTERFERENCES

An analytical interference becomes *clinically significant* (in contrast to statistically significant) when it is likely to lead to inappropriate decisionmaking. As already discussed, the degree of false elevation or depression of a result is not the only factor. In fact, if a quantitative test result is extremely altered by a drug, the clinician is more inclined to suspect an interference (despite the absence of paradoxical findings). If the result is only moderately altered, however, the interference may go unnoticed and inappropriate action may be taken. In other words, the clinician may change a drug, dosage, or case management approach because of information the affected result portends.

An interference becomes *clinically relevant* when a drug is likely to be in the blood or other specimen source during a commonly used test. For example, in acetaminophen overdose, various liver function tests including ALP probably will be run and *N*-acetylcysteine probably will be administered. As the serum concentrations of cysteine increase, however, ALP readings become falsely decreased.[12] This finding is relevant because clinicians may underestimate the degree of hepatotoxicity without other tests that also assess liver damage. Fortunately, when acetaminophen hepatotoxicity is suspected, ALT levels are usually ordered. The ALT assay is not affected by cysteine.

Relevancy increases if a drug has a history of generating spurious results with many assays. It is particularly important to consider potential interferences with such drugs, just as it is to consider seriously a drug–drug interaction in a patient on warfarin or cimetidine. Drug classes that cause the most analytical interferences include antibacterials, antihypertensives, anticonvulsants, hormones, and psychoactive agents. Some specific drugs include ascorbic acid, levodopa, methyldopa, propranolol, radiographic agents, and theophylline.

Ascorbic acid is especially relevant because many patients take large doses of it, and this vitamin interferes with numerous assays, particularly those using the peroxidase method. This method is common with multi-test reagent-impregnated strips for blood, Hgb, and glucose. On the other hand, drugs notable for their relative lack of interference include digoxin, furosemide, bumetanide, ethacrynic acid, diazepam, chlorpheniramine, propoxyphene, and nonabsorbable drugs in nonstool specimens.

## REFERENCE SOURCES ON DRUG–LABORATORY TEST INTERFERENCES

Clinicians should be familiar with sources of information—books, journals, databases, and computer services—on this topic. Then, retrospectively at least, they should be able to confirm or rule out this problem.

The widely used *Physicians' Desk Reference* includes official product information circulars. Newer monographs contain a section called "drug–lab test interferences," which is separate from the section on test result abnormalities (accurate analytical readings of a side effect seen in some patients on the drug). Monographs in *AHFS Drug Information*, published by the American Society of Health-System Pharmacists, also contain a section on lab test interferences. Although the information provided is brief, it can be used as a "screen." *Meyler's Side Effects of Drugs* gives limited background information on each interference and is referenced.

As mentioned previously, Young updated his comprehensive compilation of the effects of drugs on tests and published a 1991 supplement. Young's books are divided into two sections: a database sorted by test and a database sorted by drug. This compilation includes pharmacological and analytical effects (using primary, secondary, and tertiary references) and is the most useful tool for initial screening for suspected drug–lab test interferences.

Services that also maintain this type of information include the Iowa Drug Information Service and Drugdex. They are available on microfiche and CD-ROM computer disk. Electronic databases, such as DataStar and Medicom, are also available for computer use.

Journals that routinely cover this topic include *Clinical Chemistry, Clinical Chemistry and Clinical Biochemistry, Clinica Chimica Acta, Annals of Clinical and Laboratory Science, Clinical Biochemistry*, and *American Journal of Clinical Pathology*.

### Books and Review Articles

Dukes MNG, ed. Meyler's side effects of drugs. New York: Elsevier (most recent edition).

Hansten PD, Horn J. Drug interactions. Vancouver, WA: Applied Therapeutics (most recent edition).

Knoben JE, Anderson PO. Handbook of clinical drug data, 7th ed. Hamilton, IL: Drug Intelligence Publications; 1993.

McEvoy GK, ed. AHFS drug information. Bethesda, MD: American Society of Health-System Pharmacists (most recent edition).

Physicians' desk reference, 50th ed. Oradel, NJ: Medical Economics; 1996.

Salway JG. Drug–test interaction handbook, 1st ed. New York: Raven Press; 1990.

Tryding N, Roos K-A. Drug interferences and drug effects in clinical chemistry, 6th ed. Stockholm, Sweden: Apotekbolaget; 1992.

Wallach J. Interpretation of diagnostic tests: a synopsis of laboratory medicine, 5th ed. Boston, MA: Little, Brown; 1992.

Young DS. Effects of drugs on clinical laboratory tests, 3rd ed. Washington, DC: American Association for Clinical Chemistry Press; 1990 and supplement 1991.

## Journal Articles and Supplements

Kabat HF, Constantino NV. Drug-induced modifications of laboratory test values. *Am J Hosp Pharm.* 1973; 30:24–71.

Kroll MH, Elin RJ. Interference with clinical laboratory analyses. *Clin Chem.* 1994; 40:1996–2000.

National Committee for Clinical Laboratory Standards. Interference testing in clinical chemistry: proposed guidelines. NCCLS publication EP7-P. Villanova, PA: National Committee for Clinical Laboratory Standards; 1986 (or most recent edition).

Sher PP. Drug interferences with clinical laboratory tests. *Drugs.* 1982; 24:24–63.

Yosselson-Superstine S. Drug interference with clinical tests performed by a 20-channel computerized autoanalyzer. *Am J Hosp Pharm.* 1982; 39:848–9.

## Information/Computer Services

DataStar. Plaza Suite, 114 Jermyn St., London SW1Y 9HJ, England.

Drugdex Information System. Micromedex, 660 Bancock St., Denver, CO 80204-4506.

Iowa Drug Information Service (IDIS), University of Iowa, Oakdale, IA 52319.

Medicom micro clinical laboratory test interference database. Professional Drug Systems, 2388 Schuetz Rd., Suite A-56, St. Louis, MO 63146.

## SUMMARY

Most drug effects on laboratory tests reflect a true physiological change caused by a pharmacological action. However, drug–laboratory test interferences do occur and should be suspected when an inconsistency exists among related test results or between test results and the clinical picture.

This chapter explores ways to identify and evaluate potential interferences. Because the possible combinations and permutations of laboratory test interference by drugs are in the millions, only the most clinically relevant ones can be remembered. Newer assays usually are more specific and, therefore, less affected by drugs than were older methods. Thus, it is essential to understand the mechanisms of interferences of laboratory tests and to be able to recognize paradoxical chemical–clinical findings.

## REFERENCES

1. Norfleet RG, Rhodes RA, Saviage K. False-positive Hemoccult reaction with cimetidine. *N Engl J Med.* 1980; 302:467. Letter.
2. Schentag JJ. False-positive Hemoccult reaction with cimetidine. *N Engl J Med.* 1980; 303:110. Letter.
3. Hauser A, Quigley ML, Driever CW, et al. More on false-positive Hemoccult reaction with cimetidine. *N Engl J Med.* 1980; 303:847–8. Letter.
4. Pickering LK, Rutherford I. Effect of concentration and time upon inactivation of tobramycin, gentamicin, netilmicin, and amikacin by azlocillin, carbenicillin, mecillinam, mezlocillin and piperacillin. *J Pharmacol Exp Ther.* 1981; 217:345–9.
5. Chow MS, Quintiliani R, Nightingale CH. In vivo inactivation of tobramycin by ticarcillin. *JAMA.* 1982; 247:658–9.
6. Thompson MI, Russo ME, Saxon BJ, et al. Gentamicin inactivation by piperacillin or carbenicillin in patients with end stage renal disease. *Antimicrob Agents Chemother.* 1982; 21:268–73.
7. Bryan CS, Stone WJ. Comparably massive penicillin G therapy in renal failure. *Ann Intern Med.* 1975; 82:189–95.
8. Young DS, Pestaner C, Gibberman V. Effects of drugs on clinical laboratory tests. *Clin Chem.* 1975; 21:1D–432D.
9. Young DS. Effects of drugs on clinical laboratory tests, 3rd ed. Washington, DC: American Association for Clinical Chemistry Press; 1990.
10. National Committee for Clinical Laboratory Standards. Interference testing in clinical chemistry: proposed guidelines, vol. 6. NCCLS publication EP7-P. Villanova, PA: National Committee for Clinical Laboratory Standards; 1986:259–366.
11. Galteau MM, Siest G. Guidelines for evaluation of analytical interference. *Ann Biol Clin (Paris).* 1984; 42:137–44.
12. Letellier G, Desjarlais F. Analytical interference of drugs in clinical chemistry: I. Study of 20 drugs on seven different instruments. *Clin Biochem.* 1985; 18:345–51.

## Chapter 4

# Drugs of Abuse Testing

*Gregory N. Hayner*

Testing of individuals for various drugs of abuse is now one of the most common types of biological testing. Such tests are used by government agencies and private corporations. In the legal arena, not only criminal defendants but also parties to divorce actions and child dependency cases may be tested for their use of drugs and alcohol.

To promote worker safety and to avoid financial losses due to employee substance use, many companies now require preemployment drug testing as a hiring condition. The drugs of concern range from illicit street drugs (e.g., heroin and cocaine) to prescription medications prone to abuse when taken inappropriately. Additional testing, either randomly or due to suspicion of drug use, also may be required during employment. Such testing is based in part on estimates that as many as one in six members of the U.S. federal work force uses illicit drugs or abuses prescription drugs regularly. Reportedly, one-third of the applicants to the New York Transit Authority have had positive drug tests on preemployment screening.[1]

Health practitioners also may perform drug and alcohol testing when making a differential diagnosis. Numerous physical and psychiatric illnesses may be caused, in part, by substance use or withdrawal. In addition, many symptoms of such use mimic other conditions, making it prudent to rule out this cause of patient complaints.[1]

Furthermore, the Federal Government, with the issuance of Executive Order 12564, mandated the maintenance of a drug-free federal workplace in September 1986. This order stipulates that all federal employees must refrain from illegal drug use both on and off the job.[2] Since that time, such testing has been extended to private employers who receive government contracts or subsidies.

As a consequence, many health professionals probably will be asked to interpret drug screen results. This chapter is written to facilitate an understanding of this deceptive and complex topic.

## OBJECTIVES

Upon completion of this chapter, the reader should be able to

1. List the testing methods used in drug and substance abuse screening and discuss their limitations.
2. Discuss the difference between screening and confirmatory testing of urine samples and recognize the need for both.
3. Discuss the significance of a positive drug screen in a population with a high incidence of substance use versus a population with a low incidence (i.e., predictive value of the test result).
4. Discuss why ingestion of interfering substances can cause both false-negative and false-positive results of screening tests.
5. Recognize the adulterants commonly added to a urine sample and discuss how each affects the test outcome.
6. Discuss the effects of various blood alcohol concentrations on physical and mental performance.

## TESTING METHODS

Various methods of testing biological samples for drug use have been developed, primarily for screening purposes. These methods involve hair samples,[3,4] saliva,[5] perspiration stains,[6] blood stains, and semen[7] in addition to urine. Nevertheless, urinalysis is the only testing method recognized by the Food and Drug Administration (FDA) and the National Institute on Drug Abuse (NIDA) for employee testing[2] because

➤ Sample collection is relatively noninvasive in nature.

➤ Well-recognized and accepted methods of quality assurance are possible.

Therefore, the discussion will focus mainly on urine testing.

### Urine Testing

As a waste product, urine contains substances that were in the body *some time in the past*. However, the urine may not accurately reflect the presence of these substances in the body at the time the sample is taken. Furthermore, the presence of a drug and/or its metabolites in urine does not necessarily imply drug intoxication at the time the sample is obtained. Urinary drug and metabolite concentrations may be due to a large drug dose taken even days before sample collection or to a small dose taken recently. Attempts to use actual urinary concentrations may be influenced by such things as

> The time of day when the sample is obtained.
> Sample pH.
> The individual's state of hydration.

In addition, one must be aware of the analyte detected by a specific test. High concentrations of a metabolite say nothing about drug intoxication at the sampling time. Metabolites of drugs, such as tetrahydrocannabinol, with long clearance half-lives may be excreted long after the last use of a substance.[8]

Urine testing, therefore, is best looked at as a snapshot of drug use during the previous few hours or past several days. It gives no information as to the pattern or chronicity of an individual's drug use, unless the test is repeated over time.

As discussed later, substances other than drugs of abuse may interfere with the test or indicate prescription drug use. Hence, the Federal Government requires that a medical review officer—a physician with knowledge of substance abuse disorders as well as the pharmacology and toxicology of illicit drugs—evaluates the findings before accepting raw data and reporting results to an employer.[2] This medical review officer must interpret positive results in the context of the test itself, the subject's medical history, the chain of custody of the sample, and the clinical evidence of illicit drug use. In this way, alternative medical or scientific explanations are explored before action is taken on the basis of a positive test result.[2]

There also are statistical reasons for not taking all test results at face value. *No method of detection has absolute accuracy.* Even very low rates of error can be important if enough people are tested and/or the incidence of drug use is very low. Predictive value plays an important role in drug screening.

To illustrate this concept, Osterloh and Becker[9] cited a hypothetical test specificity of 99.9% (i.e., 0.1% or 0.001 false-positive rate) for 1000 people being tested for marijuana and phencyclidine (PCP) use. In such a case, one false-positive result is expected for every 1000 tests run due to the limitations of the test itself. Now, if the actual incidence of PCP use is very low in this group while marijuana use is relatively high, one person out of the 1000 will actually have PCP in the urine while 100 of the 1000 will have the marijuana metabolite. In this case, the predictive value of the test results would vary widely. If two tests are positive for PCP, then only one result may be considered valid, meaning that the test has a 50% reliability even though the specificity is still 99.9%.

In the case of marijuana, however, with 101 positive test results, 100 can be considered valid with one false positive. Here, the test is 99% reliable, even with a specificity identical to that for PCP. For PCP in this example, the expected rates of true and false positives are identical, making the test result meaningless by itself. Thus, random testing for a drug with very low incidence of use in a particular population is not cost effective or predictive of actual usage among that group.

## Hair Analysis

Of the nonurine methods, hair analysis has received the most attention despite ongoing problems. Since drugs and their metabolites are incorporated into the hair shaft from the circulatory system,[3] this test, in theory at least, should have some advantages. Its proponents believe that[10]

> Hair testing expands the window of detection of abused drugs from a few days to several months.
> Hair samples are less invasive and much less embarrassing to collect than urine samples.
> Contamination or adulteration of a hair sample is much more difficult than with a urine sample.
> Hair samples require no special storage conditions and do not pose a threat of disease transmission.
> Reproducible hair samples are obtainable for retesting if necessary.

Despite these attractive features, serious questions about this technique remain. Studies have investigated the time course and dose–response relationship between drug dosage and hair drug concentration.[5,11] There is, however, disagreement concerning drug deposition in the hair of people of different races, sexes, and ages. For example, the coarse black hair of some African Americans may absorb proportionally more cocaine than the hair of Caucasians.[11–13] Studies to elucidate this phenomenon remain to be performed, leaving open the question of racial bias in hair analysis.

Furthermore, the detection of drugs found in low concentrations in hair presents technical problems. Up to 1000 times greater test sensitivity is needed to analyze the drug content of hair as compared to urine. This demanding requirement stretches the sensitivity limits of most analytical techniques.[14] In addition, such common hair treatments as shampooing and conditioning, not to mention bleaching, can reduce the drug concentrations present even further.[15]

For these reasons and others, the FDA does not accept hair analysis as a proven procedure supported by scientific literature or clinical trials. Radioimmunoassay (RIA), the most commonly used technique for hair analysis, is "not generally recognized by qualified experts as reliable" when applied to hair.[16] Therefore, despite its allure as a test sample capable of providing a linear drug use map for a particular individual, hair analysis has yet to prove itself in situations involving serious consequences. Its use by employers or the courts must be approached with caution.

## Alcohol Testing

Alcohol testing is treated separately because results are usually quantitative rather than qualitative. Qualitative results, however, may be used in special circumstances (e.g., alcohol treatment programs) when consumption rather than impairment is in question.

Blood alcohol concentrations are routinely used to determine a person's ability to drive safely. In addition, physicians may use such concentrations to evaluate changes in consciousness in a patient smelling of alcohol. Alcohol intoxication also can affect the body's response to various drugs. Often, this effect is due to augmented central nervous system depression, leading to possible overdose. The major impetus for testing alcohol concentrations, however, continues to be the high rate of motor vehicle accidents and traffic deaths attributable, at least in part, to drinking.

Testing for alcohol takes several forms. Breath analysis has been used since the 1930s and is still common. With this method, expired air is collected and analyzed for its alcohol content. This number is then used to calculate an equivalent blood alcohol content. This calculation may be accomplished with an Alcometer that uses a fuel cell to oxidize the alcohol present. Electrical current generated by this process then activates one of three colored lights, providing a quantitative estimate of blood alcohol concentrations.

Alternatively, saliva may be tested using various simple devices.[17,18] A Breathalyser, used in the laboratory, relies on color changes in a vial of chromic acid. The color changes occur as alcohol is oxidized. An intoximeter, another laboratory device, uses infrared spectroscopy.

Blood alcohol determinations are accomplished using gas chromatography, enzymatic oxidation with alcohol dehydrogenase, chromic acid oxidation, and osmometry. Of these methods, gas chromatography is the most specific.[19]

## Test Limitations

The primary controversy surrounding drug testing involves the limitations of passive exposure. This controversy has centered primarily around marijuana testing, partly due to the large numbers of people using this drug as well as its wide acceptance as an innocuous activity. Passive exposure can confound test results and produce false positives.

### Urine Testing

The urine test of particular concern in passive exposure is the 20-ng/mL enzyme-multiplied immunoassay technique (EMIT); it is favored by many companies whose employees work under potentially hazardous conditions. This assay treats urinary concentrations of tetrahydrocannabinol of 20 ng/mL or more as "positive." Hayden reviewed the literature concerning this subject and found that experimental conditions varied widely.[20]

In the most extreme case, subjects were placed in an area, roughly the size of a 4-ft³ packing crate, and exposed to the smoke of four marijuana cigarettes over a 30-min period.[20]

When tested, these subjects indeed showed urinary concentrations of tetrahydrocannabinol at or above 20 ng/mL on the day of the experiment (maximum of 30 ng/mL). Moreover, they were extremely uncomfortable due to the high smoke levels.[20]

The most realistic study placed subjects in a room, $10 \times 10 \times 8$ ft, and exposed them to the smoke of four marijuana cigarettes over a 1-hr period. Samples taken 20–24 hr after exposure were all less than 6 ng/mL.[20]

Therefore, Hayden concluded that only unrealistically high concentrations of smoke yield urinary concentrations at even a 20-ng/mL cutoff, let alone the 100 ng/mL at which most people are tested. As one might expect, these conditions also are associated with subjective effects of intoxication. Claims that ambient exposure to marijuana smoke has yielded a positive urine screen can now be firmly discounted, at least at a cutoff concentration of 100 ng/mL. Also, testing at 20 ng/mL is affected only under conditions that are not clinically relevant.

### Hair Analysis

A serious problem with hair analysis is that washing hair samples may not be sufficient to remove surface drug contamination and to avoid falsely elevated concentrations. In one study, the external contamination of samples was often undetectable, nor were attempts at decontamination successful.[21] Due to this effect, externally applied PCP yielded a false-positive result because the drug bound tightly to the hair sample.[22] As a consequence, passive exposure to drugs may be problematic with this testing method.

## SCREENING VERSUS CONFIRMATORY TESTS

To safeguard against test inaccuracy and false accusations, a two-tiered testing system is employed:

1. A screening test is conducted.
2. A confirmatory assay is performed.

The second test should use a different methodology than

the screening test so that substances responsible for false-positive results can be eliminated.

## Screening Tests

The usual screening test is an immunoassay. Three types are in common use:

> ➤ EMIT—used by all NIDA-certified laboratories.
> ➤ RIA—used for urine testing for nonforensic purposes.
> ➤ Fluorescence polarization immunoassay (FPIA).

Thin layer chromatography also may be employed when an inexpensive, wide-spectrum screen is desired. Although this method can detect several drugs simultaneously, the technician must have great skill and experience because substances can cause similar color changes in close proximity on the plate.[23]

These tests are employed to screen out urine samples that contain either none of the drug in question or concentrations representing negative results. Positive samples require further testing to determine the exact substance causing the result. The principles and mechanisms of such test technologies are discussed in Chapter 2.

## Confirmatory Tests

Confirmatory testing should be done on urine samples having positive results on initial screening. The major flaw of immunoassay screening tests—low specificity but high sensitivity for analytes at very low concentrations—must be avoided. Analytes with structures similar to drugs of abuse also interact with antibodies contained in screening and give false-positive results.

A classic example is the interaction of various sympathomimetic amines, some of which are in nonprescription medications, with the tests for amphetamines.[24] The introduction of monoclonal antibody tests cannot completely avoid this problem. Antibodies can recognize only a particular part of a molecule. Side chains on other parts of a molecule may drastically change its pharmacological effects and yet be detected as the parent drug by such tests. As a result, antibody testing, while inexpensive and rapid, cannot stand alone as the definitive test for the presence of drugs of abuse in urine.

An examination of Figure 1 shows how close some "amphetamine-like" structures are to each other. Labetalol, for example, contains a phenyl ring with a carbon side chain and might be considered a depressant of some bodily functions. However, interpreting a positive result simply from the presence of this substance in the urine would be a grave error. Nevertheless, one would want to know if an employee listing this medication as a prescription was also consuming amphetamines. The only truly reliable information is to be found in confirmatory testing.

The best method for confirming a positive screening test result is gas chromatography–mass spectrometry (GC–MS). As opposed to immunoassays, this method is both highly specific and sensitive. By its very nature, GC–MS is not *as susceptible* to cross-reactivities. When interference does occur, it is usually caused by chemical reactions taking place during testing or by the physical properties of the cross-reactant. The major drawbacks of GC–MS are that it

> ➤ Is expensive.
> ➤ Is time consuming.
> ➤ Can be performed only by highly trained technologists with supervision by certified toxicologists.

This method, therefore, is unsuitable as a screening tool when many samples must be analyzed within a relatively short period.[23]

High performance liquid chromatography (HPLC) also may be used to verify screening results for nonforensic purposes. Gas-liquid chromatography (GLC) is helpful for the detection of alcohol and volatile inhalants in blood and urine.[23] Neither method, however, is specific enough to satisfy federal guidelines.[2]

## TEST INTERPRETATION

### Drug Testing Procedures

Federal guidelines specify testing for marijuana and cocaine use as a minimum requirement. Testing for opiates, amphetamines, and PCP is optional.

As shown in Table 1, standard cutoff concentrations have been set for each drug group, both for immunoassay and GC–MS confirmation. These concentrations represent the minimum that must be present in a urine sample before it is reported positive for a particular drug. A positive result gives no indication of how high the actual urine drug concentration is. Conversely, a negative result simply means that illicit drugs, if present, are not in high enough concentrations to register as positive.

Table 2 (page 46) demonstrates that these numbers do not represent the lower limits of detection or sensitivity for these tests.[25] Rather, these concentrations represent a balance between the desire to detect actual drug use and the desire to minimize false-positive results. False-positive results become more likely when a test is stretched to its detection limits.

Positive results from immunoassays are referred to as presumptive positives; confirmation testing still must verify the presence of drugs in the urine. As discussed later, various substances other than illicit drugs may cross react with the antibodies of the immunoassays. This cross-reactivity causes the most fear in subjects being tested; they are afraid of being accused of illicit drug use because of innocent medication use or food ingestion.

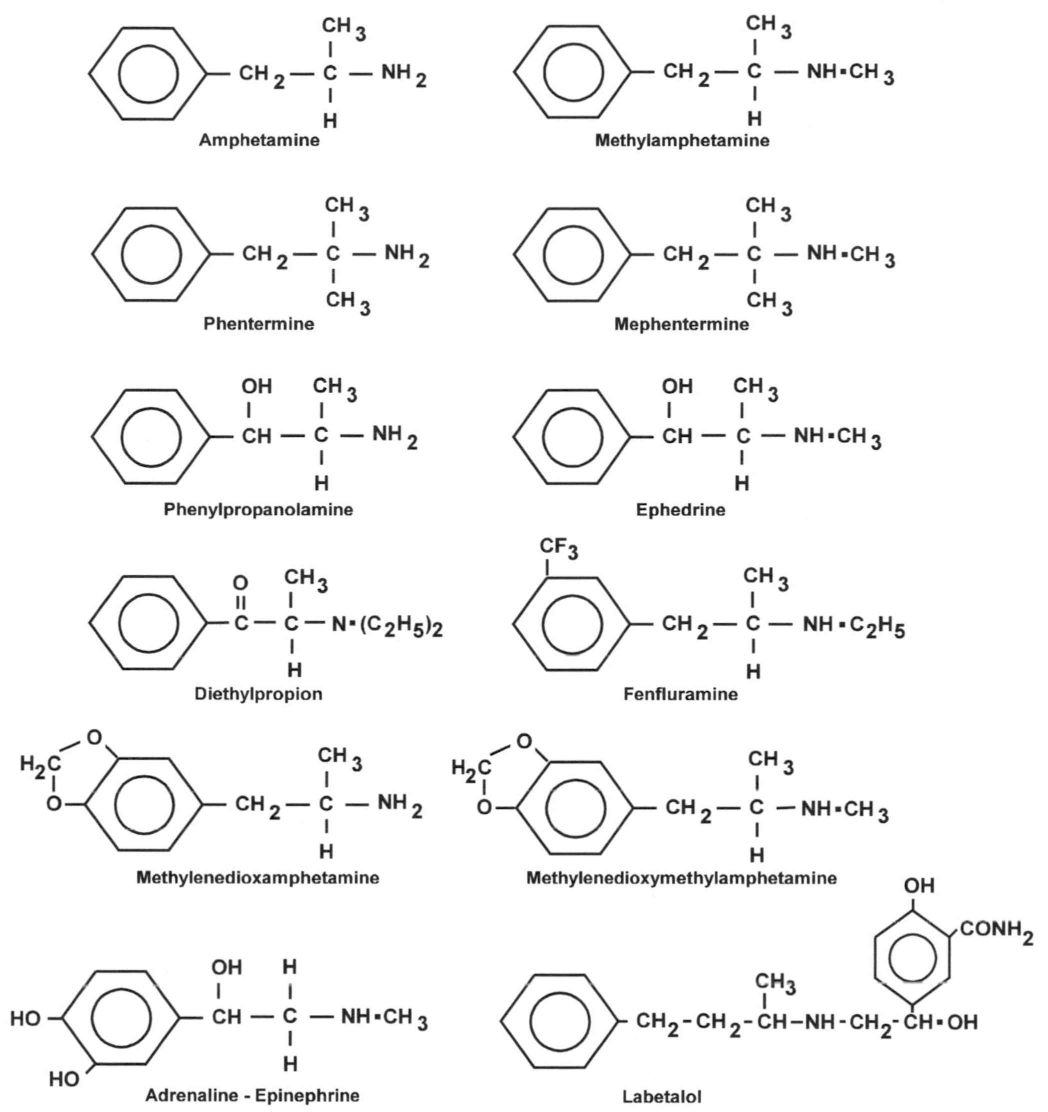

**FIGURE 1.** Structures of amphetamine and analogs that may cross-react in immunoassay tests. (Reproduced, with permission, from Reference 24.)

**TABLE 1.** NIDA Drug Testing Panel[a]

| Drug | Immunoassay Screening Level (ng/ml) | GC–MS Confirmatory Cutoff (ng/ml) |
| --- | --- | --- |
| Cannabinoids ($\Delta^9$-tetrahydrocannabinol-9-carboxylic acid) | 100 | 15 |
| Cocaine (benzoylecgonine) | 300 | 150 |
| Opiates (morphine, codeine, 6-acetyl-morphine) | 300 | 300 |
| PCP | 25 | 25 |
| Amphetamines (amphetamine and meth-amphetamine) | 1000 | 500 |

[a]*Adapted, with permission, from Fretthold DW. Drug-testing methods and reliability. J Psychoactive Drugs. 1990; 22:420.*

**TABLE 2.** Sensitivity of Commonly Used Drug Urinalysis Methods[a,b]

| Drug Group | Chromatography | | | Immunoassay | |
|---|---|---|---|---|---|
| | TLC[c] | GLC | GC–MS | EMIT[d] | RIA[e] |
| Amphetamines | 0.5 µg/mL | 0.7 µg/mL | 10 ng/mL | 0.7 µg/mL | 1 µg/mL |
| Barbiturates | 0.5 µg/mL | 0.5 µg/mL | 0.5 µg/mL | 0.5 µg/mL | 0.1 µg/mL |
| Benzodiazepines | | | 0.5 µg/mL | 0.5 µg/mL | |
| Cannabinoids | | | 1 ng/mL | 100 ng/mL | 100 ng/mL |
| Cocaine | 2 µg/mL | 0.75 µg/mL | 5 ng/mL | 0.75 µg/mL | 5 µg/mL |
| Methadone | 1 µg/mL | 0.5 µg/mL | 5 ng/mL | 0.5 µg/mL | |
| Heroin and morphine | 0.5 µg/mL | | 0.5 µg/mL | 0.5 µg/mL | 25 ng/mL |
| PCP | 0.5 µg/mL | 150 ng/mL | 5 ng/mL | 150 ng/mL | 100 ng/mL |

[a]Adapted, with permission, from Reference 25.
[b]The values listed are not precise, because many variables alter the sensitivity of the test in a particular laboratory.
[c]Thin-layer chromatography.
[d]SYVA Company, Palo Alto, California.
[e]Radioimmunoassay levels listed are the lower limit of detection.

Presumptive positive results are then subjected to confirmation by GC–MS. Due to the high specificity of this method, most cross-reactants should be eliminated as the cause of a positive result.[19] Of course, with the exception of PCP, all other test categories have legitimate therapeutic uses. Therefore, part of the confirmation process by a medical review officer is

1. To determine if there is some legitimate reason for a substance being in the urine.
2. To report the urine sample result as negative if such a reason exists.

Whether the clinician considers such a result as negative depends on the situation and the reason for testing. If an employee is tested "for cause" (i.e., suspicion of intoxication on the job or investigation following an industrial accident), one might want to know if the person is positive for drugs regardless of whether the drugs are prescribed. If, on the other hand, the clinician is interested in whether the employee uses illegal substances or is a potential drug abuser, a negative result is proper. Employees should be able to keep information concerning medical treatment confidential unless their ability to perform their jobs are adversely affected.

Table 3 lists the amount of time after drug usage that urine testing remains positive for various drugs. These times become longer with higher doses. With tetrahydrocannabinol and cocaine, this time depends on the duration of use. If it is prolonged, these drugs are stored and deposited in tissue. Testing does not pick up results from sporadic usage that fall outside of these ranges—leading to one criticism of urine testing. Furthermore, the results do not indicate the chronicity of use. Drug use detected by random testing is just as likely to represent first time use as chronic abuse. In other words, all one can say is that a drug was used to some extent within a narrow time period.

## Signs and Symptoms of Street Drug Use and Abuse

Identifying a person's behavior as symptoms of recent drug use is important when assessing urine test results. This information can help to determine if an employee at a worksite is a problem. Such information is often available before urine testing and, indeed, can help to determine if drug testing is even appropriate. Furthermore, observations of a subject's behavior by coworkers also can corroborate urine test results.

Table 4 lists easily observed symptoms of street drug use—signs that may be picked up by casual observation. Therefore, symptoms such as increased blood pressure and

**TABLE 3.** Detection Periods of NIDA Drug Testing Panel[a]

| Drug | Detection Period |
|---|---|
| Cannabinoids (Δ⁹-tetrahydrocannabinol-9-carboxylic acid) | 2 days–4 weeks |
| Cocaine (benzoylecgonine) | 2–10 days[26] |
| Opiates (morphine, codeine, 6-acetylmorphine) | 2–4 days |
| PCP | Several weeks[27] |
| Amphetamines (amphetamine and methamphetamine)[b] | 2–4 days |

[a]Adapted from Fretthold DW. Drug-testing methods and reliability. J Psychoactive Drugs. 1990; 22:420.
[b]Amphetamine also must be present at a concentration of at least 200 ng/mL before a methamphetamine is reported positive.[27]

heart rate secondary to stimulant use are omitted here but may be found in pharmacology texts. While more complete information might add to one's confidence in ascribing a drug origin to observed behavior, the symptoms in Table 4 should provide enough clues for a firm diagnosis when combined with urinalysis results (Minicase 1). Nonmedical personnel (e.g., work supervisors) also may use this table to document suspected drug use.

Of course, some of the symptoms listed in Table 4 may not be caused by drug use at all. Rapid speech and irritability, for example, may be due to anger instead of cocaine or methamphetamine. Injected conjunctiva, in addition to other symptoms for marijuana, may result from allergies and the use of antihistamines.

As with preliminary urine testing, behavioral evidence is only *suggestive* of drug use or abuse. Neither piece of information is conclusive by itself and cannot be relied on without additional confirmatory testing.

## Test Interference—Morphine, Codeine, and Cocaine

### Foodstuffs

Interpretation of test results for opiates (morphine and codeine) and cocaine requires special consideration because their sources are varied. These substances may be obtained from foodstuffs. Although drugs from food may be present in a person's urine, their concentrations in blood are too low to impart a "high." Moreover, they do not cause problems with physical or mental performance. To the true drug abuser, such foods provide an excuse for drug-positive urine. If opioids are found in random testing, their source is still a question.

Ingestion of poppyseeds has resulted in the detec-

---

> ### ✎ Minicase 1
>
> Following an industrial accident, Shelly E., an employee of a large automobile manufacturer, was seen by the company physician. Shelly E. had no history of drug abuse. In addition to a laceration on Shelly E.'s left arm, the following observations were made:
>
> ◆ Pupil size of 1–2 mm.
> ◆ Dry mouth.
> ◆ Bilateral ptosis.
> ◆ Fresh punctate lesions on left antecubital fossa.
>
> The rest of the physical exam was unremarkable. Shelly E. denied eating poppyseeds or taking any medication.
>
> The physician suspected heroin use and ordered a urine drug test for opiates. One week later, the laboratory report was positive for morphine, codeine, and 6-acetylmorphine, in order of prevalence.
>
> *Has this employee used a drug or substance that would impair her ability to work? What, if any, substance is it?*
>
> **Discussion:** This employee has indeed used heroin, probably within several hours of her industrial accident. As evidence, several findings are consistent with opiate intoxication. In addition, her urine is positive for 6-acetylmorphine. (Since this metabolite is only found in urine following heroin use, its presence eliminates other opiates as possible causes of this person's symptoms.)

tion of both morphine and codeine in urine. These seeds may contain approximately 60 µg/g of morphine and 28–54 µg/g of codeine.[28,29] These amounts are enough to give positive urine results for a person eating poppyseed cake, rolls, bagels, or muffins. Morphine predominates in the urinalysis results. Since heroin is not a natural constitu-

---

**TABLE 4.** Pharmacological and Toxic Effects of Drugs of Abuse[a]

| Drug | Route of Administration | Observed Pharmacological Effects | Observed Toxic Effects |
|---|---|---|---|
| Heroin | Intravenous (IV), intramuscular (IM), intranasal (IN) | Drowsiness, ptosis, pinpoint pupils, slurred speech, dry mouth, facial and flank pruritis | Respiratory depression, coma, death |
| Cocaine or methamphetamine | IV and smoke | Rapid speech, irritability, dry mouth, dilated pupils, short attention span, mood swings | Tremor, paranoia, auditory and visual hallucinations, fornication |
| Marijuana | Smoke and oral | Injected conjunctiva, dry mouth, short attention span, poor muscle coordination, "munchies" | Paranoia, anxiety attacks, flashbacks |
| PCP | IV, oral, smoke | Blank stare, agitation, visual and auditory hallucinations, violent outbursts, delayed verbal response | Seizures and coma |
| Lysergic acid diethylamide (LSD) | Oral | Visual changes, obsessive and delusional thinking, dilated pupils, diaphoresis, giddiness | Flashbacks and persistent psychosis |

[a]*Adapted from Jaffe JH. Drug addiction and drug abuse. In: Gilman AG, Rall TW, Nies AS, et al., eds. Goodman and Gilman's The Pharmacological Basis of Therapeutics. New York: Pergamon Press; 1990:522–73.*

ent of these seeds, a finding of 6-acetylmorphine is reason to conclude heroin use in the tested individual.

Cocaine is a natural constituent of the coca leaf, formerly sold in health food stores as a tea. Although now classified as a controlled substance in the United States, the coca leaf is still available in some South American countries as a tonic beverage. Consequently, recent visitors to these countries may have consumed this tea. For example, visitors to Lima, Peru, are served it to combat the ill effects of coming to a high altitude.

Coca leaf tea can produce detectable amounts of benzoylecgonine in the urine while having insignificant pharmacological effects. Peak urinary concentrations of this metabolite may exceed 1000 ng/mL following ingestion of a single cup of tea.[27] Furthermore, studies to understand the effects of cocaine found that experimental intravenous administration of less than pharmacologically active doses of pure cocaine (25 mg) produced positive urine tests.[26]

### *Prescriptions*

The interpretation of an opiate-positive test may be further complicated by persons having a prescription for these substances. Also, some opiates are metabolized to other opiates. Heroin, for example, is rapidly metabolized to 6-acetylmorphine and then to morphine following administration. Morphine, in turn, is metabolized by conjugation to morphine glucuronide and by demethylation to normorphine. Small amounts of codeine also may be present in street heroin and occur as a minor product of morphine metabolism. Codeine is further metabolized to codeine glucuronide and by *O*-demethylation to norcodeine and morphine.

As a result, a person using heroin has morphine, codeine, and possibly 6-acetylmorphine present in the urine, in order of prevalence. Morphine users test positive for morphine primarily, with lesser amounts of codeine detected. Codeine, because of its metabolism, produces the converse result (i.e., codeine with lesser amounts of morphine present).[2,28] Therefore, the relative concentrations of detected analytes must be noted as well as the contents of a positive sample.

Table 5 presents several scenarios that might be encountered by a health care provider or medical review officer when interpreting opioid urine results. A number of these hypothetical patients blame poppyseed ingestion for positive results. However, this possible interference is usually ruled out by the combination of

> Urine results.
> Signs of intoxication.
> Other indicia of abuse.
> Lack of a legitimate prescription that might explain the findings.

Clinical judgment, in any case, is necessary to determine the true meaning of a positive urine result.

Minicases 2–4 are expansions of selected cases listed in Table 5.

## Test Cross-Reactivity

As mentioned earlier, cross-reactivity is a problem inherent to immunoassay analyses. It occurs, in part, because the antibodies used are not specific to a particular compound but to a family of compounds with similar structures (e.g., amphetamines).[24] To a certain extent, this cross-reactivity is desirable. For example, a subject might be taking amphetamine or methylenedioxymethamphetamine, a similar compound to methamphetamine. If the assay is too specific, especially as a screening test, some drugs that people use would be missed.

Table 6 (page 50) lists some of the most commonly offending drugs resulting in false positives. Most substances that cross-react with tests for amphetamines possess structures similar to these compounds (Figure 1). In most cases, this cross-reactivity is not a problem if GC–MS confirmation is carried out on positive samples. False positives also can occur because not all medications taken by a given individual have been tested for cross-reactivity. New interferences are discovered as time passes and new drugs come to market.

---

### ✎ Minicase 2

Kathy L. was a checker at the local supermarket. Her supervisor thought that she was making too many errors, and her cash drawer was short by $100 for 3 days in a row. Moreover, her coworkers complained that Kathy L. looked sleepy all day and fell asleep on break. She was then sent to the company nurse. After noting a small pupil size, marked drowsiness, and facial scratching, the nurse asked her for a urine sample. Kathy L. was placed on administrative leave pending the outcome of the urine screen.

When the urine sample report came back, it was positive for codeine and a small amount of morphine. When interviewed, Kathy L. denied taking any medications. She also claimed that, at the time of the urine collection, she had been up at night with a sick child. She explained that the opiates in her urine were due to the poppyseed muffins she had eaten for breakfast on the day of the test.

*Has this employee used a drug or substance that would impair her ability to work? What, if any, substance is it?*

**Discussion:** The nurse can conclusively state that this employee is abusing codeine. First, Kathy L. has physical symptoms suggesting opiate use, including the itchy face, a common reaction to systemic histamine release triggered by opiate use. Second, the amounts of codeine and morphine in poppyseed muffins are not enough to cause intoxication. Third, morphine usually predominates over codeine in urine after poppyseed pastries are eaten.

**TABLE 5.** Medical Review Officer's Conclusions in Complex Opioid Cases[a]

| Urinalysis Findings | Presents Prescription | Employee Claims Poppyseed Eating | Shows Signs of Abuse | Medical Review Officer's Conclusion or Probable Explanation |
|---|---|---|---|---|
| 6-Monoacetylmorphine with or without other findings | Not relevant | Not relevant | Not relevant | Urinary confirmation of heroin abuse |
| Morphine | Morphine | Not relevant | Not relevant | No urinary confirmation of opioid abuse |
| Morphine | None | Yes | Yes | Urinary confirmation of heroin or morphine abuse |
| Predominately morphine with some codeine | Morphine | Not relevant | Not relevant | No urinary confirmation of opioid abuse |
| Predominately morphine with some codeine | Codeine | No | Yes | Urinary confirmation of morphine or heroin abuse |
| Predominately morphine with some codeine | Codeine | Yes | Not relevant | No urinary confirmation of opioid abuse |
| Predominately codeine with some morphine | Codeine | Not relevant | Not relevant | No urinary confirmation of opioid abuse |
| Predominately codeine with some morphine | None | Yes | Yes | Urinary confirmation of codeine abuse |
| Predominately codeine with some morphine | None | Yes | None | No urinary confirmation of opioid abuse |
| Negative | None | No | Yes; extreme | No urinary confirmation of opioid abuse |
| Hydromorphine | None | Yes | None | Urinary confirmation of hydromorphone abuse |
| Methadone | Methadone | No | Yes | No urinary confirmation of opioid abuse |
| Methadone and morphine | Methadone | Yes | Yes | No urinary confirmation of morphine or heroin abuse |
| Methadone | None | Yes | Not relevant | Urinary confirmation of methadone abuse |

[a]Adapted from Reference 2.

Similarly, the positive cutoff concentration should not be set too low or too high. If too low, progressively weaker cross-reactive compounds can interact with the assay. A prohibitively large number of "positive" samples then have to be confirmed. If too high, the cutoff may not recognize samples that would be deemed positive by GC–MS. Thus, the cutoff concentrations in Table 1 represent a compromise between these extremes.

As mentioned previously, confirmation testing must employ an analytical method that is different from the screening test. By design, a screening test always produces some false positives. Results at this stage can only be viewed as presumptively positive. If a different assay methodology is not used for confirmation, screening test cross-reactivities are likely to recur, giving an erroneous "confirmed positive" result.

Aaron R., a 35-year-old male, applied for a job at a car dealership. He was urine tested as a condition of employment. His urine sample showed predominantly morphine with some codeine. He had a prescription for codeine for some dental work performed 3 days beforehand, but he also claimed to have eaten a poppyseed bagel for lunch on the day of the testing. A call to his former employer revealed that Aaron R. was an average worker with no known history of drug use. A check with the state police was negative for any criminal record.

*Has Aaron R. used a drug or substance that should prevent him from employment? What, if any, substance is it?*

**Discussion:** Clinical judgment is vitally important in interpreting the urine results in this case. If the last codeine tablet taken was several days before the test, low urinary codeine concentrations could result. Poppyseeds eaten on the day of the test could also account for the predominance of morphine. The practitioner reviewing this applicant's case might well give him the benefit of the doubt in concluding that the urine results are not indicative of opioid abuse.

Alternatively, however, Aaron R. could be retested at least 96 hr after the last reported use of codeine. Of course, the applicant should be reminded to avoid foods containing poppyseeds before the second test.

If a false-positive result is suspected, even after confirmation testing, the practitioner may wish to follow the procedure recommended in Chapter 3 when a test interference is suspected. This procedure includes testing the urine of another subject taking the suspected drug to confirm the cross-reaction. Compendia are also available for reference.

### Chemical Reactions

Cross-reactivities can occur with GC–MS due to chemical reactions during the test procedure. For example, ibuprofen causes false-negative results in some confirmatory tests for marijuana metabolites. To test a urine sample by GC–MS, a derivatizing agent must be used to convert tetrahydrocannabinol metabolites to a volatile form. When ibuprofen is in such a sample, it probably consumes the derivatizing agent, thereby preventing these substances from being detected.[9]

Another example involves false-positive methamphetamine results for specimens containing high concentra-

**TABLE 6.** Cross-Reactants Causing False Positives[a]

| Substance | RIA | FPIA | EMIT | References |
|---|---|---|---|---|
| Chlorpromazine | | | Amphetamines | 24 |
| Dextromethorphan | | | Opiates | 16 |
| Fenfluramine HCl | Amphetamines | Amphetamines | Amphetamines | 23 |
| Fluconazole | | Cocaine | Cocaine | 30 |
| Ibuprofen | | Barbiturates and benzo-diazepines | | 9 |
| Labetalol | | Amphetamines | | 24 |
| 1-Me-3-phenylpropan-olamine | Amphetamines | Amphetamines | Amphetamines | 24 |
| Phenethylamine | Amphetamines | Amphetamines | Amphetamines | 24 |
| Phenmetrazine HCl | Amphetamines | Amphetamines | Amphetamines | 23 |
| Phentermine | Amphetamines | Amphetamines | Amphetamines | 23, 24 |
| Phenylpropanolamine | Amphetamines | Amphetamines | Amphetamines | 23, 24 |
| Propylhexedrine | Amphetamines | Amphetamines | Amphetamines | 23 |
| Pseudoephedrine | Amphetamines | Amphetamines | Amphetamines | 23 |
| Theophylline containing bronchodilators | Amphetamines | Amphetamines | Amphetamines | 23 |
| Trimethobenzamide | Amphetamines | Amphetamines | Amphetamines | 30 |

[a]*Not usually a problem with GC–MS.*

Charlotte M., a supervisor for a large utility company, conducted a site inspection at a nuclear power plant. She then left for a 2-week vacation with her boyfriend. On returning to work, she was asked to submit a urine sample per company policy. A week later, the sample results were reported as positive for cocaine metabolite. Charlotte M. was then asked to report to the company physician's office. During the subsequent interview, she denied illicit drug use but stated that she had a tooth filled and had received procaine HCl (Novocain) for analgesia.

*What caused the positive test result for cocaine?*

**Discussion:** This case illustrates a common excuse offered to explain a positive urine screen for benzoylecgonine. Many people wrongly believe that any substance name ending in "caine" must share structural similarity with cocaine, leading to a false-positive result. While such interference is not unheard of, it does not occur with local anesthetics. With the exception of coca leaf tea, foodstuffs as a source of interference also may be eliminated.

tions of ephedrine or pseudoephedrine. Depending on the chemicals used to derivatize the sample, methamphetamine may form at the injection port of the machine due to the heat used for vaporization. This formation leads to contamination.[29]

### Physical Properties

A recently discovered test interference due to physical properties concerns fluconazole in the benzoylecgonine assay. First, it was discovered that fluconazole cross-reacts with benzoylecgonine antibodies in both EMIT and FPIA. Then fluconazole was found to exhibit an identical chromatographic retention time to benzoylecgonine. At therapeutic doses, fluconazole prevents the detection of benzoylecgonine even in drug-spiked samples. Therefore, patients who take fluconazole may be able to mask continued cocaine use.

Previously, this interference problem was not large; fluconazole was taken primarily by human immunodeficiency virus (HIV) patients with a history of cocaine abuse. However, this drug is now used to treat vaginal yeast infections. Potentially, this problem can be dealt with by asking for verification of a fluconazole prescription. Nevertheless, fluconazole causes false-positive screening tests and false-negative confirmation by GC–MS,[30] a fact that will become common knowledge given enough time.

### Sample Handling and Storage

Phenethylamine is normally found in urine but at concentrations too low to interfere with immunoassay results at normal cutoff concentrations. If, however, the urine sits after collection at room temperature or is in transit to an offsite laboratory for 1–2 days, concentrations increase

as a result of putrefaction. A false-positive screening result can then occur. Therefore, urine collected for analysis should be refrigerated or frozen with sodium fluoride 1% as a preservative until tested.[8]

## Sample Adulteration

Some individuals who use drugs try to interfere with their test results—a goal easily accomplished through sample adulteration. Therefore, various strategies have been developed to combat adulteration, including

- ➤ Direct observation of sample collection.
- ➤ Sample collection in a bathroom with only cold tap water and blue-dyed toilet water to prevent sample dilution.

Direct observation is often not used, however, because it embarrasses both the subject and the observer. With the other approach, some chemical still may be added to the urine sample. The temperature of the sample should be at body temperature ($98.6 \pm 36$ °F or $37 \pm 2$ °C) when accepted by the tester.

Tables 7 and 8 (pages 52 and 53) list the most common and readily available substances for direct adulteration of urine samples. A number of these substances interact with RIA and EMIT (the most widely used screening assay). Fewer adulterants affect FPIA. Adulteration is especially important if it leads to false negatives, since only those samples found to be positive on initial screening are retested with GC–MS.

Of the agents listed, most interfere with the enzymes used in screening tests. Some of these adulterants, however, may themselves cause false-positive results (Table 7), particularly with RIA and FPIA. Therefore, people being tested might actually avoid closer scrutiny if they do not adulterate their samples.

Fortunately for employers, most cases of adulteration are detectable.[34] Some adulterants must be in such high concentrations to affect the tests that undissolved material remains in the container (e.g., table salt or Golden Seal). Other adulterants alter sample pH or temperature (e.g., bleach). Still others require the assaying of a control specimen to detect tampering.

To manipulate sample results, some people also overhydrate to dilute their urine samples. This practice is common, particularly if the testing agency takes precautions to inhibit sample tampering. In addition, employers may encourage water loading to help an employee produce a sample.

Klonoff and Jurow[35] reported a case of water intoxication by a flight attendant; she apparently was unable to provide a sample due to anxiety about a possible laboratory error. Although she consumed 3 L of water over 3 hr, she was still unable to urinate and was sent home. Later that night, she was admitted to the hospital exhibiting

**TABLE 7.** Adulterants Causing False Positives due to Cross-Reactions

| Substance | RIA | FPIA | EMIT | GC–MS | References |
|---|---|---|---|---|---|
| Ammonia | Marijuana metabolite | | | | 31 |
| Ascorbic acid | Marijuana metabolite | | | | 31 |
| Bleach | | Benzodiazepines | | | 32 |
| Dimetapp | | | PCP | | 23 |
| Drano | Cocaine[a] | | | | 32 |
| Hordenine | Opiates | | | | 33 |
| Lime Away | Marijuana metabolite | | | | 32 |
| Peroxide | | Benzodiazepines | | | 32 |
| Rondec | | | PCP | | 23 |
| Soap | Marijuana metabolite | | | | 32 |
| Sodium bicarbonate | Benzodiazepines | Amphetamines, barbiturates, benzodiazepines | | | 32 |
| Sodium phosphate | Barbiturates, marijuana metabolite, opiates | | | | 31 |
| Thioridazine | | | PCP | | 8 |

[a]*High concentrations.*

confusion, slurred speech, and ataxia. Although rare in patients not having histories of chronic psychiatric or neurological disease, paruresis (the inability to urinate due to a lack of privacy) may occur occasionally in 25% of women and 30% of men.[36]

## Alcohol Test Interference

As with other types of testing, blood alcohol concentration determinations are not foolproof. Breath analysis relies on an accepted blood–breath partition coefficient of 2100:1 to calculate blood alcohol concentrations. In other words, 2100 mL of air at 90 °F (34 °C), saturated with water vapor, is considered to contain the same amount of alcohol as 1 mL of circulating pulmonary arterial blood with an average hematocrit (Hct). The actual values, however, vary from 1900:1 to 2400:1.[19]

If sampling is done too soon after alcohol ingestion, falsely high readings result. To guard against alcohol remaining in the mouth, tests should be delayed 20–30 min. Belching or vomiting also may falsely elevate readings due to residual alcohol in the stomach contents. Furthermore, fever can elevate the alcohol content of breath.

In practice, therefore, breath analysis determinations of blood alcohol concentrations involve multiple potential errors based on assumptions about

➤ A person's health.

➤ Conformance to average values of partition coefficient.

➤ Conformance to average values of Hct.

A lowered Hct tends to increase the proportion of plasma in the circulating blood, giving an abnormally high reading.[18]

Blood analysis, especially if performed using gas chromatography, avoids these problems but is not error free. Since the effects on an individual are most pronounced when alcohol concentrations are rising, the clinician must know if a given concentration represents the preabsorption or postabsorption state. Furthermore, if sampling is delayed because the subject has to be taken to a hospital or clinic, estimation of the blood alcohol concentration at the time the person was driving, for instance, may be difficult. In addition, interindividual variations in alcohol metabolism rates are considerable and depend on the (1) hepatic metabolic rate, (2) chronicity and amount drunk, and (3) nutritional state.

In general, a person's blood alcohol concentration drops by 0.015%/hr (18 mg/dL/hr). However, this rate may range from 10 to 25 mg/dL/hr.[37]

After-the-fact estimation of blood alcohol concentrations is based on the assumption that everyone tested conforms to certain population averages. By definition, however, this assumption cannot be true. False assump-

**TABLE 8.** Adulterants Causing False Negatives due to Cross-Reactions

| Substance | RIA | FPIA | EMIT | GC–MS | References |
|---|---|---|---|---|---|
| Ascorbic acid | | Cocaine | | | 34 |
| Bleach | Amphetamines, marijuana metabolite, opiates | Amphetamines, marijuana metabolite, opiates, PCP | Amphetamines, barbiturates, cocaine, marijuana metabolite, opiates | | 31, 34 |
| Blood | | | Marijuana metabolite | | 31 |
| Bogus urine | a | a | a | a | |
| Detergent | Cocaine | | | | 31 |
| Drano | Cocaine | | Amphetamines, barbiturates, cocaine, marijuana metabolite, opiates | | 31, 34 |
| Flagyl | | | All test drugs | | 34 |
| Fluconazole (oral) | | | | Cocaine | 9 |
| Fluorescein dye | | All test drugs | | | 9, 34 |
| Golden Seal | Marijuana metabolite | | Marijuana metabolite | | 31, 34 |
| Lime Away | Amphetamines, opiates | | | | 31 |
| Sample dilution | a | a | a | a | |
| Soap | | | Barbiturates, benzodiazepines, marijuana metabolite, PCP | | 31, 34 |
| Sodium bicarbonate | | PCP | Opiates | | 32 |
| Sodium chloride | Marijuana metabolite | | All test drugs | | 31, 32 |
| Sodium phosphate | Cocaine | | | | 31 |
| Vanish | Amphetamines, marijuana metabolite, opiates | | | | 31 |
| Vinegar | Marijuana metabolite | | | | |
| Visine | Marijuana metabolite | Marijuana metabolite | Benzodiazepines, marijuana metabolite | | 32–34 |

a*Cross-reacts with assay.*

tions may be critical in forensic cases where guilt or innocence hinges on such calculations.

Urine testing for alcohol can be done on a *qualitative* basis only due to the poor correlation of urine to blood concentrations. Furthermore, microorganisms in the sample may ferment glucose in the urine and lead to false-positive results (Minicase 5, next page).[37]

Interpretation of alcohol concentrations is more straightforward than for other drugs. Table 9 (page 55) lists the expected impairments at various blood alcohol concentrations. In relatively linear fashion, increases in the blood alcohol concentration lead to progressive impairment. However, there is considerable overlap in the blood alcohol concentrations listed in Table 9 and their associated symptoms.

Regular intake of alcohol does, of course, lead to varying degrees of tolerance to its effects. Care must be taken, therefore, in predicting associated behavior. Research has shown, however, that as tasks become unfamiliar or more complex or when events become unpredictable, even the

---

**✎ Minicase 5**

Lisa S., a 34-year-old white female nurse, was under probation by the Board of Registered Nursing. She was required to submit results of urine drug testing monthly to the Board. After 6 months of clean urine samples, her test came back positive for alcohol; the Board then considered further disciplinary action. However, there had been no evidence of abnormal behavior or physical impairment either on her job or in regular counseling sessions.

Lisa S. protested that the testing was in error, but another sample also was positive for alcohol. After continuous protests, the drug clinic personnel looked into the matter further. A review of the patient's medical chart revealed that Lisa S. was diabetic. Her serum glucose concentrations had been over 200 mg/dL. She also claimed to have a yeast infection.

When this patient's urine was sent to the laboratory a third time, it was found to contain glucose and some alcohol, which was quantified. The sample was then allowed to sit at room temperature for 2 days before being retested. The alcohol concentration on retesting was even higher than it had been when received at the laboratory.

*What caused these results? Does the Board have evidence for pursuing further disciplinary action?*

**Discussion:** This case illustrates why clinical judgment is important when interpreting urine test results. Yeast in the urine sample was fermenting the glucose present. If the clinic staff had not taken Lisa S.'s claim seriously, the Board could have falsely accused her of relapse. The staff's knowledge of potential interferents, the discrepancy between test results and behavior, and the patient's progress in treatment prompted further investigation. Unfortunately, a breath analysis would not have avoided Lisa S.'s anguish since alcohol concentrations in blood decline before they decline in urine, making urine the preferred mode of testing.

Because the Board had zero tolerance for the presence of alcohol, a direct blood alcohol concentration determination also may be inadequate in this case. According to one critique, specimens that contained *no* alcohol were sent to 355 laboratories; their assay results ranged from 0 to 23 mg/dL (from 0 to 0.023%), with a mean value of 8.9 mg/dL. If a result in the upper range of these figures had been reported, the individual would have lost his or her license as a disciplinary action.[37]

---

tolerant alcoholic shows impairment at blood alcohol concentrations where performance of simple tasks appear normal.[37]

## SUMMARY

On the surface, screening urine for drugs of abuse appears straightforward. A sample is collected and submitted for testing, and a result is received as to the presence or absence of drugs. Positive results are confirmed by GC–MS which, as the "gold standard" method of sample analysis, should give unequivocal final results. In practice, however, test interpretation requires more judgment before a final assessment is made.

Controversies will likely continue to surface and come to bear on the final assessment. When interpreting urine tests, one must be aware of issues affecting their reliability as well as things the test subject may do to manipulate results. Foodstuffs and medications can cause false-positive results, while some assay interference mechanisms can cause false negatives. These various factors must be considered when clinically interpreting raw test data.

## REFERENCES

1. Miller NS, Giannini AJ, Gold MS, et al. Drug testing: medical, legal, and ethical issues. *J Subst Abuse Treat.* 1990; 7:239–44.
2. National Institute on Drug Abuse. Medical review officer manual: a guide to evaluating urine drug analysis. Washington, DC: U.S. Government Printing Office; 1988.
3. Baumgartner WA, Hill VA, Blahd WH. Hair analysis for drugs of abuse. *J Forensic Sci.* 1989; 34:1433–53.
4. Baumgartner AM, Jones PF, Baumgartner WA, et al. Radioimmunoassay of hair for determining opiate-abuse histories. *J Nucl Med.* 1979; 20:748–52.
5. Cone EJ. Testing human hair for drugs of abuse. 1. Individual dose and time profiles of morphine and codeine in plasma, saliva, urine, and beard compared to drug-induced effects of pupils and behavior. *J Anal Toxicol.* 1990; 14:1–7.
6. Smith FP, Liu RH. Detection of cocaine metabolite in blood stains, perspiration stains, and hair. *J Forensic Sci.* 1986; 31:1269–73.
7. Smith FP, Pomposini DA. Detection of phenobarbital in blood stains, semen, seminal stains, saliva stains, perspiration stains and hair. *J Forensic Sci.* 1981; 26:582–6.
8. Aziz K. Drugs-of-abuse testing: screening and confirmation. *Clin Lab Med.* 1990; 10:493–502.
9. Osterloh JD, Becker CE. Chemical dependency and drug testing in the workplace. *J Psychoactive Drugs.* 1990; 22:407–17.
10. Mieczkowski T, Landress HJ, Newell R, et al. Testing hair for illicit drug use. In: National Institute of Justice Research in Brief. Washington, DC: U.S. Department of Justice; Jan 1993:1–5.
11. Nakahara Y, Ochiai T, Kikura R. Hair analysis for drugs of abuse. V. The facility in incorporation of cocaine into hair over its major metabolites, benzoylecgonine and ecgonine methyl ester. *Arch Toxicol.* 1992; 66:446–9.
12. Holden C. Hairy problems for new drug testing method. *Science.* 1990; 24:1099–1100.
13. Cone EJ, Darwin WD, Wang WL. The occurrence of cocaine, heroin and metabolites in hair of drug abusers. *Forensic Sci Int.* 1993; 63(1–3):55–68.
14. Strang J, Black J, Marsh A, et al. Hair analysis for drugs: technological break-through or ethical quagmire? *Addiction.* 1993; 88:163–6.
15. Welch MJ, Sniegoski LT, Allgood CC, et al. Hair analysis for drugs of abuse: evaluation of analytical methods, environmental issues, and development of reference materials. *J Anal Toxicol.* 1993; 17:389–98.
16. Notices. *Fed Regist.* June 13, 1990; 55:No. 114.

**TABLE 9.** General Effects of Ethanol[a]

| Blood Concentrations | Nominal Stage |
|---|---|
| 10–50 mg/dL (0.01–0.05%)<br>    No apparent influence; nearly normal by ordinary observation; special tests may detect<br>    slight changes | Subclinical |
| From 30–50 to 120–150 mg/dL (from 0.03–0.05 to 0.120–0.150%)<br>    Beginning of sensory impairment<br>    Mild muscular incoordination<br>    Slowed reaction time<br>    Diminution of attention, judgment, control<br>    Visual impairment<br>    Emotional lability, talkativeness, decreased inhibitions<br>    Exhilaration, sociability, increased self-confidence<br>    Slowed information processing | Euphoria |
| From 90–150 to 250–300 mg/dL (from 0.09–0.150 to 0.250–0.300%)<br>    Emotional instability and loss of critical judgment<br>    Incoordination and impaired balance<br>    Slurred speech<br>    Reduced visual acuity, peripheral vision, glare recovery<br>    Drowsiness<br>    Mild sensory loss—impairment of perception, memory, comprehension<br>    Increased (lengthened) reaction time | Excitement |
| 180–300 mg/dL (0.180–0.300%)<br>    Disorientation, mental confusion, dizziness<br>    Exaggerated emotional states (fear, rage, sorrow)<br>    Disturbance of vision (e.g., diplopia) and perception of color, form, motion, dimensions<br>    Increased pain threshold<br>    Increased muscular incoordination, staggering gait, slurred speech<br>    Apathy and lethargy | Confusion |
| ≥250 mg/dL (≥0.250%)<br>    General inertia, approaching loss of motor functions<br>    Marked decreased response to stimuli, impaired consciousness, sleep<br>    Marked muscular incoordination and inability to stand or walk<br>    Vomiting and incontinence of urine and feces | Stupor |
| ≥350 mg/dL (≥0.350%)<br>    Complete unconsciousness and anesthesia<br>    Depressed or absent reflexes<br>    Respiratory depression<br>    Vascular collapse<br>    Hypothermia<br>    Incontinence of urine and feces<br>    Possible death | Coma |
| ≥450 mg/dL (≥0.450%)<br>    Death from respiratory arrest | Death |

[a]*Adapted, with permission, from Reference 37.*

17. Cone EJ. Saliva testing for drugs of abuse. *Ann NY Acad Sci.* 1993; 694:91–127.

18. Christopher TA, Zeccardi JA. Evaluation of the Q.E.D. saliva alcohol test: a new, rapid, accurate device for measuring ethanol in saliva. *Ann Emerg Med.* 1992; 21:1135–7.

19. Montague M, Pugh CB, Fink JL III. Testing for drug use, part 1: analytical methods. *Am J Hosp Pharm.* 1988; 45:1297–1305.

20. Hayden JW. Passive inhalation of marijuana smoke: a critical review. *J Subst Abuse* 1991; 3:85–90.

21. Blank DL, Kidwell DA. External contamination of hair by cocaine: an issue in forensic interpretation. *Forensic Sci Int.* 1993; 63(1–3):145–60.

22. Kidwell DA. Analysis of phencyclidine and cocaine in human hair by tandem mass spectrometry. *J Forensic Sci.* 1993; 38:272–84.

23. Schwartz RH. Urine testing in the detection of drugs of abuse. *Arch Intern Med.* 1988; 148:2407–12.

24. Turner GT, Colbert DL, Choudry BE. A broad spectrum immunoassay using fluorescence polarization for the detection of amphetamines in urine. *Ann Clin Biochem.* 1991; 28:588–94.

25. Seymour RB, Smith DE. Identifying and responding to drug abuse in the workplace: an overview. *J Psychoactive Drugs.* 1990; 22:383–405.

26. Osterloh J. Testing for drugs of abuse. Pharmacokinetic considerations for cocaine in urine. *Clin Pharmacokinet.*

1993; 24(5):355–61.

27. Goldberger BA, Cone EJ. Confirmatory tests for drugs in the workplace by gas chromatography—mass spectrometry. *J Chromatogr.* 1994; 647:73–86.

28. Lo DS, Chua TH. Poppy seeds: implications of consumption. *Med Sci Law.* 1992; 32(4):296–302.

29. Selavka CM. Poppy seed ingestion as a contributing factor to opiate-positive urinalysis results: the pacific perspective. *J Forensic Sci.* 1991; 36:685–96.

30. More screening test problems. *Forensic Drug Advisor.* 1993; 5(8):57–8.

31. Cody JT, Schwarzhoff RH. Impact of adulterants on RIA analysis of urine for drugs of abuse. *J Anal Toxicol.* 1989; 13:277–84.

32. Warner A. Interference of common household chemicals in immunoassay methods for drugs of abuse. *Clin Chem.* 1989; 35:648–51.

33. Singh AK, Granley K, Misrha U, et al. Screening and confirmation of drugs in urine: interference of hordenine with the immunoassays and thin layer chromatography methods. *Forensic Sci Int.* 1992; 54:9–22.

34. Reported methods for urine sample tampering in drug testing. Morristown, NJ: Franklin Diagnostics; 1989.

35. Klonoff DC, Jurow AH. Acute water intoxication as a complication of urine drug testing in the workplace. *JAMA.* 1991; 265:84–5.

36. Rees B, Leach D. The social inhibition of micturation (paruresis): sex similarities and differences. *J Am Coll Health Assoc.* 1975; 23:203–5.

37. Gerson B. Alcohol. *Clin Lab Med.* 1990; 10:355–74.

## QuickView—Δ⁹-Tetrahydrocannabinol-9-carboxylic acid (Marijuana Metabolite)

| Parameter | Description | Comments |
|---|---|---|
| **Critical value** | Positive | Interferents must be checked and result confirmed with GC–MS |
| **Location** | | |
| Absorption | Gastrointestinal tract and lungs | |
| Metabolism/storage | Metabolized by liver; extensively stored throughout body as parent drug | |
| Secretion/excretion | Urine | |
| **Major causes of . . .** | | |
| Positive results | Ingestion<br>Inhalation | May be caused by sodium phosphate tried as adulterant; may be due to prescription; not caused by ambient exposure |
| Associated signs and symptoms | May be none at time of test | |
| **After use, time to . . .** | | |
| Positive result | 20 min | |
| Negative result—light, sporadic use | 7–10 days | Washout; time from discontinuing use |
| Negative result—chronic use | 6–8 weeks | Washout; time from discontinuing use |
| **Causes of spurious results with EMIT** | Drano and bleach | False negative |

## QuickView—Urine Benzoylecgonine Screen (Cocaine Metabolite)

| Parameter | Description | Comments |
|---|---|---|
| **Critical value** | Positive | Interferents must be checked and result confirmed with GC–MS |
| **Location** | | |
| Absorption | Mucous membranes and lungs; injected | |
| Metabolism/storage | Metabolized by liver and plasma esterases; unknown storage sites for parent drug | |
| Secretion/excretion | Urine | |
| **Major causes of . . .** | | |
| Positive results | Ingestion<br>Topical application<br>Inhalation<br>Injection of cocaine | May be no signs of intoxication at time of sample collection with heavy or chronic use |
| Associated signs and symptoms | May be none at time of test | |
| **After use, time to . . .** | | |
| Positive result | 20 min | Assumes episodic use |
| Negative result—light, sporadic use | 48–72 hr | Washout; time from discontinuing use |
| Negative result—chronic use | 12–14 days | Washout; time from discontinuing use |
| **Causes of spurious results with EMIT** | Fluconazole<br>Coca leaf tea | False positive<br>False positive |
| **Causes of spurious results with GC–MS** | Fluconazole | False negative |

## QuickView—Opiates

| Parameter | Description | Comments |
|---|---|---|
| **Critical value** | Positive | Interferents must be checked and result confirmed with GC–MS |
| **Location** | | |
|     **Absorption** | Mucous membranes and lungs; injected | |
|     **Metabolism/storage** | Metabolized by liver; not stored | |
|     **Secretion/excretion** | Urine | |
| **Major causes of . . .** | | |
|     **Positive results** | Ingestion<br>Nasal application<br>Inhalation<br>Injection | May be due to legitimate medication |
|     **Associated signs and symptoms** | May be none at time of test | |
| **After use, time to . . .** | | |
|     **Positive result** | 20 min | Assumes episodic use |
|     **Negative result—light, sporadic use** | 48–72 hr | Washout; time from discontinuing use |
|     **Negative result—chronic use** | 48–72 hr | Washout; time from discontinuing use |
| **Causes of spurious results with EMIT** | Poppyseeds and dextromethorphan | False positive |

## QuickView—PCP

| Parameter | Description | Comments |
|---|---|---|
| **Critical value** | Positive | Interferents must be checked and result confirmed with GC–MS |
| **Location** | | |
|     **Absorption** | Gastrointestinal tract and lungs | |
|     **Metabolism/storage** | Metabolized by liver; extensively stored throughout body as parent drug | |
|     **Secretion/excretion** | Urine | |
| **Major causes of . . .** | | |
|     **Positive results** | Ingestion<br>Inhalation<br>Injection | Possible interfering substances: Dimetapp, Rondec, and thioridazine |
|     **Associated signs and symptoms** | May be none at time of test | |
| **After use, time to . . .** | | |
|     **Positive result** | 20 min | |
|     **Negative result—light, sporadic use** | 7–10 days | Washout; time from discontinuing use |
|     **Negative result—chronic use** | Weeks or months | Washout; time from discontinuing use |
| **Causes of spurious results with EMIT** | None known | |

## QuickView—Methamphetamine and Amphetamine

| Parameter | Description | Comments |
|---|---|---|
| **Critical value** | Positive | Interferents must be checked and result confirmed with GC–MS |
| **Location** | | |
| Absorption | Mucous membranes and lungs; injected | |
| Metabolism/storage | Metabolized by liver; not stored | |
| Secretion/excretion | Urine | Clearance pH dependent (i.e., faster in acidic urine) |
| **Major causes of . . .** | | |
| Positive results | Intranasal application<br>Inhalation<br>Injection | |
| Associated signs and symptoms | May be none at time of test | |
| **After use, time to . . .** | | |
| Positive result | 20 min | |
| Negative result—light, sporadic use | 72–120 hr | Washout; time from discontinuing use |
| Negative result—chronic use | 72–120 hr | Washout; time from discontinuing use |
| **Causes of spurious results with EMIT** | Sympathomimetic amines<br>Drano and bleach | False positive<br>False negative |

## QuickView—Barbiturates and Benzodiazepines

| Parameter | Description | Comments |
|---|---|---|
| **Critical value** | Positive | Interferents must be checked and result confirmed with GC–MS |
| **Location** | | |
| Absorption | Gastrointestinal tract; rarely injected | |
| Metabolism/storage | Metabolized by liver; not stored | |
| Secretion/excretion | Urine | |
| **Major causes of . . .** | | |
| Positive results | Ingestion (rarely injected) | No interfering substances with either EMIT or GC–MS |
| Associated signs and symptoms | May be none at time of test | |
| **After use, time to . . .** | | |
| Positive result | 20 min | |
| Negative result—light, sporadic use | 1–2 weeks | Washout; time from discontinuing use |
| Negative result—chronic use | 1–2 weeks | Washout; time from discontinuing use |
| **Causes of spurious results with EMIT** | Possibly caused by adulteration with bleach, Drano, metronidazole, soap, sodium chloride, or Visine | False negative |

## QuickView—Lysergic Acid Diethylamide (LSD)

| Parameter | Description | Comments |
|---|---|---|
| **Critical value** | Positive | Result confirmed with GC–MS |
| **Location** | | |
| Absorption | Buccal mucosa, gastrointestinal tract, occular | Not well absorbed topically |
| Metabolism/storage | Metabolized by liver; not stored | |
| Secretion/excretion | Urine | |
| **Major causes of . . .** | | |
| Positive results | Ingestion<br>Eye drops | |
| Associated signs and symptoms | May be none at time of test | |
| **After use, time to . . .** | | |
| Negative result—light, sporadic use | 24–48 hr | Usually used in this manner; washout |
| Negative result—chronic use | 24–48 hr | |
| **Causes of spurious results with EMIT** | None known | |

# Chapter 5

# Interpretation of Serum Drug Concentrations

*Scott L. Traub*

Proper ordering and interpretation of serum drug concentrations fall under the purview of the physician, pharmacist, nurse, and other practitioners who are involved with drug therapy or monitoring. Therapeutic drug monitoring connotes those activities developed around the technology of serum drug concentration measurements and subsequent dosage adjustments.[1]

Because a working knowledge of basic pharmacokinetics is necessary for proper interpretation of serum drug concentrations, this chapter begins with this discussion. Proper planning, selection, usefulness, and evaluation of serum drug concentrations are then discussed in the context of common confounding occurrences. Only some basic aspects of pharmacokinetic dosing are mentioned briefly because the topic is beyond the scope of this book. For a more indepth discussion of dosing, the reader should consult the literature listed in the references and bibliography.

## OBJECTIVES

Upon completion of this chapter, the reader should be able to

1. Discuss the importance of pharmacokinetics in proper prescribing and therapeutic drug monitoring.

2. Compare the therapeutic range of serum drug concentrations with the normal range of other laboratory tests.

3. Discuss how distribution, protein binding, elimination rate, and clearance interrelate and affect a drug's serum concentration.

4. Explain how knowing a drug's half-life can assist with estimating the time to steady state when a loading dose is not given.

5. Compare and contrast linear, nonlinear, and Michaelis–Menten pharmacokinetic behavior.

6. Explain why availability and first-pass effect must be considered when interpreting serum drug concentrations and altering drug therapy.

7. Describe the prerequisite conditions and indications for using serum drug concentrations.

8. List and discuss the information needed when planning and evaluating serum drug concentrations.

9. For drugs whose serum concentrations are commonly monitored, describe how the drug's serum concentration relates to its effectiveness and toxicity.

10. Given a serum drug concentration that is inconsistent with the clinical picture, identify potentially confounding factors from a patient's medical data, including possible assay interference.

## CLINICAL PHARMACOKINETIC PRINCIPLES AND CONCEPTS

Pharmacokinetic equations attempt to describe the relationship between drug dosages and the serum drug concentrations attained. As a bioscience, pharmacokinetics is defined as the study of the (1) time course of drug and metabolite concentrations in different fluids, tissues, and excreta, and (2) mathematical relationships used to develop models for interpretation of the serum concentration pattern observed in a given patient.[2] In the purest sense, pharmacokinetics is more than the study of how a drug is absorbed, distributed, metabolized, and excreted.

When a clinician makes certain assumptions and accepts some estimation error, kinetic principles can be useful in designing optimal dosage regimens and minimizing the serum samples required for drug monitoring. The clinician should be familiar with the following principles and concepts:

➤ Therapeutic range.
➤ Volume of distribution (Vd), apparent distribution mass, and plasma protein binding.
➤ Elimination rate constant (Ke) and total clearance ($Cl_T$).
➤ Half-life (t½) and steady state.
➤ Linear versus nonlinear (first- versus zero-order) kinetic behavior.
➤ Systemic availability and first-pass effect.

## Therapeutic Range

The terms *serum*, *plasma*, and *blood*—as they relate to drug concentrations—are often used synonymously in practice (their true meanings can be found in the Glossary). Technically, they should not be used interchangeably. However, for most analytes, including drugs, the therapeutic range is essentially the same for serum and plasma.[3]

The concept of therapeutic range is a way of describing the desirable range of drug concentrations in the serum or plasma. In fact, the therapeutic range is derived using methods similar to those used in determining ranges for endogenous analytes such as sodium (Chapter 1). Therefore, the limits of the range are not absolute. The therapeutic range of a given drug includes those serum concentrations between which the desired pharmacological response is most likely to occur. For most drugs, concentrations above this range are associated with an increasing risk of toxicity; concentrations below this range are associated with an increasing probability of inadequate response. The optimal therapeutic range may depend on the

➤ Disease being treated and its severity.
➤ Alterations in tissue or receptor responsiveness.
➤ Degrees of plasma protein binding and unbound drug.
➤ Electrolyte concentrations.

Figure 1 demonstrates a likely, but theoretical, association of serum theophylline concentrations with effectiveness and toxicity (therapeutic range: 10–20 mg/L or 55–110 µmol/L). Although the therapeutic range would be different for other drugs, this concept applies to many widely used and monitored drugs. The likelihood of effectiveness, with or without toxicity (solid line in Figure 1), increases with increasing serum concentrations up to 20 mg/L. After 20 mg/L, effectiveness increases at a slower rate. The risk of toxicity (long dashed line) is small at 10 mg/L but starts to climb quickly at concentrations above 20 mg/L. Therefore, theophylline's effectiveness without toxicity (gray line) theoretically peaks at 70% in patients with a serum concentration of 18 mg/L. In practice, the goal of therapy is to achieve the serum drug concentration with the greatest effectiveness and least risk of toxicity.

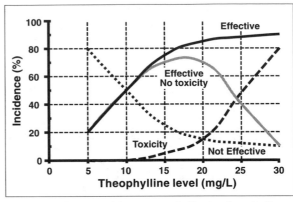

**FIGURE 1.** Theoretical frequency of effective theophylline therapy with and without toxicity as a function of the serum concentration. (Concept taken from Rowland M, Tozer TN. Clinical pharmacokinetics: concepts and applications. Philadelphia, PA: Lea & Febiger; 1980:159.)

Figure 2 depicts a typical drug concentration–time curve for a single, oral, nonsustained-release product whose elimination is more dependent on excretion of (unchanged) drug than on metabolism. The amount of drug or metabolites in various parts of the body is expressed as a percentage of the dose administered. The magnitude and duration of the distribution phase parallel those of absorption for most drugs. However, lithium and digoxin are notable exceptions; for practice purposes, several hours are required for their absorption and distribution to be complete. The true peak serum drug concentration and the "practical" peak also are shown in Figure 2. In practice, the blood for a peak is often drawn after the true peak.

After intramuscular (IM) injection, peak concentrations occur after 30–60 min. After nonsustained-release oral dosage forms, peak concentrations occur 1–2 hr following ingestion. For sustained-release oral products, the time to peak concentrations can vary greatly (4–10 hr in nonoverdose situations or up to 18 hr with massive ingestions). Moreover, the peaks are blunted relative to

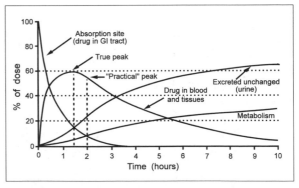

**FIGURE 2.** A typical drug concentration–time curve for an oral, nonsustained-release product. (Adapted and redrawn from Rowland M, Tozer TN. Clinical pharmacokinetics: concepts and applications. Philadelphia, PA: Lea & Febiger; 1980:14.)

the concentrations seen with nonsustained-release counterparts. The clinician must research drug products to determine their usual pharmacokinetic behavior.

Figure 3 is a schematic presentation of a typical drug concentration–time curve for multiple oral doses and a continuous infusion, including the therapeutic (10–20 mg/L), subtherapeutic (<10 mg/L), and toxic (>20 mg/L) ranges. The kinetics shown here are representative of nonsustained-release oral theophylline and aminophylline infusion. Because of the interpatient response variation seen in clinical practice for given serum concentrations, the lines representing the limits of the therapeutic range would be best depicted with ambiguous, graduated borders.

*Peak* ($C_{max}$) and *trough* ($C_{min}$, sometimes called valley) concentrations also are indicated in Figure 3. The peak is the highest drug concentration occurring within a dosing interval. In this example, the peak concentration at steady state is 18 mg/L. If desirable (e.g., improved breathing) or undesirable (e.g., nausea and tachycardia) signs and symptoms occur repeatedly or most intensely during the anticipated peak, then they are probably due to the drug. The true peak generally occurs immediately *after* a rapid (over 1 min) or slow (over 30–60 min) intravenous (IV) infusion, although the *true* peak is not always used in pharmacokinetics (Figure 2).

For clinical purposes, trough serum concentrations for a given interval occur just before administration of the next dose. However, the drug concentration may decline a small amount below the measured trough if there is a time lag before the next dose reaches the bloodstream. This phenomenon is more pronounced for solid dosage forms with slow disintegration or absorption. At the time of the true trough concentration, the signs and symptoms of the disorder being treated would most likely reappear.

One way to avoid trough and peak fluctuations is to administer drugs by constant IV infusion (e.g., at 40 mg/

hr). This technique is usually applied with drugs that have relatively short half-lives (e.g., procainamide, heparin, and lidocaine) and/or narrow therapeutic ranges (e.g., theophylline). In these cases, continuous infusion decreases the chance of concentrations becoming toxic or subtherapeutic.

An exception, based more on tradition than scientific evidence, is that parenteral antibiotics are almost always administered on an intermittent schedule despite their short half-lives. This technique has been successful, possibly due to the "postantibiotic effect," a property of fluoroquinolone and aminoglycoside antibiotics. Although controversial, increasing evidence shows that constant infusion is at least as effective as intermittent infusion in certain situations.[4] However, some constantly infused antibiotics (e.g., aminoglycosides) may be associated with a greater risk of nephrotoxicity.[5]

## Drug Distribution and Plasma Protein Binding

The relationship between the amount of drug in the body and the serum drug concentration, after the absorption and distribution phases are complete, is expressed by a proportionality constant called the apparent volume of distribution (Vd). This pharmacokinetic parameter can also be thought of as the volume of the body into which a given amount of drug distributes. The Vd does not represent a real body space, but it correlates roughly with body tissue.

Mathematically, the Vd is estimated on the basis of some form of body mass (the simplest is the patient's actual weight in kilograms). The Vd is often calculated by using the formula

$$Vd = C \times body\ mass$$

where Vd is in liters and C is a proportionality constant that can be found in the literature. (For theophylline, an average C is 0.45.) The Vd in the above equation represents primarily the volume of the bloodstream or central compartment ($Vd_c$). In the calculation of loading doses, the $Vd_c$ usually yields the best accuracy; the Vd at steady state ($Vd_{ss}$) should be used for maintenance doses. (Sources in the bibliography contain more information on Vd types.)

Drugs with low Vd values distribute largely to the plasma (central compartment) and less into the deeper tissues. These drugs are often highly plasma protein bound and cannot easily escape from the bloodstream to peripheral tissues. For example, warfarin is extensively bound to albumin and has a Vd of 0.1 L/kg. In contrast, drugs with large Vd values are more apt to distribute into the deeper tissues (e.g., lungs, brain, and heart). One example is digoxin, which becomes highly bound to tissue protein (e.g., heart muscle).

Important drug interactions related to protein-binding displacement may occur with drugs that are exten-

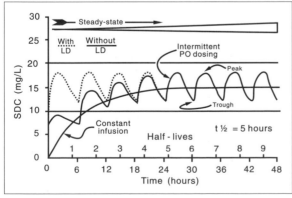

**FIGURE 3.** Typical serum drug concentration–time curve for oral intermittent dosing with (dashed line) and without (solid line) an oral loading dose (LD) and for constant intravenous infusion. The relationship between t½ and steady state also is illustrated.

sively (>90%) bound to serum proteins, although the changes in serum drug concentration are often transient.[6] Tables 1 and 2 list common drugs that are highly and poorly plasma protein bound, respectively. Unfortunately, many drugs (e.g., amitriptyline, propranolol, and digoxin) are exceptions because of a large degree of tissue binding. Numerous drugs that are extensively bound to plasma proteins still have high Vd values and vice versa.

The Vd is a function of the anatomical and physiological features of tissue as well as the chemical properties of the drug. Larger tissue masses and those with high blood flow (e.g., liver and kidneys) will have relatively more drug distributed to them. In addition to plasma protein binding, factors that affect a drug's distribution include its

> ➢ Molecular size.
> ➢ Polarity.
> ➢ Lipid solubility.

Aminoglycosides are poorly lipid-soluble (i.e., hydrophilic) drugs, and heparin is highly polar. These drugs do not have large Vd values, primarily because they have difficulty traversing lipids in cell membranes.

In practice, the Vd is often estimated using study population data and presented in liters per kilogram of body weight. For example, the Vd of tobramycin is 0.26 L/kg. A problem arises when formulas derived from subjects with normal somatotypes must be applied to patients with excessive fat mass (obese), especially for drugs that do not distribute readily to adipose tissue. For obese persons, some authors suggest using estimations of some form of apparent distribution mass. It is usually a derivative of lean or ideal body mass.[7,8] Estimates should be more representative of the patient's true Vd when drug

**TABLE 1.** Drugs that Are Highly Plasma Protein Bound

| Drug | Plasma Protein Bound (%) | Vd (L/kg) |
|---|---|---|
| Amitriptyline | 96 | 8.3[a] |
| Diazepam | 99 | 1.1 |
| Furosemide | 96 | 0.1 |
| Indomethacin | 99 | 1.0 |
| Losartan | 99 | 0.5 |
| Phenylbutazone | 98 | 0.2 |
| Phenytoin | 89 | 0.6 |
| Propranolol | 93 | 3.9[a] |
| Tolbutamide | 93 | 0.2 |
| Warfarin | 99 | 0.1 |

[a]*High degree of tissue binding.*

**TABLE 2.** Drugs that Are Poorly Plasma Protein Bound

| Drug | Plasma Protein Bound (%) | Vd (L/kg) |
|---|---|---|
| Cimetidine | 20 | 2.1 |
| Digoxin | 25 | 7.0[a] |
| Gentamicin | 20 | 0.25 |
| Metformin | <1 | 9.0 |
| Procainamide | 16 | 1.9 |

[a]*High degree of tissue binding.*

distribution to fat is assumed to be much less than to other tissues of the body. [Table 5 (discussed later) and Reference 7 offer help in deciding which drugs need dose and Vd adjustments in overweight patients.]

## Elimination Rate Constant (Ke) and Total Clearance (Cl$_T$)

For drugs with linear kinetic behavior, the Cl$_T$ represents a constant fraction of the Vd. The constant fraction that is eliminated per unit of time is known as the Ke and

$$Cl_T = Ke \times Vd$$

or

$$Ke = \frac{Cl_T}{Vd}$$

where Cl$_T$ is commonly in units of liters per hour, Ke is in hours$^{-1}$, and Vd is in liters. Half-life (t½) also is related to the Ke in that

$$t\frac{1}{2} = \frac{0.693}{Ke}$$

where 0.693 is the natural log of 2. A combination of these equations yields

$$t\frac{1}{2} = \frac{Vd \times 0.693}{Cl_T}$$

The t½ is not only mathematically related to both Vd *and* Cl$_T$ but is also physiologically related. If it is assumed that the Cl$_T$ remains constant, as the Vd becomes larger, the t½ becomes prolonged. This relationship is readily apparent in obese individuals. Although their ability to clear the drug may be typical, because obese patients have a dramatically increased Vd secondary to large body mass, their t½ will be unusually prolonged. Exemplary cases have been described elsewhere.[9] If the Vd does not change, the t½ becomes shorter (smaller) as the Cl$_T$ becomes faster (higher).

If both the Vd and Cl$_T$ increase or decrease in equal magnitude, the t½ does not change. For example, if a drug's Cl$_T$ decreases due to a drug interaction (e.g., theophylline and cimetidine) but the patient has become hypovolemic from a gastrointestinal (GI) hemorrhage (which decreases the Vd), the t½ and theophylline concentration may not change. However, when one of these confounding factors is removed (e.g., Vd is increased after blood transfusions), the t½ will increase along with the theophylline concentration and reveal the drug interaction. The Vd and $Cl_T$ are not biologically related to or dependent on each other, even though they are related mathematically. In other words, a change in the Vd does not directly influence the $Cl_T$ and vice versa.

The $Cl_T$ and Ke are often divided into their renal and nonrenal components. Population data for the components are found in the literature and are frequently applied to patient situations. For example, the following equation has been used to estimate the Ke for gentamicin:

$$Ke \ (hr^{-1}) = 0.021 + 0.00249(CrCl)$$

where CrCl is creatinine clearance. The 0.021 is the nonrenal component and the 0.00249(CrCl) is the renal component, which is dependent on the patient's CrCl (Chapter 7). As with gentamicin, any drug that is excreted mainly unchanged via glomerular filtration (i.e., minimal secretion) will have a larger renal component, and the renal portion will depend on the CrCl. In the previous example, more elimination will be renal than nonrenal as long as the CrCl is greater than 9 mL/min/ 1.73 $m^2$ (i.e., unless the patient is on the verge of total renal shutdown). When the CrCl is 9 mL/min/1.73 $m^2$, then $0.00249 \times 9 = 0.022$. This figure is slightly greater than 0.021—the nonrenal elimination component. If an average-sized patient's CrCl is 50 mL/min/1.73 $m^2$, the Ke will be 0.1455 $hr^{-1}$ and the t½ will be 0.693/0.1455 or 4.76 hr. This information can be used to determine dosing and estimate serum concentrations at various time points and to estimate the time before which toxic concentrations will return to the therapeutic range in overdose situations.

## Half-Life (t½) and Steady State

The *elimination* t½ of a drug is the time required for a 50% decrease in its serum concentration relative to the initial concentration. Technically, the elimination t½ should reflect concentrations that are not under the influence of absorption or distribution. These influences are most pronounced early in the dosing interval (Figure 2) but may continue throughout the interval with certain drugs and sustained-release dosage forms.

If the serum concentration of theophylline is currently 20 mg/L, the elimination t½ is 6 hr, and no additional drug is given, the concentration should drop to 10 mg/L in 6 hr. Of course, this example assumes that absorption and distribution phases are complete. Although other types of t½ (i.e., absorption and distribution) are described in kinetics, the elimination t½ is most commonly applied in dosing adjustments because it is usually highly correlated with the duration of pharmacodynamic effect. In fact, it is the primary factor in determining a proper dosing interval for nonsustained-release drugs.

For drugs that follow first-order kinetics (described later), the elimination t½ is not affected by the dose, interval, serum drug concentration, route of administration, or dosage form. For those drugs, t½ is mainly dependent on the functional status of the patient's organs of elimination (i.e., kidneys and liver). Therefore, t½ refers only to elimination half-life in this chapter.

Figure 4 shows the concept of t½ with a drug that follows first-order (linear) pharmacokinetic behavior. An IV dose is quickly "pushed" into the bloodstream. The drug's t½ is 1 hr because every hour the serum drug concentration falls another 50% (e.g., from 25 to 12.5 mg/L).

If the drug concentration axis is drawn in a logarithmic scale, the curve will become a straight line (hence, the term *linear*) and t½ can be estimated more readily and accurately.

*Steady state*, an important kinetics concept, is directly influenced by t½. From the first dose, a drug continues to accumulate in the body until its rate of elimination equals its rate of administration (Figure 3). Even with continued dosing, however, steady state is theoretically never reached. Nonetheless, in practice, steady state is said

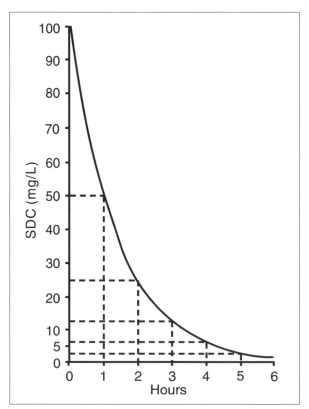

**FIGURE 4.** Serum drug concentration (SDC) and elimination t½ of a drug that follows first-order (linear) pharmacokinetics.

to be achieved after five to seven half-lives have passed.

For the drug in Figure 3, with a t½ of approximately 5 hr, concentrations will not reach steady state for 25–35 hr (five to seven half-lives). Once steady state is achieved with intermittent dosing, the peaks and valleys remain relatively constant from one dosing interval (6 hr) to the next. With a constant infusion, the curve reaches a plateau or levels off. At this time, the serum drug concentration is directly proportional to the drug's t½. If an IV (not illustrated) or oral loading dose is given (dashed lines in Figure 3), a steady state can be achieved "immediately" as long as the loading dose brings the concentration up to the desired level and proper maintenance doses follow. A proper maintenance dose replaces the amount of drug eliminated during the dosing interval.

According to pharmacokinetic theory, after one t½, 50% of steady state is achieved; after two, 75%; after three, 88%; after four, 94%; and, after five, 97%. Prerequisites for this theory are that the patient must be receiving the drug at both a fixed dose and dosing interval or at a constant infusion rate and that the patient's drug elimination has not changed (usually implies no change in renal or hepatic function). Whenever either the dose or interval changes, one must wait another five to seven half-lives before a new steady state is attained. Some practitioners draw levels after only three to five half-lives because of their need to make urgent decisions. After three half-lives, predictions will be off by 12% (100 – 88), but the direction of variation is not known. In other words, the drug concentration measured at that time may be 12% higher or lower than what it will be at full steady state.

Pharmacokinetic methods can predict steady-state concentrations from serum drug concentrations obtained after a first dose, even before a steady state is reached. Unfortunately, the method is complex and the needed expertise is not available in most institutions. Without such methods, a concentration drawn prior to steady state is usually of less prognostic value and may lead to inappropriate dosing decisions. This situation is described in

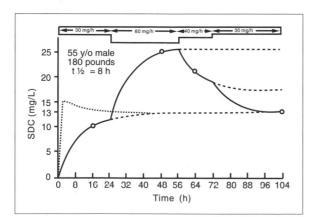

**FIGURE 5.** Example of how nonsteady-state theophylline concentrations can lead to inappropriate dosing decisions (described in detail in text).

---

### Minicase 1

Charles W., a 56-year-old male asthmatic patient with a t½ of 8 hr, was started on an aminophylline infusion of 30 mg/hr at 3 p.m. (day 1). His doctor ordered a drug level "in the morning." The laboratory drew the blood at 7 a.m. (after two half-lives) and reported a concentration of 10 mg/L at 3 p.m. (day 2). The rate was increased to 60 mg/hr because of poor clinical response and a low theophylline concentration. In the past, Charles W. required serum drug concentrations in the high therapeutic range to suppress his bronchospasm. His doctor assumed that doubling the dose would double the concentration.

At 3 p.m. on day 3, Charles W. complained of nausea, palpitations, and jitteriness; his heart rate (HR) was at 110. Therefore, the doctor ordered a stat theophylline level. The laboratory called back 2 hr later with a "critical value" of 25.5 mg/L, but the doctor did not become informed until 11 p.m. that night (day 3). At this point, the doctor decreased the rate to 40 mg/hr and ordered a level in the morning. The laboratory drew blood at 7 a.m. (after one t½) and reported a concentration of 21.5 mg/L at 3 p.m. that afternoon (day 4), at which time the rate was decreased to the original 30 mg/hr. A level drawn 32 hr later was 13 mg/L.

*Why did the original rate of 30 mg/hr not yield a serum theophylline concentration of 13 mg/L as it did at the end of the case? What could have been done to avoid the bouncing concentrations and side effects?*

**Discussion:** This type of "tail-chasing" scenario commonly occurs when the concept of steady state is not appreciated or applied. The dashed lines in Figure 5 represent the concentrations if no changes in infusion rates had been made. Given more time (about 16 hr), the initial infusion rate would have brought the concentration into the therapeutic range and might have been adequate for the hospital course. Fewer costly levels would have been needed, and morbidity could have been avoided.

Another alternative would have been to give a loading dose (dotted line in Figure 5), followed by the constant infusion. A loading dose would have minimized the difference between the first level drawn and the ultimate steady-state concentration. The report to the doctor would have shown a concentration of 14 mg/L (78 µmol/L) instead of 10 mg/L (55 µmol/L), which might have prevented the initial inappropriate response.

---

Minicase 1 and also shown in Figure 5. Dashed lines in Figure 5 represent concentrations if no changes in infusion rates had been made. Dotted lines represent concentrations if a loading dose and then a 30-mg/hr infusion had been given. For the concentration to remain constant or "plateaued," the infusion rate must equal the clearance.

As stated previously, one way (theoretically) to reach steady state "instantaneously" is to administer the perfect loading dose. If the loading dose raises the serum drug concentration to where it continues to peak during subsequent dosing intervals (assuming a proper maintenance dose is given), then steady state is reached immediately. This situation does not happen in practice because the calculated loading dose is never exactly on target. But even a loading dose that is somewhat off the mark may decrease the time before meaningful concentrations can be drawn because a "reasonable closeness" to steady state is achieved earlier.

Loading doses are given when an immediate pharmacological response is needed. They are especially useful with drugs that have long half-lives. If the patient's Vd is known, the loading dose (LD) can be estimated using the following equation:

$$LD = C_{max} \text{ desired} \times Vd$$

where the LD is in milligrams, $C_{max}$ is the peak serum drug concentration desired in milligrams per liter, and Vd is in liters. For example, if the desired initial peak is 15 mg/L and the patient's Vd for theophylline is 35 L, then the LD is 15 mg/L × 35 L or 525 mg of theophylline. If the drug is given as a salt of the active ingredient (e.g., theophylline *ethylenediamine*), the right side of the equation must be divided by the fraction that is the active ingredient. For theophylline, it is about 80% or 0.80. Therefore, the LD becomes

$$\frac{525 \text{ mg}}{0.80} = 656 \text{ mg}$$

which would be rounded off to 650 mg of aminophylline and given IV over 15–30 min. For oral products, the right side must also be divided by the fraction absorbed (e.g., 0.73).

As illustrated in the above example, the loading dose is almost always given as a single dose. However, to minimize risks of toxicity and to allow for accurate interpretation of the serum drug concentration, the loading dose may be divided into two or three doses or infused over a longer period when a drug is slow to distribute to its target organ (e.g., digoxin and lidocaine to the myocardium).

For the serum drug concentration to remain at steady state, a *maintenance dose* must be given. It replaces the amount of drug lost during the previous dosing interval. For constant infusions, the practitioner uses infusion rates (milligrams per minute) as the dose, and the term *plateau* replaces consistency of peaks and troughs.

## Linear versus Nonlinear Kinetic Behavior

As mentioned previously, inherent kinetic behavior of a drug can be classified as linear (first order), nonlinear (zero order), or a mixture of the two (Michaelis–Menten). At common dosages, most drugs used today follow first-order kinetics. Their $Cl_T$, t½, and Vd are independent of the dose or serum drug concentration. The steady-state serum drug concentration is directly proportional to the dose. For example, if a 50-mg/hr infusion of aminophylline results in a serum drug concentration of 20 mg/L, decreasing the infusion to 25 mg/hr should result in a concentration of 10 mg/L (if a new steady state has been reached when the levels are drawn).

The *rate* of change of the serum drug concentration varies continuously with the concentration of the drug. In other words, it is not a fixed *amount* of drug that is eliminated per hour but a fixed *percentage* of the remaining drug (Ke). In an intermittent dosing schedule, more drug is eliminated during the first half of the interval than during the last. More drug is remaining earlier, but the same percentage of the amount left is eliminated throughout the interval. This fact explains why a logarithmic curve is generated when serum drug concentration versus time is plotted on a Cartesian axis (Figure 4).

Nonlinear pharmacokinetics are not encountered much in clinical practice. Drugs that behave nonlinearly include aspirin, phenytoin, and ethanol. Infrequently, heparin, theophylline, and quinidine also do so. Until enzyme systems responsible for their metabolism, or excretion sites responsible for their elimination become saturated (i.e., working at their maximum capacity), all of these drugs display the simpler first-order (linear) behavior. Beyond saturation, the t½ is prolonged (and the percent clearance is decreased) as the dose and serum drug concentration increase.

Some authors described these drugs as following "capacity-limited" kinetics. For example, if 4 g/day of aspirin results in a trough serum concentration of 12 mg/L, increasing the daily dose by one 325-mg tablet could result in a concentration of 20 mg/L. In other words, no linear relationship exists between the dose and serum drug concentration. At the upper end of the therapeutic range, the consequences of a seemingly small dosage increase could be serious.

## Systemic Availability and First-Pass Effect

Systemic availability is the extent to which a drug reaches the general circulation. When a drug is given IV, systemic availability is absolute or complete. When the same drug is given IM or orally, however, less than 100% of the dose reaches the bloodstream. With the latter two routes, a lag time also is seen before an appreciable serum drug concentration can be measured. Therefore, there is a lag in the appearance of the therapeutic effect.

With solid oral products, a lag time exists because several preliminary processes must occur before the drug reaches the bloodstream. These processes include

1. Disintegration of the tablet or capsule.
2. Dissolution of the dosage form particles.
3. Absorption of the drug from the GI tract to the blood perfusing the intestinal tissue (mesenteric blood flow).

The dissolution time is usually the rate-limiting step. Stomach-emptying time, intestinal transit time, and pH of the GI tract fluid also influence the rate and extent of absorption.

For oral drugs, *bioavailability* or fraction absorbed (F) is the major determinant of systemic availability. It is an important variable used in evaluating the quality of generic drugs. The F value of a drug given orally would be 1 if the area under the serum drug concentration versus time curve is equal to the area under the curve when the drug is given IV (i.e., all ingested drug is absorbed). In practice, this equality is not common. The area under the curve of a generic product could also be compared with that of an innovator's brand name product to determine relative bioavailability. Differences among products are more likely to be clinically significant with drugs that are

> ➤ Given in small doses (e.g., digoxin).
> ➤ Have a narrow therapeutic index.
> ➤ Follow Michaelis–Menten kinetic behavior within common dosage ranges.

From the mesenteric bloodstream, the oral drug must travel through the hepatic (or portal) vasculature before reaching the general venous circulation. Drug passage through and metabolism by the liver (or intestinal wall) is called the first-pass effect and is another major determinant of systemic availability for certain drugs. Common drugs that are extensively inactivated (in the liver) by the first-pass effect include isoproterenol, terbutaline, diltiazem, losartan, omeprazole, propranolol, metoprolol, hydralazine, imipramine, nortriptyline, verapamil, nifedipine, lidocaine, morphine, meperidine, pentazocine, propoxyphene, and nitrate derivatives.

Clinicians must be especially careful with these drugs when converting oral to IV dosages because parenteral doses are much smaller than oral ones. For example, a usual oral dose of propranolol is 20–40 mg, whereas a therapeutically equivalent IV dose is about 1 mg. Less than 5% of an oral dose reaches the systemic circulation unmetabolized. Furthermore, patients with severe liver dysfunction or congestive heart failure (CHF) (decreased liver perfusion) may have an exaggerated response to a typical oral dose if their diminished first-pass metabolic capabilities lead to increased bioavailability.

## CLINICAL USEFULNESS OF SERUM DRUG CONCENTRATIONS

Clinicians must always remember what they should be determining from a serum drug concentration: the concentration of drug available to receptors and the subsequent intensity of effect from that concentration. Although it is not practical, the concentration of *free* drug should be measured at the site of action (usually receptors). This measurement probably could help to determine the percent of receptors that have been "turned on" by the drug. Instead, clinicians usually measure the concentration of *total* drug in the blood. Thus, several important prerequisites must be met before the serum drug concentration can furnish meaningful, interpretable information.

### Prerequisites for Use of Serum Drug Concentrations

The following are prerequisites for the use of serum drug concentrations:

> ➤ The intensity of the pharmacological action or response must be proportional to the concentration of free drug at the receptor site (or site of action).
> ➤ The concentration of free drug at the receptor site must be consistently proportional to the concentration in the serum.
> ➤ The degree of serum protein and tissue binding must remain relatively constant. In other words, the percentage of free to bound drug must not fluctuate much under common clinical conditions.

This last situation must be present because results reported by a laboratory routinely are measurements of total drug, a combination of bound and unbound drug in the serum. To use total drug concentrations in dosage adjustment decisions, it is assumed that the ratio of free to total drug is fixed. A more direct measurement or predictor of intensity of pharmacological response is unbound or free serum drug concentrations, an assay that is more complex, costly, and time consuming.

Unfortunately, many drugs produce their desirable or undesirable effects in a relationship that does not directly correspond to their concentration in the blood.[10] A list of these drugs is impractical. However, if serum drug concentration monitoring is not routinely performed on a specific drug, the concentration versus effect relationship (mentioned above) probably is not strong. Serum drug concentrations should not be used to monitor or adjust doses of these drugs.

### Indications for Serum Drug Concentrations

There is no consensus on when to obtain a serum drug concentration. As with any laboratory test, a serum drug level should not be performed if the result will not affect future related actions or decisions. Many practitioners agree that drug concentrations are most useful in the following situations: (1) the drug has complex kinetics (e.g., nonlinear, as with phenytoin); (2) the drug has a narrow therapeutic margin (e.g., lithium); (3) the drug's effect cannot be easily quantified clinically (e.g., gentamicin); (4) the dose–response relationship varies widely (e.g., procainamide); (5) a drug that alters the kinetics of other drugs is added to the regimen (e.g., digoxin–quinidine interaction); (6) the patient experiences a major change in weight, fluid status, or renal or liver function; (7) an overdose is suspected; and (8) a patient compliance or absorption problem is suspected.

### Complex Kinetics

The metabolism and clearance of certain drugs (e.g., phenytoin) are dependent on the dose and serum concentration at any given time. The concentration can change dramatically with only slight changes in dose or in rate of metabolism. Therefore, concentrations of these drugs should be checked after each dosage change (preferably after a new steady state is reached).

### Narrow Therapeutic Margin

For drugs such as lithium, gentamicin, digoxin, and phenytoin, there is either little difference or even overlap between the concentrations associated with therapeutic effects and those associated with toxicity. Therefore, levels might be obtained to ensure that they are in the desired part of the therapeutic range.

### Drug Effect Not Easily Quantified Clinically

The therapeutic effects of phenytoin are difficult to measure because the goal of therapy is usually absence of a phenomenon. It is also sometimes not easy to distinguish between a sign or symptom of a disease and a side effect of a drug treating that disease. For example, both digoxin toxicity and CHF can cause nausea, anorexia, and arrhythmias. A serum digoxin concentration may help to identify the cause. Similarly, both gentamicin toxicity and Gram-negative septicemia can lead to renal damage. Although the temporal relationships of other related factors (hypotension) may help to identify the cause of renal damage, a drug level also may be helpful.

### Dose–Response Relationship Varies Widely

The metabolism of drugs such as procainamide depends on the patient's acetylator status (fast or slow). The same dose in two patients can lead to quite different drug concentrations. Because acetylator status is usually unknown, serum procainamide and its active metabolite (*N*-acetylprocainamide) concentrations are needed to guide therapy. Again, the therapeutic goal is absence of a phenomenon (i.e., arrhythmias). Some clinicians can roughly determine whether a patient is a slow or fast metabolizer by giving the drug, measuring two serum concentrations, and determining the clearance. This information may help to ascertain the patient's risk of developing procainamide-induced lupus.

### Drug Interactions

When quinidine or quinine is added to the regimen of a patient who is stabilized on digoxin, digoxin concentrations may increase substantially over the next few days due to decreased digoxin clearance. Digoxin levels drawn 2–3 days after the addition of quinidine would indicate the significance of the interaction in a particular patient. Obtaining levels may also be prudent in a patient who has been on both drugs but is being withdrawn from quinidine. Digoxin concentrations would fall if a reverse kinetic drug interaction occurred.

### Major Change in Weight, Fluid Status, or Renal or Liver Function

Weight and fluid status can change the volume of distribution while renal and liver function can change the elimination of a drug. Therefore, these factors can change a patient's serum drug concentration. Significant weight changes usually occur over months, but changes in the other parameters can occur over a few days. Under normal conditions, renal function gradually (years) declines with age, but acute renal failure can happen within 1–2 days. Patients who have been on the same dose of digoxin from ages 55 to 75 may become toxic because kidney function declines with age. Serum creatinine (SCr) may not change to reflect the dysfunction (Chapter 7).

### Suspected Overdose

When prompted by signs and symptoms of overdose consistent with one or more drugs, drug levels can determine whether the suspected agent is the culprit. Drug levels may also offer some therapeutic and prognostic information. For example, serial acetaminophen concentrations offer some prognostic information with respect to risk for liver damage. A patient who takes theophylline and presents with tachycardia, nausea, and vomiting should have a theophylline level drawn. In overdose situations, steady state is not usually reached but is not needed for diagnostic (or prognostic and therapeutic) purposes. A level drawn during a suspected overdose often reveals whether the signs and symptoms are from a particular drug.

### Suspected Patient Compliance or Absorption Problem

Patients may intentionally or unintentionally not take their medication as directed. It may be causing bothersome side effects, they may not have enough money to purchase it (but are embarrassed to admit it), or they may have gotten it mixed up with another medication. Whatever the cause, if the medicine is crucial and does not seem to be working as expected, drug levels may help to identify compliance problems. Likewise, some patients have GI absorption problems; concentrations that are significantly lower after oral than IV or IM administration prove drug malabsorption.

## INFORMATION NEEDED FOR PLANNING AND EVALUATING SERUM DRUG CONCENTRATIONS

The prognostic usefulness and cost–benefit of a serum drug concentration improve while the evaluation of concentrations becomes easier and more accurate if a careful, logical plan is developed. As with most laboratory results, a serum drug concentration is just one piece of information to be interpreted in light of the patient's entire database. From this database, decisions are made and a plan is developed. A serum drug concentration is seldom pathognomonic by itself. In general, the clinician should usually give more credence to the patient's symptoms and clinical signs and accept or act on the serum drug concentration only if it is consistent with these factors, other test results [e.g., electrocardiogram (ECG)], and other patient data.

Table 3 can help the clinician in a systematic assimilation of the data needed for serum drug concentration planning and evaluation. The information is classified into

> Demographics.
> History and physical examination.
> Serum drug concentration history.
> Other laboratory tests.
> Drug and dosing history.

Although each area is discussed here, not all of this information may be necessary or obtainable for every case.

### Demographics

Demographic variables are used to generate initial estimates of volume of distribution, body surface area, CrCl, half-life, apparent distribution mass, and dosing suggestions. To ensure proper interpretation of serum drug concentrations, measured (as opposed to reported) weight and height should be used whenever possible.

### History and Physical Examination

History and physical examination findings are customarily acquired from the patient but can be obtained from other practitioners or the medical record. Diagnoses currently under consideration may have to be factored into the interpretation. For example, a patient with mania has been controlled at home on 900 mg/day of lithium with average 12-hr serum concentrations of around 1 mEq/L (1 mmol/L). If this patient is hospitalized with possible acute renal failure, one should anticipate increased lithium concentrations and suggest that lithium measurements be obtained.

### Serum Drug Concentration History

Serum drug concentration history is important because it suggests what concentrations should be expected for a given dose. It may also reveal at what serum concentra-

**TABLE 3.** Information Needed to Plan and Evaluate Serum Drug Concentrations[a]

| Type of Data | Specific Data | Reason for Obtaining Information or Comments |
|---|---|---|
| Demographics | Age, sex, height, weight, race | For initial estimates of half-life, volume of distribution, clearance time to steady state, loading dose, and maintenance dose |
| History and physical examination | Active diseases and nutritional status<br><br>Presence of edema, jaundice, or dehydration<br><br>Smoking and alcohol history | Focus on kidney, liver, and heart disease and major fluid status problems; may impact volume of distribution, clearance, protein binding, and percent of free drug |
| Serum drug concentration history | Previous dose–response, date and time of serum levels, serum drug concentration results | Was serum drug concentration drawn at steady state? Does it represent peak, trough, average, or other concentration? Was it drawn after absorption and distribution phase (if drawing peak)? |
| Other laboratory tests | BUN, SCr, CrCl, urine output | Assess kidney function (renal clearance) |
| | Bilirubin, SGPT or alanine aminotransferase, SGOT or aspartate aminotransferase, alkaline phosphatase, LDH, prothrombin time, albumin | Assess liver function (metabolic clearance) |
| | Thyroid function tests (TSH, $T_4$, etc.) | May affect clearance (e.g., digoxin) |
| Drug and dosing history | Amount of drug, date, and time of each dose | Ensure that time recorded is time given and infusion period is as ordered |
| | Kinetic drug interactions | Have interacting drugs been changed? |

[a]*BUN = blood urea nitrogen; LDH = lactate dehydrogenase; TSH = thyroid-stimulating hormone; $T_4$ = thyroxine. (Adapted from Reference 11.)*

tion the patient experienced a therapeutic or toxic effect. Recent serum drug concentrations are better predictors than older ones because recent changes in volume of distribution, clearance, or half-life are less likely to have occurred due to numerous factors (e.g., pathophysiology, drugs, and weight changes). The clinician must evaluate a serum drug concentration relative to a dose and degree of steady state. A wait of three to five half-lives (depending on urgency) is recommended. Half-life can be estimated based on the literature, demographic data, recent serum drug concentrations, and/or dosing history (if available).

## Other Laboratory Tests

Laboratory data related to the patient's ability to eliminate drugs may be needed for serum drug concentration assessment. For drugs primarily excreted by the kidneys, blood urea nitrogen (BUN), SCr, and CrCl should be obtained or estimated (Chapter 7). For drugs metabolized by the liver, tests might include (Chapter 11)

- Albumin.
- Prothrombin time.
- Bilirubin.
- Aspartate aminotransferase (AST or SGOT).
- Alanine aminotransferase (ALT or SGPT).
- Alkaline phosphatase.

Because these so-called liver function tests (LFTs) do not correlate as well with metabolism as CrCl does with renal excretion of drugs, the former are not as useful. Therefore, some clinicians obtain LFTs only if moderate to severe liver disease is suspected.

## Drug and Dosing History

The drug and dosing history is quintessential for proper interpretation of a serum drug concentration. Some reasons why accurate documentation is important have already been mentioned. Additionally, interactions of drugs whose concentrations are commonly monitored and whose kinetics (mainly elimination) are altered by other drugs can be identified from a careful drug history. Discussion of the interactions is outside the scope of this book. However, Table 4 provides examples of the common pharmacokinetic interactions in order of frequency.

When a serum drug concentration is used to monitor for a potential interaction, increased concentrations may not be apparent immediately. For example, if quinidine is added to the regimen of a patient stabilized on digoxin, the time to the new steady-state peak is 3–7 days. Therefore, unless the patient manifests toxicity earlier, a digoxin level should not be obtained until several days after the addition of quinidine. In this situation, some clinicians might monitor for the interaction using ECGs or clinical signs and symptoms. ECGs are expensive and uncomfortable for the patient, but they may be needed for other reasons; the monitoring of signs and symptoms is less specific than a digoxin level.

**TABLE 4.** Top 12 Pharmacokinetic Drug Interactions at Mercy Hospital (Springfield, MA), January–June: 1988 versus 1990[a]

| 1988 | | 1990 | |
|---|---|---|---|
| **Interacting Drugs** | **Frequency** | **Interacting Drugs** | **Frequency** |
| Digoxin–verapamil | 68 | Digoxin–verapamil | 27 |
| Digoxin–quinidine/quinine | 46 | Digoxin–quinidine/quinine | 23 |
| Digoxin–thyroid product | 36 | Theophylline–ciprofloxacin | 22 |
| Theophylline–erythromycin | 28 | Digoxin–thyroid product | 17 |
| Theophylline–phenytoin | 28 | Theophylline–erythromycin | 10 |
| Lidocaine–beta blocker | 17 | Theophylline–phenytoin | 7 |
| Phenobarbital–steroid | 14 | Phenobarbital–steroid | 5 |
| Phenytoin–trimethoprim/sulfamethoxazole | 13 | Warfarin–thyroid product | 3 |
| Theophylline–cimetidine | 12 | Lithium–diuretic | 2 |
| Phenytoin–cimetidine | 10 | Phenytoin–warfarin | 2 |
| Theophylline–ciprofloxacin | 10 | Carbamazepine–erythromycin | 1 |
| Phenytoin–warfarin | 9 | Theophylline–cimetidine | 1 |

[a]*Kinetic interactions involve one or more drugs whose serum drug concentration is commonly measured and can be altered by another drug. Frequency denotes the number of computer interaction alerts that were followed up by pharmacist notes to prescribers. Frequencies in 1990 may be lower in part due to concurrent, persistent prescriber education since 1988.*

Ted N., a 65-year-old, 200-lb, 65-in-tall male, had a history of urinary incontinence and chronic obstructive pulmonary disease controlled by theophylline (sustained release), inhaled cromolyn, ipratropium, and albuterol. He was brought to the hospital's emergency department (from a nursing home) with dyspnea, nausea, and vomiting that had worsened over the past 3 days. Ted N. had been admitted 3 months ago with theophylline toxicity (peak of 30 mg/L), probably caused by inadvertent excessive dosing (300 mg three times a day versus twice a day). During that visit, his theophylline concentration dropped from 20 to 10 mg/L in about 6 hr on the day of admission. History and physical examination revealed dehydration, tachycardia (HR 110), a fever of 102.2 °F (39 °C), and a cough productive of yellow-green viscous sputum but no rigors, tremors, jaundice, chest pain, or peripheral edema. A chest X-ray showed a new right upper-lobe infiltrate, consistent with bacterial pneumonia.

Ted N.'s test results that were higher than recent ones from the nursing home included sodium 148 mEq/L (136–145 mEq/L), chloride 104 mEq/L (96–106 mEq/L), hemoglobin (Hgb) 15 g/dL (14–18 g/dL), glucose 190 mg/dL (70–110 mg/dL fasting), white blood cell (WBC) count $18 \times 10^3$ cells/mm³ ($4.8$–$10.8 \times 10^3$ cells/mm³), and BUN 30 mg/dL (8–20 mg/dL). SCr was 1.1 mg/dL (0.7–1.5 mg/dL), his usual normal. LFTs and enzymes were within normal limits and relatively unchanged from previous measurements. Arterial blood gases were compatible with increased outflow obstruction. The theophylline concentration drawn 12 hr after the patient's last dose was 17 mg/L. In the past, valley concentrations of 10–12 mg/L were reported to prevent unacceptable bronchospasm while he was otherwise healthy (on 300 mg twice a day), but concentrations of 14–18 mg/L were required during prior exacerbations.

The nursing home referral report stated that Ted N. had taken all of his drugs as prescribed, including erythromycin (500 mg every 6 hr) which was started 3–4 days earlier for a suspected upper respiratory tract infection. It also stated that he had not vomited within 3 hr of theophylline ingestions, except for one time 3–4 hr after his last dose. No pill particles were observed in the vomitus.

*What information from this case would be useful in planning or interpreting serum drug concentrations? How would it be used?*

**Discussion:** *Demographics.* Age and history are helpful in roughly estimating a theophylline half-life of about 6 hr based on population data. If a minimal change is assumed, Ted N.'s theophylline half-life is confirmed by historical serum drug concentration data. His theophylline concentration dropped 50% (20 to 10 mg/L) in 6 hr during a period not influenced by absorption and distribution (after overdose without drug administration). The dose per apparent distribution mass (based on height in this

overweight man) would usually place theophylline concentrations within the therapeutic range, as it did here. With a half-life of 6 hr, it should take 24–30 hr to reach a new steady state after any regimen change or abrupt change in clearance (as from a drug interaction).

*History and physical examination.* Because Ted N. had been vomiting and had an increased HR (both consistent with theophylline toxicity), a theophylline concentration should be ordered. A theophylline concentration of 17 mg/L is not usually associated with nausea, vomiting, and significant tachycardia; however, this concentration is a "valley" (discussed below). Positive chronotropic effects of albuterol also may be a contributing factor; however, information on intensity of use is not available. Dehydration, as well as stress and fever from the pneumonia, also is a likely cause of the increased HR. Dehydration also may affect interpretation for other reasons (discussed below). Finally, Ted N. probably had not lost any theophylline in his vomitus while at the nursing home since vomiting occurred after the tablets should have been well into the small intestine.

*Serum drug concentration history.* Although current and past theophylline concentrations are within the therapeutic range (except for the overdose), they are troughs. The current trough (17 mg/L) is higher than those previously seen on the same dose (10–12 mg/L). Even though theophylline is a sustained-release product and its peaks are relatively blunted, Ted N.'s recent peaks (prior to admission) were probably above the therapeutic range. He was already near the upper limit of the therapeutic range (20 mg/L) on admission, and this level was drawn 12 hr after the last dose.

*Other laboratory tests.* Ted N.'s sodium, chloride, Hgb, and BUN were probably elevated from hemoconcentration (Chapters 1 and 6), confirming the clinical impression of dehydration. Even if the regimen and draw time are not changed, the theophylline concentration may decrease as fluid is replaced. On the other hand, no change occurs if intravascular fluid repletion increases clearance (increased hepatic blood flow) to the same degree (but opposite direction) as it causes hemodilution. In clinical practice, it is difficult to ascertain which variable plays a stronger role in affecting serum drug concentrations. The LFTs are probably not needed since acute liver dysfunction (another theoretical cause or contributor to theophylline toxicity) is not suspected.

*Drug and dosing history.* Because the usual time course fits the picture, erythromycin probably has caused theophylline concentrations to increase over the past 2–3 days, contributing to Ted N.'s symptoms. The clinician should try to ascertain whether peak nausea, vomiting, or tachycardia coincided with peak theophylline concentrations. Of course, erythromycin, which can cause GI distress, was started around the same time.

Minicase 2 illustrates the importance and usefulness of the information listed in Table 3 for planning and interpreting serum drug concentrations. For clarity, discussion is separated by category as much as possible. In practice, all types of data must be simultaneously and mutually weighed and analyzed.

## INTERPRETATION OF SERUM CONCENTRATIONS OF RELEVANT DRUGS

Table 5, a compilation of pharmacokinetic data and issues on drugs commonly monitored with serum drug concentrations, provides the practitioner with some information needed to plan and interpret those concentrations. The data relate to therapeutic (as opposed to overdose) situations in adults. Only side effects that may be related to serum drug concentrations are listed.

Each drug (class) is discussed below, with emphasis on the relationships among usual doses, serum drug concentrations, efficacy, and toxicity. The therapeutic range is not listed in the heading of each drug because the range appears in Table 5 (next page). Appendix A (at the end of this book) is a table of therapeutic ranges of commonly assayed drugs in standard units and International System (SI) units, along with respective conversion factors.

## Aminoglycosides (Broad Spectrum, Parenteral)

Drugs in this group (e.g., gentamicin, tobramycin, amikacin, and netilmicin) are all bactericidal antibiotics used to treat serious, systemic, Gram-negative infections. Because of poor oral bioavailability, these drugs must be administered by injection. Their kinetics are very similar, as are their inherent antimicrobial activities (with a few exceptions). Serum drug concentrations cannot be used as a guide for treating central nervous system (CNS) infections because distribution into cerebrospinal fluid is poor (<25%) and variable.

Dosages commonly required to attain safe and effective serum drug concentrations in patients without renal failure are 50–150 mg every 8 hr (5–6 mg/kg/day) for gentamicin, tobramycin, and netilmicin and 250–500 mg every 8 hr (15–20 mg/kg/day) for amikacin. A trend toward once-daily dosing is increasing, based on studies showing that efficacy and safety appear to be similar to those seen with divided daily doses.[13,14] Typically, doses of 4–5 mg/kg of gentamicin and tobramycin are given once daily and lead to peak concentrations (drawn 1 hr after the start of a 30–60-min infusion) of 16–24 mg/L. With netilmicin, a single daily dose of 4–6 mg/kg achieves a peak of about 20–28 mg/L. Extended-interval amikacin regimens use 15 mg/kg every day, and peaks are about 25–60 mg/L.

In most single daily dosing studies, it is not clear whether total weight or apparent distribution mass was used to calculate the dose. Despite many studies, it is also not clear what optimal target peaks and troughs are for maximum efficacy and minimal toxicity. Some institutions suggest measuring a trough concentration within 2 hr of the next dose and using a target of less than 1 mg/L. However, some assays cannot accurately measure concentrations that may be encountered 24 hr after a dose in a patient with normal clearance. A meta-analysis of 16 studies, which included 1224 patients, revealed no statistically significant difference in efficacy and toxicity between the extended-interval and traditional dosing groups.[15]

Lower doses (e.g., 1–2 mg/kg/day for gentamicin and tobramycin) are sufficient in simple lower urinary tract infections because the drugs concentrate in the urine (80–100 times the concurrent serum concentration). Because serum and urine concentrations do not match, serum drug concentrations are of little value in such infections. Lower doses are also required for renal failure and are adjusted based on CrCl.[11] Higher dosages may be needed to achieve therapeutic serum concentrations in patients who have cystic fibrosis or burns or who undergo major surgery.[16] In overweight patients, dosing should be based on apparent distribution mass.[7,8,11,17]

When the traditional dosing interval with gentamicin is used, peak serum drug concentrations greater than 5 mg/L for bacteremia and greater than 8 mg/L for pneumonia have been advocated. The higher the ratio of peak serum drug concentration to minimal inhibitory concentration (MIC), the higher is the therapeutic success. For example, if a suspected pathogen has an MIC (Chapter 16) of 2 mg/L, the peak serum concentration should be 8–10 mg/L to have a substantial chance of success with sepsis.[18] The basis for these recommendations has been criticized,[19] but most clinicians are comfortable with them.

The two most serious side effects of aminoglycosides, ototoxicity (especially vestibular) and nephrotoxicity, are probably related to serum drug concentration. With traditional split dosing, troughs rising above 2 mg/L are considered a warning sign of nephrotoxicity,[20] which is usually reversible.[21] A deep-tissue (gamma) elimination half-life of 150–200 hr may be associated with the risk of nephrotoxicity;[22] however, this phase is becoming less important as hospital stays and treatment durations are shortening. The risk of ototoxicity, which is usually irreversible, historically was thought to increase when troughs remain higher than 4 mg/L for longer than 10 days. Controversial evidence suggests that the risk is independent of the serum drug concentration but related to the duration of therapy and other factors.[23,24] The fact that high peaks achieved with extended-interval dosing do not appear to increase the likelihood of ototoxicity[25] supports this claim.

Aminoglycosides are inactivated in vitro by extended-spectrum penicillins such as carbenicillin and piperacillin. Degradation, which is dependent on time, temperature, and penicillin concentration, causes artifactually low aminoglycoside concentrations.[26] Amikacin is least affected. Inactivation also may be important in vivo in patients with renal failure, but interpretation of affected concentrations is unclear.[27] Aminoglycoside samples should be frozen immediately or penicillinase should be added to the tube if an interacting beta-lactam antibiotic is present. Drawing serum aminoglycoside concentrations when penicillin concentrations are lowest also should minimize this interference. (Details are discussed in Chapter 3.)

## Carbamazepine

Like phenytoin, carbamazepine is useful for trigeminal neuralgia and all seizures except absence type. This drug

**TABLE 5.** Pharmacokinetic Data on Drugs Whose Serum Concentrations Provide Clinically Useful Information[a]

| Drug | t½, Usual / In ESRD | Time[b] to Peak (hr) / Route | Therapeutic Range, Traditional / SI | F (%) | Vd (L/kg) ADM | Serum Drug Concentration–Related Toxicity and Comments |
|---|---|---|---|---|---|---|
| Amikacin | 2–3 hr / 30–60 hr | 1[c] / IV | 20–30 mg/L / No SI units | 100 | 0.25 / ADM | Attempt to keep valley levels <10 mg/L and peaks 20–30 mg/L. Dose with adjusted weight. Of aminoglycosides, least degraded by penicillins. *Toxicity:* kidneys, ototoxicity (e.g., dizziness and hearing loss) |
| Carbamazepine | 15–20 hr / 15–20 hr | 8–12 / Oral | 4–12 mg/L / 17–51 µmol/L | 80 | 1.4 / Wgt | Epoxide metabolite responsible for most neurotoxicity and may cross-react with carbamazepine assay if epoxide levels are increased[3]. *Toxicity:* nystagmus, ataxia, sedation, blurred vision |
| Cyclosporine | 10–27 hr / 10–27 hr | 3.5 / Oral | 100–200 ng/mL / 80–160 nmol/L | 30 | 3.5–13 / Wgt | Range is for whole blood HPLC assay just before next dose (24-hr trough). Oral absorption erratic, levels suggested. *Toxicity:* nephrotoxicity |
| Digoxin | 36–48 hr / 100–120 hr | 6–8[d] / Oral | 0.9–2.2 ng/mL / 1.2–2.8 nmol/L | 75[e] | 7.3 / IBM | Low potassium and magnesium and elevated calcium and age, as well as heart disease, predispose to toxicity. Only unbound levels interpretable after Digibind. Assay interferences discussed later in chapter. *Toxicity:* nausea, visual and mental disturbances, dysrhythmias |
| Ethosuximide | 55 hr / 60 hr | 4 / Oral | 40–100 mg/L / 280–710 µmol/L | 100 | 0.7 / Wgt | *Toxicity:* does not correlate well with serum drug concentrations |
| Gentamicin | 2–3 hr / 30–60 hr | 1[c] / IV | 4–10 mg/L / No SI units | 100 | 0.25 / ADM | Dose with adjusted weight. Inactivated by carbenicillin and other penicillins in vivo (in severe renal failure) and in vitro. *Toxicity:* nephrotoxicity may increase with peaks >12 mg/L and valleys >2 mg/L but controversial, especially in light of new data on extended-interval, high-dose regimens. Usual MIC = 0.1–3 mg/L |
| Lidocaine | 1.7 hr[f] / 1.3–3 hr | NA / IV | 1–5 mg/L / 5–22 µmol/L | 100 | 1.3 / Wgt | IV only; volume of distribution = 0.9 in CHF and 2.3 in cirrhosis. Initial volume of distribution = 0.5. *Toxicity:* dizziness, confusion, blurred vision, seizures |
| Lithium | 20–24 hr / 50 hr | 0.5–3 / Oral | 0.5–1.5 mEq/L / 0.5–1.5 µmol/L | 100 | 0.7 / Wgt | Levels increase with renal failure, diuretics, low sodium diets, pregnancy, and infection. Target serum drug concentration = 0.6–1 mEq/L for maintenance. Obtain level before first morning dose (>12 hr after last evening dose). *Toxicity:* lethargy, fatigue, tremor, nausea, abdominal pain |
| Nortriptyline | 30 hr / 15–66 hr | 10–15 / Oral | 50–150 ng/mL / 190–570 nmol/L | 66 | 17 / Wgt | Slow equilibrium. Collection tube caps may falsely lower levels. Cyclobenzaprine may cause false elevations.[12] F is systemic availability after first-pass effect. *Toxicity:* blurred vision, tachycardia, sedation, prolongation of QT interval |
| Phenobarbital | 3–5 days / 5–7 days | 5 / Oral | 15–40 mg/L / 65–172 µmol/L | 95 | 0.7 / Wgt | Tolerance lessens value of levels. Sodium accounts for 10% of dose. *Toxicity:* ataxia, decreased CNS and cognitive skills; highly variable |

**TABLE 5** *(continued)*

| Drug | $t_{1/2}$, Usual / In ESRD | Time[b] to Peak (hr) / Route | Therapeutic Range, Traditional / SI | F (%) | Vd (L/kg) / ADM | Serum Drug Concentration-Related Toxicity and Comments |
|---|---|---|---|---|---|---|
| Phenytoin | 18–30 hr[g] / 30 hr | 6 / Oral | 10–20 mg/L / 40–80 µmol/L | 100 | 0.65 / Wgt | Sodium salt accounts for 8% of capsule or injectable dose. Slow absorption (Dilantin); valleys are best for monitoring<br>*Toxicity:* nystagmus, ataxia, confusion; possibly gingival hyperplasia |
| Primidone | 7–10 hr / 12 hr | 2 / Oral | 4–12 mg/L / 18–55 µmol/L | 100 | 0.6 / Wgt | Active metabolite phenobarbital should be measured. Usually valleys are monitored<br>*Toxicity:* similar to phenobarbital |
| Procainamide | 3 hr / 6 hr | 1.5–2 / Oral | 4–8 mg/L / 17–34 µmol/L | 85 | 2 / ADM | Also measure *N*-acetyl active metabolite. Sum of drug and metabolite >20–30 mg/L is often associated with toxicity. Hydrochloride salt accounts for 13% of dose<br>*Toxicity:* nausea, weakness, mild hypotension, ECG changes |
| Quinidine | 6–7 hr / 4–14 hr | 1.5–2 / Oral | 2–6 mg/L[h] / 5–18 µmol/L | 72 | 2.8 / Wgt | Sulfate salt is 82% quinidine base; gluconate is 62%. Volume of distribution and clearance decreased in CHF<br>*Toxicity:* ECG changes, nausea, tinnitus, headache |
| Salicylates | 5–9 hr[g] / 5–9 hr | 2 / Oral | 15–25 mg/dL / 1.1–1.8 mmol/L | 100 | 0.2 / Wgt | Therapeutic range for rheumatoid arthritis. Consider salt. Lethal >60 mg/dL. May take on nonlinear behavior, especially at higher levels<br>*Toxicity:* tinnitus, nausea, possibly GI bleed |
| Theophylline | 5–8 hr / 5–8 hr | 1.5–2[i] / Oral | 10–20 mg/L / 55–110 µmol/L | 100 | 0.45 / Wgt / ADM | Aminophylline is 80% theophylline. Choledyl is 64% theophylline. Half-life = 18–24 hr in cirrhosis. Many interactions. Use ADM only for maintenance dose; wgt for loading dose<br>*Toxicity:* nausea, tachycardia, arrhythmias, seizures |
| Tobramycin | 2–3 hr / 30–60 hr | 1[c] / IV | 4–10 mg/L / No SI units | 100 | 0.25 / ADM | *Toxicity:* see gentamicin comments. Netilmicin very similar. Usual MIC = 0.1–3 mg/L |
| Vancomycin | 7 hr / 7 days | 1 / IV | 10–40 mg/L / No SI units | <5 | 0.7 / Wgt | Little absorbed when given orally to treat pseudomembranous colitis. Cannot treat systemic infection with oral route. Desired peak = 30–40 mg/L; trough = 5–15 mg/L<br>*Toxicity:* ototoxicity; nephrotoxic potential much less than previously reported |

[a]*ESRD = end-stage renal disease; NA = not applicable; ADM = apparent distribution mass; Wgt = actual weight; HPLC = high performance liquid chromatography; IBM = ideal body mass; MIC = minimal inhibitory concentration; CNS = central nervous system.*

[b]*This time does not necessarily represent a "true" peak; it may be representative of an "average" serum drug concentration for those drugs whose concentration is slow to reach equilibrium with the tissue (target receptor) concentration. The actual time to peak after IV administration depends on the infusion time. Theoretically, it occurs just after the dose is infused.*

[c]*Traditionally, peaks are drawn 30 min after a 30-min infusion. The actual time to peak after IV administration depends on the infusion time. Theoretically, it occurs just after the dose is infused.*

[d]*Peak is actually a reflection of peak tissue (myocardium) concentration. Therapeutic range and time to "peak" are not relevant for single daily dosing.*

[e]*For tablets. F is 95% with capsules and 85% with elixir.*

[f]*Alpha half-life = 8 min.*

[g]*Nonlinear kinetics; concentration-dependent half-life. Half-life of salicylate is 15–20 hr in patients taking 10–20 g of aspirin per day.*

[h]*Depends on type of assay performed.*

[i]*Time to peak varies greatly (3–12 hr) with sustained-release products.*

has also been used in refractory bipolar affective disorders. Doses required to achieve anticonvulsant and anti-manic–depressive serum concentrations in adults are 800–1200 mg/day or 10–20 mg/kg/day, given in two to four divided doses. Because autoinduction of enzymes occurs, the half-life of carbamazepine (5–27 hr) shortens over the first month, requiring gradually increasing dosages and making serum drug concentration monitoring before that time of less prognostic value.[28] Usual daily doses for trigeminal neuralgia are 400–800 mg.

The addition of phenytoin or phenobarbital may lead to lower carbamazepine concentrations due to enzyme induction. However, increases in the active epoxide metabolite along with the additive anticonvulsant activity of the second drug may paradoxically improve seizure control. The addition of cimetidine, erythromycin, isoniazid, verapamil, and possibly diltiazem—but not nifedipine—may result in increased serum carbamazepine concentrations and toxicity. Ataxia, nystagmus, drowsiness, and blurred vision are related to the serum drug concentration, but the relationship has significant inter- and intra-patient variability. Concentrations above 20 mg/L (85 μmol/L) are associated with seizures. The most serious side effects, blood dyscrasias and liver damage, are rare and not related to the serum drug concentration.

## Cyclosporine

Cyclosporine is an immunosuppressant that prolongs organ transplant survival by inhibiting delayed hypersensitivity without causing bone marrow suppression. It primarily inhibits T-helper cell function and number. High performance liquid chromatography (HPLC) is the gold standard assay method, but radioimmunoassay (RIA) is most commonly used.

Although no serum drug concentration goal is definitive, many practitioners use a *whole blood* 24-hr trough concentration of 100–200 ng/mL (80–160 nmol/L) with the newer immunoassays that utilize very specific monoclonal antibodies and measure only the parent drug (not metabolites). Some authors use higher target concentrations.[29] Older RIAs were not as specific, and the ranges reported were about twofold higher because metabolites were measured. Although some metabolites have minor activity, their importance is not yet elucidated. *Plasma* concentrations range from 20 to 50% of whole blood concentrations.

Because assays vary considerably, practitioners should check with their clinical laboratory before ordering levels and interpreting results. Regardless of the assay type, after 6 months of therapy, concentrations lower than the initial therapeutic range are often effective in preventing rejection. Serial levels should be drawn at the same time of day since there is some diurnal variation. Collection tubes containing ethylenediamine tetraacetic acid (anticoagulant) should be used, and blood should not be drawn

through tubing previously used for the drug.[30]

Cyclosporine is lipophilic and, therefore, distributes well beyond the blood volume. Within the blood, about 36% is in plasma, 6% in lymphocytes, 8% in granulocytes, and 50% in erythrocytes. In plasma, 90% is bound to proteins (mainly lipoproteins).

Doses required to attain "therapeutic" serum concentrations for prevention of transplant rejection vary by route. Absorption of oral forms depends on the presence of bile salts and is low and erratic. Average absolute bioavailability is about 30% and is usually decreased in patients with diarrhea. Peak blood concentrations occur at 3.5 hr. The whole blood peak achieved is about 1.5–3.0 ng/mL/mg ingested.

Cyclosporine is usually given 4–12 hr prior to transplantation in a single, oral 15-mg/kg dose. A dose of 10–14 mg/kg/day is continued for 1–2 weeks and then tapered by 5% per week to a maintenance dose of 5–10 mg/kg/day. Although the dose is tapered, concentrations may not decline. The injection is given in a similar manner but at one-third of the oral dose. Corticosteroids are routinely coadministered. Doses for treatment of autoimmune diseases, such as refractory rheumatoid arthritis, are lower; therefore, serum concentrations mainly require monitoring only when a significant pharmacokinetic interaction is likely.[31,32]

The elimination half-life in adults is approximately 20 hr. Children clear cyclosporine twice as fast as adults. The drug is metabolized by the liver and eliminated primarily via the biliary tract, with only 6% of the dose excreted in the urine. Thus, its clearance may be reduced in patients with liver disease. The addition of azole antifungal agents (e.g., fluconazole), erythromycin, colchicine, calcium channel blockers (e.g., verapamil), danazol, bromocriptine, metoclopramide, and steroids (routinely given with cyclosporine) as well as ingestion of grapefruit juice may increase concentrations. Phenytoin, phenobarbital, carbamazepine, rifampin, isoniazid, and nafcillin may decrease concentrations. An important drug–laboratory interference involves cycloserine, a second-line antitubercular agent. The HPLC assay may read cycloserine as cyclosporine.[33]

The principal adverse effects from cyclosporine are

> Tremor.
> Hirsutism.
> Hypertension.
> Gum hyperplasia.
> Renal dysfunction.

At least some forms of renal dysfunction appear to be related to serum concentrations since elevations of BUN and SCr have been responsive to dosage reduction. This dysfunction manifests as a stoppage in normalization of high preoperative BUN and SCr concentrations 2–3 months post-transplant at concentrations around 35–45

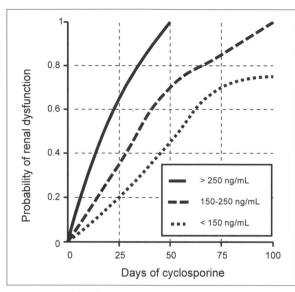

**FIGURE 6.** Risk of kidney dysfunction by serum drug concentration and duration of cyclosporine therapy after bone marrow transplantation. [Redrawn (step data smoothed), with permission, from Yee GC, Lennon TP, Gmur DG, et al. Clinical pharmacology of cyclosporine in patients undergoing bone marrow transplantation. *Transplant Proc.* 1986; Dec 18 (6 Suppl 5):153–9.]

mg/dL (12.5–16 mmol/L) and 2.0–2.5 mg/dL (177–221 μmol/L), respectively. Nephrotoxicity at a given serum concentration is also related to duration of therapy. As seen in Figure 6, the risk of nephrotoxicity increases with blood concentration and duration of "therapy."

Hepatoxicity, manifested by elevated "hepatic" enzymes and bilirubin, occurs in 4–7% of patients during the first month of therapy when doses are higher. Because elevations often decrease with dosage reduction, hepatotoxicity may be related to the serum drug concen-

tration. Minicase 3 demonstrates the role of serum drug concentrations in cyclosporine therapy.

## Digoxin

Digoxin is used to treat patients with CHF and atrial tachydysrhythmias. It is most useful for CHF associated with dilated ventricles and poor ejection fractions ($S_3$ sound may be present) and less beneficial with elevated filling pressures from decreased ventricular compliance but preserved systolic function.[34] The drug acutely and chronically decreases pulmonary capillary wedge pressure and HR but increases cardiac output both at rest and during exercise.

Digoxin is variably absorbed, and 60–80% is excreted unchanged in the urine in normal patients. Oral absorption averages 60–75% with tablets, 85% with elixir, and 95% with capsules. Bioavailability differences must be considered when switching dosage forms. Cholestyramine, colestipol, kaolin-pectin, sulfasalazine, and neomycin decrease digoxin absorption, while omeprazole increases bioavailability (by decreasing acid breakdown in the stomach).

Patients stabilized on digoxin who carry intestinal *Eubacterium lentum* (about 5–10% of patients) are at risk of developing toxic digoxin concentrations several days after starting antibiotics. In these patients, the bacterium metabolizes digoxin to dihydrodigoxin, an inactive metabolite. If the bacteria are killed off by oral antibiotics such as tetracycline and erythromycin, digoxin does not undergo this metabolism and clearance declines.[35,36]

Because digoxin does not distribute well to adipose tissue,[37] apparent distribution mass should be used for dosing calculations. Loading doses of 10–15 μg/kg are given in three divided doses over the first 24 hr. Mainte-

---

**✎ Minicase 3**

Teresa R., a 37-year-old female with chronic renal failure from long-term use of amphotericin B for a previous fungal infection, recently underwent a kidney transplant. She received an oral loading dose of cyclosporine (14 mg/kg) and then oral maintenance doses of cyclosporine (8 mg/kg/day), prednisone (1.5 mg/kg/day), and azathioprine (1 mg/kg/day). Eight days after the transplant, she developed urosepsis from *Escherichia coli* and was given gentamicin and piperacillin. She was hemodynamically stable, but 3 days later her kidney function declined (BUN from 25 to 50 mg/dL and urine output from 1000 to 400 mL per day). Gentamicin troughs had been only slightly above (3 mg/L) the desired target of about 2 mg/L. The cyclosporine 24-hr trough concentration was low at 75 ng/mL (whole blood, specific assay). Her kidney biopsy revealed signs of early rejection.

Teresa R. was taken off of gentamicin and piperacillin and switched to ceftriaxone because it is cleared by nonrenal routes and not associated with nephrotoxicity. She was given boluses of methylprednisolone (15 mg/kg/

day) for 2 days, and her cyclosporine was increased to 10 mg/kg/day. Over the next 7 days, her renal function improved. At the end of that period, her valley cyclosporine concentration was 135 ng/mL. Teresa R. was discharged and experienced no complications for a long time.
*What role did cyclosporine concentrations play here?*

**Discussion:** Early rejection was suspected to be the cause of decreasing renal function as opposed to gentamicin toxicity, given low gentamicin concentrations and only 3 days of therapy. Low initial cyclosporine concentrations were consistent with this hypothesis, and a biopsy confirmed it. Rejection was probably related to low cyclosporine concentrations. An appropriate increase in dosage led to concentrations in the desired range, which was associated with long-term graft survival. If Teresa R.'s cyclosporine concentration had been greater than 300 ng/mL and her biopsy showed no signs of rejection, cyclosporine nephrotoxicity would have been diagnosed and her dosages reduced.

nance doses required to achieve therapeutic serum concentrations are 0.125–0.5 mg/day with normal renal function. In renal failure, doses may be given every 3–5 days. Higher serum drug concentrations are often required to treat atrial fibrillation (1.5–2.2 ng/mL or 1.9–2.8 nmol/L) than those needed for CHF (0.9–1.8 ng/mL or 1.2–2.3 nmol/L).

Hypercalcemia, hypokalemia, hypomagnesemia, acidosis, hypoxia, and, possibly, hypothyroidism may increase tissue sensitivity to and toxicity from digoxin. In fact, a decrease in serum potassium from 3.5 to 3.0 mEq/L (3.5–3.0 mmol/L) will lead to an increase in sensitivity to digoxin by about 50%. Thus, potassium concentrations should be measured with every digoxin level[38] (Minicase 4). Addition of the following drugs may cause significant gradual increases in digoxin concentrations:

> ➤ Amiodarone.
> ➤ Cyclosporine.
> ➤ Diltiazem.
> ➤ Indomethacin.

> ➤ Quinidine.
> ➤ Quinine.
> ➤ Spironolactone.
> ➤ Verapamil.

A week of close serum concentration and/or clinical monitoring might be started 2–3 days after adding these drugs.

Actual peak serum concentrations occur within 1–2 hr but are not used because they are not proportionate to peak concentrations at the site of action (myocardium) and, therefore, do not reflect pharmacologic activity. Serum concentrations drawn about 6 hr after a dose are in equilibrium with myocardial tissue concentrations. Levels drawn after absorption but before equilibrium (1–4 hr after oral dose) may be very high but are clinically unimportant.

Digoxin-like immunoreactive substances may interfere with proper serum concentration interpretation in certain subpopulations (Assay Interferences section). Serum concentrations should always be interpreted in light of clinical measures of success. For example, for CHF

---

### ✎ Minicase 4

Alfred F., a 57-year-old male with chronic asthma, hypertension, and diabetes, was hospitalized because of palpitations associated with occasional dizziness. ECG monitoring during the first 24 hr revealed atrial fibrillation with a ventricular rate of 160 beats/min. Physical maneuvers and two doses of IV verapamil were unsuccessful in converting the tachyarrhythmia to normal sinus rhythm.

Alfred F. was given 0.5 mg of digoxin IV but had no chronotropic response. Six hours later, he was given digoxin 0.25 mg IV, which brought his ventricular rate to 105. A digoxin concentration drawn 2 hr after the 0.25-mg dose was 4.2 ng/mL. Because the patient might have been in digoxin toxicity (although his ECG had not changed), the planned third 0.25-mg dose was held. He was also taking chlorthalidone, glyburide, nifedipine, and alternate-day prednisone. Alfred F. was not using any β-adrenergic or anticholinergic drugs or theophylline and did not consume caffeine.

Alfred F.'s glucose and electrolytes were normal except for potassium, which was low at 3.0 mEq/L (3.5–5.0 mEq/L). His SCr was 0.7 mg/dL (0.7–1.5 mg/dL). Over the next 3 days, he received digoxin tablets 0.25 mg daily and was sent home with a ventricular rate of around 100. His digoxin concentration at discharge was 1.2 ng/mL 8 hr after his last dose. His potassium concentration was still low at 3.1 mEq/L, so he was given a potassium chloride supplement to take at home.

Two days later, Alfred F. was back in the emergency department with symptomatic atrial fibrillation and a ventricular rate of 180. He was not dehydrated. His digoxin concentration 6 hr after his dose was 1.4 ng/mL. His SCr was 0.9 mg/dL, and his potassium was 4.0 mEq/L.

*Why was Alfred F.'s digoxin concentration 4.2 ng/mL on the first day? Why did his digoxin not continue to control his ventricular rate?*

**Discussion:** The digoxin concentration of 4.2 ng/mL was

obtained before the distribution phase was complete; therefore, equilibrium had not been reached between the serum and tissues (myocardium). The level was drawn too soon after the dose and is uninterpretable. For peaks, digoxin levels should be drawn 6–8 hr after ingestion of tablets. Even if this level had been done, a full steady state had not been achieved. In this patient, at least 5 days of constant dosing would be required to reach steady state. Therefore, future concentrations (drawn at the same time relative to the dose) may not be similar values. Alfred F.'s peak concentration at discharge (1.2 ng/mL) was also probably not at steady state, although the concentration would be (at most) 25% away from the true steady-state concentration (3 days = two half-lives = 75% of steady state) with an assumed half-life of 36 hr. Actually, because of the loading dose, the concentration was probably less than 25% away from steady state.

Because Alfred F.'s potassium concentration was low, a more intense response would be expected at lower digoxin concentrations. Two reasons may explain why his ventricular rate broke through 2 days after discharge:

1. He was started on potassium supplements, which elevated his potassium concentration enough to suppress digoxin's activity on the AV node.
2. A peak concentration of 1.4 ng/mL is often not sufficient to control atrial fibrillation with a normal potassium concentration, and this value was his "highest" concentration of the day. His trough concentrations were probably well below 1.0 ng/mL (1.3 nmol/L).

Furthermore, verapamil may cause digoxin concentrations to increase; however, it is unclear (and probably unlikely) if two boluses on day 1 would impact Alfred F.'s digoxin kinetics significantly. His hypokalemia could have been caused by his diuretic and steroids, and potassium concentrations may fluctuate more in diabetic patients.

patients, success is decreased peripheral or pulmonary edema (chest X-ray clearing or decreased dyspnea or rales), increased urine output, and disappearance of S$_3$ gallop. For atrial fibrillation, a slowing of ventricular rate (ECG or pulse reading) indicates successful treatment.

The appearance of suspected side effects warrants acquisition of digoxin levels. Most side effects of digoxin are related to serum drug concentrations but occur at different concentrations in different patients. Side effects include premature ventricular beats and atrioventricular (AV) nodal heart block and other dysrhythmias, as well as nausea, vomiting, anorexia, disorientation, lethargy, weakness, agitation, and visual disturbances.[34,39]

## Ethosuximide

Ethosuximide is the drug of choice for absence seizures. It is given orally and almost completely absorbed. About 10–20% of the dose is excreted unchanged in the urine. Daily doses required to attain therapeutic concentrations are 20–40 mg/kg, and they are given in two divided doses or as a single dose. Single doses are associated with more nausea.

Serum ethosuximide concentrations do not correlate well with toxicity. Nausea, drowsiness, and dizziness diminish with time; therefore, serum drug concentrations should be used mainly for guiding doses for seizure control or for ensuring patient compliance.

## Lidocaine

Lidocaine, an antiarrhythmic in the same class (IB) as mexiletine, phenytoin, and tocainide, is usually given IV to treat or prevent serious ventricular arrhythmias. It also has local anesthetic activity and inhibits cellular sodium channels. Lidocaine is often used after a myocardial infarction to treat

> Greater than six ventricular premature beats (VPBs)/min.
> Closely coupled VPBs (R on T phenomenon).
> Multiform VPBs.
> Salvos (three or more) of VPBs.
> Ventricular tachycardia or fibrillation resistant to electrical defibrillation.

Routine prophylactic use in postmyocardial infarction patients, without any of the above indications, does not produce clear benefit and causes relatively frequent side effects.[40,41]

Because of the urgency of treatment, loading doses (100 mg or 1–1.5 mg/kg) are used. Lidocaine's effects last only about 20 min; therefore, constant infusions of 2–4 mg/min are required to maintain serum drug concentrations in the therapeutic range. Almost exclusively metabolized by the liver, lidocaine undergoes extensive first-pass extraction. Thus, clearance is decreased in CHF

and liver disease. Cimetidine and propranolol also may decrease lidocaine clearance by reducing hepatic metabolism and blood flow, respectively.[42]

One of lidocaine's metabolites, glycinexylidide, has much less antiarrhythmic activity but possesses neurotoxic activity. Glycinexylidide is 50% cleared by the kidneys, and its CNS side effects (e.g., headache and mental changes) manifest in renal failure patients. Lidocaine's side effects related to serum concentrations include numbness, drowsiness, confusion, dizziness, twitching, diplopia, bradycardia, hypotension, and seizures. Cardiovascular and respiratory depression, and seizures are associated with concentrations greater than 7–9 mg/L (30–38 µmol/L).

Lidocaine infusions are generally adjusted by clinical response. Serum concentrations are most useful in patients with symptoms consistent with lidocaine toxicity (e.g., confusion and seizures) who are receiving other drugs or have disease processes that may cause these symptoms. Serum drug concentrations are also useful when clearance should be dramatically decreased (e.g., uncontrolled CHF or severe liver disease).

McCollam and Bauman[43] recommended that an isolated "therapeutic" serum drug concentration be made the endpoint of antiarrhythmic "therapy" when the drug is used prophylactically (e.g., as with lidocaine). Otherwise, these authors and other researchers found that "targeting" patient-specific serum drug concentrations is successful.[44] Targeting is done by drawing a concentration when a definable efficacy endpoint (from electrophysiological testing and Holter monitor criteria) is reached. Chronic therapy is then initiated at doses required to maintain the serum drug concentration at or above the target value. This technique assumes that the threshold for effectiveness does not change with time. Since factors that affect the threshold for arrhythmias are not static (e.g., electrolyte changes and acid–base balance), this assumption is often invalid.[45]

## Lithium

In patients with manic–depressive disorders, the therapeutic goal is to minimize mood swings. Serum lithium concentrations have been shown to correlate well with efficacy and CNS toxicity. Maintenance doses of the carbonate salt range from 900 to 1500 mg/day (18.4–40.6 mEq/day). A loading regimen of 30 mg/kg, given in three divided doses, usually achieves the desired serum concentrations within 12 hr.[46] Lithium is eliminated almost entirely in the urine, with its clearance approximately equal to 25% of the CrCl. Its half-life averages 20–24 hr but varies among patients and may become prolonged with chronic therapy.

Although lower maintenance lithium concentrations (0.4–0.8 mEq/L) have been suggested to reduce nephrotoxicity, one study indicated that levels drawn 12 hr after a dose should be targeted for the narrow range of 0.8–1.0

mEq/L.[47] In this study, the group with lower serum drug concentrations (0.4–0.6 mEq/L) experienced relapse more often and side effects (tremor, diarrhea, urinary frequency, weight gain, and metallic taste) less often than the other group. Serum lithium concentrations should generally be monitored every 5–7 days during initiation of therapy and every 1–2 months thereafter. In patients stabilized on maintenance therapy, every 6–12 months is adequate, unless a factor known to influence lithium kinetics is apparent.

Initial transient side effects and minor toxicity (e.g., hand tremor, headache, nausea, mild polyuria, and muscle weakness) can occur with serum concentrations of 1.5 mEq/L or less. Nausea and tremor are sometimes minimized by initiating therapy with divided daily doses (two or three times a day). Moderate toxicity (e.g., coarse tremor, twitching, slurred speech, vertigo, confusion, lethargy, and hyperreflexia) occurs with concentrations of 1.6–2.5 mEq/L. Finally, severe toxicity (e.g., ataxia, stupor, extrapyramidal symptoms, coma, seizures, shock, and death) occurs with serum concentrations greater than 2.5 mEq/L.[48,49]

Unfortunately, concentrations do not always correlate with the types of toxicity listed above. There can be much overlap. Furthermore, concentrations peak in the CNS up to 24 hr later than in the serum, which can delay the expected onset of neurotoxicity or delay (weeks) its offset following dose reduction after chronic intoxication.[49,50]

Lithium causes notable side effects probably not related to serum drug concentrations. Reversible hypothyroidism [i.e., elevated thyrotropin or decreased free thyroxine ($T_4$)] occurs in 10–20% of patients on chronic therapy, with 4% requiring levothyroxine.[48] A 10–30% increase in total WBC count (usually in the range of 14,000–24,000 cells/mm³) with a normal differential (Chapter 14) occurs after 3–7 days and normalizes after withdrawal. Nephrogenic diabetes insipidus (Chapter 12) occurs in about 30–50% of patients shortly after starting therapy. Usually unimportant, reversible T-wave depressions on ECG, which are seen in about 15% of patients, are related to the lithium atom's ability to alter the myocardial conduction system by incomplete substitution for cardioactive cations (i.e., sodium and potassium).

The addition of thiazide diuretics, nonsteroidal antiinflammatory agents (aspirin and sulindac may be exceptions), or angiotensin-converting enzyme inhibitors (e.g., captopril) can significantly increase serum drug concentrations. Loop diuretics, such as furosemide and amiloride, usually do not impact lithium concentrations to a clinically significant degree. Interactions with thiazides are clinically relevant, since they are frequently used to treat lithium-induced polyuria. Amiloride also is used to treat the polyuria and may be a better choice. The addition of theophylline or sodium can decrease lithium concentrations.[50]

## Nortriptyline and Tricyclic Antidepressants (TCAs)

Serum concentrations of TCAs correlate well with CNS tissue concentrations, but the correlation between serum TCA concentrations and efficacy varies with the drug.[51] In 1985, the American Psychiatric Association stated that serum concentrations of imipramine, desipramine, and nortriptyline are useful in patients who are not responding to usual doses, are experiencing side effects, are receiving drug combinations, are suspected to be noncompliant, or are elderly.[52]

Without serum drug concentration adjustment of TCA dosages, approximately 65% of depressed patients respond to treatment; with it, 80–85% respond.[53] Nortriptyline, which has been studied more than any other TCA, is emphasized here; however, Table 6 lists the accepted therapeutic ranges for other TCAs. The value of serum concentrations of TCAs also has been studied in nonpsychiatric disorders (e.g., idiopathic functional nocturnal enuresis in children).[54]

Like most TCAs, nortriptyline is completely absorbed, heavily protein and tissue bound, and metabolized by the liver. Because of extensive but variable first-pass liver extraction, interpatient dose–serum concentration relationships vary greatly (F = 66%).[55] (African Americans usually have 50% higher concentrations than Caucasians on the same dose.) Usual maintenance doses are 75–150 mg/day. Nortriptyline steady-state serum concentrations above 50 ng/mL (190 nmol/L) but below 150 ng/mL (570 nmol/L) are associated with efficacy. The reason for the upper limit for efficacy is not known. Steady state is typically reached after 1–2 weeks of constant TCA dosing.

Side effects include anticholinergic symptoms and sedation (which are often transitory), tremor, postural hypotension, glucose alterations, weight gain, and allergic reactions. Serum concentrations do not correlate well with these signs and symptoms. Widening of the QRS interval, which stems from the inherent quinidine-like activity of the TCA, is related to the serum drug concentration. An ECG with widened QRS interval warrants a dosage reduction despite achieving the desired clinical response or serum concentration. Heart block (or asystole) is a serious risk in patients with a history of conduction

**TABLE 6.** Therapeutic Ranges for TCAs

| Antidepressant | Therapeutic Range | |
|---|---|---|
| | ng/mL | nmol/L |
| Amitriptyline | 75–175 | 180–720 |
| Desipramine | 100–160 | 170–700 |
| Imipramine | 200–250 | 180–710 |
| Nortriptyline | 50–150 | 190–570 |

problems, even at "therapeutic" serum concentrations.

TCA concentrations may be increased by the addition of phenothiazines, fluoxetine, hydrocortisone, methylphenidate, or cimetidine (enzyme inhibition); oral contraceptives, verapamil, labetalol, or diltiazem (decreased first-pass extraction);[56,57] and phenylbutazone, phenytoin, or aspirin (protein displacement). Serum concentrations may be decreased (slow onset) secondary to enzyme induction by barbiturates, carbamazepine,[58] phenytoin, chloral hydrate, and smoking.

## Phenobarbital and Primidone

Phenobarbital is used mainly as an anticonvulsant, especially for febrile seizures. With a half-life of about 5 days in adults, maintenance doses of 2 mg/kg/day (usually given orally) will achieve therapeutic steady-state serum concentrations in 2–3 weeks. The half-life in children is 2–3 days. An oral loading dose of 5 mg/kg can be given every 8 hr for the first day. It can also be given as a single 15-mg/kg IV dose, if needed. As with phenytoin, clearance may increase during pregnancy. Alkalinization of urine increases renal clearance (usually 10–30% of the total). Clearance may decrease in patients with hepatic cirrhosis and in those on valproic acid.

Hyperactivity and behavioral disturbances, which occur in 40–50% of treated pediatric patients, are not related to serum drug concentrations.[59] Sedation is common and dose related; however, tolerance usually develops with continued therapy. Ataxia, nystagmus, and dysarthria are likely at serum drug concentrations above 40 mg/L (172 µmol/L); coma is likely above 70 mg/L (300 µmol/L) in nontolerant patients.

Primidone is useful for complex partial and generalized tonic–clonic seizures. Up to 53% of primidone and 81% of phenylethylmalonamide, its active metabolite, are excreted unchanged in the urine.[60] Doses required to achieve a serum concentration in the therapeutic range are 125–250 mg three or four times a day. Loading doses are not used because of increased toxicity related to high starting doses.

Concomitant phenytoin may increase the amount of primidone that is converted to phenobarbital, its other active metabolite, and may cause excessive CNS depression. Urine acidification may decrease excretion and increase concentrations. Primidone toxicity includes sedation, vertigo, visual disturbances, and nausea, which may or may not be related to serum drug concentrations because they can be minimized or avoided with gradual dosage increases. If an unusual relationship between serum primidone concentrations and efficacy or toxicity is suspected, testing for phenylethylmalonamide and phenobarbital concentrations may shed some light.

## Phenytoin

Phenytoin is used primarily to suppress partial (psycho-

motor or focal) or generalized (grand mal) seizures. In most epileptic patients, seizures occur infrequently and irregularly; therefore, a reduction in frequency is not an easy clinical endpoint to measure. Phenytoin levels should still be obtained since most clinicians,[11] but not all,[61] think that a good relationship exists between serum concentrations and suppression of seizures. In most patients, the daily doses required to achieve desired concentrations are 200–500 mg in one to three divided doses. Children often require dosing more than once daily because their average half-life is shorter (about 12 hr) than adults (18–30 hr). Because the half-life is variable and long, clinicians should try to wait 10–14 days before drawing what is assumed to be *steady-state* levels.

A loading dose of 15 mg/kg is sometimes given. If given, a "practical" steady state is reached within 5–7 days. Peak serum concentrations are not seen for 6–14 hr after a large (900-mg) oral loading dose. (Table 5 shows salt equivalencies of dosage forms.) Phenytoin follows Michaelis–Menten kinetics, and small dose increases may lead to large increases in serum concentrations. Figure 7 depicts the nonlinearity of phenytoin's dose–serum concentration curve in various patients. Because the enzyme systems responsible for phenytoin's metabolism are "exhausted" at different phenytoin concentrations in different patients, it is difficult to predict when a small increase in dose will lead to a disproportionately large increase in the serum concentration. For most patients, linearity is lost within the therapeutic range (gray area) of 10–20 mg/L (40–80 µmol/L).

Phenytoin's pharmacodynamics may be affected by

> Renal and liver dysfunction.
> Pregnancy.
> Viral infections.
> Drugs.

Protein binding is altered with hypoalbuminemia and

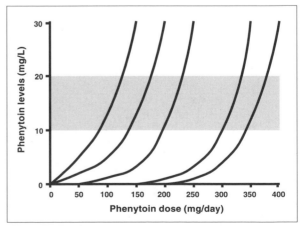

**FIGURE 7.** Phenytoin dose–serum concentration curves in various patients. The therapeutic range (gray area) is 10–20 mg/L (40–80 µmol/L).

renal failure such that there is more free drug (Factors Confounding Interpretation of Drug Concentrations section). In patients with a CrCl of less than 10 mL/min, a total serum phenytoin concentration of 5–10 mg/L (20–40 µmol/L) would be pharmacologically equivalent to the usual range of 10–20 mg/L (40–80 µmol/L). Similarly, 6–12 mg/L (24–48 µmol/L) of total phenytoin would be the adjusted "therapeutic range" with CrCl values between 10 and 25 mL/min.[62]

Total and free serum phenytoin concentrations will rise when the liver is damaged, because the drug is extensively metabolized in the liver. Total phenytoin concentrations may decrease by 60% due to increased clearance during pregnancy.[63] But, because free concentrations decline much less (18%),[64] other mechanisms may be involved. Infectious mononucleosis also may decrease phenytoin concentrations. Phenobarbital and valproic acid may increase or decrease phenytoin concentrations. Chloramphenicol, cimetidine, amiodarone, isoniazid, metronidazole, and omeprazole may increase phenytoin concentrations; carbamazepine, folic acid, and rifampin may decrease serum phenytoin concentrations (Minicase 5).

Phenytoin concentrations are also helpful in differentiating phenytoin-induced neurological side effects from those caused by neurological disorders that commonly accompany phenytoin use (e.g., stroke). These side effects are related to the serum concentration. Dizziness, ataxia, nystagmus, slurred speech, blurred vision, and, rarely, choreiform movements are seen at concentrations of 20–40 mg/L (80–160 µmol/L). Mood changes and confusion develop above 40 mg/L. Gingival hyperplasia, which occurs in about 20–45% of treated patients, is possibly related to serum drug concentration.[65,66] Folate deficiency, peripheral neuropathy, acne, and hirsutism are probably not concentration related.

## Procainamide

Procainamide is an antiarrhythmic agent mainly used to suppress atrial tachycardias that have been converted to normal sinus rhythm. It is in the same class (IA) as quinidine and disopyramide. It depresses the automaticity and excitability of the myocardium, slows conduction, and prolongs the refractory period.

Maintenance doses required for therapeutic serum concentrations are 1–6 g given in six to eight divided doses or three or four doses with sustained-release products. Infusions usually run at 1.5–5 mg/min or 20–80 µg/kg/min. Loading doses of 1–2 g can be given orally (75–95% absorbed) or IV (<20 mg/min). Doses should be lower in liver or renal disease but not in CHF.[67] Historically, the therapeutic range for the sum of procainamide plus its *N*-acetylated metabolite (NAPA) has been 10–25 mg/L. Some authors feel that the sum should not be used because NAPA has less inherent activity.[43]

Following NAPA concentrations (normal serum drug concentrations: 4–10 mg/L or 14–36 µmol/L) is important in patients with renal failure (mostly renal elimina-

---

### ✎ Minicase 5

Daniel I., a 45-year-old male, had been taking phenytoin 300 mg at bedtime for 12 years for control of tonic–clonic seizures that first occurred after head trauma in a motor vehicle accident. He was started on omeprazole 10 days ago for esophageal reflux refractory to famotidine 40 mg/day. In the past year, his only other medications were nontherapeutic multivitamins and occasional ibuprofen for tendinitis.

Today, his wife called the doctor's office because Daniel I. had become increasingly confused, lethargic, and dizzy over the past 3–4 days and complained today of visual disturbances (diplopia). His reflux had improved greatly. On examination, nystagmus on lateral gaze was present. He was told to stop taking omeprazole and phenytoin (for 3 days) and was placed back on famotidine 40 mg twice a day with antacids prn. A phenytoin concentration drawn at the office 12 hr after his last dose was 36 mg/L (144 µmol/L). After 1 week, his signs and symptoms disappeared. Daniel I. restarted his phenytoin at 300 mg daily after 3 days; after 14 more days, his concentration drawn 12 hr after his dose was 14 mg/L (55 µmol/L). He was seizure free.

*What was the probable cause of the patient's elevated phenytoin concentration? What signs and symptoms were related to phenytoin toxicity?*

**Discussion:** The probable cause of Daniel I.'s elevated concentration was the addition of omeprazole, which inhibits the enzymes involved in phenytoin's metabolism. A reversal of elevated concentrations and symptoms after withdrawal of omeprazole confirms the interaction. The onset of the drug interaction is typical. Even if metabolizing enzymes were abruptly and absolutely inhibited, it would take 2–3 days before phenytoin concentrations increased to the point of toxicity. Because enzyme systems are only partially inhibited over time, signs and symptoms may not manifest for 5–7 days (as in this case).

The sign of toxicity here is nystagmus; the symptoms are confusion, lethargy, dizziness, and double vision. Their appearance is expected at an average concentration of 36 mg/L (143 µmol/L). Altered protein binding was not suspected. Although some folic acid may be in the vitamins, it has the potential to *increase* phenytoin clearance at therapeutic doses (the dose was probably insufficient here). For a year, Daniel I. had been on folate and his clearance *decreased*. Although cimetidine may increase phenytoin concentrations, famotidine does not. The concentrations reported are averages, drawn halfway through the dosing interval. Concentrations may have been slightly higher earlier and slightly lower later in the dosing interval. Daniel I.'s wife could have been asked whether there was any pattern in the degree of signs and symptoms during the dosing interval.

tion) or major GI or visual side effects that may be more related to NAPA.[43] Ratios of NAPA to procainamide of 1.2 or 0.8 (using traditional units) are seen in rapid or slow acetylators, respectively. (About 85% of Asians are fast acetylators.) Procainamide-induced lupus (arthritis, rash, etc.), which occurs in 30% of patients, occurs more rapidly in slow acetylators. About 50–80% of patients develop a positive antinuclear antibody test (Chapter 17).[68]

Adverse effects that are likely to occur at procainamide concentrations above 10 mg/L include ECG changes (e.g., prolonged PR, QT, or QRS intervals of ECG reading), nausea, weakness, and mild hypotension.

## Quinidine

Quinidine's antiarrhythmic activity is similar to procainamide. The therapeutic range varies slightly, depending on the assay and clinical endpoint used.[11,43] Oral doses of the sulfate salt (83% base) required to maintain therapeutic serum drug concentrations are 200–600 mg every 6 hr (commonly) to 8 hr. Loading doses of 200 mg every 2 hr for five or six doses also can be given. The polygalacturonate (60% base) and sustained-release gluconate (62% base) salts are usually dosed every 8 and 12 hr, respectively. Quinidine undergoes an extensive first-pass effect (two active metabolites); therefore, lower initial doses should be used in patients with CHF and liver disease. Only 10–20% is excreted unchanged in urine.[69] Quinidine's normal half-life of 6–7 hr is prolonged only in chronic liver disease.

Urinary clearance may decrease and serum concentrations may increase when drugs that alkalinize urine (e.g., acetazolamide and sodium bicarbonate) are added. Concentrations may also increase (about 33%) after amiodarone is begun. Serum concentrations may decrease if enzyme inducers (e.g., phenobarbital and phenytoin) are added. With high concentrations, cinchonism—manifested by nausea, tinnitus, blurred vision, headache, and mental changes—may occur. The risk of paroxysmal ventricular fibrillation is related to the serum quinidine concentration. On ECGs, serum drug concentration-related cardiotoxicity is revealed by conduction defects (50% widening QRS interval, complete AV block, and frequent premature ventricular contractions).

## Salicylates

Aspirin, the prototypical salicylate, has antipyretic, anti-inflammatory, analgesic, antiplatelet, and uricosuric (>4–5 g/day) properties. Serum salicylate concentrations are monitored mainly when high doses are required, such as in rheumatoid arthritis where the therapeutic range is 15–25 mg/dL (1.1–1.8 mmol/L). For perspective, only about 3–6 mg/dL (0.22–0.44 mmol/L) is needed to treat a headache. With serum salicylate concentrations as a guide, the therapeutic goal in rheumatoid arthritis is amelioration or elimination of morning stiffness and the number of painful or swollen joints as well as improvement in the range of motion, time to onset of fatigue, and possibly erythrocyte sedimentation rate (Chapter 17).

Doses required to maintain serum drug concentrations in the therapeutic range for rheumatoid arthritis are 3–6 g/day in adults. In pediatrics, the dose is 90–130 mg/kg/day in divided doses. The onset of anti-inflammatory action occurs within 1–4 days of continuous therapy; optimal effects depend on attainment and maintenance of adequate serum concentrations and may not be experienced for several weeks.

Absorption of salicylate products is excellent. Although older, enteric-coated products had problems, most of these current products have reliable absorption. In most rheumatoid arthritis patients, about 15–30% of salicylate is unbound to plasma proteins. Uremia and hypoalbuminemia may lead to increased fractions of unbound salicylate without affecting the total serum concentration measured by the laboratory. However, uremic samples in one study contained only 17–26% of unbound salicylate, which is within the range for nonuremic rheumatoid arthritis patients.[70] These patients should still be monitored closely because they may experience toxicity despite serum concentrations in the therapeutic range.

Many side effects are related to serum drug concentrations and have been studied extensively. CNS-induced nausea and vomiting occur at concentrations above 27 mg/dL (1.9 mmol/L), but nausea and vomiting from local gastric irritation occur frequently at lower concentrations. Tinnitus, the most frequent adverse effect in adults, usually occurs only if serum salicylate concentrations are above 20 mg/dL (1.4 mmol/L) and is almost always present at concentrations above 30 mg/dL (2.2 mmol/L).

Hepatotoxicity, which most often occurs after 1–4 weeks of therapy, is more likely with serum concentrations exceeding 20 mg/dL. Elevations in aminotransferases (Chapter 11) normalize within 1–2 weeks of dosage reduction; they may also decline without any dosage adjustment. Salicylate-induced noncardiogenic pulmonary edema occurs when salicylate concentrations exceed 40 mg/dL (2.9 mmol/L). In children, the most frequent manifestations of chronic intoxication (concentrations >30 mg/dL) are hyperventilation with metabolic acidosis and respiratory alkalosis (Chapter 8), hypoglycemia, giddiness, drowsiness, and behavioral changes.

Salicylate's half-life is dose dependent, averaging

> ➤ 2.4 hr after 250 mg.
> ➤ 5 hr after 1 g.
> ➤ 19 hr after 10–20 g.

Because the drug follows Michaelis–Menten kinetics, small increases in doses may lead to disproportionately large increases in concentrations. Urine alkalinization, which can occur from systemic and "nonsystemic" antacids, can increase renal clearance and decrease serum salicylate concentration dramatically.[71] Sulfinpyrazone may increase salicylate concentrations, and corticosteroids and acetazolamide may decrease them.

## Theophylline

Theophylline, a xanthine analog, is used principally for its bronchorelaxation properties in asthma and chronic obstructive lung disease. Although it may have minor anti-inflammatory activity,[72] theophylline improves the bronchoconstrictive component of airway obstruction in asthma more than mucosal edema/swelling and mucus plugging. If all three components were improved by the drug, spirometric measurement of forced expiratory volume (FEV$_1$) (Chapter 9)—which reflects all three—could be used to monitor theophylline.[73]

In acute situations, an IV loading dose of 5–6 mg/kg (total body weight) in noninfants is given if no circulating drug is assumed. Each 1 mg/kg (1.25 mg/kg aminophylline) results in a 2-mg/L increase in the serum drug concentration. Except in patients with uncompensated CHF or severe liver disease, aminophylline infusion rates of 0.5–0.8 mg/kg/hr maintain concentrations in the therapeutic range in adults and older children. In children 1–9 years, a rate of 1 mg/kg/hr is needed. Apparent distribution mass, as opposed to actual weight, should be used for maintenance doses in overweight patients. Usual oral doses are 200–300 mg three or four times a day.

Because of wide interpatient variability, the above guidelines should not be used blindly without serum drug concentration monitoring. In the hospital setting, these concentrations should be obtained daily until they are rather steady. With constant infusions, draw time is unimportant after steady state is reached (usually after 24–48 hr). A steady state is not required with sophisticated calculator or computer methods to predict patient-specific kinetics and adjust doses, but two or more theophylline concentrations are needed during the first day. Moreover, followup serum drug concentrations are still recommended.

Theophylline is almost entirely cleared via liver metabolism. Many diseases and drugs alter usual clearance and must be considered when interpreting serum concentrations. Clearance is decreased in patients with active CHF, hypothyroidism, and severe liver dysfunction (Chapter 11) where half-life may be longer than 24 hr. Clearance is also decreased with acute pulmonary edema, acute viral infections, and febrile illnesses. The increased clearance seen in tobacco or marijuana smokers (1.5 to 2 times that of nonsmokers) may persist for 3–24 months after cessation of smoking. Rifampin, carbamazepine, phenytoin, and phenobarbital may increase theophylline's clearance. In contrast, cimetidine, erythromycin, ciprofloxacin, oral contraceptives, interferon, methotrexate,

mexiletine, and thiabendazole decrease its clearance.[74,75]

The H$_2$-antagonists other than cimetidine (e.g., famotidine) do not affect theophylline concentrations significantly. Nonlinear kinetics, seen within the therapeutic range in some children, should be suspected when dosage increases lead to disproportionate serum concentration increases and toxicity. Similarly, very prolonged half-lives are seen in the *early* phase of some overdose patients.

Toxicity is related to serum drug concentrations and, in order of usual increasing concentrations, includes

- Nausea.
- Vomiting.
- Diarrhea.
- Headache.
- Tachycardia.
- Dysrhythmias.
- Seizures.

Unfortunately, the above sequence does not always occur in that order, and seizures (often associated with brain damage) may be the first and only sign of excessive theophylline.

## Vancomycin

Vancomycin is a bactericidal antibiotic used against resistant Gram-positive organisms (e.g., methicillin-resistant *Staphylococcus aureus*) as well as for enterococci. Vancomycin is also useful for patients allergic to first-line drugs such as beta-lactams. Additionally, vancomycin is used orally to treat antibiotic-associated pseudomembranous colitis (Chapter 11). Because the drug has poor bioavailability, serum vancomycin concentrations need not be measured in oral administration cases.

The dose required to achieve the therapeutic range in most patients without renal dysfunction is 1 g every 12 hr (20–30 mg/kg/day). Lower doses or prolonged dosing intervals (1–2 weeks in hemodialysis patients) are used in patients with renal failure[76] and are adjusted based on CrCl.[11] The fluorescence polarization immunoassay (FPIA) overestimates vancomycin concentrations in patients with renal failure compared with enzyme-multiplied immunoassay technique (EMIT) measured values, possibly because the former measures accumulated metabolites. Higher doses may be needed in patients with burns since their volume of distribution and clearance are increased.[77]

The MIC for susceptible staphylococci is less than 5 mg/L and is easily achieved with a 1-g dose in the average patient. Therefore, valley concentrations of 5–10 mg/L are recommended to ensure adequate penetration and kill while avoiding toxicity. Although some authors feel that routine peak concentrations do not provide any valuable information in most patients,[78] many clinicians target peaks at 20–40 mg/L. In a recent retrospective "outcomes" study of patients with Gram-positive bacteremia,[79] no association between peak or trough vancomycin concentrations and mortality was found. However, patients were more likely to become afebrile within 72 hr if peaks and troughs were at least 20 and 10 mg/L, respectively.

Ototoxicity has been reported with peaks above 50 mg/L; it is likely above 80 mg/L.[76] The relationship between vancomycin and nephrotoxicity is even weaker. In one retrospective study, nephrotoxicity did not develop until trough concentrations reached 20 mg/L.[79] In a prospective study,[80] reversible nephrotoxicity occurred in 5% of patients receiving the drug alone. In another study, concomitant aminoglycosides were associated with an incidence of 22–35% nephrotoxicity.[81]

A "red neck" syndrome that manifests secondary to histamine release may occur with the first dose. The syndrome and hypotension are more likely to occur when vancomycin is infused quickly (>500 mg over 30 min). Other side effects that are not related to serum vancomycin concentration include urticaria, eosinophilia, and neutropenia. These effects occur less frequently with the newer, purer products compared to the original products.[81]

For most patients, a trough concentration obtained on day 2 (usually when culture and susceptibility data become available and the decision to continue treatment is made) allows for proper initial dosage adjustment. Before that time, toxicity or clinically significant underdosing is unlikely. In renal dialysis patients, timing is not important and random serum concentrations can be drawn every 3–4 days to ensure that they are above 5 mg/L.

## Antipsychotics

Although relationships between serum concentrations and therapeutic and toxic effects of certain antipsychotics (e.g., chlorpromazine, fluphenazine, perphenazine, thiothixene, and haloperidol) have been postulated, clear guidelines are not widely accepted.[82] Therefore, these serum concentrations should not be used routinely and will not be discussed here.[83] However, Table 7 provides the accepted therapeutic ranges for select antipsychotics. (References

82–85 provide discussions on the application and interpretation of these serum drug concentrations.)

## FACTORS CONFOUNDING INTERPRETATION OF DRUG CONCENTRATIONS

### Clinical Factors

Clinicians commonly face serum drug concentrations that appear illogical or intuitively "off," based on the information in Tables 3 and 5. The most common factors that confound evaluation of serum drug concentrations are delineated in Table 8 (next page).

Mistakes involve

➤ Drug administration and blood-drawing logistics.
➤ Application of pharmacokinetic principles.
➤ Laboratory "error."

Some of these errors are discussed later in this section; others are discussed elsewhere in this chapter. Because of the importance and complexity of errors, interference with serum drug concentration assays and laboratory errors are discussed in later sections.

No matter what the suspected cause, clinicians should always doublecheck calculations, dosing, and administration times. One can also request that the specimen be run through the assay again to check for errors in technologist performance or methodology. This step may not be necessary in some laboratories that automatically re-run samples yielding results significantly outside the normal range.

#### Steady-State–Serum Drug Concentration Relationship Ignored

One common error by ordering clinicians is obtaining serum drug concentrations before a steady state is attained. Unless a steady state exists, the serum drug concentration will not be proportionate to the dose over time. The potential outcome of this error was discussed previously (Figure 5 and related text).

#### Dose–Serum Drug Concentration Draw Time Ignored

The most common logistics error relates to the serum concentration being drawn at the wrong time relative to the dose being administered. This error is more likely to occur when the nursing staff is very busy or when the

TABLE 7. Therapeutic Ranges for Select Antipsychotic Agents

| Generic Name | Usual Daily Dose (mg) | Therapeutic Range (ng/mL) | Therapeutic Range (SI Units) |
|---|---|---|---|
| Chlorpromazine | 25–150 | 50–300 | 150–950 nmol/L |
| Clozapine | 200–600 | 450–?[a] | 1.38–? µmol/L |
| Fluphenazine | 2.5–10 | 0.5–2.5 | 5.3–21 nmol/L |
| Haloperidol | 5–20 | 5–15[b] | 13–40 nmol/L |
| Perphenazine | 5–20 | 0.8–2.4 | 2–6 nmol/L |

[a]The upper limit has not been established. Seizures have occurred above 1000 ng/mL (3 µmol/L).
[b]Other suggested ranges are 7–25 ng/mL (19–67 nmol/L) and 15–38 ng/mL (40–101 nmol/L) for patients receiving the drug for months and years, respectively.[86]

**TABLE 8.** Common Factors that Confound Interpretation of Serum Drug Concentrations

> **Related to drug administration or blood-drawing logistics**
> Wrong dose administered and/or dispensed
> Dose skipped (e.g., patient undergoing procedure or refused medication; nursing error)
> Dose given at wrong time; blood drawn as ordered
> Dose given at right time; blood not drawn at right time
> Infusion time too fast or slow
> Infusion held prior to draw to give another IV drug (in patients with limited venous access)
> Infusion rate increased prior to draw to "catch up" with schedule
> Blood drawn from same vein into which drug is infused
>
> **Related to pharmacokinetics**
> *General*
> Levels ordered before steady state is reached (Figure 5 and Minicase 1)
> Levels ordered without respect to dosing time
> Active metabolites not considered (e.g., NAPA)
>
> *Related to absorption and distribution*
> Absorption problems with oral (postsurgical) or IM (severely hypotensive patients) route
> Drawing levels before distribution to site of effect is complete (e.g., digoxin)
>
> *Related to volume of distribution*
> Dramatic fluid status changes (e.g., volume overload, dehydration/hypovolemia, and "third spacing")
> Inappropriate apparent distribution mass (weight) used in dosing (obese patients; Table 5)
> Significant nonfluid weight loss or gain (affects long-term outpatient therapeutic drug monitoring)
>
> *Related to elimination*
> Significant changes in function of liver, heart, or kidneys (Table 3)
> Significant changes in percentages of free and bound drug (hypoalbuminemia); may also affect volume of distribution
> Change in metabolizing enzyme saturation threshold (Figure 7)
>
> *Pharmacokinetic drug interactions*
> Change in drug regimen or dosing history for drugs that alter kinetics (mainly elimination) of other medications (Table 4)
>
> **Related to laboratory**
> Improper performance of assay
> Laboratory transcription or computer-entry error
> Active metabolites not measured
> Assay interference by drugs or other substances
> Improper specimen collection or storage (Test Tubes, Stoppers, and Postphlebotomy Storage Conditions section)

patient is undergoing a procedure (e.g., computer-assisted tomography scan) at the scheduled dosing time. If the clinician is unaware of this deviation from orders, a peak may be interpreted as a trough or vice versa. Nurses should always inform the blood drawer and the person responsible for any dosing schedule of administration changes, especially if serum drug concentrations have been ordered in that dosing interval.

A similar problem arises when the order is for an unqualified "peak" or "valley," leaving draw time decisions up to the nurse. This type of error may also occur because the serum drug concentration is ordered at an improper time in the first place.

The factors that involve the relative timing of dose-to-serum drug concentration draws are most significant for drugs with short half-lives (e.g., aminoglycosides), including those given by constant infusion (e.g., lidocaine and procainamide). These drugs are so susceptible because the serum concentration can change more quickly, even with short interruptions or delays in drug administration.

### Inappropriate Dosing Weight Used

Another common confounding factor involves the use of an inappropriate weight for dosing. Certain drugs should be dosed on the basis of an adjusted body mass as opposed to actual weight.[7,8] If, for example, a 150-kg male is given a 4-mg/kg (600-mg) daily extended-interval dose of gentamicin, his peak concentration may reach 32 mg/L if total body weight is used in the calculation. This high concentration theoretically places the patient at higher risk for ototoxicity. If the patient's apparent distribution mass (dosing weight) of 100 kg is used, a 400-mg dose would yield a peak of 21.4 mg/L, which is closer to the peaks seen in extended-interval regimen studies that show no increased risk for ototoxicity.[13] This principle should be applied to other drugs identified in Table 5.

### Free versus Bound Drug Ignored

In the presence of hypoalbuminemia, the therapeutic range of some drugs must be adjusted to maintain the relationship between drug bound or unbound to albumin and pharmacological response. Phenytoin, for example, usually has only 10% of its total concentration unbound. In other words, the therapeutic range for *unbound* drug would be 1–2 mg/L instead of 10–20 mg/L. If albumin can bind only 80% of the drug, then *total* concentrations of 10–20 mg/L would reflect *free* concentrations of 2–4 mg/L, and the patient may manifest signs and symptoms of toxicity despite a total serum phenytoin concentration in the "therapeutic range." To adjust quantitatively for this apparent discrepancy, the following formula was proposed:[11]

$$C_{p\text{-NB}} = \frac{C_p{}'}{(1-a)\left(\dfrac{P'}{P_{NL}}\right) + a}$$

where $C_{p\text{-NB}}$ is the total phenytoin concentration that would have been reported if the patient's albumin concentration had been normal (i.e., NB or normal binding), $C_p{}'$ is the total phenytoin concentration reported by the laboratory, a is the normal free fraction of the drug (0.1), $P'$ is the patient's albumin concentration (in grams per deciliter), and $P_{NL}$ is an average, normal albumin concentration (4.4 g/dL).

A patient with an albumin concentration of 2 g/dL and a reported total phenytoin concentration of 15 mg/L would have a pharmacological response expected from a concentration of about 29 mg/L had his or her albumin been normal at 4.4 g/dL. The therapeutic range for phenytoin also must be interpreted differently in patients with renal failure because of changes in the amount and affinity of binding and in patients receiving valproic acid (Anticonvulsants section).[11]

## Assay Interferences

Clinicians generally feel that serum drug concentration reports from the laboratory are accurate. Their confidence comes from assuming that the laboratory has ongoing internal and external quality controls. In some situations, however, quality controls may be insufficient or the cause of error cannot be controlled for by technologists or technicians (e.g., when it is not related to performance of the assay). For example, errors may be due to improper collection of specimens or inaccurate transcription. An external error may be due to substances in the patient's serum or in the collection tube that interfere with the chemical reactions or the reading of the assay. This type of error is discussed in Chapter 3, except for interference with serum drug concentrations (discussed below). Because of the clinician's need to refer to original studies for proper case analysis, the following discussion is heavily referenced.

The subject of drug interferences with serum drug concentration determinations was reviewed in 1984.[87] For details on reports before 1984, one should refer to that article or the original articles listed therein. These reports are summarized here along with more recent reports. Nondrug causes of false serum drug concentration results also are discussed. Because commercially available assays are occasionally modified, their specificity can change. Therefore, the clinician should check with the laboratory periodically to obtain information on the assays used. (General guidelines on preventing, identifying, circumventing, and resolving interferences with laboratory tests are discussed in Chapter 3.)

### Aminoglycosides

As noted previously, microbiological assays for aminoglycosides can be influenced by other aminoglycosides and antibacterials, including certain "antibiotic" antineoplastic agents (bleomycin, daunorubicin, and doxorubicin). For patients with renal failure who are switched from one aminoglycoside to another, the clinician should consider the impact of the residual antibiotic. If the therapeutic ranges of the two are similar, the additive effectiveness and risk of toxicity may be underestimated because only a percentage of the first aminoglycoside would be detected. This factor is significant with netilmicin and gentamicin, because they cross-react with one another in the EMIT and fluorescence-based assays. Fortunately, the simultaneous administration of two systemically available aminoglycosides is rare. Amikacin and tobramycin do not significantly cross-react with other aminoglycosides. One exception is that kanamycin may cross-react with tobramycin tested with a fluorescent immunoassay (TDA, Miles).

Heparin in concentrations as low as 5–10 U/mL may cause falsely low measurements of tobramycin and netilmicin with the EMIT system. The gentamicin assay is less affected (500–1000 U/mL of heparin required).[88] Concentrations of 5–10 U/mL should not be achievable in patients (therapeutic concentrations are 0.2–0.4 U/mL), but they may occur in the specimen tube if the (1) two drugs are infused through a common tubing, (2) specimen collection tube contains heparin, or (3) blood is sampled through a heparin lock. The RIA and FPIA (TDx, Abbott) assays are not affected.[89]

### Digoxin

Because only small nanogram amounts must be detected (i.e., high sensitivity required), digoxin is usually measured by RIA. Although this assay and the other two immunoassays cannot always distinguish digoxin from digitoxin at therapeutic concentrations, the clinical frequency of this problem is low because digitoxin is rarely used today. This limitation would be important if a patient had been switched from digitoxin to digoxin within 1–2 weeks of the test. Cross-reactivity has been highest (40%) with the enzyme-linked immunosorbent assay.[90]

In contrast, spironolactone is often prescribed concomitantly with digoxin. Spironolactone interference appears to be related to dose and serum concentration in most immunoassay studies. Persons receiving 75–200 mg/day commonly had spurious digoxin concentration increases of 0.5–1.5 ng/mL. Most investigators used the RIA. However, an in vitro investigation of a fluoroimmunoassay revealed no effect. According to some authors, canrenone (an active metabolite with a longer half-life) may be responsible for the interference.[91] Another drug with a structure similar to digoxin, prednisolone, also has been shown to interfere with some assays.

It is uncommon for patients to present with severe, symptomatic digoxin toxicity (serum concentration >3 ng/mL) requiring treatment with digoxin fab antibodies. Within minutes of administration, fab antibodies cause *total* serum digoxin concentrations to increase 10–30 fold. They also decrease unbound digoxin in plasma from 75–90% to only 0–5%. Common assays (because they measure *total* digoxin) show a dramatically elevated serum drug concentration. However, most of it is bound to antibody fragments and, therefore, pharmacologically inactive.

These results should be ignored; in fact, the test should not have been ordered because the results are uninterpretable. Assays that measure only *free* digoxin should be employed. Several commercial assays purport to measure only unbound digoxin accurately; however, one study found that only ultrafiltered samples tested with the FPIA (TDx) gave accurate results.[92] Measurement of free digoxin concentrations can help the clinician to determine how much (if any) additional fab antibodies are needed and when digoxin may be restarted.

*Nondrug substances* also interfere with immunoassays. Digoxin-like immunoreactive substances have been found in the sera of patients with liver[93] or renal[94] failure, in newborns, and in pregnant women.[95] Some investigators postulated that these substances have a role in the timely onset of labor.[96] About 7% of children less than 6 years old may appear to have therapeutic digoxin concentrations even though none is in their serum. Digoxin-like immunoreactive substances are read as if they were digoxin. RIAs can differ with respect to vulnerability to these substances.

RIANEN-Digoxin I[125] (Du Pont) exhibited large cross-reactivity with digoxin-like immunoreactive substances and was withdrawn from the market in January 1990. Immophase (Corning),[97] EMIT C-B (Syva), and BDS (Baxter Dade Stratus) are much less susceptible.[93,98] Neonates on digoxin therapy are uncommon (i.e., seen only in cases of congenital heart disease), but this group shows the most interference.[99] In patients with liver disease, false-positive digoxin concentrations measured with FPIA and RIA also have been reported.

Reformulation of assay reagents has led to confusion. The older TDx method (Digoxin I) is minimally affected by digoxin-like immunoreactive substances compared with the newer TDx method (Digoxin II).[99,100] However, the antibody pool for Digoxin II has been changed.[101] A comparison of Digoxin II with an affinity column-mediated immunoassay (ACMIA), in a patient with moderate renal dysfunction (CrCl of 28 mL/min), revealed that the ACMIA assay yielded values four to five times higher than those from the TDx system.[101] The TDx assay following ultrafiltration is not affected by digoxin-like immunoreactive substances, probably because they are extensively protein bound and readily removed by ultrafiltration.[102]

The digoxin-like immunoreactive substances have not been identified specifically, although some investigators speculate that they are primitive hormones close in structure to ouabain. The metabolites dihydrodigoxin and digoxigenin are known to cross-react with digoxin assays, and digoxin metabolites may account for up to 40% of the measurement with immunoassays.[103] However, it is unlikely that digoxin-like immunoreactive substances are solely metabolites of digoxin; they are seen in patients who have not been receiving the cardiac glycoside. Furthermore, the amount of metabolites in the serum is about the same for patients with normal and minimal renal function.[104]

In summary, the degree of false elevations (0.25–1.0 ng/mL)[98] from digoxin-like immunoreactive substances is not enough for clinicians to suspect interference but may be enough to encourage inappropriate dosage changes. Because of the vast differences in specificities among the digoxin assays and because commercially available assays are continually modified to improve specificity, clinicians have to become familiar with assay- and product-specific interferences. Technologists should be asked to inform practitioners whenever an assay is modified. Some clinicians obtain a digoxin level before starting the drug in high-risk patients to determine the extent of baseline digoxin-like immunoreactive substances. This value can be subtracted from steady-state digoxin concentrations to get a more accurate reading of the true digoxin concentration.

### Procainamide

There are few reports of interferences with procainamide assays. HPLC methods are influenced (false increases) by caffeine and metronidazole (NAPA is not affected) if blood is drawn during the peak of these substances.[105] NAPA readings may be altered by quinidine metabolites with the HPLC assay, but most laboratories use an immunoassay for this antidysrhythmic agent. Procaine cross-reacts with the EMIT system at concentrations greater than 10 mg/L, an unlikely concentration in clinical practice. NAPA can be measured separately with the EMIT assay, which is not affected by the parent drug.

### Quinidine

Quinidine is usually measured with an HPLC or immunoassay. Several drugs or their metabolites can lead to false increases in quinidine concentrations with the HPLC method. These drugs include chlordiazepoxide, disopyramide, propranolol, primaquine, and quinine. In therapeutic doses, quinine may cause false increases with the EMIT assay. Quinine concentrations greater than 40 mg/L are required to give a response equal to that of 0.5 mg/L of quinidine.[106] An active metabolite, dihydroquinidine, contributes 5–10% to the assayed value.

### Anticonvulsants

Immunoassays are most commonly used to measure phenobarbital and phenytoin. In general, cross-reactivity may occur if the patient is on another drug in the same chemical class (e.g., mephobarbital with the phenobarbital assay), but such an event rarely happens today. Carbamazepine measurements by the immunoassays have no reported cross-reactions. These drugs have been tested with others that are likely to be given simultaneously or that might be expected to cross-react because of structural similarity.

Patients with renal failure may retain phenytoin metabolites such as 5-(*p*-hydroxyphenyl)-5-phenylhydantoin (HPPH), which are measured as parent drug by certain assays. Concentrations may appear to be 20, 60, and 80% higher than the true value using the FPIA, enzyme immunoassay, and rate nephelometric inhibition immunoassay, respectively.[107] Roberts and Rainey[108] found that in patients with SCr greater than 13 mg/dL (>1149 μmol/L), the TDx FPIA overestimated both free and total phenytoin concentrations by as much as 100%, whereas the aca (Du Pont) and EMIT (Syva) assays yielded results close to those measured by HPLC. The cross-reactive substance was not the HPPH metabolite.

HPPH may also diminish phenytoin binding to albumin, leading to higher free drug concentrations. Therefore, free phenytoin concentrations should be obtained in patients with renal failure.

### Theophylline

Many spectrophotometric theophylline assays are disturbed by numerous drugs. To avoid the interferences, most assays can be slightly modified. Dimenhydrinate has been shown to interfere with one HPLC and one RIA method. Metronidazole has been reported to interfere with an HPLC assay.[109] In contrast, some investigators found that the usual clinical concentrations of pentoxifylline do not interfere with the TDx, EMIT, and HPLC assays for theophylline.[110] (Pentoxifylline was studied because of its structural similarity to theophylline.)

Other investigators showed that four likely interferents (pentoxifylline, 1-methylxanthine, allopurinol, and oxypurinol) at clinically achievable serum concentrations did not interfere with an assay based on theophylline oxidase (GDS Diagnostics).[111] Concentrations of caffeine, attainable by drinking large amounts of coffee, can interfere with some immunoassays if blood is drawn near the caffeine peak (i.e., shortly after drinking). In this situation, interpretation is difficult because high concentrations of either drug lead to similar signs and symptoms.

### Test Tubes, Stoppers, and Postphlebotomy Storage Conditions

Evacuated blood collection systems are now state of the art. Although these closed systems have many advantages, interferences with assays from a plasticizer in the rubber stoppers were identified in the late 1970s and early 1980s. The plasticizer reduced drug binding to $\alpha_1$-acid glycoprotein. A redistribution of drug in whole blood took place, resulting in an increase of drug uptake by the red blood cells and a decrease of the total serum concentration. This effect occurred primarily with the red-stoppered Vacutainers[112] and was most important with lidocaine, quinidine, and the TCAs. Since then, a blue-stoppered Vacutainer without plasticizers has replaced the old one, and the problem appears to be solved. Other tube producers have followed suit.

Other potential problems with collection tubes relate to the stabilizers, anticoagulants, and separation gels within them. For example, although measurement of concentrations of these drugs is not common, beta-blockers, benzodiazepines, antidepressants, anticancer agents, and neuroleptics can have their concentrations altered by the presence of serum separator gels. The drugs are adsorbed to the gel in a time-dependent manner.[3] Thus, these tubes should not be used for drug concentration analysis. Clinicians should suspect laboratory methods, machinery, or equipment (including rubber stoppers) if certain assay results *consistently* appear too high or low relative to doses or clinical response.

One final consideration relating to interpretation of serum drug concentrations is the possibility of improper storage after the blood sample is drawn. Investigators evaluated the stability of eight commonly monitored drugs in both whole blood and plasma at 4 and 25 °C over 72 hr. The data suggest that meticulous postphlebotomy handling of blood samples containing vancomycin, gentamicin, theophylline, lidocaine, procainamide, digoxin, quinidine, and phenytoin is probably not essential to obtain accurate concentrations.[113] Despite these findings, it is safer to have the sample assayed as soon as possible after collection.

Many substances can interfere with determinations of serum drug concentrations. As the substances are identified, assays are modified to avoid the alteration. Because most interferences are assay specific, practitioners need to be familiar with the specificity of the assay used in their setting. If results are inconsistent with pharmacokinetic estimates or clinical response, assay interference should be investigated. If any potential interferences are identified, a different type of assay might be run.

## SUMMARY

Clinicians responsible for ordering or monitoring drugs that have commonly available assays must understand applied pharmacokinetics to avoid the pitfalls that lead to faulty decisions. Even with this understanding, accurate and thorough patient, drug, and assay data are necessary for optimal planning and interpretation of serum drug concentrations.

The therapeutic range is the range of serum drug concentrations associated with a high likelihood of effectiveness and the least chance of toxicity. Peak and trough (valley) concentrations are the highest and lowest drug concentrations, respectively, occurring within a dosing interval. The Vd is the apparent volume of blood or other tissue into which a given amount of drug distributes. The clearance ($Cl_T$) of a drug represents the clearance of a constant fraction of the Vd. The constant fraction that is eliminated per unit of time is known as the elimination rate constant (Ke), which is related to the half-life (t½). The half-life is the time required for a 50% decrease in the serum drug concentration relative to the initial concentration. Practically speaking, steady state is achieved after five to seven half-lives have passed. When a loading dose is given, steady state is reached when the serum drug concentration raises to where it would continue to peak during subsequent dosing intervals.

For serum drug concentrations to be useful, (1) the intensity of the pharmacological action or response must be proportional to the concentration of free drug at the site of action, (2) the concentration of free drug at the site of action must be consistently proportional to the concentration in the serum, and (3) the degree of serum protein and tissue binding must remain relatively constant. Serum drug concentrations are often ordered when the drug has complex kinetics or a narrow therapeutic margin, the drug effect cannot be easily quantified clinically, the dose–response relationship varies widely, a drug interaction is possible, a suspected change in distribution or metabolism exists, or overdose or noncompliance is suspected.

Information needed to plan or interpret serum drug concentrations properly includes demographics, history and physical examination, serum drug concentration history, other laboratory tests, and drug and dosing history. Table 5 (pages 74 and 75) contains the most pertinent drug information needed for proper interpretation of serum drug concentrations. Factors that confound interpretation of these concentrations are related to drug administration or blood drawing logistics, pharmacokinetics, laboratory procedures, and interferences with serum drug concentration assays.

## REFERENCES

1. McCleod DC, Taylor WJ. Therapeutic drug monitoring as a standard of care. *Drug Intell Clin Pharm.* 1985; 19:473–4.
2. Wagner JG. Fundamentals of clinical pharmacokinetics. Hamilton, IL: Drug Intelligence Publications; 1976.
3. McCoy HG, Labrosse KR. State of the art: measurement of drug concentrations for therapeutic drug monitoring. *J Pharm Pract.* 1989; 2:335–46.
4. Craig WA. The rationale for continuous-infusion dosing of beta-lactams. *Infect Med.* 1992; 9(Suppl B):6–9.
5. Danziger LH. Controversies in antimicrobial therapy: innovative methods of administration. *Am J Hosp Pharm.* 1986; 43:646–52.
6. Hansten PD, Horn JR. Mechanisms of drug interactions: protein binding displacement. *Drug Interact Newslett.* 1986; 6:9–12.
7. Traub SL. Pharmacokinetics and apparent distribution mass. *Clin Pharmacokinet Newslett.* 1985; 2:1–4.
8. Traub SL, Kichen L. Estimating ideal body mass in children. *Am J Hosp Pharm.* 1983; 40:107–10.
9. Koup JR, Vawter TK. Theophylline pharmacokinetics in an extremely obese patient. *Clin Pharm.* 1983; 2:181–3.
10. Brown GR, Miyata M, McCormack JP. Drug concentration monitoring: an approach to rational use. *Clin Pharmacokinet.* 1993; 24:187–94.
11. Winter ME. Basic clinical pharmacokinetics, 2nd ed. Spokane, WA: Applied Therapeutics; 1988.
12. Taylor EH, Eudy S, Pappas AA. False positive identification of a tricyclic antidepressant due to cyclobenzaprine (Flexeril). *Clin Chem.* 1988; 34:1262.
13. Preston SL, Briceland LL. Single daily dosing of aminoglycosides. *Pharmacotherapy.* 1995; 15:297–316.
14. Bates RD, Nahata MC. Once-daily administration of aminoglycosides. *Ann Pharmacother.* 1994; 28:757–66.
15. Galloe AM, Graudal N, Christensen HR, et al. Aminoglycosides: single or multiple daily dosing? A meta-analysis on efficacy and safety. *Eur J Clin Pharmacol.* 1995; 48:39–43.
16. Yee GC, Evans WB. Reappraisal of guidelines for pharmacokinetic monitoring of aminoglycosides. *Pharmacotherapy.* 1981; 1:55–75.
17. Bauer LA, Blouin RA, Griffen WO Jr, et al. Amikacin pharmacokinetics in morbidly obese patients. *Am J Hosp Pharm.* 1980; 37:519–22.
18. Moore RD, Leitman PS, Smith CR. Clinical response to aminoglycoside therapy: implication of the ratio of the peak concentration to MIC. *J Infect Dis.* 1987; 155:93–9.
19. McCormack JP, Jewesson PJ. A critical reevaluation of the "therapeutic range" of aminoglycosides. *Clin Infect Dis.* 1992; 14:320–39.
20. Cimino MA, Rotstein C, Slaughter RL, et al. Relationship of serum antibiotic concentrations to nephrotoxicity in cancer patients receiving concurrent aminoglycoside and vancomycin therapy. *Am J Med.* 1987; 83:1091–7.
21. Sawyers CL, Moore RD, Lerner SA, et al. A model for predicting nephrotoxicity in patients treated with aminoglycosides. *J Infect Dis.* 1986; 153:1062–8.
22. Schentag JJ, Jusko WJ. Renal clearance and tissue accumulation of gentamicin. *Clin Pharmacol Ther.* 1977; 22:364–70.
23. Moore RD, Smith CR, Leitman PS. Risk factors for the development of auditory toxicity in patients receiving aminoglycosides. *J Infect Dis.* 1984; 149:23–30.
24. Evans DA, Buring J, Mayrent S, et al. Qualitative overview of randomized trials of aminoglycosides. *Am J Med.* 1986; 80(Suppl 6B):39–43.
25. Mattie H, Craig WA, Pecheve JC. Determinants of efficacy and toxicity of aminoglycosides. *J Antimicrob Chemother.* 1989; 24:281–93.
26. Pickering LK, Rutherford I. Effect of concentration and time upon inactivation of tobramycin, gentamicin, netilmicin, and amikacin by azlocillin, carbenicillin, mecillinam, mezlocillin, and piperacillin. *J Pharmacol Exp Ther.* 1981; 217:345–9.
27. Chow MSS, Quintiliani R, Nightingale CH. In vivo inactivation of tobramycin by ticarcillin. *JAMA.* 1982; 247:658–9.
28. Bertilsson L, Hojer B, Tybring G, et al. Autoinduction of carbamazepine metabolism in children examined by stable isotope technique. *Clin Pharmacol Ther.* 1980; 27:83–8.
29. Lindholm A, Kahan BD. Influence of cyclosporine pharmacokinetics, trough concentrations, and AUC monitoring on outcome after kidney transplantation. *Clin Pharmacol Ther.* 1993; 54:205–18.
30. Reynolds DJM, Aronson JK. ABC of monitoring drug therapy: cyclosporin. *Br Med J.* 1992; 305:1491–4.
31. Speed C. Monitoring cyclosporin treatment. *Br Med J.* 1993; 306:396. Letter.
32. Dijkmans BAC, Van Rijthoven AWAM, Goeithe HS, et al. Cyclosporine in rheumatoid arthritis. *Semin Arthritis Rheum.* 1992; 22:30–6.
33. Arroyo J. Potential interference of cycloserine in assay for cyclosporine. *Clin Infect Dis.* 1993; 17:142. Letter.
34. Smith TW. Digitalis: mechanisms of action and clinical use. *N Engl J Med.* 1988; 318:358–65.
35. Dobkin JF, Saha JR, Butler VP, et al. Digoxin-inactivating bacteria: identification in human gut flora. *Science.* 1983; 220:325–7.
36. Lindenbaum J, Rund DG, Butler VP Jr, et al. Inactivation

of digoxin by gut flora: reversal by antibiotic therapy. *N Engl J Med.* 1981; 305:789–94.

37. Ewy GA, Groves BM, Ball MF, et al. Digoxin metabolism in obesity. *Circulation.* 1971; 44:810–4.

38. Aronson JK, Hardman M. ABC of monitoring drug therapy: digoxin. *Br Med J.* 1992; 305:1149–52.

39. Smith TW, Antman EM, Friedman PL, et al. Digitalis glycosides: mechanisms and manifestations of toxicity: III. *Prog Cardiovasc Dis.* 1984; 27:21–56.

40. Zehender M, Kasper W, Just H. Lidocaine in the early phase of acute myocardial infarction: the controversy over prophylactic or selective use. *Clin Cardiol.* 1990; 13:534–9.

41. Gunnar RM, Passamani ER, Bourdillon PD, et al. Guidelines for the early management of patients with acute myocardial infarction. A report of the American College of Cardiology/American Heart Association Task Force on Assessment of Diagnostic and Therapeutic Cardiovascular Procedures. *J Am Coll Cardiol.* 1990; 16:249–92.

42. Berk SI, Gal P, Bauman JL, et al. The effect of oral cimetidine on total and unbound serum lidocaine concentrations in patients with suspected myocardial infarction. *Int J Cardiol.* 1987; 14:91–4.

43. McCollam PL, Bauman JL. New concepts in antiarrhythmic drug monitoring. *J Pharm Pract.* 1989; 2:393–402.

44. McCollam PL, Bauman JL, Beckman KJ, et al. A simple method of monitoring antiarrhythmic drugs during short- and long-term therapy. *Am J Cardiol.* 1989; 63:1273–5.

45. Brown GR, Miyata M, McCormack JP. Drug concentration monitoring: an approach to rational use. *Clin Pharmacokinet.* 1993; 24:187–94.

46. Kook KA, Stimmel GL, Wilkins JN, et al. Accuracy and safety of a prior lithium loading. *J Clin Psychiatry.* 1985; 46:49–51.

47. Gelenberg AJ, Kane JM, Keller MB, et al. Comparison of standard and low serum levels of lithium for maintenance treatment of bipolar disorder. *N Engl J Med.* 1989; 321: 1489–93.

48. Saklad SR, Kastenholz KV. Bipolar affective disorders. In: Young LY, Koda-Kimble MA, eds. Applied therapeutics: the clinical use of drugs. Vancouver, WA: Applied Therapeutics; 1988:1255–75.

49. Price LH, Heninger GR. Lithium in the treatment of mood disorders. *N Engl J Med.* 1994; 331:591–8.

50. Morton WA, Sonne SC, Lydiard RB. Lithium side effects in the medically ill. *Int J Psychiatry Med.* 1993; 23:357–82.

51. Perry PJ, Pfohl BM, Hostad SG. The relationship between antidepressant response and tricyclic antidepressant plasma concentrations: a retrospective analysis of the literature using logistic regression analysis. *Clin Pharmacokinet.* 1987; 13:381–92.

52. American Psychiatric Association Task Force on the Use of Laboratory Tests in Psychiatry. TCA blood level measurements and clinical outcome: an APA Task Force report. *Am J Psychiatry.* 1985; 142:155–62.

53. Morin A, Stoukides CA. Use of tricyclic antidepressant concentrations to determine individual response. *Ann Pharmacother.* 1993; 27:896–7.

54. Fritz GK, Rockney RM, Yeung AS. Plasma levels and efficacy of imipramine treatment for enuresis. *J Am Acad Child Adolesc Psychiatry.* 1994; 33:60–4.

55. Brown CS, Bryant SG. Drug treatment of depression. *J Pharm Pract.* 1990; 2:252–61.

56. Hermann DJ, Krol TF, Dukes GE, et al. Comparison of verapamil, diltiazem and labetolol on the bioavailability and metabolism of imipramine. *J Clin Pharmacol.* 1992;

32:176–83.

57. Feldman MD. Therapeutic blood monitoring of tricyclic antidepressants. *South Med J.* 1994; 87:101. Letter.

58. Jerling M, Bertilsson L, Sjöqvist F. The use of therapeutic drug monitoring data to document kinetic drug interactions: an example with amitriptyline and nortriptyline. *Ther Drug Monit.* 1994; 16:1–12.

59. Wolf SM, Forsythe A. Behavior disturbance, phenobarbital, and febrile seizures. *Pediatrics.* 1978; 61:728–31.

60. Pisani F, Richens A. Pharmacokinetics of phenylethylmalonamide after oral and intravenous administration. *Clin Pharmacokinet.* 1983; 8:272–6.

61. Schumacher GE, Barr JT, Brownie TR, et al. Test performance characteristics of the serum phenytoin concentration (SPC): the relationship between SPC and patient response. *Ther Drug Monit.* 1991; 13:318–24.

62. Liponi DF, Winter ME, Tozer TN. Renal function and therapeutic concentrations of phenytoin. *Neurology.* 1984; 34:395–7.

63. Levy RH, Yerby MS. Effects of pregnancy on antiepileptic drug utilization. *Epilepsia.* 1985; 28(Suppl 1):S52–7.

64. Tomson T, Lindbom U, Ekqvist B, et al. Epilepsy and pregnancy: a prospective study of seizure control in relation to free and total plasma phenytoin concentrations of carbamazepine and phenytoin. *Epilepsia.* 1994; 35:122–30.

65. Butler RT, Kalwarf KL, Kaldahl WB. Drug-induced gingival hyperplasia: phenytoin, cyclosporine and nifedipine. *J Am Dent Assoc.* 1987; 114:56–60.

66. Kapur RN, Girgis S, Little TM, et al. Diphenylhydantoin-induced gingival hyperplasia: its relationship to dose and serum level. *Dev Med Child Neurol.* 1973; 15:483–7.

67. Kessler KM, Kayden DS, Estes DM, et al. Procainamide pharmacokinetics in patients with acute myocardial infarction or congestive heart failure. *J Am Coll Cardiol.* 1986; 7:1131–9.

68. Mongey AB, Donovan-Brand R, Thomas TJ, et al. Serological evaluation of patients receiving procainamide. *Arthritis Rheum.* 1992; 35:219–23.

69. Ochs HR, Greenblatt DJ, Woo E. Clinical pharmacokinetics of quinidine. *Clin Pharmacokinet.* 1980; 5:150–68.

70. Borga O, Odar-Cederlof I, Ringberger V-A, et al. Protein binding of salicylate in uremic and normal plasma. *Clin Pharmacol Ther.* 1976; 20:464–75.

71. Dahl SL. Rheumatic disorders. In: Young LY, Koda-Kimble MA, eds. Applied therapeutics: the clinical use of drugs. Vancouver, WA: Applied Therapeutics; 1988:1775–1802.

72. Stoloff SW. The changing role of theophylline in pediatric asthma. *Am Fam Physician.* 1994; 49:839–44.

73. Aronson JK, Hardman M, Reynolds DJM. ABC of monitoring drug therapy: theophylline. *Br Med J.* 1992; 305: 1355–6.

74. Jonkman JHG, Upton RA. Pharmacokinetic drug interactions with theophylline. *Clin Pharmacokinet.* 1984; 9:309–34.

75. Hendeles L, Weinberger M, Szefler S, et al. Safety and efficacy of theophylline in children with asthma. *J Pediatr.* 1992; 120:177–83.

76. Matzke GR, Zhanel GG, Guay DRP. Clinical pharmacokinetics of vancomycin. *Clin Pharmacokinet.* 1986; 11: 257–82.

77. Rybak MJ, Albrecht LM, Berman JR, et al. Vancomycin pharmacokinetics in burn patients and intravenous drug abusers. *Antimicrob Agents Chemother.* 1990; 34:792–5.

78. Freeman CD, Quintiliani R, Nightingale CH. Vancomycin therapeutic drug monitoring: is it necessary? *Ann Pharmacother.* 1993; 27:594–8.

79. Zimmermann AE, Katona BG, Plaisance KI. Association

of vancomycin serum concentrations with outcomes in patients with gram-positive bacteremia. *Pharmacotherapy.* 1995; 15:85–91.

80. Rybak MJ, Albrecht LM, Boike SC, et al. Nephrotoxicity of vancomycin, alone and with an aminoglycoside. *J Antimicrob Chemother.* 1990; 25:679–87.

81. Farber BF, Moellering RC. Retrospective study of the toxicity of preparations of vancomycin from 1974–1981. *Antimicrob Agents Chemother.* 1983; 23:138–41.

82. Dahl S. Plasma level monitoring of antipsychotic drugs. *Clin Pharmacokinet.* 1986; 11:36–61.

83. Seifert RD. Therapeutic drug monitoring: psychotropic drugs. *J Pharm Pract.* 1989; 2:403–16.

84. Ereshefsky L, Richards A. Psychoses. In: Young LY, Koda-Kimble MA, eds. Applied therapeutics: the clinical use of drugs. Vancouver, WA: Applied Therapeutics; 1988:1189–1230.

85. Balant-Gorgia AE, Balant LP, Andreoli A. Pharmacokinetic optimisation of the treatment of psychosis. *Clin Pharmacokinet.* 1993; 25:217–36.

86. Santos JL, Cabranes JA, Vazquez C, et al. Clinical response and plasma haloperidol levels in chronic and subchronic schizophrenia. *Biol Psychiatry.* 1989; 26:381–8.

87. Yosselson-Superstine S. Drug interferences with plasma assays in therapeutic drug monitoring. *Clin Pharmacokinet.* 1984; 9:67–87.

88. Matzke GR, Piveral K, Halstenson CE, et al. Heparin interferes with tobramycin serum concentration determinations by EMIT. *Drug Intell Clin Pharm.* 1984; 18:517–9.

89. O'Connell MB, Heim K, Halstenson C, et al. Heparin interference with tobramycin, netilmicin, and gentamicin concentrations determined by EMIT. *Drug Intell Clin Pharm.* 1984; 18:503–4. Abstract.

90. Scherrmann JM, Bourdon R. Cross-reactivity of digitoxin in radioimmunoassay and enzyme-linked immunoassay for digoxin in plasma. *Clin Chem.* 1980; 26:670–1.

91. Al-Hakiem MHH, Nargess RD, Pourfarzaneh M, et al. Fluoroimmunoassay of digoxin in serum. *J Clin Chem Clin Biochem.* 1982; 20:151–6.

92. Ujhelyi MR, Green PJ, Cummings DM, et al. Determination of free serum digoxin concentrations in digoxin toxic patients after administration of digoxin fab antibodies. *Ther Drug Monit.* 1992; 14:147–54.

93. Frisolone J, Sylvia LM, Gelwan J, et al. False-positive serum digoxin concentrations determined by three assays in patients with liver disease. *Clin Pharm.* 1988; 7:444–9.

94. Gault MH, Vasdev S, Vlasses P, et al. Interpretation of serum digoxin values in renal failure. *Clin Pharmacol Ther.* 1986; 39:530–6.

95. Graves SW, Valdes R, Brown BA, et al. Endogenous digoxin immunoreactive substance in human pregnancies. *J Clin Endocrinol Metab.* 1984; 58:748–51.

96. Yapar EG, Ayhan A. The influence of tocolytic therapy on serum digoxin-like immunoreactive substance concentration. *Gynecol Obstet Invest.* 1994; 37:10–3.

97. Valdes R. Endogenous digoxin-like immunoreactive factors: impact on digoxin measurements and potential physiological implications. *Clin Chem.* 1985; 31:1525–32.

98. Skogen WF, Rea MR, Valdes R Jr. Endogenous digoxin-like immunoreactive factors eliminated from serum samples by hydrophobic silica-gel extraction and enzyme immunoassay. *Clin Chem.* 1987; 33:401–4.

99. Soldin SJ, Stephey C, Giesbrecht E, et al. Further problems with digoxin measurement. *Clin Chem.* 1986; 32:1591.

100. Gault MH, Vasdev S, Longerich L. Higher values for digitalis-like factors with TDx Digoxin II. *Clin Chem.* 1986; 32:2000–1. Letter.

101. Karboski JA, Godley PJ, Frohna PA, et al. Marked digoxin-like immunoreactive factor interference with an enzyme immunoassay. *Drug Intell Clin Pharm.* 1988; 22:703–5.

102. Christenson RH, Studenberg SD, Beck-Davis S, et al. Digoxin-like immunoreactivity eliminated from serum by centrifugal ultrafiltration before fluorescence polarization immunoassay of digoxin. *Clin Chem.* 1987; 33:606–8.

103. Gault MH, Longerich L, Loo JCK, et al. Digoxin biotransformation. *Clin Pharmacol Ther.* 1984; 35:74–82.

104. Gault MH, Vasdev S, Vlasses P, et al. Interpretation of serum digoxin values in renal failure. *Clin Pharmacol Ther.* 1986; 39:530–6.

105. Gannon RH, Phillips LR. Metronidazole interference with procainamide HPLC assay. *Am J Hosp Pharm.* 1982; 39:1966–7.

106. Collins C, Hu M, Crowl C, et al. A homogeneous enzyme immunoassay for quinidine in serum. *Clin Chem.* 1979; 25:1093.

107. Haughey DB, Matzke GR, Halstenson CE, et al. Analytical specificity of commercially available methods for serum phenytoin determination. *J Anal Toxicol.* 1984; 8:106–11.

108. Roberts WL, Rainey PM. Interference in immunoassay measurements of total and free phenytoin in uremic patients: a reappraisal. *Clin Chem.* 1993; 39:1872–7.

109. Garfinkel D, Glazener F, Hoffman BB. Metronidazole interferes with theophylline measurements. *Ann Intern Med.* 1987; 106:170. Letter.

110. Cohen IA, Johnson CE, Wesolowicz L, et al. Effect of pentoxifylline and its metabolites on three theophylline assays. *Clin Pharm.* 1988; 7:457–61.

111. Vaughan LM, Gotteher A. Effect of xanthine-related compounds on a theophylline assay using theophylline oxidase. *Ann Pharmacother.* 1992; 26:1576–9.

112. Janknegt R, Lohman JJHM, Hooymans PM, et al. Do evacuated blood collection tubes interfere with therapeutic drug monitoring? *Pharm Weekbl.* 1983; 5:287–90.

113. Colucci RD, Halpern NA, Levy E, et al. The effects of various postphlebotomy storage conditions on drug levels. *J Clin Pharmacol.* 1988; 28:762–6.

## BIBLIOGRAPHY

DiPiro JT, Blouin RA, Pruemer JM. Concepts in clinical pharmacokinetics: a self-instructional course. Bethesda, MD: American Society of Hospital Pharmacists; 1988.

Evans WE, Schentag JJ, Jusko WJ, eds. Applied pharmacokinetics: principles of therapeutic drug monitoring, 2nd ed. Spokane, WA: Applied Therapeutics; 1986.

Gibaldi M, Levy G. Pharmacokinetics in clinical practice. *JAMA.* 1976; 235:1864–7.

Greenblatt DJ, Shader RI. Pharmacokinetics in clinical practice. Philadelphia, PA: W. B. Saunders; 1985.

Morley PC, Strand LM. Critical reflections on therapeutic drug monitoring. *J Pharm Pract.* 1989; 2:327–34.

Mungall DR, ed. Applied clinical pharmacokinetics. New York: Raven Press; 1983.

Pleasants RA, Gadsden RH. A short course on drug assay methods. *US Pharmacist.* 1986; (May):H1–16.

Rowland M, Tozer TN. Clinical pharmacokinetics: concepts and applications. Philadelphia, PA: Lea & Febiger; 1980.

Schumacher GE. Choosing optimal sampling times for therapeutic drug monitoring. *Clin Pharm.* 1985; 4:84–92.

Chapter 6

# Electrolytes, Other Minerals, and Trace Elements

*Arasb Ateshkadi and Mitchell A. Pelter*

This chapter covers the clinical interpretation and significance of serum electrolytes, other minerals, and certain trace elements. Since disorders of electrolytes frequently are encountered and cross over almost every area of clinical practice, clinicians should remember normal ranges and understand the physiological significance of each electrolyte, mineral, and trace element. This chapter should be particularly interesting to clinicians involved in nutritional support, because therapy with hyperalimentation solutions must include careful attention to the balances of these substances. The increased use of parenteral nutrition demands it. Table 1 shows the normal daily dietary intake of electrolytes, minerals, and trace elements. Practitioners in critical care, cardiology, and nephrology also rely heavily on serum electrolyte and mineral values; their patients often have multiorgan failure,

resulting in acute and chronic disturbances.

Most deficiencies in trace elements occur because of (1) decreased intake, (2) increased utilization, and/or (3) increased excretion. Since clinical signs and symptoms take months to develop, trace element deficiencies commonly are not observed in acute care settings. Nonetheless, the clinician needs to be aware of such abnormalities so that appropriate preventive and therapeutic interventions may be taken.

In practice, the first three tests (sodium, potassium, and chloride) usually are labeled as electrolytes; other minerals (magnesium, calcium, and phosphate) are included as part of serum chemistries. Calcium and phosphate metabolism sometimes are discussed in the context of the endocrine system because of their strong relationship with vitamin D and parathyroid hormone. Serum carbon dioxide content, often grouped with electrolytes, is discussed in Chapter 8 because its interpretation involves abnormalities of arterial pH.

Although serum concentrations of trace elements are not routinely measured, close monitoring of patients on chronic enteral and parenteral nutrition requires the clinician to be familiar with clinical manifestations of imbalances. Finally, clinicians should appreciate the interplay among minerals and electrolytes and consider all laboratory values in a patient rather than evaluate each as a separate, independent entity.

**TABLE 1.** Normal Dietary Intake of Electrolytes, Other Minerals, and Trace Elements

| Nutrient | Normal Daily Dietary Intake |
|---|---|
| Sodium | Highly variable; average 5.6–7.2 g (243–355 mEq) |
| Potassium | 50–100 mEq |
| Chloride | Varies with potassium and sodium intakes |
| Magnesium | 300–400 mg |
| Calcium | ~1000 mg |
| Phosphate | 700–800 g |
| Copper | 2–5 mg |
| Zinc | 4–14 mg |
| Manganese | 3–4 mg |
| Chromium | 50–100 µg |

## OBJECTIVES

Upon completion of this chapter, the reader should be able to

1. Describe homeostatic mechanisms involved in plasma sodium and water balance and distinguish between hyponatremia and hypernatremia.

2. Describe the physiology of intracellular and ex-

tracellular potassium equilibrium and the signs and symptoms of hypokalemia and hyperkalemia.

3. List common causes of serum chloride abnormalities.

4. List common conditions resulting in serum magnesium abnormalities and describe signs and symptoms of hypomagnesemia and hypermagnesemia.

5. Describe the relationship among the metabolism of calcium, phosphate, parathyroid hormone (PTH), and vitamin D.

6. List common conditions resulting in serum calcium abnormalities and describe signs and symptoms of hypocalcemia and hypercalcemia.

7. List common conditions resulting in serum copper, zinc, manganese, and chromium abnormalities and describe the signs and symptoms associated with them.

8. In the context of a clinical case description, including history and physical examination, interpret the results of laboratory tests used to assess sodium, potassium, chloride, calcium, phosphate, magnesium, copper, zinc, manganese, and chromium.

## ELECTROLYTES

The International System (SI) units for electrolytes, as well as other substances discussed in this chapter, are listed in Table 2.

### Sodium
*Normal range: 136–145 mEq/L or 136–145 mmol/L*

Sodium is the most abundant cation in extracellular fluid. As such, it is the major contributor to serum osmolality, which is important in the control of water movement between the extracellular (i.e., intravascular and interstitial) and intracellular fluid spaces. Thus, any discussion of sodium must include a discussion of water.[1] The reader should consider disorders of sodium as water imbalances. Once the physiology of sodium and water is mastered, abnormalities in serum sodium are easy to understand.

### *Physiology*

The principal role of sodium is the regulation of serum osmolality as well as fluid and acid–base balance. Sodium is also needed for maintaining the appropriate transmembrane electric potential for neuromuscular functioning.[2] Figure 1

summarizes the physiology of water and sodium. (Chapter 12 discusses serum osmolality.)

Water intake primarily is determined by thirst. Under normal circumstances, thirst is the most important homeostatic mechanism controlling body water.[3] The typical American diet contains 10 g of salt, although less than 1 g is needed for normal physiological functions. Therefore, inadequate salt intake usually is not a cause of sodium imbalance. Once sodium is in the gastrointestinal (GI) tract, it is actively absorbed and water passively follows along the osmotic gradient.

The kidneys are the primary organs responsible for controlling body sodium and water. When abnormalities occur, the kidneys usually are involved. The glomeruli receive and filter about 180 L of water and 600 g (nearly 26,000 mEq) of sodium per day. Less than 2 L of water and 0.1–40 g of sodium end up in the urine, depending on the fluid status. Most filtered water and sodium are reabsorbed in the proximal tubules of the kidneys. However, the major areas of water and sodium control are the distal and collecting tubules. Aldosterone acts at these two sites, while antidiuretic hormone (ADH) primarily acts at the collecting tubules.[3]

*Antidiuretic hormone effects.* ADH is released from the posterior pituitary gland in response to signals from the hypothalamus. The hypothalamus contains cells that detect the osmolality of blood in the brain. When osmolality is high (i.e., either serum sodium is high or serum water is low), ADH output increases and urine output decreases. If serum sodium is high but blood volume is normal, the baroreceptors (in the left atrium and carotid sinus) override the release of ADH, thus preventing hypervolemia.[3]

ADH increases the permeability of the collecting ducts to water, resulting in a more concentrated urine. In

**TABLE 2.** Conversion Factors to SI Units

| Nutrient | Traditional Units | Conversion Factors to SI Units | SI Units |
|---|---|---|---|
| Sodium | mEq/L | 1 | mmol/L |
| Potassium | mEq/L | 1 | mmol/L |
| Chloride | mEq/L | 1 | mmol/L |
| Magnesium | mEq/L | 0.5 | mmol/L |
| Calcium | mg/dL | 0.25 | mmol/L |
| Phosphate | mg/dL | 0.3229 | mmol/L |
| Copper | µg/dL | 0.1574 | µmol/L |
| Zinc | µg/dL | 0.1530 | µmol/L |
| Manganese | µg/L | 18.2 | µmol/L |
| Chromium | µg/L | 18.3 | nmol/L |

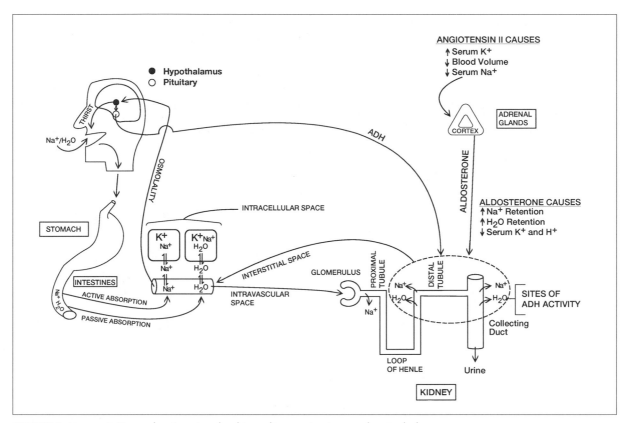

**FIGURE 1.** Homeostatic mechanisms involved in sodium, potassium, and water balance.

the syndrome of inappropriate ADH secretion (SIADH), an abnormally high quantity of ADH is present. This condition results in increased water reabsorption, a low serum sodium concentration (dilutional effect), and a very concentrated urine. Conversely, *central* diabetes insipidus occurs when an inadequate amount of ADH is synthesized or released.

In some situations, the kidneys fail to respond to normal or high quantities of circulating ADH. This condition is called *nephrogenic* diabetes insipidus. In central or nephrogenic diabetes insipidus (Chapter 12), little water reabsorption occurs, resulting in a large urine output. However, thirst usually causes persons to consume the quantity of water needed to replenish their diminished blood volume.[3] (Chapter 7 offers an indepth discussion of the effects of other diseases on urine composition.)

*Aldosterone effects.* Aldosterone affects the distal tubular reabsorption of sodium rather than water.[4] This hormone is released from the adrenal cortex in response to various dietary and neurohormonal factors, including low serum sodium, high serum potassium, low blood volume, and angiotensin II. Aldosterone increases the urinary secretion of potassium from the distal tubules in exchange for sodium reabsorption.

Aldosterone's effect on serum potassium is profound, but the effect on serum sodium is minor. As serum so-

dium increases, so does water reabsorption following the osmotic gradient.[3] Renal arteriolar blood pressure (BP) then increases, which increases the glomerular filtration rate (GFR). Ultimately, more water and sodium pass through the distal tubules, overriding the initial effect of aldosterone.[3,4]

*Osmolality effects.* The last homeostatic mechanism for water and sodium involves the equilibrium among intravascular, interstitial, and intracellular spaces.[3] The net movement of water is from an area of low osmolality to one of high osmolality. This effect can be readily observed in patients with a low serum osmolality due to either a low serum sodium concentration or high serum water. In these patients, water moves toward the higher osmolality in the interstitial space to equalize the osmolar gap.[3] In the presence of high hydrostatic and oncotic pressure gaps across capillary walls, the net effect is excessive interstitial water accumulation and edema formation.[3,4]

Sodium moves among cells, interstitial spaces, and intravascular spaces. It may be easiest to interpret serum sodium values by conceptualizing the amount of sodium ion in the blood as fixed and the volume of water as variable. In this way, interpretation focuses on determining the causes of excessive or diminished serum water. Serum sodium is reported per liter of plasma water; as such, this value reflects not only sodium but also water. Consequently, when interpreting abnormal sodium values, the practitioner must determine if the problem is due to a sodium and/or water imbalance.

### Hyponatremia

Hyponatremia is defined as a serum sodium concentration less than 136 mEq/L (<136 mmol/L). In general, hyponatremia involves defects in the kidneys' diluting capacity, such as SIADH secretion in the presence of low serum osmolality. Since serum sodium reflects total body water rather than total body sodium, hyponatremia may occur in the presence of low, normal, or high total body sodium.

When presented with a low serum sodium concentration, the clinician must determine if the value reflects an abnormal accumulation of water in the intravascular space (dilutional hyponatremia), a decline in both extracellular water and sodium, or a reduction in total body sodium, with the water balance remaining normal. Serum sodium alone cannot answer this question; therefore, the clinician must also consider a patient's history, physical exam, and other lab values. Moreover, fluid intake and urine output should be monitored.

When encountering an asymptomatic patient with moderately severe hyponatremia, the clinician should suspect a laboratory error. Hyponatremic signs and symptoms probably are due to cellular swelling and cerebral edema and usually do not occur until serum sodium is in the low 120s (Table 3). However, patients may vary in their tolerance for a reduced serum sodium concentration.

As with any electrolyte disorder, the chronicity of the imbalance is a major determinant of the severity of signs and symptoms. For example, a patient with hyponatremia due to long-standing congestive heart failure (CHF) is less likely to be symptomatic than a patient who is hyponatremic due to rapid infusion of a hypotonic solution. The most common hyponatremic symptom is confusion, which may be mistaken for senility in elderly patients. If sodium continues to fall, seizure, coma, and death may result.[3–6]

*Hyponatremia associated with low total body sodium.* Hyponatremia associated with low total body sodium reflects a reduction in total body water, with an even larger reduction in total body sodium. This condition is caused

**TABLE 3.** Signs and Symptoms of Hyponatremia

| Signs | Symptoms |
|---|---|
| Abnormal sensorium | Agitation |
| Cheyne-Stokes respiration | Anorexia |
| Depressed deep-tendon reflexes | Apathy |
| Hypothermia | Disorientation |
| Seizures | Lethargy |
| | Muscle cramps |
| | Nausea |

primarily by depletion of extracellular fluid volume, which stimulates ADH release even at the expense of hypoosmolality. Some common causes include vomiting; diarrhea; intravascular fluid losses due to burns, peritonitis, and pancreatitis; hypoaldosteronism (Addison's disease); and certain forms of renal failure (e.g., salt-wasting nephropathy).[3] This type of hyponatremia may also occur in patients treated too aggressively with diuretics who receive sodium-free solutions (e.g., dextrose 5% in water) as replacement fluid.

Low serum sodium can also result when a large quantity of an osmotically active substance enters the bloodstream.[3] Physiologically, water follows the osmotic gradient, resulting in a dilutional hyponatremia. This situation can occur with mannitol infusions and hyperglycemia. In hyperglycemia, slow but continuous intracellular penetration of glucose creates an osmolar gap. This gap leads to a shift of water into the intravascular space, diluting the serum sodium concentration and creating the impression of hyponatremia.[3,5]

Additionally, the hyperglycemia leads to an osmotic diuresis. Hence, hyponatremia occurs as long as the rate of water moving from the cells into the blood is greater than the volume of water excreted through the urine. The serum sodium increases in hyperglycemia by 1 mEq/L for every 62-mg/dL increase in serum glucose concentration above normal. As cellular water diminishes and diuresis continues, the patient progresses from hyponatremia to hypernatremia.[3,5]

Patients with hyponatremia associated with low total body sodium often exhibit signs and symptoms of dehydration. These manifestations include thirst, dry mucous membranes, weight loss, sunken eyes, diminished urine output, and diminished skin turgor.[3]

*Hyponatremia associated with normal total body sodium.* Also called euvolemic or dilutional hyponatremia, this condition refers to impaired water excretion without any alteration in sodium excretion. Etiologies include any mechanism that enhances ADH secretion or potentiates its action at the collecting tubules. This condition can occur during states of glucocorticoid deficiency, severe hypothyroidism, administration of water to a patient with impaired water excretion capacity, and SIADH.[3,5]

As the name implies, SIADH is a disorder in which continued ADH secretion occurs in spite of low serum osmolality. Secretion may be drug induced; therefore, the clinician should consider potential causative agents. These agents generally can be divided into two categories (Table 4):

➢ Drugs that act centrally to cause ADH release.
➢ Drugs that have ADH-like action or potentiate ADH's effect at the collecting tubules.

Patients with SIADH have a high urine osmolality

**TABLE 4.** Drugs Associated with Dilutional Hyponatremia

---

**Drugs that increase ADH secretion**
- Carbamazepine
- Chlorpropamide
- Clofibrate
- Cyclophosphamide
- Diuretics
- Narcotics
- Nicotine
- Vincristine

**Drugs that have ADH-like action or potentiate ADH renal effect**
- Acetaminophen
- ADH analogs
- Chlorpropamide
- Cyclophosphamide
- Diuretics
- Nonsteroidal anti-inflammatory drugs (NSAIDs)

---

(i.e., concentrated urine) and urine sodium; normal renal, adrenal, and thyroid function; and no evidence of volume abnormalities.[3,5]

*Hyponatremia associated with high total body sodium.* This condition, the most common form of hyponatremia, implies an increase in total body sodium with a larger increase in total body water. Hyponatremia perhaps is most frequently observed in edematous states such as CHF, cirrhosis, nephrotic syndrome, and chronic renal failure. In these conditions, water and sodium excretion from the kidneys is impaired. Edema is one hallmark sign of hyponatremia with increased total body sodium.[3,5]

### Fractional Excretion of Sodium ($FE_{Na}$)
#### Normal range: 1–2%

When a serum sodium value is abnormal, the clinician should identify possible etiologies by determining whether the abnormality is associated with low, normal, or high total body sodium. A urine sample (preferably from a 24-hr urine collection) is needed to determine renal handling of sodium. Then $FE_{Na}$, the measure of the percentage of filtered sodium excreted in the urine (Chapter 7), must be calculated:

$$FE_{Na}(\%) = \frac{U_{Na}}{S_{Na}} \div \frac{UCr}{SCr} \times 100$$

where $U_{Na}$ and $S_{Na}$ are urine and serum sodium in milliequivalents per liter or millimoles per liter, and UCr and SCr are urine and serum creatinine in milligrams per deciliter or micromoles per liter.

Values greater than 2% indicate that the kidneys are excreting a higher than normal fraction of the filtered sodium. Conversely, $FE_{Na}$ values less than 1% indicate renal sodium retention. Since acute diuretic therapy can increase the $FE_{Na}$ to 20% or more, urine samples should be obtained at least 24 hr after diuretics have been discontinued.[3] Minicase 1 demonstrates how to calculate $FE_{Na}$.

---

**✎ Minicase 1**

Alice W., a 74-year-old white female, had a history of coronary artery disease, CHF, and insulin-dependent diabetes mellitus (IDDM). She was brought to the emergency room by her daughter, who complained about her mother's increasing disorientation over the past week. Medications at the time of admission were benazepril 10 mg oral daily, digoxin 0.125 mg oral daily, furosemide 40 mg oral twice a day, nitroglycerin patch 0.2 mg/hr, diphenhydramine 25 mg every bedtime, NPH plus regular insulin subcutaneously twice a day, and acetaminophen 650 mg prn. She last took these medications the morning before admission. Alice W. also drank many cans of diet cola every day.

A review of systems revealed lethargy and apathism with no apparent distress. Vital signs showed a sitting BP of 110/75 (standing BP not measured), a regular heart rate of 96, and a rapid and shallow respiratory rate of 36. Alice W.'s physical examination was pertinent for bilaterally depressed deep-tendon reflexes. Her laboratory findings were unremarkable, except for a serum sodium of 120 mEq/L (136–145 mEq/L) and a serum glucose of 185 mg/dL (70–110 mg/dL). A urine collection was started on admission to the hospital. Her 24-hr collection showed: urine volume, 2280 mL (<2000 mL); SCr, 1.0 mg/dL (0.7–1.5 mg/dL); urine creatinine, 32 mg/dL; and urine sodium, 12 mEq/L.

*What subjective and objective data for Alice W. are* consistent with a diagnosis of hyponatremia? What are the potential etiologies of hyponatremia in this patient?*

**Discussion:** Aside from her low serum sodium concentration, Alice W. is exhibiting symptoms of hyponatremia [e.g., lethargy, apathy, and rapid and shallow breathing (Cheyne-Stokes respiration)] and diminished deep-tendon reflexes. A clinician must determine volume status when assessing a patient with sodium abnormality. However, Alice W. currently does not exhibit any signs or symptoms of dehydration or fluid overload. To identify possible etiologies, a determination must be made as to whether the hyponatremia is associated with low, normal, or high total body sodium. Since Alice W. last took her diuretic yesterday morning, her 24-hr urine collection may be used for calculating $FE_{Na}$:

$$0.3\% = \frac{12\ mEq/L}{120\ mEq/L} \div \frac{32\ mg/dL}{1.0\ mg/dL} \times 100$$

Therefore, Alice W. is trying to preserve sodium in the presence of her hyponatremia, which implies a deficit in total body water with a larger deficit in total body sodium. This condition may be due to aggressive furosemide treatment, with replacement of her lost body fluid with a low sodium or sodium-free solution (e.g., dextrose 5% in water or free water).

### Blood Urea Nitrogen (BUN): Serum Creatinine (SCr) Ratio
*Normal range: <20:1*

The BUN:SCr ratio is another useful parameter. When this ratio is higher than 20, it can indicate dehydration. As extracellular fluid volume is diminished, the kidneys increase their reabsorption of urea but not creatinine. Therefore, BUN increases by a larger magnitude than the SCr concentration in dehydrated individuals, leading to a rise in the BUN:SCr ratio. (Chapter 7 offers a more indepth discussion.)

### Hypernatremia

Hypernatremia is defined as a serum sodium concentration greater than 145 mEq/L (>145 mmol/L). It is less common than hyponatremia. High serum sodium concentrations are most common in patients with either an impaired thirst mechanism (e.g., neurohypophyseal lesion—common after strokes) or an inability to replace water depleted through normal insensible losses (i.e., uncontrollable water loss through respiration or skin) or from renal or GI losses. Like hyponatremia, hypernatremia may occur in the presence of high, normal, or low total body sodium content.[3,4,6]

The clinical manifestations of hypernatremia primarily involve the neurological system (Table 5). These manifestations are the consequence of cellular dehydration, particularly in the brain. In adults, acute elevation in serum sodium above 160 mEq/L (>160 mmol/L) is associated with a 75% mortality. Unfortunately, neurological sequelae are common even in survivors. Elevated urine specific gravity, indicating concentrated urine, is uniformly observed. Hematocrit values may not be useful because changes in total body water also can affect erythrocyte water.[3-6]

*Hypernatremia associated with low total body sodium.* Hypernatremia with low total body sodium results when both sodium and water losses occur, but water is lost to a greater extent.[3] The thirst mechanism generally increases water intake, but this adjustment is not always possible (e.g., institutionalized elderly patients). This condition may also be iatrogenic when hypotonic fluid losses (e.g., profuse sweating and diarrhea) are replaced with an inadequate quantity of water and salt. In these circumstances, fluid losses should be replaced with dextrose 5% in water or sodium chloride 0.45%.[3,5]

These patients have high urine osmolalities (>800 mOsm/L, roughly equivalent to a specific gravity of 1.023) and low urine sodium concentrations (<10 mEq/L), indicating that the renal concentrating mechanisms are intact. Patients often exhibit orthostatic hypotension, flat neck veins, tachycardia, poor skin turgor, and dry mucous membranes. In addition, the BUN:SCr ratio may be greater than 20, indicating dehydration.[3,5]

*Hypernatremia associated with normal total body sodium.* Also called euvolemic hypernatremia, this condition refers to a general water loss without sodium loss.[3] Because of water redistribution between the intracellular and extracellular fluid, no volume contraction usually is evident unless water loss is substantial (Minicase 2). Etiologies include increased insensible water loss (e.g., fever, extensive burns, and mechanical ventilation) and central and nephrogenic diabetes insipidus. The clinician should be aware of drugs that may cause nephrogenic diabetes insipidus (Table 6).[3,5] (Chapter 12 covers diabetes insipidus in more detail.)

*Hypernatremia associated with high total body sodium.* This form of hypernatremia is the least common, since sodium homeostasis is maintained indirectly through the control of water and defects in the system usually affect total body water more than total body sodium.[3] This form of hypernatremia usually is due to exogenous administration of high sodium-containing solutions such as

> ➤ Resuscitative efforts using hypertonic sodium bicarbonate.
> ➤ Inadvertent intravenous (IV) infusion of hypertonic saline (i.e., solutions >0.9% sodium chloride).
> ➤ Inadvertent dialysis against high sodium-containing solution.
> ➤ Sea-water near-drowning.

Primary hyperaldosteronism and Cushing's disease also may cause this form of hypernatremia. Large quanti-

**TABLE 5.** Signs and Symptoms of Hypernatremia

| | |
|---|---|
| Thirst | Seizures |
| Restlessness | Hyperreflexia |
| Irritability | Coma |
| Lethargy | Death |
| Muscle twitching | |

**TABLE 6.** Drugs that Can Cause Nephrogenic Diabetes Insipidus

| | |
|---|---|
| Acetohexamide | Loop diuretics |
| Amphotericin B | Methicillin |
| Angiographic dyes | Methoxyflurane |
| Cisplatin | Norepinephrine |
| Colchicine | Osmotic diuretics |
| Demeclocycline | Propoxyphene |
| Foscarnet | Thiazide diuretics |
| Gentamicin | Tolazamide |
| Glyburide | Vinblastine |
| Lithium | |

---

### Minicase 2

Todd M., a 21-year-old male, was admitted to the neurosurgical service for a complete hypophysectomy to reduce an expanding pituitary tumor affecting his optic nerve. He was otherwise in good health and on no chronic medication. His postoperative medications included morphine (administered in a patient-controlled analgesia pump) and cefazolin 1 g every 8 hr.

Within 3 hr after surgery, Todd M.'s urine output reached 4.5 L. His physical exam was unremarkable, and his vital signs were stable. Clinical laboratory tests included serum sodium 152 mEq/L (136–145 mEq/L), potassium 3.8 mEq/L (3.5–5.0 mEq/L), chloride 102 mEq/L (96–106 mEq/L), carbon dioxide content 24 mEq/L (24–30 mEq/L), glucose 98 mg/dL (70–110 mg/dL), serum phosphate 2.9 mg/dL (2.6–4.5 mg/dL), BUN 9 mg/dL (8–20 mg/dL), and SCr 0.9 mg/dL (0.7–1.5 mg/dL). Urine specific gravity was 1.003 (1.010–1.020). On day 2, his urine volume reached 14 L, and he complained of excessive thirst.

*What subjective and objective data for Todd M. are consistent with a diagnosis of hypernatremia? What are the potential etiologies of hypernatremia in this patient?*

**Discussion:** Aside from his serum sodium concentration and excessive thirst, Todd M. is not exhibiting any sign or symptom specific to hypernatremia. The first step in identifying possible etiologies usually is determining whether the hypernatremia is associated with low, normal, or high total body sodium (i.e., calculating $FE_{Na}$ and measuring urine osmolality and specific gravity). However, Todd M.'s urine specific gravity may be used as a surrogate marker since $FE_{Na}$ and urine osmolality were not measured.

Because this problem is acute, potential causes must be considered so that appropriate interventions can be made. Given the rapid onset of polyuria shortly after Todd M.'s complete hypophysectomy, a lack of circulating ADH probably caused his sodium–water imbalance. Todd M.'s hypernatremia is associated with a normal total body sodium (also called euvolemic hypernatremia) since ADH affects only the excretion of water. If his urine had been tested, his urine osmolality probably would be low, indicating production of dilute urine. This supposition is indirectly supported by his low urine specific gravity. His condition, therefore, probably is due to a general water loss without sodium loss. Since this abnormality was detected early, Todd M.'s only clinical manifestations were polyuria and polydipsia.

IV fluid replacement with dextrose 5% is adequate for correcting his hypernatremia. However, vasopressin (ADH) or its analog will be needed for long-term therapy.

---

ties of sodium can be found in these patients' urine. Signs and symptoms include diminished skin turgor and elevated plasma proteins.[3,5]

## Potassium
*Normal range: 3.5–5.0 mEq/L or 3.5–5.0 mmol/L*

Potassium is the major cation in intracellular space, with an average concentration in the intracellular fluid of 140 mEq/L (140 mmol/L). The major physiological role of potassium is in regulating muscle and nerve excitability. Other roles include control of intracellular volume (similar to sodium's control of extracellular volume), protein synthesis, enzymatic reaction, and carbohydrate metabolism.[7,8]

### Physiology

The most important aspect of potassium physiology is its effect on muscle and nervous tissue excitability.[2] In disorders of potassium, the cardiovascular system is of principal concern. Like other muscle tissues, the function of cardiac muscle cells depends on their ability to change their resting-state electrical potentials when presented with the proper stimulus. This change leads to muscle contraction and nerve conduction.[7,8]

One important aspect of potassium homeostasis is its distribution equilibrium. In a 70-kg man, total body potassium is about 4000 mEq; of that amount, only 60 mEq is located in the extracellular fluid. The average daily Western diet contains 50–100 mEq of potassium, which is completely and passively absorbed in the upper GI tract.

To enter cells, potassium must first pass through the extracellular compartment. If serum potassium concentrations rise above 6 mEq/L (>6 mmol/L), symptomatic hyperkalemia may occur; extreme cases can include cardiac arrhythmias.[6,9]

Abnormalities in potassium homeostasis usually are related to problems with insulin, aldosterone, acid–base balance, renal function, or GI and skin losses. These factors can be altered by various pathological states and drug therapy. Although potassium influences tissues throughout the body, its effect on the cardiac muscle is most important due to the life-threatening nature of arrhythmias caused by either high or low serum potassium concentrations.[4,6–10]

*Renal homeostasis.* The body essentially has two ways of reducing a high serum potassium concentration. One quick way is to shift the potassium into the cells; the other, slower mechanism is renal elimination.[10] The kidneys are the primary organs involved in the control and elimination of potassium. Potassium is freely filtered at the glomerulus and almost completely reabsorbed before the filtrate reaches the distal tubules. Approximately 10% of the filtered potassium is secreted from the distal and collecting tubules into the urine. Therefore, virtually all urinary potassium is due to tubular secretion rather than glomerular filtration.[7]

Several mechanisms are involved in sodium–potassium exchange in the distal tubule. This exchange results in renal potassium secretion and sodium reabsorption. Aldosterone is an important factor since it increases po-

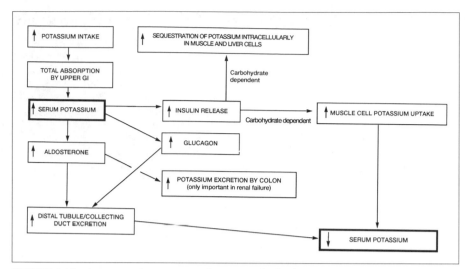

**FIGURE 2.** The homeostatic sequence of events in the body to maintain serum potassium within a narrow concentration range.

tassium secretion into the urine[10] (Figures 1 and 2). Aldosterone release by the adrenal glands is directly stimulated by high potassium concentrations. Potassium secretion and its subsequent elimination are stimulated by the delivery of large quantities of sodium and fluid to the distal tubules, as evidenced by the hypokalemia observed with diuretics.[11] When sodium and fluid delivery are decreased, potassium secretion declines.

The presence of anions in the distal tubules, which are relatively permeable to reabsorption, can increase potassium loss in the urine because the negatively charged anions attract the positively charged potassium ions. This mechanism is responsible for hypokalemia due to renal tubular acidosis and administration of high doses of a penicillin (e.g., carbenicillin).[10] Potassium secretion is also influenced by the potassium concentration in distal tubular cells. When the intracellular potassium concentration rises, as with dehydration, potassium secretion into the urine increases.

Several additional points should be mentioned:

1. Although the kidney is the primary route of elimination, potassium secretion into the colon becomes important in patients with advanced renal failure.[10]
2. Unlike sodium, the kidneys are not totally able to arrest potassium's secretion into the urine. In hypokalemia, the urinary potassium concentration may be as low as 5 mEq/L, but potassium excretion does not completely cease.
3. The kidneys may take hours to adjust serum potassium when drastic, acute changes take place.

Therefore, in the short term, the body must rely on extrarenal mechanisms for keeping serum potassium within tight limits.

*Arterial pH homeostasis.* Another potentially relevant factor influencing renal potassium secretion is arterial pH. When arterial pH increases due to metabolic—but not respiratory—alkalosis, there is a compensatory shift of hydrogen ions out of the cells and into the extracellular fluid (bloodstream).[7] To maintain the electropotential gradient, potassium moves intracellularly. Although total body potassium experiences no immediate change, this movement results in an increased cellular potassium content (primarily in muscle tissues). This movement also occurs in distal tubular cells in the kidneys, which leads to increased potassium secretion into the urine if the alkalemia persists. Therefore, in the early phase of metabolic alkalosis, serum potassium drops. This decline is due to intracellular potassium movement without a change in total body concentration. Chronically, total body potassium decreases as a result of increased renal loss.

Metabolic acidosis has the opposite effect. Decreased arterial pH results in an extracellular shift of potassium, causing an elevated serum potassium concentration.[7] Since the potassium content of distal tubular cell potassium is decreased, secretion of potassium in the urine is diminished. Chronically, however, the potassium loss gradually increases in the urine due to unknown mechanisms.

When a severe metabolic acid–base abnormality exists, the serum potassium concentration should be corrected to reflect the change in transcellular shifting (redistribution) of potassium. For every 0.1-U reduction in arterial pH less than 7.4, roughly 0.6 mEq/L (range: 0.2–1.7 mEq/L) should be added to the serum potassium value:

$$K_{corr} = [(7.4 - pH)/0.1 \times 0.6 \text{ mEq/L}] + K_{uncorr}$$

where $K_{corr}$ is the corrected serum potassium concentration and $K_{uncorr}$ is the uncorrected serum potassium concentration (Minicase 3).[7]

Although total body potassium does not change abruptly in alkalemia or acidemia, arrhythmias can occur if the serum potassium concentration changes drastically. Even a small percentage change in intracellular potassium can produce a clinically significant change in extracellular concentrations.

*Acute homeostasis.* Figure 2 summarizes the acute homeostatic mechanism involved in potassium distribution. In hyperkalemia, along with the release of aldosterone, increased glucagon and insulin release also contributes to reducing the serum potassium concentration. Glucagon stimulates potassium secretion into the distal tubules and collecting ducts, while insulin helps to drive potassium intracellularly. This insulin–potassium interaction is completely independent of transcellular glucose transport. Although insulin is not a major controlling factor in potassium homeostasis, it is an important agent in the emergency treatment of hyperkalemia.[7,12]

Another factor affecting the transcellular equilibrium of potassium is the pharmacological stimulation of ß$_2$-adrenergic receptors, which leads to the movement of potassium from extracellular fluid to the intracellular fluid compartment. This mechanism serves as the rationale for treating certain hyperkalemic patients with a ß$_2$-adrenergic agonist (e.g., albuterol).[7–9]

### Hypokalemia

Hypokalemia is defined as a serum potassium concentration less than 3.5 mEq/L (<3.5 mmol/L). It may indicate true or apparent potassium deficit, although the signs and symptoms are indistinguishable.[10] To interpret low potassium values, the clinician should determine whether hypokalemia is due to intracellular shifting of potassium (apparent deficit) or increased loss from the body (true deficit) (Table 7, next page).

Intracellular shifting occurs with metabolic alkalosis or administration of dextrose, insulin, or ß$_2$-adrenergic agonists.[9,13] Hyperalimentation solutions can drive potassium intracellularly due to their high glucose, insulin,

---

### 🖎 Minicase 3

Andrew D., a 65-year-old, 150-lb male, was admitted to University Hospital for surgical management of acute urinary retention due to long-standing bladder outlet obstruction. His past medical history was significant for hypertension and diet-controlled noninsulin-dependent diabetes mellitus. His medications included propranolol 120 mg oral twice a day, furosemide 80 mg oral twice a day, and enalapril 10 mg oral every morning.

A review of Andrew D.'s systems was unremarkable, except for his inability to urinate. Vital signs included respiratory rate 25, pulse 60 and regular, and BP 190/98–190/102 mm Hg. Positive physical findings included an audible S$_4$ heart sound and decreased deep-tendon reflexes bilaterally. The only other abnormal clinical finding was an indurated, fixed prostate gland. Abnormal clinical laboratory tests included serum potassium 5.6 mEq/L (3.5–5.0 mEq/L), serum carbon dioxide 16 mEq/L (24–30 mEq/L), glucose 237 mg/dL (70–110 mg/dL), phosphate 6.4 mg/dL (2.6–4.5 mg/dL), BUN 56 mg/dL (8–20 mg/dL), and SCr 3.3 mg/dL (0.7–1.5 mg/dL). A presurgery arterial blood gas showed pH 7.30 (7.36–7.44), partial pressure of carbon dioxide (pCO$_2$) 17 mm Hg (36–44 mm Hg), and partial pressure of oxygen (pO$_2$) 99 mm Hg (80–100 mm Hg).

Due to postsurgical complications, Andrew D. was placed on a daily peripheral vein hyperalimentation solution containing dextrose 5%, amino acids 3%, sodium chloride 50 mEq, potassium chloride 30 mEq, potassium phosphate 40 mEq (based on potassium), calcium gluconate 4.6 mEq, magnesium sulfate 16.2 mEq, and multivitamin supplements 10 mL. Over the next several days, Andrew D. complained of muscle weakness, and his urine output dropped to 20 mL/hr. His pulse was 40 and irregular, and his BP was 130/65 mm Hg. His electrocardiogram (ECG) showed flat P waves, tall T waves, and widened QRS intervals. A repeat serum chemistry revealed a serum potassium concentration of 7.1 mEq/L (3.5–5.0 mEq/L).

*What subjective and objective data for Andrew D. are consistent with a diagnosis of hyperkalemia? What are the potential etiologies of hyperkalemia in this patient?*

**Discussion:** Aside from his high serum potassium concentration, Andrew D. is exhibiting signs and symptoms of hyperkalemia (e.g., muscle weakness, rhythm disturbances, worsening of bradycardia, and reduced BP).

Andrew D. has several predisposing factors that may have contributed to his hyperkalemia. First, he has mild metabolic acidosis. This condition resulted in an extracellular shifting of potassium, causing an elevated serum potassium concentration. Although clinically insignificant, his serum potassium value may be corrected for his acidosis to reflect his extracellular potassium status more accurately. The serum potassium value must be corrected as follows:

$$K_{corr} = [(7.4 - pH)/0.1 \times 0.6\ mEq/L] + K_{uncorr}$$

$$K_{corr} = [(7.4 - 7.3)/0.1 \times 0.6\ mEq/L] + 7.1 = 7.7\ mEq/L$$

This correction implies that if acidemia is corrected, serum potassium will increase by 0.6 mEq/L without any addition of potassium to the body. This equation becomes more significant during severe metabolic acid–base disorders.

Second, although the potassium balance usually is not disturbed until the GFR falls to less than 10 mL/min, Andrew D.'s renal impairment contributed to his hyperkalemia. His creatinine clearance is about 22 mL/min (Chapter 7). Since angiotensin-converting enzyme inhibitors decrease urine potassium excretion by inhibiting the renin–angiotensin–aldosterone system, enalapril also may have contributed to this patient's hyperkalemia (decreased output). Although β$_2$-adrenergic receptors potentiate the movement of potassium from extracellular fluid to the intracellular fluid compartment, propranolol (a β$_1$- and β$_2$-adrenergic receptor inhibitor) does not appear to have a clinically significant effect on serum potassium concentrations.

Finally, the potassium content of Andrew D.'s hyperalimentation solution is 70 mEq. Although this value is consistent with the average Western diet (50–100 mEq), this quantity may be inappropriately high (increased intake) given his renal impairment.

**TABLE 7.** Etiologies of Hypokalemia

---

**Apparent deficit—intracellular shifting of potassium**
  Alkalosis
  $\beta_2$-Adrenergic stimulation
  Insulin
**True deficit**
  Decreased intake
    "Tea and toast" diet
    Alcoholism
    Indigence
    Potassium-free IV fluids
    Anorexia nervosa
    Bulimia
  Increased output
    Extrarenal
      Vomiting
      Diarrhea
      Laxative abuse
      Intestinal fistulas
    Renal
      Corticosteroids
      Amphotericin B
      Diuretics
      Hyperaldosteronism
      Cushing's syndrome
      Licorice abuse

---

and amino acid content (potassium, an intracellular cation, is taken up during the formation of new cells). Potassium loss usually can occur from the kidneys or GI tract. Increased renal loss occurs from decreased potassium reabsorption in the proximal tubules or increased secretion in the distal tubules and collecting ducts.[10]

*Amphotericin B.* Proximal tubular damage can occur with amphotericin B therapy, resulting in renal tubular acidosis. Reabsorption of potassium, magnesium, and bicarbonate is simultaneously affected by amphotericin B, leading to hypokalemia, hypomagnesemia, and metabolic acidosis.[7,13]

Potassium balance strongly depends on magnesium homeostasis. Magnesium maintains the sodium–potassium–adenosine triphosphate (ATP) pump activity and facilitates renal preservation of potassium. Therefore, if a hypokalemic patient is also hypomagnesemic, he or she may not respond to potassium replacement therapy unless the magnesium balance is restored.[7,8,12]

*Diuretics.* The most common class of drugs associated with renal potassium wasting is diuretics. Although their mechanism of natriuretic action differs, diuretic-induced hypokalemia is caused primarily by increased secretion of potassium at the distal sites in the nephron in response to an increased load of exchangeable sodium. Diuretics increase the distal urinary blood flow by inhibiting sodium reabsorption. This increase leads to more fluid and sodium in the distal portions of the nephron, which attempts to reabsorb this excess sodium. To maintain a neutral electropotential gradient in the lumen, potassium is excreted as sodium is reabsorbed. Therefore, any diuretic-inhibiting sodium absorption prior to or at the distal tubules can increase potassium loss. Additionally, when nonabsorbable anions are present, potassium is attracted to the urine.

Due to the high potency of loop diuretics (e.g., furosemide), they waste the most potassium, followed by thiazides (e.g., hydrochlorothiazide). However, a common misconception is that thiazide diuretics always lead to hypokalemia. In antihypertensive doses ($\leq$50 mg/day), severe hypokalemia is rare. The fifth report of the Joint National Committee on Detection, Evaluation and Treatment of High Blood Pressure recommended diuretics as first-line agents for the treatment of hypertension.[14]

At least part of the criticism about this recommendation was concern for hypokalemia and subsequent arrhythmias. However, no statistically significant correlation exists between thiazide-induced hypokalemia and ventricular ectopy and sudden death. While hydrochlorothiazide in doses of less than or equal to 50 mg/day can reduce serum potassium concentrations by 0.4 mEq/L (0.4 mmol/L), intracellular potassium concentrations and serum magnesium concentrations usually are unaffected. These agents can be safely administered to most patients, but monitoring serum potassium is recommended, especially in the elderly, patients with ischemic heart disease, and patients concomitantly receiving digoxin.[15–17]

Spironolactone, triamterene, and amiloride do not cause potassium loss; in fact, they cause retention of potassium due to their effects on aldosterone-dependent (spironolactone) and aldosterone-independent (triamterene and amiloride) exchange sites in the collecting tubules. These agents are also magnesium sparing.[11,18]

*Other causes.* Conditions that cause hyperaldosteronism, either primary (e.g., adrenal tumor) or secondary to other causes (e.g., renovascular hypertension), can produce hypokalemia.[13] Cushing's syndrome leads to increased circulation of mineralocorticoids such as aldosterone. Corticosteroids with a strong mineralocorticoid activity (e.g., cortisone) also can cause hypokalemia.[10]

GI loss of potassium can be important. Aldosterone influences not only renal potassium handling but also that of the intestines.[10] A decrease in extracellular volume increases aldosterone secretion, resulting in renal and colonic potassium wasting. Diarrhea can contain 20–120 mEq/L (20–120 mmol/L) of potassium; consequently, profuse diarrhea can rapidly lead to a potassium imbalance. Since the vomitus contains only 0–32 mEq/L (0–32 mmol/L) of potassium, an imbalance is unlikely to be significant. However, with severe vomiting, the resultant metabolic alkalosis may lead to hypokalemia due to intracellular shifting of potassium. Finally, patients receiving potassium-free parenteral fluids can become hypokalemic if not monitored properly.[7,10]

**TABLE 8.** Signs, Symptoms, and Other Effects of Hypokalemia

> **Cardiovascular**
> Decrease in T-wave amplitude
> Development of U waves
> Hypotension
> Increased risk of digoxin toxicity
> PR prolongation (with severe hypokalemia)
> Rhythm disturbances
> ST segment depression
> QRS widening (with severe hypokalemia)
>
> **Metabolic/endocrine (mostly serve as compensatory mechanisms)**
> Decreased aldosterone release
> Decreased insulin release
> Decreased renal responsiveness to ADH
>
> **Neuromuscular**
> Areflexia (with severe hypokalemia)
> Cramps
> Loss of smooth muscle function (ileus and urinary retention with severe hypokalemia)
> Weakness
>
> **Renal**
> Inability to concentrate urine
> Nephropathy

*Clinical diagnosis.* Signs and symptoms of hypokalemia involve many physiological systems; however, the primary concern surrounds the cardiovascular system (i.e., cardiac rhythm). Hypokalemia-induced arrhythmias are of particular concern in patients receiving digoxin. Both digitalis glycosides and hypokalemia inhibit the cardiac cell's sodium–potassium–ATP pump. Together, they can deplete intracellular potassium, which may lead to fatal arrhythmias. The signs and symptoms of hypokalemia are listed in Table 8. Skeletal muscle weakness is often seen, with severe depletion leading to decreased reflexes and paralysis. Death can occur from respiratory muscle paralysis.[7,9,19]

## Hyperkalemia

Hyperkalemia is defined as a serum potassium concentration greater than 5.0 mEq/L (>5.0 mmol/L). As with hypokalemia, hyperkalemia may indicate a true or apparent potassium imbalance, although the signs and symptoms are indistinguishable.[10] To interpret a high serum potassium value, the clinician should determine whether hyperkalemia is due to an apparent excess caused by extracellular shifting of potassium or to a true potassium excess in the body caused by increased intake with diminished excretion (Table 9).[4,6,9,11]

*Causes.* Since renal excretion is the major route of potassium elimination, renal failure is the most common cause of hyperkalemia. However, potassium handling by the nephrons is well preserved until the GFR falls to less than 10% of normal. Therefore, many patients with renal impairment maintain a near-normal serum potassium concentration. These patients are still prone to hyperkalemia, however, if too much potassium is given and/or renal disease progresses.[9,12]

Increased potassium intake rarely is a problem in the absence of significant renal impairment. Increased intake leads to increased potassium excretion and redistribution in persons with normal renal function, because the body can use insulin and aldosterone to shift potassium intracellularly and to increase renal excretion, respectively. Interference with either mechanism can cause hyperkalemia. Decreased aldosterone can occur with Addison's disease or other defects affecting the hormone's adrenal output.[7,12]

Potassium-sparing diuretics can cause hyperkalemia, especially when potassium supplements (including potassium-rich salt substitutes) are coadministered and/or the patient has renal impairment. Pathological changes affecting the proximal or distal renal tubules also can lead to hyperkalemia.[7,12]

Finally, like hypokalemia, hyperkalemia can result from transcellular shifting of potassium. During severe metabolic acidosis, potassium shifts from the extracellular to the intracellular component. This shift leads to a clinically significant increase in the serum potassium concentration.[10]

*Clinical diagnosis.* The hyperkalemic signs and symptoms of principal concern involve the cardiovascular system. They include cardiac rhythm disturbances, bradycardia, hypotension, and, in severe cases, cardiac arrest. Muscle weakness may occur before cardiac manifestations are observed.

Potassium is the principal component of cardioplegic

**TABLE 9.** Etiologies of Hyperkalemia

> **Apparent excess—extracellular shifting of potassium**
> Metabolic acidosis
>
> **True excess**
> Increased intake
> Endogenous
> Hemolysis
> Rhabdomyolysis
> Muscle crush injuries
> Burns
> Exogenous
> Salt substitutes
> Drugs (e.g., penicillin potassium)
> Decreased output
> Chronic or acute renal failure
> Drugs
> Potassium-sparing diuretics
> Angiotensin-converting enzyme inhibitors
> NSAIDs
> $\beta_2$-Adrenergic antagonists
> Heparin
> Trimethoprim
> Deficiency of adrenal steroids
> Addison's disease

solutions used to arrest the function of the heart during cardiac surgeries.[7,9,12]

*Causes of spurious laboratory results.* Clinicians must be aware of fictitious hyperkalemia in which a high serum concentration is not associated with clinical manifestations. Erythrocytes, like other cells, are rich in potassium. When they are allowed to hemolyze in the specimen collection tube (e.g., too small a needle is used to draw the sample, tourniquet is too tight, or specimen stands too long or is mishandled), red cells release potassium into the specimen in quantities large enough to produce misleading results. If hyperkalemia is present without associated signs and symptoms, another serum potassium concentration should be obtained.[6,7,10]

A similar phenomenon also can occur when the specimen is allowed to clot (when nonheparinized tubes are used), because platelets and white cells also are potassium rich. In patients with leukemia or thrombocytosis, the potassium concentration should be obtained from plasma rather than serum samples. However, the normal plasma potassium concentration is 0.3–0.4 mEq/L lower than serum values.

# Chloride
*Normal range: 96–106 mEq/L or 96–106 mmol/L*

## Physiology

Chloride is the most abundant extracellular anion; however, its intracellular concentration is small (about 4 mEq/L). Chloride is absorbed passively from the upper small intestine. In the distal ileum and large intestine, its absorption is coupled with bicarbonate ion secretion. Chloride is regulated primarily by the renal proximal tubules, where it is exchanged for bicarbonate ions. Throughout the rest of the nephron, chloride passively follows sodium and water.

Chloride is influenced by the extracellular fluid balance and acid–base balance.[19,20] Although homeostatic mechanisms do not directly regulate chloride, they indirectly regulate it through changes in sodium and bicarbonate. The role of chloride is primarily passive. It balances out positive charges in the extracellular fluid and, by passively following sodium, helps to maintain extracellular osmolality. Finally, chloride fills in electronegative voids created by bicarbonate ion depletion.

## Hypochloremia and Hyperchloremia

Serum chloride values are used as confirmatory tests to identify fluid balance and acid–base abnormalities.[21] Like sodium, a change in the serum chloride concentration does not necessarily reflect a change in total body content. Rather, it indicates an alteration in fluid status and/or acid–base balance. Chloride has the added feature of being influenced by bicarbonate. Therefore, it would be expected to decrease to the same proportion as sodium when serum is diluted with fluid and to increase to the same proportion as sodium during dehydration. However, when a patient is on acid-suppressive therapy (e.g., cimetidine or omeprazole), has had nasogastric suction, or is profusely vomiting, a greater loss of chloride than sodium can occur because gastric fluid contains 1.5–3 times more chloride than sodium. Gastric outlet obstruction, protracted vomiting in alcoholism, and self-induced vomiting also can lead to hypochloremia.

*Drug and parenteral nutrition causes.* Even though drugs can influence serum chloride concentrations, they rarely do so directly. For example, although loop diuretics (e.g., furosemide) and thiazide diuretics (e.g., hydrochlorothiazide) inhibit chloride uptake at the loop of Henle and distal nephron, respectively,[18] the hypochloremia that may result is due to the concurrent loss of sodium and contraction alkalosis.[21] Since chloride passively follows sodium, salt and water retention can transiently raise serum chloride concentrations. This effect occurs with corticosteroids, guanethidine, and NSAIDs such as ibuprofen. Also, parenteral nutrition solutions with a chloride:sodium ratio greater than 1 are associated with an increased risk of hyperchloremia. Acetate or phosphate salts used in place of chloride salts (e.g., potassium chloride) reduce this risk. Acetazolamide also can cause hyperchloremia.

*Acid–base status and other causes.* The acid–base balance is partly regulated by renal production and excretion of bicarbonate ions. The proximal tubules are the primary regulators of bicarbonate. These cells exchange bicarbonate with chloride to maintain the intracellular electropotential gradient. (The production of bicarbonate and hydrogen ions is discussed in more detail in Chapter 8.) The clinician must understand that the renal excretion of chloride increases during metabolic alkalosis, resulting in a reduced serum chloride concentration.

The opposite situation also may be true—metabolic or respiratory acidosis results in an elevated serum chloride concentration. Hyperchloremic metabolic acidosis is not common but may occur when the kidneys are unable to conserve bicarbonate, as in interstitial renal disease (e.g., obstruction, pyelonephritis, and analgesic nephropathy), GI bicarbonate loss (e.g., cholera and staphylococcal infections of the intestines), and acetazolamide-induced carbonic anhydrase inhibition. Falsely elevated chloride rarely occurs from bromide toxicity due to a lack of distinction between these two halogens by the laboratory's chemical analyzer.

(Since the signs and symptoms associated with hyperchloremia and hypochloremia are related to fluid status or the acid–base balance and underlying causes, rather than to chloride itself, the reader is referred to discussions in Chapter 8.)

# OTHER MINERALS

## Magnesium

*Normal range: 1.5–2.2 mEq/L or 0.75–1.1 mmol/L*

### Physiology

Magnesium has a widespread physiological role in neuromuscular functions and enzymatic systems. This cation functions as a cofactor in all enzyme reactions of phosphate transfer utilizing ATP as a substrate. Magnesium is also vital for binding macromolecules to organelles [messenger ribonucleic acid (RNA) to ribosomes].

Magnesium's bodily regulation is not well understood. The average 70-kg adult body contains 2000 mEq of magnesium with the following distribution:

> ➤ 50% in bone (about 30% is slowly exchangeable with extracellular fluid).
> ➤ 45% in intracellular fluid.
> ➤ 5% in extracellular fluid (one-third is plasma protein bound).

Normal intake is 20–40 mEq/day. Approximately 30% of ingested magnesium is absorbed from the jejunum and ileum by an active process that is coupled to calcium absorption. When magnesium intake is low, calcium absorption from the intestines is increased. Magnesium is excreted primarily by the kidneys, where unbound serum magnesium is freely filtered at the glomerulus. All but about 3–5% of filtered magnesium is normally reabsorbed.

Physiological mechanisms that maintain serum magnesium homeostasis are not quite as rigid as for some electrolytes. For example, hypomagnesemia does not necessarily cause magnesium to move outward from intracellular stores. When interpreting an abnormal serum magnesium concentration, clinicians must remember that regulation of serum magnesium is only controlled by GI absorption and renal excretion.

Factors affecting calcium homeostasis also affect magnesium homeostasis.[22] A decline in serum magnesium concentration stimulates the release of PTH, which increases serum magnesium by increasing both its release from bone stores and its renal reabsorption. Hyperaldosteronism causes increased magnesium renal excretion, while insulin does not appear to affect magnesium homeostasis. Excretion of magnesium is influenced by serum calcium and phosphate concentrations. Magnesium movement generally follows that of phosphate (i.e., if phosphate declines, magnesium also declines) and is the opposite of calcium.[21,22]

### Hypomagnesemia

Hypomagnesemia is defined as a serum magnesium concentration less than 1.5 mEq/L (<0.75 mmol/L). Since serum magnesium deficiency can be offset by magnesium release from bone, muscle, and heart stores, serum values may not be a useful indicator of cellular depletion and complications (e.g., arrhythmias). However, low serum magnesium usually indicates low cellular magnesium, as long as the patient has a normal extracellular fluid volume.[22,23]

*Causes.* Magnesium deficiency is more common than magnesium excess. Depletion usually results from excessive loss from the GI tract or kidneys (e.g., diuresis). Depletion commonly is not the result of decreased intake, because the kidneys can cease magnesium elimination in 4–7 days to conserve the ion. With chronic alcohol consumption, however, deficiency can occur from a combination of poor intake, poor GI absorption (e.g., vomiting or diarrhea), and increased renal elimination. Depletion can also occur from poor intestinal absorption (e.g., small-bowel resection). Diarrhea can be a source of magnesium loss because diarrhea stools may contain as much as 14 mEq/L (7 mmol/L) of magnesium.

Urinary loss may result from osmotic diuresis or tubular defects, such as the diuretic phase of acute tubular necrosis. Some patients with hypoparathyroidism may exhibit low magnesium serum concentrations from renal loss and, possibly, decreased intestinal absorption. Other conditions associated with magnesium deficiency include hyperthyroidism, primary aldosteronism, diabetic ketoacidosis, and pancreatitis. Magnesium deficiency in these states may be particularly dangerous because they often are associated with potassium and calcium deficiencies. Most diuretics lead to magnesium depletion; however, thiazide diuretics do not cause hypomagnesemia, especially at lower doses (≤50 mg/day). Furthermore, potassium-sparing diuretics (spironolactone, triamterene, and amiloride) also are magnesium sparing and are clinically useful in diuretic-induced hypokalemia and hypomagnesemia.[22,24]

*Clinical diagnosis.* Magnesium depletion usually is associated with neuromuscular symptoms such as weakness, muscle fasciculation with tremor, tetany, and increased reflexes.[22] They occur because the release of acetylcholine to motor endplates is affected by the presence or absence of magnesium. Motor endplate sensitivity to acetylcholine also is affected. When serum magnesium decreases, acetylcholine release increases, resulting in increased muscle excitation.

Magnesium also affects the central nervous system (CNS). Magnesium depletion can cause personality changes, disorientation, convulsions, psychosis, stupor, and coma.[22,25] Severe hypomagnesemia may result in hypocalcemia due to intracellular cationic shifts. Many symptoms of magnesium deficiency are due to decreased calcium.

Perhaps the most important effects of magnesium imbalance are on the heart. Decreased magnesium in cardiac cells may manifest as a prolonged QT interval (increased risk of arrhythmias).[25] Moderately decreased concentrations can cause ECG abnormalities similar to those observed with hypokalemia. In addition, vasodilation may occur by a direct effect on blood vessels and ganglionic blockade.

One published method of diagnosing true magnesium deficiency concluded that if the serum concentration is low or normal initially and a deficiency is suspected, a 24-hr urine magnesium should be obtained. If the value is normal, the patient is not considered deficient as long as serum magnesium also is normal. If serum magnesium is normal but the 24-hr urine is low, magnesium replacement (30 mmol/500 mL dextrose 5% in water over 8–12 hr) is administered and urine is collected for another 24-hr period. If greater than 60% of the dose is excreted, magnesium stores are normal. If less than 50% of the dose is excreted, the patient is magnesium deficient. If the serum magnesium concentration is low and the 24-hr urinary magnesium is decreased, the patient probably has depleted magnesium stores. If the 24-hr urine magnesium is high but the serum magnesium concentration is low, renal loss probably is the cause of hypomagnesemia.[26]

### Hypermagnesemia

Hypermagnesemia is defined as a serum magnesium concentration greater than 2.2 mEq/L (>1.1 mmol/L).

*Causes.* Hypermagnesemia commonly is caused by increased magnesium intake in the presence of renal dysfunction. The magnesium content of antacids and laxatives should be considered when a patient has renal disease (Minicase 4). Rapid infusions of IV solutions containing large amounts of magnesium, such as those given for myocardial infarction, can cause symptomatic hypermagnesemia. Other causes of symptomatic hypermag-

**TABLE 10.** Signs and Symptoms of Hypermagnesemia

| 2–5 mEq/L | Bradycardia, flushing, sweating, sensation of warmth, nausea, vomiting. Decreased serum calcium and decreased clotting mechanisms |
| 6 mEq/L | Drowsiness and decreased deep-tendon reflexes |
| 10–15 mEq/L | Flaccid paralysis and increased PR and QRS intervals |
| >15 mEq/L | Respiratory distress and asystole |

nesemia include hepatitis and Addison's disease.[22,27]

*Clinical diagnosis.* Serum magnesium concentrations below 5 mEq/L (<2.5 mmol/L) rarely are symptomatic. As with hypomagnesemia, magnesium excess is associated with neuromuscular signs and symptoms. However, the opposite manifestations also are observed (Table 10).[22,24,27]

## Calcium
*Normal range: 8.5–10.8 mg/dL or 2.1–2.7 mmol/L for adults*

### Physiology

Calcium plays an important role in the propagation of neuromuscular activity, regulation of endocrine functions (e.g., pancreatic insulin release and gastric hydrogen secretion), blood coagulation including platelet aggregation, and bone and tooth metabolism.[2,28]

The serum calcium concentration is closely regulated by a complex interaction among PTH, serum phosphate, vitamin D system, and target organ (Figure 3). About one-third of the ingested calcium is actively absorbed from the proximal area of the small intestine, facilitated by 1,25-dihydroxycholecalciferol (1,25-DHCC or calcitriol), the

---

### ✎ Minicase 4

Minicase 3 described the case of Andrew D., a 65-year-old male with hyperkalemia, metabolic acidosis, and renal impairment. His hyperalimentation solution contained an inappropriately high amount of potassium for his condition. When the potassium content was reduced to 30 mEq, his signs and symptoms of hyperkalemia resolved. However, Andrew D. developed severe pneumonia and required intubation and mechanical ventilation. To reduce gastric pH and the likelihood of stress ulcers, he received 30 mL of aluminum–magnesium hydroxide antacid every 2 hr through his nasogastric tube.

Three days after his intubation, Andrew D. developed bradycardia again and appeared drowsy. His bedside neurological exam revealed bilaterally depressed deep-tendon reflexes. Andrew D.'s vital signs included respiratory rate 26, pulse 45 and regular, and BP 145/78 mm Hg. Abnormal clinical laboratory tests included serum potassium 5.3 mEq/L (3.5–5.0 mEq/L), serum carbon dioxide content 17 mEq/L (24–30 mEq/L), phosphate 6.9 mg/dL (2.6–4.5 mg/dL), BUN 60 mg/dL (8–20 mg/dL), SCr 3.5

mg/dL (0.7–1.5 mg/dL), and magnesium 7.2 mEq/L (1.5–2.2 mEq/L).

*What subjective and objective data for Andrew D. are consistent with a diagnosis of hypermagnesemia? What are the potential etiologies of hypermagnesemia in this patient?*

**Discussion:** Aside from his high serum magnesium concentration, Andrew D. is exhibiting signs and symptoms of hypermagnesemia, including drowsiness, bradycardia, and depressed deep-tendon reflexes.

Hypermagnesemia commonly is associated with severe renal impairment; however, it may be due to increased magnesium intake and decreased magnesium output. Although magnesium balance usually is not disturbed until the GFR falls below 10 mL/min, Andrew D.'s renal impairment is a contributing factor. Another factor is the daily magnesium dose that he receives from his hyperalimentation solution and the antacid (increased intake).

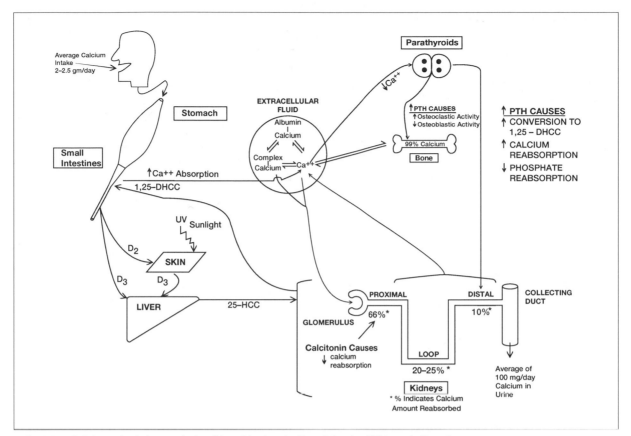

**FIGURE 3.** Calcium physiology: relationship with vitamin D, calcitonin, PTH, and albumin.

most active form of vitamin D. Passive intestinal absorption is negligible with intakes of less than 2 g/day.

The normal adult body contains about 1000 g of calcium, with only 0.5% found in the extracellular fluid; 99.5% is integrated in the bones. The average daily intake of calcium is 2–2.5 g/day. Tissue concentration of calcium is small. Since bone is constantly remodeled by osteoblasts and osteoclasts, a small quantity of bone calcium is in equilibrium with the extracellular fluid. Extracellular calcium exists in three forms:

> Complex bound (6%).
> Protein bound, mostly to albumin (40%).
> Ionized or free fraction (54%).

The equilibrium among these three forms determines the homeostasis of calcium.

*Intracellular calcium.* In the acute care setting, muscle contraction and nerve action potential are major concerns with calcium imbalances.[28] Calcium concentration is low intracellularly. The calcium that is attracted into the negatively charged cell is either actively pumped out or sequestered by mitochondria or the endoplasmic reticulum. This difference in intracellular concentration allows calcium to be used for transmembrane signaling. In response to stimuli, calcium is either allowed to enter a cell or released from internal cellular stores, where it interacts with

specific intracellular proteins to regulate cellular functions or metabolic processes.[2,26,27] Calcium enters cells through calcium channels. Three have been identified: T (transient or fast), N (neuronal), and L (long lasting or slow). Subsets of these channels may exist. Calcium channel-blockers likely affect the L channels.[29]

In muscle, calcium is released from the intracellular sarcoplasmic reticulum. The released calcium binds to troponin and stops troponin from inhibiting the interaction of actin and myosin. This interaction results in muscle contraction. Muscle relaxation occurs when the calcium is pumped back into the sarcoplasmic reticulum. In cardiac tissue, calcium's role becomes important during phase 2 of the action potential. During this phase, fast entry of sodium stops and calcium entry through slow channels begins (Figure 4, next page). Contraction occurs during this slow intracellular movement.

During repolarization, calcium is actively pumped out of the cell.[2] Calcium channel-blocking drugs (e.g., nifedipine, diltiazem, and verapamil) inhibit the movement of calcium into muscle cells, thus decreasing the strength of contraction. The areas most sensitive to these effects appear to be the sinoatrial and atrioventricular nodes and vascular smooth muscles (which explains nifedipine's hypotensive effects).

*Extracellular calcium.* Complex-bound calcium usually

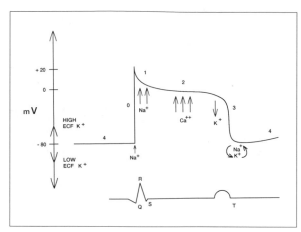

**FIGURE 4.** Cardiac intracellular potential and its relationship to the ECG.

accounts for less than 1 mg/dL (<0.25 mmol/L) of blood calcium. The complex usually is formed with bicarbonate, citrate, or phosphate. It can occur with sulfate in chronic renal failure when sulfate is retained. Phosphate has an important role in calcium homeostasis. Under normal physiological conditions, the product of calcium concentration times phosphate concentration (the so-called calcium–phosphate product) is relatively constant, so an increase in one ion necessitates a decline in the other. In addition, many homeostatic mechanisms for controlling calcium also control phosphate. This relationship is particularly important in renal failure; the decreased phosphate excretion may ultimately lead—through a complex mechanism—to hypocalcemia, especially if the hyperphosphatemia is untreated.[30,31]

Calcium is bound primarily to serum albumin (80%) and globulins (20%). Protein-bound calcium is in equilibrium with ionized calcium, and the direction is determined by the serum anion concentration and blood pH. This equilibrium is important, since ionized calcium is the physiologically active moiety. Alkalosis increases protein binding of calcium, resulting in a lower free fraction; acidosis has the opposite effect. Signs and symptoms of hypocalcemia may become more pronounced in patients who develop respiratory or metabolic alkalosis. Conversely, signs and symptoms of hypercalcemia become more apparent in a patient with metabolic or respiratory acidosis. Therefore, total serum calcium (i.e., what is measured by the lab) is less important than the quantity of ionized calcium available. In fact, the free fraction is closely controlled by homeostatic mechanisms.

Clinically, the most important determinant of ionized calcium is the amount of serum proteins (primarily albumin) available for binding. The normal serum calcium range is 8.5–10.8 mg/dL (2.1–2.7 mmol/L) for a patient with a serum albumin of approximately 4 g/dL (40 g/L). Since a fraction of calcium will be protein bound in hypoalbuminemic patients, this normal range must be corrected based on the serum albumin concentration to reflect the additional quantity of free (active) calcium when less protein is available for binding. The following formula may be used:

$$Ca_{corr} = [(4.0 - albumin) \times 0.8 \text{ mg/dL}] + Ca_{uncorr}$$

where $Ca_{corr}$ is the corrected serum calcium concentration, and $Ca_{uncorr}$ is the uncorrected serum calcium concentration. For example, a clinician may be asked to write parenteral nutrition orders for an emaciated cancer patient. The serum albumin is 1.9 g/dL (19 g/L), and the serum calcium is 7.7 mg/dL (1.9 mmol/L) (calcium is reported as total calcium, not free or ionized fraction). At first glance, one might consider the calcium to be low. But, with the reduced serum albumin concentration, more ionized calcium is available to cells.

$$Ca_{corr} = [(4.0 - 1.9) \times 0.8] + 7.7 = 9.4 \text{ mg/dL} (2.34 \text{ mmol/L})$$

Thus, the corrected serum calcium concentration is within the normal range. In severe hypoalbuminemia, as seen in nutritionally deprived patients, an apparently low measured serum calcium may in fact be normal or even high. If such a patient were given IV albumin, the free fraction of calcium would acutely decline. Again, the clinician would need to correct measured calcium for the new albumin concentration.

Although this serum calcium correction method may be useful, the clinician must be aware of its potential for inaccuracy, especially since the correction figure of 0.8 represents an average value. Fortunately, this method may be circumvented by directly measuring serum ionized calcium concentrations (normal range: 4.6–5.2 mg/dL or 1.15–1.38 mmol/L).

Other, less important factors can influence the calcium–protein equilibrium. Sodium may affect binding and, with severe hyponatremia, one might find increased calcium–protein binding. The opposite is true for severe hypernatremia. Hypothermia also can decrease calcium binding.

*Influence of vitamin D system.* Small amounts of calcium are excreted daily into the GI tract from saliva, bile, and pancreatic and intestinal secretions; however, the primary route of elimination is filtration by the kidneys. Calcium is freely filtered at the glomerulus, where approximately 65% is reabsorbed by the proximal tubules under partial control of calcitonin and 1,25-DHCC. Roughly 25% is reabsorbed in the loop of Henle, and another 10% is reabsorbed by the distal tubules under the control of PTH.

Vitamin D is important for:

➢ Intestinal absorption of calcium.
➢ PTH-induced mobilization of calcium from bone.
➢ Calcium reabsorption in the proximal renal tubules.

Vitamin D must undergo several conversion steps before the active form, calcitriol or 1,25-DHCC, is formed. Vitamin D is absorbed by the intestines in two forms, vitamin $D_2$ (7-dehydrocholesterol) and vitamin $D_3$ (cholecalciferol). Vitamin $D_2$ is converted into vitamin $D_3$ in the skin by the sun's ultraviolet radiation. (At least one cause of childhood hypocalcemia, rickets, is caused by reduced exposure to sunlight, resulting in diminished production of vitamin $D_3$.)

Liver enzymes hydroxylate vitamin $D_3$ to calcifediol or 25-hydroxycholecalciferol (25-HCC), which is then hydroxylated by the kidneys to form the active 1,25-DHCC. This last conversion step is controlled by PTH. When PTH is increased during hypocalcemia, renal production of 1,25-DHCC increases. This rise leads to an increased intestinal absorption of calcium. PTH synthesis and secretion are closely regulated by 1,25-DHCC.[30,32]

*Influence of calcitonin.* Calcitonin is a hormone secreted from specialized "C" cells of the thyroid gland in response to a high circulating ionized calcium. Calcitonin inhibits osteoclastic activity, thereby inhibiting bone resorption and decreasing calcium reabsorption in the renal proximal tubules. This decreased reabsorption leads to increased calcium clearance.[28] Different forms of calcitonin are used in the treatment of acute hypercalcemia.

*Influence of parathyroid hormone.* PTH is the most important hormone involved in calcium homeostasis. It is secreted by the parathyroid glands (embedded in the thyroid) in direct response to low circulating ionized calcium. PTH closely regulates, and is regulated by, the vitamin D system in maintaining the serum ionized calcium concentration within a narrow range. Generally, PTH increases the serum calcium concentration. PTH stimulates renal conversion of 25-HCC to 1,25-DHCC, which enhances calcium absorption from the intestines. Conversely, 1,25-DHCC is a potent suppressor of PTH synthesis via a direct mechanism that is independent of the serum calcium concentration.[28,31] The normal reference range for serum PTH concentrations is 10–60 pg/mL.

Tubular reabsorption of calcium and phosphate at the distal nephron is controlled by PTH. PTH increases renal reabsorption of calcium and decreases the reabsorption of phosphate, resulting in lower serum phosphate and higher serum calcium concentrations. Perhaps the most important effect of PTH is on the bone. In the presence of PTH, osteoblastic activity is diminished and the bone-resorption processes of osteoclasts are increased. These effects increase serum ionized calcium, which feeds back to the parathyroid glands to decrease PTH output.[30]

The suppressive effect of 1,25-DHCC (calcitriol) on PTH secretion is used clinically in patients with chronic renal failure who commonly have excessively high serum PTH concentrations. PTH is a known uremic toxin, and its presence in supraphysiological concentrations has nu-merous adverse effects (e.g., suppressed erythropoiesis by the bone marrow and increased osteoclastic resorption of bones with replacement by fibrous tissue).[33] Figure 5 depicts the relationship between serum PTH and serum calcium concentrations.

*Abnormalities.* True abnormal serum concentrations of calcium may be due to an abnormality in any of the previously mentioned mechanisms, including

> Altered intestinal absorption.[8,30,31,34]
> Altered number or activity of osteoclast and osteoblast cells in bone.[8,30,31,34]
> Changes in renal reabsorption of calcium.[8,30,31,34]
> Calcium or phosphate IV infusions.

Since laboratories commonly measure total serum calcium as opposed to ionized calcium, normal lab results may not be a true predictor of the signs and symptoms of calcium imbalances. Therefore, as previously mentioned, one must also consider serum protein or albumin in interpreting serum calcium values.[28,31,35]

Due to several factors that interact via a complex mechanism, patients with chronic renal failure have increased serum phosphate and decreased serum calcium concentrations. These factors include decreased phosphate clearance by the kidneys, decreased renal metabolism of PTH, and decreased renal production of 1,25-DHCC. This interaction is further complicated by the metabolic acidosis of renal failure; it can increase bone resorption, resulting in decreased bone integrity in patients with chronic renal failure. This complex process is counteracted by administering calcitriol, phosphate binders, and calcium supplements to keep serum calcium and phosphate concentrations near normal and to prevent secondary hyperparathyroidism.[31,36]

### Hypocalcemia

Hypocalcemia is defined as a total serum calcium concentration less than 8.5 mg/dL (<2.1 mmol/L). The most common cause of hypocalcemia is low serum proteins; however, since the ionized calcium concentration remains

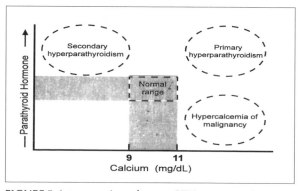

**FIGURE 5.** Interpretation of serum PTH concentrations with concomitant serum calcium concentrations.

**TABLE 11.** Common Etiologies of Hypocalcemia

---

**Diminished intake**

**Medications**
    Calcitonin
    Ethylenediaminetetraacetic acid (EDTA)
    Glucocorticoids
    Loop diuretics
    Phosphate salts
    Plicamycin

**Hyperphosphatemia**

**Hypoalbuminemia**

**Hypomagnesemia**

**Hypoparathyroidism (common)**

**Pancreatitis**

**Renal failure**

**Secondary hyperparathyroidism**

**Vitamin D deficiency (common)**

---

unaffected, patients remain asymptomatic and often no treatment is required.

The most common causes of decreased total serum calcium are disorders of vitamin D metabolism and PTH production (Table 11). Osteomalacia (in adults) and rickets (in children) can be caused by a lack of dietary calcium or vitamin D, diminished synthesis of vitamin $D_3$ from insufficient sunlight exposure, or resistance by the intestinal wall to the action of vitamin D. The reduction in serum calcium leads to secondary hyperparathyroidism, which increases bone resorption. With long-standing disease, bones lose their structural integrity and become more susceptible to fracture. The diminished serum calcium concentration sometimes gives rise to tetany.

*Diminished intake.* Although uncommon, diminished intake of calcium is an important cause of hypocalcemia, especially in patients receiving long-term hyperalimentation solutions.[37,38]

*Medications.* Excessive utilization of some drugs used to lower serum calcium by either increasing bone deposition or decreasing renal reabsorption of calcium also may lead to hypocalcemia. These drugs include plicamycin, calcitonin, glucocorticoids, loop diuretics, etidronate, pamidronate, and alendronate.

IV bicarbonate administration and hyperventilation can cause systemic alkalosis, with a resultant decrease in ionized serum calcium. This decrease usually is important only in patients who already have low serum calcium concentrations. Other drugs that may cause hypocalcemia include phenytoin, phenobarbital, antacids containing aluminum, cis-platinum, theophylline, sodium fluoride, and magnesium sulfate.

Another cause is rapid IV administration of phosphate salts (a common ingredient in hyperalimentation solutions), especially at high doses. Phosphate can bind calcium and form an insoluble product. This product can deposit into soft tissues, causing metastatic calcification or hardening of normally pliable tissues.[37,38] Soft-tissue deposition of the calcium–phosphate complex (e.g., in lungs and blood vessels) occurs when the serum solubility product of calcium times phosphate exceeds 70. The risk of deposition increases in patients who develop alkalosis. Phosphate can be absorbed into the circulation from some enema and laxative preparations (e.g., Fleet's enema).[33]

*Hypoparathyroid effects.* Hypoparathyroidism can reduce serum calcium concentrations. The most common cause of hypoparathyroidism is thyroidectomy, when the parathyroids are removed along with the thyroid glands. Since PTH is the major hormone of calcium balance, its absence significantly reduces serum calcium.[38]

*Hyperparathyroid effects.* Secondary hyperparathyroidism, which commonly is due to chronic renal failure, also causes hypocalcemia (Figure 5). The mechanism is complex and involves elevated serum phosphate concentrations. PTH acts on the bone to increase calcium and phosphate resorption. Since serum phosphate cannot be eliminated, serum calcium remains depressed. Because of high phosphate concentrations in the intestinal wall, dietary calcium is bound and absorption is impaired while phosphate absorption continues.

The metabolic acidosis usually accompanying chronic renal failure further enhances bone resorption. With prolonged severe hyperparathyroidism, osteoclastic resorption of bones increases with replacement by fibrous tissues. This condition is termed *osteitis fibrosa cystica*.[31,34,35] This diminution of bone density may lead to pathological fractures. Although serum calcium concentrations are low, patients may not show symptoms of hypocalcemia because the accompanying acidosis helps to maintain a proper balance of ionized serum calcium.

*Magnesium effects.* Much like potassium, the calcium balance strongly depends on magnesium homeostasis. Therefore, if a hypocalcemic patient is also hypomagnesemic (as occurs with loop diuretic therapy), he or she may not respond to calcium replacement therapy unless the magnesium balance is restored.

*Clinical diagnosis.* As with any electrolyte disorder, the severity of clinical manifestations of hypocalcemia depends on the acuteness of onset. In acute settings, hypocalcemia can be a medical emergency.[37,38] Symptoms primarily involve the neuromuscular system. They include fatigue, depression, memory loss, hallucinations, and, in severe cases, seizures and tetany. The earliest signs of hypocalcemia are finger numbness, tingling and burning of extremities, and paresthesia. Mental instability and confusion also can occur.

Tetany is the hallmark of severe hypocalcemia. The mechanism of muscle fasciculation of tetany is the loss of the inhibitory effect of ionized calcium on muscle proteins. In extreme cases, this loss leads to increased neuromuscular excitability that can progress to laryngospasm and tonic–clonic seizures. Chvostek's and Trousseau's signs are hallmarks of hypocalcemia. Chvostek's sign is a unilateral spasm induced by a slight tap over the facial nerve. Trousseau's sign is carpal spasm elicited when the upper arm is compressed by a BP cuff.[31,38,40]

As hypocalcemia worsens, the cardiovascular system may be affected, as evidenced by myocardial failure, cardiac arrhythmias, and hypotension.[37,38] Special attention should be given to serum calcium concentrations of patients receiving diuretics, corticosteroids, digoxin, vitamin preparations, antacids, lithium, and parenteral nutrition and in patients with renal disease. Although hypercalcemia is not as striking as hypokalemia, it can enhance the inotropic effects of digoxin, increasing the likelihood of cardiac arrhythmias.[35,37,38]

### Hypercalcemia

Hypercalcemia is defined as a total serum calcium concentration greater than 10.8 mg/dL (>2.7 mmol/L).

*Causes.* The most common causes of hypercalcemia are malignancy and primary hyperparathyroidism (Figure 5). Malignancies can increase serum calcium by several mechanisms. Osteolytic metastases can arise from breast, lung, thyroid, kidney, or bladder cancer. These tumor cells invade bone and produce substances that directly dissolve bone matrix and mineral content. Some malignancies, such as multiple myeloma, can produce factors that stimulate osteoclast proliferation and activity. Another mechanism is the ectopic production of PTH or PTH-like substances by tumor cells, resulting in a pseudohyperparathyroid state.[39,41]

In primary hyperparathyroidism, inappropriate secretion of PTH from the parathyroid gland (usually due to adenoma) increases serum calcium concentrations. The other major cause of hypercalcemia in hyperparathyroidism is the increased renal conversion of 25-HCC to the active 1,25-DHCC. As the serum calcium concentration rises, the renal ability to reabsorb calcium may be exceeded, leading to the formation of calcium–phosphate and calcium–oxalate renal stones. Typically, this condition results from parathyroid adenomas but may also be caused by primary cell hyperplasia, primary chief-cell hyperplasia, or other carcinomas.[31,41]

Approximately 2% of patients treated with thiazide diuretics may develop hypercalcemia. Patients most at risk are those with hyperparathyroidism. The mechanism appears to be multifactorial and includes enhanced renal reabsorption of calcium (decreasing urinary calcium) and decreased plasma volume.

The milk-alkali syndrome (Burnett's syndrome),

rarely observed today, is another drug-related cause of hypercalcemia.[33] This syndrome occurs from a chronic high intake of milk or calcium products combined with an absorbable antacid (e.g., calcium carbonate, sodium bicarbonate, or magnesium hydroxide). This syndrome was more common in the past when milk or cream was used to treat gastric ulcers and before the advent of nonabsorbable antacids. Renal failure can occur as the result of calcium deposition in soft tissues.[33,42]

Hypercalcemia can result from[28,40,41,43]

> ➤ Excessive administration of IV calcium salts.
> ➤ Calcium supplements.
> ➤ Chronic immobilization.
> ➤ Paget's disease.
> ➤ Sarcoidosis.
> ➤ Hyperthyroidism.
> ➤ Acute adrenal insufficiency.
> ➤ Some respiratory diseases.
> ➤ Lithium-induced renal calcium reabsorption.
> ➤ Excessive vitamin D, vitamin A, or thyroid hormone, which increases intestinal absorption.
> ➤ Tamoxifen.
> ➤ Androgenic hormones.
> ➤ Estrogen.
> ➤ Progesterone.

*Clinical diagnosis.* Like hypocalcemia and other electrolyte disorders, the severity of clinical manifestations of hypercalcemia depends on the acuteness of onset. In acute settings, hypercalcemia can be a medical emergency, especially when serum concentrations rise above 14 mg/dL (>3.5 mmol/L). Symptoms associated with this condition often consist of vague GI complaints such as nausea, vomiting, abdominal pain, dyspepsia, and anorexia. More severe GI complications include peptic ulcer disease (possibly due to increased gastrin release) and acute pancreatitis.[43,44]

Severe hypercalcemic symptoms primarily involve the neuromuscular system (e.g., lethargy, obtundation, psychosis, cerebellar ataxia, and, in severe cases, coma and death). Signs of severe hypercalcemia involve the kidneys and the cardiovascular system but may also involve other organs.[43,44]

Renal function may be affected by hypercalcemia through calcium's inhibition of the adenyl cyclase–cyclic adenosine monophosphate system that mediates the ADH effects on the collecting ducts. This inhibition results in diminished conservation of water by the kidneys. The situation is further compounded by diminished solute transport in the loop of Henle, leading to polyuria and polydipsia.[28] Other chronic renal manifestations include nephrolithiasis, nephrocalcinosis, chronic interstitial nephritis, and renal tubular acidosis.

In addition, hypercalcemia can cause vasoconstriction of the renal vasculature, with a resultant decrease in renal blood flow and GFR. If hypercalcemia is allowed to progress, oliguric acute renal failure may ensue.[28] With increased calcium–phosphate product (usually >70), soft-tissue calcification of the calcium–phosphate complex may occur. The cardiac signs of hypercalcemia are arrhythmias and an increased risk of digoxin toxicity.[43,44]

*Causes of spurious laboratory results.* False hypercalcemia can occur if the tourniquet is left in place too long. This interference occurs as a result of increased plasma-protein pooling in the phlebotomized arm. Falsely elevated calcium should be suspected if serum albumin is greater than 5 g/dL (>50 g/L). Table 12 contains the normal range values for tests related to calcium metabolism.

## Phosphate
*Normal range: 2.6–4.5 mg/dL or 0.84–1.45 mmol/L for adults*

Many factors that influence serum calcium concentrations also influence serum phosphate, either directly or indirectly. The clinician should consider calcium and phosphate together when interpreting lab results. The clinician should also be aware that some laboratories report phosphate results as phosphorus.

### Physiology

Phosphate is a major intracellular anion with several functions. It is important for intracellular metabolism of proteins, fats, and carbohydrates and is a major component in phospholipid membranes, RNAs, nicotinamide diphosphate (an enzyme cofactor), cyclic adenine and guanine nucleotides (second messengers), and phosphoproteins. Still another important function of phosphate is in the formation of high-energy bonds in ATP production, which is a source of energy for many cellular reactions. Phosphate is a component of 2,3-diphosphoglycerate (2,3-DPG), which regulates the release of oxygen from hemoglobin (Hgb) to tissues. In addition, phosphate has a regulatory role in glycolysis and hydroxylation of cholecalciferol. Phosphate is also an important acid–base buffer.[35,40]

The average daily phosphate dietary intake for an adult is 700–800 g. About two-thirds is actively absorbed from the small intestine. Absorption is increased by 1,25-

**TABLE 12.** Normal Ranges for Tests Related to Calcium Metabolism

| | |
|---|---|
| Calcium (free) | 4.6–5.2 mg/dL |
| Calcium (total) | 8.5–10.5 mg/dL |
| 1,25-DHCC | 16–42 pg/mL |
| Phosphate | 2.6–4.5 mg/dL |
| PTH | 10–60 pg/mL |
| Urine calcium | 0–300 mg/day |
| Urine hydroxyproline | 10–50 mg/day (adults) |
| Urine phosphate | average: 1 g/day |

DHCC, which also increases the intestinal absorption of calcium. However, phosphate is the first of the two to be absorbed.[40]

Diminished phosphate absorption occurs when large quantities of calcium or aluminum are in the intestines (from some antacids) due to formation of insoluble phosphate compounds. This interaction is used clinically in patients with chronic renal failure who commonly have high serum phosphate concentrations. Calcium- and aluminum-containing antacids are administered with meals to bind dietary phosphate and prevent its absorption.[45]

Phosphate is distributed widely throughout the

> Plasma.
> Extracellular fluid.
> Cell membrane structures.
> Intracellular fluid.
> Collagen.
> Bone.

Bone holds 85% of the body's phosphate. About 90% of plasma phosphate is filtered at the glomerulus, and the majority is actively reabsorbed at the proximal tubule. Some reabsorption also takes place in the loop of Henle, distal tubules, and possibly the collecting ducts.[31] Therefore, urine phosphate concentration is the net effect of filtered minus reabsorbed phosphate. An increase in plasma volume can cause increased urinary phosphate excretion. PTH can increase phosphate excretion by blocking its reabsorption throughout the nephron. Vitamin $D_3$ and its metabolites directly stimulate proximal tubular phosphate reabsorption. In all, 90% of eliminated phosphate is excreted in the urine; the remainder is secreted into the intestines.[31,35,46]

Although renal filtration and reabsorption of phosphate are similar to those of calcium, they play a more dominant role in the homeostatic mechanisms of phosphate.[31] Of the intestinally absorbed phosphate, 50% is actively absorbed under the control of vitamin D and 50% is passively absorbed with calcium. The proximal renal tubules are the primary controllers of serum phosphate concentrations. Renal phosphate transport is active, saturable, and pH and sodium ion dependent. However, most changes in serum phosphate result from changes in either the GFR or the rate of tubular reabsorption.[2,31,35]

Serum phosphate indirectly controls PTH secretion via a negative feedback mechanism. With a decrease in the serum phosphate concentration, the conversion of vitamin $D_3$ to 1,25-DHCC increases, which increases serum concentrations of both phosphate and calcium. This increase occurs by increasing intestinal absorption and phosphate renal reabsorption. The concomitant increase in serum calcium then directly decreases PTH secretion. This decrease in serum PTH concentration permits an increase in renal reabsorption of phosphate.[30,31]

A true phosphate imbalance may be due to an abnormality in any of the previously mentioned mechanisms and hormones for maintaining calcium homeostasis. These abnormalities include altered intestinal absorption, altered number or activity of osteoclast and osteoblast cells in bone, changes in renal reabsorption of calcium and phosphate, and IV infusions of calcium or phosphate salts.[35,40]

### Hypophosphatemia

Hypophosphatemia is defined as a serum phosphate concentration less than 2.6 mg/dL (<0.84 mmol/L). Whereas hyperphosphatemia primarily occurs in renal failure, hypophosphatemia can occur as a result of renal dysfunction and various other conditions. Clinically, three causes of decreased serum phosphate concentrations are common:

> ➤ Increased renal excretion.[41,47,48]
> ➤ Intracellular shifting.
> ➤ Decreased phosphate or vitamin D intake.[41,47,48]

The most common causes of hypophosphatemia are decreased intake and increased renal loss.[40] To differentiate between them, one must consider the serum and urine content of phosphate.

Low urine and serum phosphates indicate either a diminished phosphate intake or excessive use of phosphate-binding antacids. An increased urine phosphate suggests either hyperparathyroidism or renal tubular dysfunction. If the increased urine phosphate is accompanied by an elevated serum calcium, the presence of primary hyperparathyroidism or decreased vitamin D metabolism must be considered.

*Common causes.* Hypophosphatemia usually is due to altered renal reabsorption or GFR, an extracellular-to-intracellular fluid shift of phosphate, alcoholism, or malnutrition. Phosphate is required in hyperalimentation solutions to promote muscle growth and fat replacement and to replenish hepatic glycogen storage in malnourished patients. The infusion of concentrated glucose solutions increases insulin secretion from the pancreas. Insulin allows glucose and phosphate to enter cells. Phosphate is used to form phosphorylated hexose intermediates during the cellular utilization of glucose. An inadequate phosphate content in hyperalimentation solutions can decrease anabolism, glycolysis, ATP, and 2,3-DPG production.[48]

Infusion of concentrated glucose solutions, especially when accompanied by insulin, can produce hypophosphatemia by shifting phosphate intracellularly. This condition can occur in patients receiving hyperalimentation solutions with inadequate amounts of phosphate, because large amounts of phosphate are taken up by new cells during anabolism.

Hypophosphatemia can also occur when treating hyperkalemia with insulin and dextrose. In addition, aluminum- and calcium-containing antacids, as well as magnesium hydroxide, are potent binders of intestinal phosphate.[45] Overuse of these agents can severely reduce serum phosphate concentrations in patients with normal renal function. Moreover, calcitonin, glucagon, and ß-adrenergic stimulants can decrease serum phosphate concentrations. Thiazide and loop diuretics can increase phosphate renal excretion; however, this effect is clinically insignificant in otherwise healthy individuals.

Other conditions known to cause hypophosphatemia include nutritional recovery after starvation, treatment of diabetic ketoacidosis, decreased absorption or increased intestinal loss, alcohol withdrawal, diuretic phase of acute tubular necrosis, and prolonged respiratory alkalosis. To compensate for respiratory alkalosis, carbon dioxide shifts from intracellular to extracellular fluid. This shift increases the intracellular fluid pH, which activates glycolysis and intracellular phosphate trapping. Metabolic acidosis, in contrast, produces a minimal change in serum phosphate.

*Uncommon causes.* Burn patients often retain a great amount of sodium and water; as their burns heal, diuresis often ensues. This condition results in a loss of phosphate. Since anabolism also occurs during treatment, hypophosphatemia may be inevitable without proper replacement. Moderate reductions in serum phosphate can occur from prolonged nasogastric suctioning, gastrectomy, small-bowel or pancreatic disease with malabsorption, and states of impaired renal reabsorption of phosphate (multiple myeloma, Fanconi syndrome, heavy-metal poisoning, amyloidosis, and nephrotic syndrome).[47,48]

*Severe hypophosphatemia.* Severe phosphate depletion (<1 mg/dL or <0.32 mmol/L) can occur from diabetic ketoacidosis. The resultant acidosis mobilizes bone, promotes intracellular organic substrate metabolism, and releases phosphate into extracellular fluid. The glycosuria and ketonuria caused by diabetic ketoacidosis result in an osmotic diuresis that increases the urinary clearance of phosphate. This effect may produce normal serum phosphate concentrations with severe intracellular deficiency. When diabetic ketoacidosis is corrected with insulin, phosphate accompanies glucose intracellularly. Serum phosphate usually is reduced within 24 hr of treatment. With correction of acidosis, phosphate experiences even more of an intracellular shift, resulting in profound hypophosphatemia. This problem is compounded during volume repletion.

*Clinical diagnosis.* Signs and symptoms of hypophosphatemia usually are due to diminished intracellular ATP and erythrocyte 2,3-DPG concentrations. Patients with moderate reductions in serum phosphate (2–2.5 mg/dL or 0.64–0.81 mmol/L) often are asymptomatic. Neurological irritability may occur as the serum phosphate concentration drops below 2 mg/dL (<0.64 mmol/L). Severe hypophosphatemia usually is associated with muscle weakness, rhabdomyolysis, paresthesia, hemolysis, platelet dysfunction, and cardiac and respiratory failure.

CNS effects often include encephalopathy, confusion, obtundation, seizures, and, ultimately, coma. The mechanism for these effects may involve decreased glucose utilization by the brain, decreased brain cell ATP, or cerebral hypoxia from increased oxygen–Hgb affinity, secondary to diminished erythrocyte 2,3-DPG content. This decreased content results in decreased glycolysis, which leads to decreased 2,3-DPG and ATP production. The decreased contents of 2,3-DPG and ATP result in an increased affinity of Hgb for oxygen, ultimately leading to decreased tissue oxygenation. The ensuing cerebral hypoxia may explain the persistent coma often seen in patients with diabetic ketoacidosis. Hemolysis may occur but is rarely seen at serum phosphate concentrations greater than 0.5 mg/dL (>0.16 mmol/L).

### Hyperphosphatemia

Hyperphosphatemia is defined as a serum phosphate concentration greater than 4.5 mg/dL (>1.45 mmol/L). Clinically, three fundamental causes of elevated serum phosphate exist:

1. Decreased renal excretion of phosphate.
2. Shift of phosphate from intracellular to extracellular fluid.
3. Increased intake of vitamin D or phosphate products (orally, rectally, or IV).

Elevated phosphate may also result from reduced PTH secretion, increased body catabolism, and some oncological disorders (e.g., leukemias and lymphomas).[4,47,48]

*Causes.* The most common cause of hyperphosphatemia is renal dysfunction, which usually occurs as the GFR falls below 25 mL/min. Chronic renal failure can result in secondary hyperparathyroidism, which can further reduce phosphate clearance. The increase in serum phosphate concentration eventually results in the deposition of insoluble calcium–phosphate complex in soft tissues (i.e., metastatic calcification). This deposition reduces the serum concentration of ionized calcium and leads to increased PTH production and release. This process also results in bone resorption, thus severely weakening its structural integrity.[36,40]

Hyperphosphatemia can be caused by a shift of phosphate from intracellular fluid to extracellular fluid. This shift of phosphate can occur during chemotherapy for leukemia or lymphoma, in rhabdomyolysis, and in septic shock. Finally, hyperthyroidism can elevate serum phosphate by increasing bone resorption and PTH suppression and also by directly increasing tubular phosphate reabsorption.

*Clinical diagnosis.* Signs and symptoms of hyperphosphatemia primarily are due to the hypocalcemia and hyperparathyroidism that often ensue (Hypocalcemia section). Renal failure may occur if hyperphosphatemia is left untreated. If renal failure occurs, phosphate clearance is reduced. This results in an even greater increase in the serum phosphate concentration and a greater decline in the serum calcium concentration[36,40,45] (Minicase 5).

### Causes of Spurious Laboratory Results

Hemolysis can occur during phlebotomy, which may lead to a false elevation in the serum phosphate concentration. If serum is not separated soon after phlebotomy, phosphate may be falsely decreased as it is taken up by the cellular components of blood.

A phenomenon similar to that observed with potassium specimens also can occur with phosphate. When the specimen is allowed to clot (when nonheparinized tubes are used), phosphate leaches out of platelets. In patients with thrombocytosis, phosphate concentrations

---

**Minicase 5**

Paul M., a 65-year-old man, had a 1-week history of nausea, vomiting, and general malaise. His appetite had severely decreased over the past 2 months. He had a long-standing history of uncontrolled hypertension and diabetes mellitus as well as diabetic nephropathy, retinopathy, and neuropathy.

Paul M.'s current medications included levothyroxine 0.1 mg oral daily, metoclopramide 10 mg oral three times a day, and regular insulin subcutaneously twice a day. His physical examination revealed a BP of 160/99 mm Hg, diabetic retinopathic changes with laser scars bilaterally, and diminished sensation bilaterally below the knees.

Paul M.'s laboratory values were as follows: serum sodium 146 mEq/L (136–145 mEq/L), potassium 4.7 mEq/L (3.5–5.0 mEq/L), chloride 104 mEq/L (96–106 mEq/L), serum carbon dioxide content 15 mEq/L (24–30 mEq/L), SCr 7.9 mg/dL (0.7–1.5 mg/dL), BUN 92 mg/dL (8–20 mg/dL), and a random blood glucose of 181 mg/dL (70–110 mg/dL). On detection of his renal failure, additional laboratory tests were obtained: calcium 7.5 mg/dL (8.5–10.8 mg/dL), phosphate 9.1 mg/dL (2.6–4.5 mg/dL), total serum protein 5.2 g/dL (5.5–9.0 g/dL), albumin 3 g/dL (3.5–5 g/dL), and uric acid 8.9 mg/dL (3.4–7.0 mg/dL).

Paul M. was started on a daily peripheral hyperalimentation solution containing dextrose 5%, amino acids 3%, sodium chloride 50 mEq, potassium chloride 10 mEq, potassium phosphate 30 mEq (based on potassium), calcium gluconate 4.6 mEq, magnesium sulfate 8.1 mEq, and multivitamin supplements 10 mL. Over the next several days, he complained of finger numbness, tingling, and burning of extremities. Paul M. also experienced increasing confusion and fatigue. A neurological examination was positive for both Chvostek's and Trousseau's signs. Repeated laboratory tests showed substantial changes in serum cal-

should be obtained from plasma rather than serum samples.

Serum phosphate may also vary 1–2 mg/dL (0.32–0.64 mmol/L) with meals. Meals rich in carbohydrates can reduce serum phosphate, and meals high in phosphate can increase serum phosphate. Therefore, borderline patients should have their serum phosphate concentrations measured in a fasting state.

# TRACE ELEMENTS

## Copper

*Normal range: 75–150 µg/dL or 11.8–23.6 µmol/L for adults*

### Physiology

Copper is an essential trace element with multiple roles in the biological system. Many of its physiological functions are similar to those of iron. In fact, copper behaves as a companion to iron, and the two are metabolized in much the same way.[49] Copper serves as either a component of, or cofactor to, many enzymes responsible for di-

verse biological activities, including mobilization of iron from its stores for transport to the bone marrow, synthesis of norepinephrine, formation of collagen and elastin, catabolism of numerous neurotransmitters (e.g., norepinephrine, serotonin, and histamine), energy generation, regulation of plasma lipids, and protection of cells against oxidative damage.[50,51]

The normal adult daily intake of copper, from both animal and plant sources, is 2–3 mg. Plant copper is in the inorganic (free ionic) form, while meat (animal) copper is in the form of cuproproteins (copper–protein complex). Inorganic copper is absorbed in the upper portion of the GI tract (stomach and proximal duodenum) under acidic conditions. Cuproprotein copper is absorbed below the pancreatic duct after digestion.

Once absorbed, copper is bound to a mucosal copper-binding protein called metallothionein (a sulfur-rich, metal-binding protein present in intestinal mucosa). From this protein, copper is slowly released into the circulation, where it is readily taken up by the liver and other tissues.[50] Copper absorption may be reduced by a high

---

### ✎ Minicase 5 *continued*

cium (6.1 mg/dL) and phosphate (10.4 mg/dL). The patient's intact serum PTH was 280 pg/mL (10–60 pg/mL).

*What subjective and objective data for Paul M. are consistent with a diagnosis of calcium and phosphate abnormalities? What are the potential etiologies of calcium–phosphate disorder in this patient?*

**Discussion:** Paul M. has three laboratory abnormalities relating specifically to calcium–phosphate metabolism: (1) hypocalcemia, (2) hyperphosphatemia, and (3) severe hyperparathyroidism. He is exhibiting classic signs and symptoms of hypocalcemia, such as finger numbness, tingling, burning of extremities, confusion, fatigue, and positive Chvostek's and Trousseau's signs.

Chronic renal failure, as seen in Paul M., commonly is associated with hypocalcemia, hyperphosphatemia, hyperparathyroidism, and vitamin D deficiency. These calcium–phosphate abnormalities frequently lead to the secondary complication of renal osteodystrophy. As stated previously, no single mechanism is responsible for these abnormalities.

At earlier stages of his renal disease, Paul M.'s kidneys probably were retaining phosphate. As his serum phosphate concentration rose, his ionized calcium concentration fell and stimulated PTH release. This release led to secondary hyperparathyroidism. High concentrations of PTH reduced this patient's renal tubular reabsorption of phosphate and increased its excretion. Both his serum phosphate and calcium concentrations then returned to normal as a result of hyperparathyroidism (Figure 3).

As Paul M.'s renal disease worsened (GFR fell below 30 mL/min), his renal tubules ceased to respond adequately to his high serum PTH concentrations. Hyperphosphatemia developed. In response to the hypocalcemia that followed, calcium was mobilized from the bone by a PTH-mediated mechanism. However, this

compensatory response obviously was not adequate since hypocalcemia and hyperphosphatemia persisted.

Although concentrations were not measured, this persistent hyperphosphatemia probably contributed to the diminished renal conversion of 25-HCC to its biologically active metabolite l,25-DHCC. As a result, the gut absorption of dietary calcium was diminished. Vitamin D deficiency also contributed to hypocalcemia and mobilization of calcium from bone. The metabolic acidosis of renal failure potentially present in Paul M. also may contribute to a negative calcium balance in the bone.

Paul M. was relatively asymptomatic up to this point, primarily because these laboratory abnormalities developed chronically and were, therefore, better tolerated. When nausea and vomiting developed and his appetite decreased, his oral calcium intake probably was substantially reduced. This reduction potentially enhanced his malaise. During this period of malnutrition, the patient's serum albumin concentration also diminished, which further contributed to his hypocalcemia.

Since calcium is reported as total calcium and not as the free or ionized fraction, Paul M.'s total serum calcium concentration must be corrected for his serum albumin value. For every 1-g/dL reduction in serum albumin less than 4 g/dL, 0.8 mg/dL should be added to his serum calcium concentration. Therefore, when corrected for his serum albumin concentration of 3 g/dL, Paul M.'s first serum calcium value of 7.5 mg/dL is equivalent to a total concentration of 8.3 mg/dL. Likewise, his second serum calcium value of 6.1 mg/dL is equivalent to a total concentration of 6.9 mg/dL.

During hospitalization, the calcium content of Paul M.'s hyperalimentation solution was apparently not adequate for correcting or sustaining his serum calcium concentration. Therefore, the worsening of his hypocalcemia augmented his hyperparathyroidism and increased his serum phosphate concentration.

intake of zinc (>20 mg/day), ascorbic acid, and dietary fiber. Zinc may induce the synthesis of intestinal metallothionein and form a barrier to copper ion absorption.[50,51]

The normal adult body contains 75–150 mg of copper, with approximately one-third found in the liver and brain at high tissue concentrations.[52] Another one-third is located in the muscles at low tissue concentrations. The rest is found in the heart, spleen, kidneys, and blood (erythrocytes and neutrophils).[50,52]

In the liver, copper is bound by an $\alpha_2$-globulin to form ceruloplasmin, a blue copper protein.[49] In the circulation, 95% of copper is protein bound as ceruloplasmin (normal serum range: 2–15 mg/dL or 20–150 mg/L for newborns; 30–50 mg/dL or 300–500 mg/L for pediatrics and adults). The remainder is bound to albumin and amino acids or is free.[50,52] Since ceruloplasmin accounts for such a large fraction of serum copper, changes in its concentration determine serum copper concentrations.[53] Copper is eliminated mainly by biliary excretion (average 25 µg/kg/day), with only 0.5–3% of daily intake found in the urine.[50]

## Hypocupremia

Although many persons have copper intakes below the recommended level, copper deficiency is uncommon in humans.[51] Hypocupremia usually occurs in infants with chronic diarrhea or a malabsorption syndrome or those whose diet consists mostly of milk.[49,51,53] Premature infants, who typically have low copper stores, are at a higher risk for developing copper deficiency under these circumstances.[50]

In adults, copper deficiency occurs in patients receiving long-term hyperalimentation solutions low in copper. Certain malabsorption syndromes (e.g., celiac disease and ulcerative colitis), protein-losing enteropathies, and nephrotic syndrome also may cause copper deficiency; however, symptomatic deficiency is rare.[49,53] Vegetarians are at an increased risk because (1) some major food sources of copper are meat, and (2) plant sources have a high-fiber content that may interfere with copper absorption.[49]

Menkes' syndrome (also called kinky- or steely-hair syndrome) is a rare disorder that leads to defective copper absorption with accumulation in the intestinal mucosa. Patients with Menkes' syndrome have reduced copper concentrations in the blood, liver, and brain.[49,51] These patients (mostly children) suffer from slow growth and retardation, defective keratinization and pigmentation of hair, hypothermia, and degenerative changes in the aortic elastin. Paradoxically, anemia and neutropenia usually are not present.

Prolonged hypocupremia leads to a syndrome of neutropenia and iron-deficiency anemia correctable with copper.[53] The anemia is normocytic and hypochromic and

is due mainly to poor iron absorption and ineffective heme incorporation of iron.[45,52] Copper deficiency can affect any system or organ whose enzymes require copper for proper functioning. As such, copper deficiency may lead to abnormal glucose tolerance, arrhythmias, hypercholesterolemia, atherosclerosis, depressed immune function, defective connective tissue formation, demineralization of bones, and pathological fractures.[51]

## Hypercupremia

Copper excess is not common in humans and usually occurs with a deliberate attempt to ingest large quantities of copper. Acute or long-term ingestions of greater than 15 mg of elemental copper may lead to symptomatic copper poisoning.[52] Like other metallic poisonings, acute copper poisoning leads to nausea, vomiting, intestinal cramps, and diarrhea.[52] Larger ingestions leads to shock, hepatic necrosis, intravascular hemolysis, renal impairment, coma, and death.[53]

Wilson's disease, an autosomal recessive disorder, leads to excessive accumulation of copper in the liver, brain, kidneys, and cornea. Paradoxically, it is associated with decreased serum copper and ceruloplasmin concentrations. Wilson's disease is caused by an abnormal form of metallothionein that has a high binding affinity for copper. The excessive tissue content is a result of decreased biliary excretion of copper and may cause cirrhosis, neurological disorders, and renal failure. Chronic cholestasis, as seen in primary biliary cirrhosis, also may lead to hepatic copper accumulation.[49,50,53]

Patients with Wilson's disease suffer from chronic hepatitis, resting and intention tremors, choreoathetosis, dysarthria, disturbances in gait maintenance, Fanconi syndrome (a proximal renal tubular disease), and copper deposits in the cornea (called Kayser-Fleischer rings).[53]

# Zinc
*Normal range: 70–130 µg/dL or 10.7–19.9 µmol/L*

## Physiology

Next to iron, zinc is the most abundant trace element in the body. It is an essential nutrient that is a constituent of, or a cofactor to, many enzymes. These metalloenzymes participate in the metabolism of carbohydrates, proteins, lipids, and nucleic acids.[50] As such, zinc influences[50,53]

- Tissue growth and repair.
- Cell membrane stabilization.
- Bone collagenase activity and collagen turnover.
- Immune response, especially T-cell mediated response.
- Sensory control of food intake.
- Spermatogenesis and gonadal maturation.
- Normal testicular function.

The normal adult body contains 1.5–2.5 g of zinc.[51]

Food sources of zinc include meat products, oysters, and legumes.[50] Food zinc is bound largely to proteins and released below the common duct for absorption by the ileum. Ionic zinc found in zinc supplements is absorbed in the duodenum due to a lower pH in that region.[50] Body zinc stores control, to some extent, the percentage of zinc that is absorbed from food and mineral supplements. Foods rich in calcium, dietary fiber, or phytate may interfere with zinc absorption, as can folic acid supplements.[50]

After absorption, zinc is transported from the small intestine to the portal circulation, where it binds to proteins such as albumin, transferrin, and globulins.[50] Circulating zinc is bound mostly to serum proteins; two-thirds is bound loosely to albumin and prealbumin, while one-third is bound tightly to $\alpha_2$-macroglobulin.[53] Only 2–3% of zinc is either in free ionic form or bound to amino acids.[50]

Zinc distributes to many organs. Tissues high in zinc include the liver, pancreas, spleen, lungs, eyes (retina, iris, cornea, and lens), prostate, skeletal muscle, and bone. Because of their mass, skeletal muscle (60–62%) and bone (20–28%) have the highest zinc contents of body tissues.[50] Only 2–4% of total body zinc is contained in the liver. In blood, 85% is in erythrocytes, although each leukocyte contains 25 times the zinc content of an erythrocyte.[51]

A plasma zinc concentration is the best indicator of total body zinc status; however, this laboratory test has certain limitations.[50] Acute stress situations, such as infection and acute myocardial infarction, may increase distribution of zinc to the liver and lower serum zinc concentrations, even when total body zinc is normal. Conversely, serum zinc concentrations may be normal during starvation or wasting syndromes due to release of zinc from tissues and cells.[50]

Zinc undergoes substantial enteropancreatic recirculation and is excreted primarily in pancreatic and intestinal secretions. Zinc also is lost dermally through sweat, hair and nail growth, and skin shedding. Except in certain disease states, only 2% of zinc is lost in the urine.[50]

### Hypozincemia

In Western countries, zinc deficiency is rare from inadequate intake. Persons with serum zinc concentrations below 70 μg/dL (<10.7 μmol/L) are at an increased risk for developing symptomatic zinc deficiency. Given the caveats of measuring serum zinc concentrations in certain disease states, response to zinc supplements may be the only way of diagnosing this deficiency. In many chronic diseases, it is unclear whether zinc deficiency is clinical or subclinical due to reduced protein binding.[53] Conditions leading to deficiency may be divided into five classes (Table 13):[50,53]

➤ Low intake.
➤ Decreased absorption.
➤ Increased utilization.

**TABLE 13.** Etiologies of Zinc Deficiency

**Low intake**
  Anorexia
  Nutritional deficiencies
    Alcoholism
    Chronic renal failure
    Premature infants
    Some vegetarian diets
    Therapy with hyperalimentation solutions
**Decreased absorption**
  Acrodermatitis enteropathica
  Malabsorption syndromes
**Increased utilization**
  Adolescence
  Lactation
  Menstruation
  Pregnancy
**Increased loss**
  Alcoholism
  β-Thalassemia
  Cirrhosis
  Diabetes mellitus
  Diarrhea
  Diuretic therapy
  Enterocutaneous fistula drainage
  Exercise (long term, strenuous)
  Glucagon
  Loss of enteropancreatic recycling
  Nephrotic syndrome
  Protein-losing enteropathies
  Sickle cell anemia
  Therapy with hyperalimentation solutions
**Unknown causes**
  Arthritis and other inflammatory diseases
  Down's syndrome

➤ Increased loss.
➤ Unknown causes.

The most likely candidates for zinc deficiency are infants; rapidly growing adolescents; menstruating, lactating, or pregnant women; persons with low meat intake; institutionalized patients; and patients on zinc-deficient hyperalimentation solutions.[53] Acrodermatitis enteropathica is an autosomal, recessive disorder involving zinc malabsorption that occurs in infants of Italian, Armenian, and Iranian heritage. It is characterized by severe dermatitis, chronic diarrhea, emotional disturbances, and growth retardation.[50] Examples of malabsorption syndromes that may lead to zinc deficiency include Crohn's disease, ulcerative colitis, celiac sprue (gluten enteropathy), and short-bowel syndrome.

Excessive zinc may be lost in the urine (hyperzincuria), as occurs in alcoholism, ß-thalassemia, diabetes mellitus (due to hyperglycemia), diuretic therapy, nephrotic syndrome, sickle cell anemia, and therapy with hyperalimentation solutions. Excessive zinc may be lost dermally in athletes who routinely perform strenuous exercises.[50,53]

Because zinc is involved with a diverse group of en-

**TABLE 14.** Signs and Symptoms of Zinc Deficiency

**Signs**
    Acrodermatitis enteropathica
    Anemia
    Anergy to skin test antigens
    Complicated pregnancy
        Excess bleeding
        Maternal infection
        Premature or stillborn birth
        Spontaneous abortion
        Toxemia
    Decreased basal metabolic rate
    Decreased circulating thyroxine ($T_4$) concentration
    Decreased lymphocyte count and function
    Effect on fetus, infant, or child
        Congenital defects of skeleton, lungs, and CNS
        Fetal disturbances
        Growth retardation
        Hypogonadism
    Impaired neutrophil function
    Impairment and delaying of platelet aggregation
    Increased susceptibility to dental caries
    Increased susceptibility to infections
    Mental disturbance
    Pica
    Poor wound healing
    Short stature in children
    Skeletal deformities

**Symptoms**
    Acne and recurrent furunculosis
    Ataxia
    Decreased appetite
    Defective night vision
    Hypogeusia
    Hyposmia
    Impotence
    Mouth ulcers

zymes, its deficiency manifests in numerous organs and physiological systems (Table 14).[50] Hypogeusia and hyposmia are diminished taste and smell acuity, respectively. Pica is a pathological craving for specific food or nonfood substances (e.g., geophagia). Chronic zinc deficiency, as occurs in acrodermatitis enteropathica, leads to growth retardation, anemia, hypogonadism, hepatosplenomegaly, and impaired wound healing. Additional signs and symptoms of acrodermatitis enteropathica include diarrhea; vomiting; alopecia; skin lesions in oral, anal, and genital areas; paronychia; nail deformity; emotional lability; photophobia; blepharitis; conjunctivitis; and corneal opacities.[50,53]

### Hyperzincemia

Zinc is one of the least toxic trace elements.[53] Clinical manifestations of excess zinc occur with chronic, high doses of a zinc supplement. However, patients with Wilson's disease who commonly take high doses of zinc rarely show signs of toxicity. This situation may be due to stabilization of serum zinc concentrations during high-dose administration.[50] As much as 12 g of zinc sulfate (>2700 mg of elemental zinc) taken over 2 days has caused drowsiness, lethargy, and increases in serum lipase and amylase concentrations. Nausea, vomiting, and diarrhea also may occur.[50]

Serum zinc concentrations must be measured using nonhemolyzed samples. Erythrocytes and leukocytes, like many other cells, are rich in zinc. When they are allowed to hemolyze in the tube (e.g., too small a needle is used to draw the sample, tourniquet is too tight, or specimen stands too long or is mishandled), these cells release zinc into the specimen in quantities large enough to produce misleading results. This phenomenon can also occur when the specimen is allowed to clot (with nonheparinized tubes).[50]

## Manganese
*Normal range: 2–3 µg/L or 36–55 µmol/L for adults*

### Physiology

Manganese is an essential trace element that serves as a cofactor for numerous diverse enzymes involved in carbohydrate, protein, and lipid metabolism; protection of cells from free radicals; steroid biosynthesis; and metabolism of biogenic amines.[54] Interestingly, manganese deficiency does not affect the functions of most of these enzymes, presumably because magnesium may substitute for manganese in most instances.[53] In animals, manganese is required for normal bone growth, lipid metabolism, reproduction, and CNS regulation.[51]

Manganese has an important role in the normal function of the brain, primarily through its effect on biogenic amine metabolism. This effect may be responsible for the relationship between brain concentration of manganese and catecholamine.[54]

The manganese content of the adult body is 10–20 mg. Manganese homeostasis is regulated through the control of its absorption and excretion.[54] Plants are the primary source of food manganese, since animal tissues have low contents.[54] Manganese is absorbed from the small intestine by a mechanism similar to that of iron;[51] however, only 3–4% of the ingested manganese is absorbed. Dietary iron and phytate may affect manganese absorption.[49]

Human and animal tissues have a low manganese content.[54] Tissues relatively high in manganese are the bone, liver, pancreas, and pituitary gland.[49,54] Most circulating manganese is loosely bound to the ß$_1$-globulin transmanganin, a transport protein similar to transferrin.[51,53] In situations of overexposure, excess manganese accumulates in the liver and brain, causing severe neuromuscular signs and symptoms.[49]

Manganese is excreted primarily in biliary and pancreatic juices. In manganese overload, other GI routes of elimination also may be used. Little manganese is lost in urine.[53,54]

### Manganese Deficiency

Due to its relative abundance in plant sources, manganese deficiency is rare among the general population.[49] Deficiency normally occurs after several months of deliberate manganese omission from the diet.[53,54] Little information is available regarding serum manganese concentrations and disease states in humans.[53]

Information from the signs and symptoms of manganese deficiency comes from experimental subjects who intentionally followed low-manganese diets for many months. Their signs and symptoms included weight loss, slow hair and nail growth, color change in hair and beard, transient dermatitis, hypocholesterolemia, and hypotriglyceridemia.[54]

Adults and children with convulsive disorders have lower mean serum manganese concentrations than normal subjects, although a cause-and-effect relationship has not been established. However, serum manganese concentrations correlate with seizure frequency.[54] Animals deficient in manganese show defective growth, skeletal malformation, ataxia, reproductive abnormalities, and disturbances in lipid metabolism.[49,53]

### *Manganese Excess*

Manganese is one of the least toxic trace elements.[53] Its excess primarily occurs through inhalation of manganese compounds (e.g., manganese mines).[54] Since excess drug accumulates in the liver and brain, severe neuromuscular manifestations occur. They include encephalopathy and profound neurological disturbances mimicking Parkinson's disease.[49,53,54] These manifestations are not surprising since metabolism of biogenic amines is altered in both manganese excess and Parkinson's disease. Other signs and symptoms include anorexia, apathy, headache, impotence, and speech disturbances.[53] Inhalation of manganese products may lead to manganese pneumonitis.[54]

## Chromium
*Normal range: 1–5 µg/L or 18–92 nmol/L*

### *Physiology*

The main physiological role of chromium is as a cofactor for insulin.[55] In its organic form, chromium potentiates the action of endogenous and exogenous insulin, presumably by augmenting its adherence to cell membranes.[49] The organic form is in the dinicotinic acid–glutathione complex or glucose tolerance factor (GTF).[51] Chromium is the metal portion of GTF; with insulin, GTF affects the metabolism of glucose, cholesterol, and triglycerides.[53] Therefore, chromium is important for glucose tolerance, glycogen synthesis, amino acid transport, and protein synthesis. Chromium is also involved in the activation of several enzymes.[51]

The adult body contains an average of 5 mg of chromium.[53] Food sources of chromium include brewer's yeast, spices, vegetable oils, unrefined sugar, liver, kidney, beer, meat, dairy products, and wheat germ.[50,51] GTF is present in the diet and can be synthesized from inorganic trivalent chromium ($Cr^{+3}$) available in food and dietary supplements.[50] Chromium is absorbed via a common pathway with zinc; its degree of absorption is inversely related to dietary intake, varying from 0.5 to 2%.[49,50] Absorption of $Cr^{+3}$ from GTF is 10–25%, but the absorption is only 1% for inorganic chromium.[51]

Chromium circulates as free $Cr^{3+}$, bound to transferrin and other proteins, and as the GTF complex.[50,53] GTF is the biologically active moiety and is more important than total serum chromium concentration.[53] Trivalent chromium accumulates in the hair, kidneys, skeleton, liver, spleen, lungs, testes, and large intestine. GTF concentrates in insulin-responsive tissues such as the liver.[50,51]

The metabolism of chromium is not well understood for several reasons:[51]

> ➤ Low concentrations in tissues.
> ➤ Difficulty in analyzing chromium in biological fluids and tissue samples.
> ➤ Presence of different chromium forms in food.

Homeostasis is controlled by release of chromium from GTF and by dietary absorption.[50] The kidneys are the main route of elimination.[53] The urinary excretion of chromium is constant despite variability in the fraction absorbed; however, excretion increases after glucose or insulin administration.[50,53] Insulin, or a stimulus for insulin release, can mobilize chromium from its stores. This increased release in chromium then is lost in the urine. Therefore, circulating insulin controls the daily loss and requirement of chromium.[55]

### *Chromium Deficiency*

Because body chromium status cannot be reliably assessed,[50] a diagnosis of chromium deficiency is based on response to chromium supplements (e.g., improvement in glucose tolerance).[55] As with other trace elements, the risk for developing deficiency increases in patients receiving prescribed nourishment low in chromium content (e.g., hyperalimentation solutions).[55] Marginal deficiencies or defects in utilization of chromium may be present in the elderly, patients with diabetes, or patients with atherosclerotic coronary artery disease.[50] The hepatic stores of chromium decrease 10-fold in the elderly, suggesting a predisposition to deficiency. Since chromium is involved in lipid and cholesterol metabolism, its deficiency is a suspected risk factor for the development of atherosclerosis.[50,55]

Urinary losses of chromium due to hyperglycemia, coupled with marginal intake, predispose to deficiency that worsens glucose tolerance metabolism.[55] This mechanism is suspected for chromium deficiency in patients with Type II diabetes mellitus.[50,55] Finally, multiparous women are at a higher risk than nulliparous women for becoming chromium deficient because, over time, chromium intake may not be adequate to meet fetal needs and maintain a mother's stores.[55]

The main manifestation of chromium deficiency involves insulin resistance and disturbance in glucose metabolism. Such abnormalities may be divided into three stages:

1. Glucose intolerance occurs but is masked by a compensatory increase in insulin release.
2. Impaired glucose tolerance and disturbance in lipid metabolism are clinically evident.
3. Marked insulin resistance and manifestations of diabetes' unresponsiveness to insulin are evident.[55]

Therefore, chromium deficiency may contribute to many conditions that affect glucose tolerance, such as pregnancy and protein-calorie malnutrition.[50,55]

Chromium deficiency may lead to hypercholesterolemia and, as a result, serve as a risk factor for development of atherosclerotic disease.[50] Low chromium tissue concentrations have been associated with cardiovascular disease, although a cause-and-effect relationship has not been established. Likewise, a negative correlation has been established between cardiovascular morbidity and mortality and chromium intake.[55]

### *Chromium Excess*

Chromium has very low toxicity. As such, information is lacking about the clinical significance of a high body chromium content.

## SUMMARY

Hyponatremia and hypernatremia may be associated with high, normal, or low total body sodium. Hyponatremia may be due to abnormal accumulation of water in the intravascular space (dilutional hyponatremia), a decline in both extracellular water and sodium, or a reduction in total body sodium, with the water balance remaining normal. Hypernatremia is most common in patients with either an impaired thirst mechanism (e.g., neurohypophyseal lesion) or an inability to replace water depleted through normal insensible losses or from renal or GI losses. Signs and symptoms of a sodium and water imbalance mostly involve the neurological system. The most common symptom of hyponatremia is confusion; however, if sodium continues to fall, seizure, coma, and death may result. Thirst is a major symptom of hypernatremia; an elevated urine specific gravity, indicating concentrated urine, is uniformly observed.

Hypokalemia and hyperkalemia may indicate either a true or an apparent (due to transcellular shifting) potassium imbalance. Hypokalemia can occur due to excessive loss from the kidneys (diuretics) or GI tract (vomiting). The most serious manifestation involves the cardiovascular system (i.e., cardiac arrhythmias). Renal impairment,

usually in the presence of high intake, commonly causes hyperkalemia. Like hypokalemia, the most serious clinical manifestations of hyperkalemia involve the cardiovascular system.

A serum chloride concentration serves as a confirmatory test to identify fluid balance and acid–base abnormalities. Hypochloremia may be diuretic induced and is due to the concurrent loss of sodium and contraction alkalosis. Hyperchloremia may occur with parenteral nutrition solutions with a chloride:sodium ratio greater than 1. Signs and symptoms associated with these conditions are related to the fluid status or acid–base balance and underlying causes rather than to chloride itself.

Hypomagnesemia usually results from excessive loss from the GI tract (e.g., nasogastric suction, biliary loss, or fecal fistula) or from the kidneys (e.g., diuresis). Magnesium depletion usually is associated with neuromuscular symptoms such as weakness, muscle fasciculation with tremor, tetany, and increased reflexes. Increased magnesium intake in the presence of renal dysfunction commonly causes hypermagnesemia. Neuromuscular signs and symptoms opposite those caused by hypomagnesemia are observed.

The most common causes of true hypocalcemia are disorders of vitamin D metabolism and PTH production. In acute settings, hypocalcemia can be a medical emergency and lead to cardiac arrhythmias and tetany. Symptoms primarily involve the neuromuscular system.

The most common causes of hypercalcemia are malignancy and primary hyperparathyroidism. In acute settings, hypercalcemia can be a medical emergency and lead to cardiac arrhythmias. Symptoms often consist of vague GI complaints such as nausea, vomiting, abdominal pain, anorexia, constipation, and diarrhea.

The most common causes of hypophosphatemia are decreased intake and increased renal loss. Although mild hypophosphatemia usually is asymptomatic, severe depletion (<1 mg/dL or <0.32 mmol/L) typically is associated with muscle weakness, rhabdomyolysis, paresthesia, hemolysis, platelet dysfunction, and cardiac and respiratory failure. The most common cause of hyperphosphatemia is renal dysfunction, usually occurring as the GFR falls below 25 mL/min. Signs and symptoms of this condition are due primarily to the hypocalcemia and hyperparathyroidism that often ensue.

Hypocupremia is uncommon in humans but can occur in infants, especially those born prematurely, those who have chronic diarrhea or a malabsorption syndrome, or those whose diet consists mostly of milk. Prolonged hypocupremia leads to a syndrome of neutropenia and iron-deficiency anemia correctable with copper.

Copper excess is not common in humans and usually occurs with a deliberate attempt to ingest large quantities. Like other metallic poisonings, acute copper poisoning leads to nausea and vomiting, intestinal cramps, and diarrhea.

Likely candidates for zinc deficiency are infants; rapidly growing adolescents; menstruating, lactating, or pregnant women; persons with low meat intake; institutionalized patients; and patients on hyperalimentation solutions. Because zinc is involved with a diverse group of enzymes, its deficiency manifests in numerous organs and physiological systems. Zinc excess occurs with chronic, high doses of a zinc supplement. Signs and symptoms include nausea, vomiting, diarrhea, drowsiness, lethargy, and increases in serum lipase and amylase concentrations.

Manganese deficiency normally occurs after several months of deliberate omission from the diet. Signs and symptoms include weight loss, slow hair and nail growth, color change in hair and beard, transient dermatitis, hypocholesterolemia, and hypotriglyceridemia. Manganese excess primarily occurs through inhalation of manganese compounds (e.g., manganese mines). Due to excess accumulation, severe neuromuscular manifestations occur, including encephalopathy and profound neurological disturbances mimicking Parkinson's disease. Inhalation of manganese products may lead to manganese pneumonitis.

The risk for developing chromium deficiency increases in patients receiving prescribed nourishment low in chromium content (e.g., hyperalimentation solutions). The main manifestations of deficiency involve insulin resistance and disturbance in glucose metabolism.

## REFERENCES

1. Sterns RH, Spital A. Disorders of water balance. In: Kokko JP, Tannen RL, eds. Fluids and electrolytes, 2nd ed. Philadelphia, PA: Harcourt Brace Jovanovich; 1990:139–94.
2. Guyton AC, ed. Textbook of medical physiology, 8th ed. Philadelphia, PA: W. B. Saunders; 1991.
3. Berl T, Schrier RW. Disorders of water metabolism. In: Schrier RW, ed. Renal and electrolyte disorders, 4th ed. Boston, MA: Little, Brown; 1992:1–87.
4. Rose BD, ed. Clinical physiology of acid-base and electrolyte disorders, 4th ed. New York: McGraw-Hill; 1994.
5. Briggs JP, Sawaya BE, Schnermann J. Disorders of salt balance. In: Kokko JP, Tannen RL, eds. Fluids and electrolytes, 2nd ed. Philadelphia, PA: Harcourt Brace Jovanovich; 1990:70–138.
6. Halperin ML, Goldstein MB, eds. Fluid, electrolyte, and acid-base physiology: a problem-based approach, 2nd ed. Philadelphia, PA: W. B. Saunders; 1994.
7. Zull DN. Disorders of potassium metabolism. *Emerg Med Clin North Am.* 1989; 7:771–94.
8. Oh MS, Carroll HJ. Electrolyte and acid-base disorders. In: Chernow B, ed. The pharmacologic approach to the critically ill patient, 3rd ed. Baltimore, MD: Williams & Wilkins; 1994:957–68.
9. Gabow PA, Peterson LN. Disorders of potassium metabolism. In: Schrier RW, ed. Renal and electrolyte disorders, 4th ed. Boston, MA: Little, Brown; 1992:231–85.
10. Tannen RL. Potassium disorders. In: Kokko JP, Tannen RL, eds. Fluids and electrolytes, 2nd ed. Philadelphia, PA: Harcourt Brace Jovanovich; 1990:195–300.
11. Rose BD. Diuretics. *Kidney Int.* 1991; 39:336–52.
12. Williams ME. Endocrine crises. Hyperkalemia. *Crit Care Clin.* 1991; 7:155–74.
13. Freedman BI, Burkart JM. Endocrine crises: hypokalemia. *Crit Care Clin.* 1991; 7:143–53.
14. The fifth report of the Joint National Committee on Detection, Evaluation, and Treatment of High Blood Pressure (JNC V). *Arch Intern Med.* 1993; 153:154–83.
15. Siegel D, Hulley SB, Black DM, et al. Diuretics, serum and intracellular electrolyte levels, and ventricular arrhythmias in hypertensive men. *JAMA.* 1992; 267:1083–9.
16. Moser M. Current hypertension management: separating fact from fiction. *Cleve Clin J Med.* 1993; 60:27–37.
17. Papademetriou V, Burris JF, Notargiacomo A, et al. Thiazide therapy is not a cause of arrhythmia in patients with systemic hypertension. *Arch Intern Med.* 1988; 148:1272–6.
18. Ellison DH. Diuretic drugs and the treatment of edema: from clinic to bench and back again. *Am J Kidney Dis.* 1994; 23:623–43.
19. Shapiro JI, Kaehny WD. Pathogenesis and management of metabolic acidosis and alkalosis. In: Schrier RW, ed. Renal and electrolyte disorders, 4th ed. Boston, MA: Little, Brown; 1992:161–210.
20. Kaehny WD. Pathogenesis and management of respiratory and mixed acid-base disorders. In: Schrier RW, ed. Renal and electrolyte disorders, 4th ed. Boston, MA: Little, Brown; 1992:211–30.
21. Koch SM, Taylor RW. Chloride ion in intensive care medicine. *Crit Care Med.* 1992; 20:227–40.
22. Alfrey AC. Normal and abnormal magnesium metabolism. In: Schrier RW, ed. Renal and electrolyte disorders, 4th ed. Boston, MA: Little, Brown; 1992:371–404.
23. Salem M, Munoz R, Chernow B. Hypomagnesemia in critical illness: a common and clinically important problem. *Crit Care Clin.* 1991; 7:225–52.
24. Cronin RE. Magnesium disorders. In: Kokko JP, Tannen RL, eds. Fluids and electrolytes, 2nd ed. Philadelphia, PA: Harcourt Brace Jovanovich; 1990:631–45.
25. Ghamdi SM, Cameron EC, Sutton RA. Magnesium deficiency: pathophysiologic and clinical overview. *Am J Kidney Dis.* 1994; 24:737–52.
26. Berkelhammer C, Bear RA. A clinical approach to common electrolyte problems: hypomagnesemia. *Can Med Assoc J.* 1985; 132:360–8.
27. Van-Hook JW. Endocrine crises: hypermagnesemia. *Crit Care Clin.* 1991; 7:215–23.
28. Pak CYC. Calcium disorders: hypercalcemia and hypocalcemia. In: Kokko JP, Tannen RL, eds. Fluids and electrolytes, 2nd ed. Philadelphia, PA: Harcourt Brace Jovanovich; 1990:596–630.
29. Zelis R, Moore R. Recent insights into the calcium channels. *Circulation.* 1989; 80(Suppl IV):14–6.
30. DeLuca HF, Krisinger J, Darwish H. The vitamin D system: 1990. *Kidney Int.* 1990; 29(Suppl 8):S2–8.
31. Slatopolsky E, Hruska K, Klahr S. Disorders of phosphorus, calcium, and magnesium metabolism. In: Schrier RW, Gottschalk CW, eds. Diseases of the kidney, 5th ed. Boston, MA: Little, Brown; 1993:2599–644.
32. Slatopolsky E, Lopez-Hilker S, Delmez J, et al. The parathyroid-calcitriol axis in health and chronic renal failure. *Kidney Int.* 1990; 29(Suppl 7):S41–7.
33. Ateshkadi A, Johnson CA. Chronic renal failure. In: Young LY, Koda-Kimble MA, eds. Applied therapeutics: the clinical use of drugs, 6th ed. Vancouver, British Columbia: Applied Therapeutics, Inc.; 1995:1–29.
34. Slatopolsky E, Berkoben M, Kelber J, et al. Effects of calcitriol and non-calcemic vitamin D analogs on secondary hyperparathyroidism. *Kidney Int.* 1992; 38(Suppl

9):S43–9.

35. Zaloga GP, Chernow B. Divalent ions: calcium, magnesium, and phosphorus. In: Chernow B, ed. The pharmacologic approach to the critically ill patient, 3rd ed. Baltimore, MD: Williams & Wilkins; 1994:777–804.

36. Ritz E, Matthias S, Seidel A, et al. Disturbed calcium metabolism in renal failure—pathogenesis and therapeutic strategies. *Kidney Int.* 1992; 42(Suppl 38):S37–42.

37. Zaloga GP. Hypocalcemic crisis. *Crit Care Clin.* 1991; 7:191–200.

38. Zaloga GP. Hypocalcemia in critically ill patients. *Crit Care Med.* 1992; 20:251–62.

39. Mundy GR. Hypercalcemia of malignancy. *Kidney Int.* 1987; 31:142–55.

40. Popovtzer MM, Knochel JP, Kumar R. Disorders of calcium, phosphorus, vitamin D, and parathyroid hormone activity. In: Schrier RW, ed. Renal and electrolyte disorders, 4th ed. Boston, MA: Little, Brown; 1992:287–369.

41. Hall TG, Schaiff RA. Update on the medical treatment of hypercalcemia of malignancy. *Clin Pharm.* 1993; 12:117–25.

42. Randall RE, Straus MB, McNeely WF, et al. The milk-alkali syndrome. *Arch Intern Med.* 1961; 107:63–81.

43. Bilezikian JP. Management of acute hypercalcemia. *N Engl J Med.* 1992; 326:1196–1203.

44. Davis KD, Attie MF. Management of severe hypercalcemia. *Crit Care Clin.* 1991; 7:175–90.

45. Delmez JA, Slatopolsky E. Hyperphosphatemia: its consequences and treatment in patients with chronic renal disease. *Am J Kidney Dis.* 1992; 19:303–17.

46. Lau K. Phosphate disorders. In: Kokko JP, Tannen RL, eds. Fluids and electrolytes, 2nd ed. Philadelphia, PA: Harcourt Brace Jovanovich; 1990:505–95.

47. Peppers MP, Geheb M, Desai T. Endocrine crises: hypophosphatemia and hyperphosphatemia. *Crit Care Clin.* 1991; 7:201–14.

48. Halevy J, Bulvik S. Severe hypophosphatemia in hospitalized patients. *Arch Intern Med.* 1988; 148:153–5.

49. Williams SR, ed. Nutrition and diet therapy. St. Louis, MO: C. V. Mosby; 1993.

50. Flodin N, ed. Pharmacology of micronutrients. New York: Alan R. Liss; 1988.

51. Robinson CH, Lawler MR, Chenoweth WL, et al., eds. Normal and therapeutic nutrition, 7th ed. New York: Macmillan; 1990.

52. Grant JP, Ross LH. Parenteral nutrition. In: Chernow B, ed. The pharmacologic approach to the critically ill patient, 3rd ed. Baltimore, MD: Williams & Wilkins; 1994:1009–33.

53. Lindeman RD. Minerals in medical practice. In: Halpern SL, ed. Quick reference to clinical nutrition, 2nd ed. Philadelphia, PA: J. B. Lippincott; 1987:295–323.

54. Hurley LS. Clinical and experimental aspect of manganese in nutrition. In: Prasad AR, ed. Clinical, biochemical, and nutritional aspects of trace elements, 1st ed. New York: Alan R. Liss; 1982:369–78.

55. Mertz W. Clinical and public health significance of chromium. In: Prasad AS, ed. Clinical, biochemical, and nutritional aspects of trace elements, 1st ed. New York: Alan R. Liss; 1982:315–23.

## QuickView—Sodium

| Parameter | Description | Comments |
|---|---|---|
| **Common reference ranges** | | |
| Adults | 136–145 mEq/L (136–145 mmol/L) | Measure of water status |
| Pediatrics | 130–140 mEq/L (130–140 mmol/L) | Premature |
| | 135–145 mEq/L (135–145 mmol/L) | Older |
| **Critical value** | >160 or <120 mEq/L (>160 or <120 mmol/L) | Acute changes more dangerous than chronic abnormalities |
| **Natural substance?** | Yes | Most abundant cation in extracellular fluid |
| **Inherent activity?** | Yes | Maintenance of transmembrane electric potential |
| **Location** | | |
| Storage | Mostly in extracellular fluid | |
| Secretion/excretion | Filtered by kidneys, mostly reabsorbed; some secretion in distal nephron | Closely related to water homeostasis |
| **Major causes of . . .** | | |
| High results | Multiple (discussed in text) | Can occur with low, normal, or high total body sodium |
| Associated signs and symptoms | Mostly neurological | Table 4 |
| Low results | Multiple (discussed in text) | Can occur with low, normal, or high total body sodium |
| Associated signs and symptoms | Mostly neurological | Table 2 |
| **After insult, time to . . .** | | |
| Initial elevation or positive result | Hours to years, depending on chronicity | The faster the change, the more dangerous the consequences |
| Peak values | Hours to years, depending on chronicity | |
| Normalization | Days, if renal function is normal | Faster with appropriate treatment |
| **Drugs often monitored with test** | Diuretics, angiotensin converting enzyme inhibitors (ACE) inhibitors, ADH analogs | Any drug that affects water homeostasis |
| **Causes of spurious results** | None | |

## QuickView—Potassium

| Parameter | Description | Comments |
|---|---|---|
| **Common reference ranges** | | |
| Adults and pediatrics | 3.5–5.0 mEq/L (3.5–5.0 mmol/L) | >10 days old |
| **Critical value** | >7 or <2.5 mEq/L (>7 or <2.5 mmol/L) | Acute changes more dangerous than chronic abnormalities |
| **Natural substance?** | Yes | Most abundant cation; 98% in intracellular fluid |
| **Inherent activity?** | Yes | Control of muscle and nervous tissue excitability, acid–base balance, intracellular fluid balance |
| **Location** | | |
| Storage | 98% in intracellular fluid | |
| Secretion/excretion | Mostly secreted by distal nephron | Some via GI tract secretion |

*continued*

## QuickView—Potassium *continued*

| Parameter | Description | Comments |
|---|---|---|
| **Major causes of . . .** | | |
| High results | Renal failure (GFR <10 mL/min) | Usually with increased intake |
| Associated signs and symptoms | Mostly cardiac | ECG changes, bradycardia, hypotension, cardiac arrest |
| Low results | Decreased intake or increased loss | Usually combination of the two |
| Associated signs and symptoms | Involves many physiological systems | Table 6 |
| **After insult, time to . . .** | | |
| Initial elevation or positive result | Hours to years, depending on chronicity | The faster the change, the more dangerous the consequences |
| Peak values | Hours to years, depending on chronicity | |
| Normalization | Days, if renal function is normal | Faster with appropriate treatment |
| **Drugs often monitored with test** | Diuretic, ACE inhibitors, amphotericin B, *cis*-platinum | Potassium-containing preparations if renal failure present |
| **Causes of spurious results** | Hemolyzed samples (falsely elevated) | High potassium content in erythrocytes |

## QuickView—Chloride

| Parameter | Description | Comments |
|---|---|---|
| **Common reference ranges** | | |
| Adults and pediatrics | 96–106 mEq/L (96–106 mmol/L) | |
| **Critical value** | | Depends on underlying disorder |
| **Natural substance?** | Yes | |
| **Inherent activity?** | Yes | Primary anion in extracellular fluid and gastric juice, cardiac function, acid–base balance |
| **Location** | | |
| Storage | Extracellular fluid | Most abundant extracellular anion |
| Secretion/excretion | Passively follows sodium and water | Also influenced by acid–base balance |
| **Major causes of . . .** | | |
| High results | Dehydration<br>Acidemia | |
| Associated signs and symptoms | Associated with underlying disorder | |
| Low results | Nasogastric suction<br>Vomiting<br>Serum dilution<br>Alkalemia | |
| Associated signs and symptoms | Associated with underlying disorder | |
| **After insult, time to . . .** | | |
| Initial elevation or positive result | Hours to years, depending on chronicity | The faster the change, the more dangerous the consequences |
| Peak values | Hours to years, depending on chronicity | |
| Normalization | Days, if renal function is normal | Faster with appropriate treatment of underlying disorder |
| **Drugs often monitored with test** | Same as with sodium | |
| **Causes of spurious results** | Bromides; iodides (falsely elevated) | |

## QuickView—Magnesium

| Parameter | Description | Comments |
|---|---|---|
| **Common reference ranges**<br>  **Adults and pediatrics** | 1.5–2.2 mEq/L (0.75–1.1 mmol/L) | |
| **Critical value** | >5 or <1 mEq/L (>2.5 or <0.5 mmol/L) | Acute changes more dangerous than chronic abnormalities |
| **Natural substance?** | Yes | |
| **Inherent activity?** | Yes | Enzyme cofactor, thermoregulation, muscle contraction, nerve conduction, calcium and potassium homeostasis |
| **Location**<br>  **Storage** | 50% bone, 45% intracellular fluid, 5% extracellular fluid | |
|   **Secretion/excretion** | Filtration by kidneys | 3–5% reabsorbed |
| **Major causes of . . .**<br>  **High results** | Renal failure | Usually in presence of increased intake |
|   **Associated signs and symptoms** | Neuromuscular manifestations | Table 9 |
|   **Low results** | Excessive loss from GI tract or kidneys<br>Decreased intake | Alcoholism and diuretics |
|   **Associated signs and symptoms** | Neuromuscular and cardiovascular manifestations including weakness, muscle fasciculations, tremor, tetany, increased reflexes, and ECG abnormalities | More severe with acute changes |
| **After insult, time to . . .**<br>  **Initial elevation or positive result** | Hours to years, depending on chronicity | The faster the change, the more dangerous the consequences |
|   **Peak values** | Hours to years, depending on chronicity | |
|   **Normalization** | Days, if renal function is normal | Faster with appropriate treatment |
| **Drugs often monitored with test** | Diuretics and magnesium-containing antacids | |
| **Causes of spurious results** | Hemolyzed samples (falsely elevated) | |

## QuickView—Calcium

| Parameter | Description | Comments |
|---|---|---|
| **Common reference ranges**<br>  **Adults** | 8.5–10.8 mg/dL (2.1–2.7 mmol/L) | Approximately half is bound to serum proteins; only ionized (free) calcium is physiologically active |
|   **Pediatrics** | 8–10.5 mg/dL (2–2.6 mmol/L) | |
| **Critical value** | >14 or <7 mg/dL (>3.5 or <1.8 mmol/L) | Also depends on serum albumin and pH values |
| **Natural substance?** | Yes | |
| **Inherent activity?** | Yes | Preservation of cellular membranes, propagation of neuromuscular activity, regulation of endocrine functions, blood coagulation, bone metabolism, phosphate homeostasis |

*continued*

**QuickView—Calcium** *continued*

| Parameter | Description | Comments |
|---|---|---|
| **Location** | | |
|     **Storage** | 99.5% in bone and teeth | Very closely regulated |
|     **Secretion/excretion** | Filtration by kidneys | Small amounts excreted into GI tract from saliva, bile, and pancreatic and intestinal secretions |
| **Major causes of . . .** | | |
|     **High results** | Malignancy<br>Hyperparathyroidism | Also thiazide diuretics, lithium, vitamin D, and calcium supplements |
|       **Associated signs and symptoms** | Vague GI complaints and neurological, cardiovascular, and renal signs | More severe with acute onset |
|     **Low results** | Vitamin D deficiency<br>Hypoparathyroidism<br>Hyperphosphatemia<br>Pancreatitis<br>Loop diuretics<br>Calcitonin<br>Renal failure<br>Hypoalbuminemia | Hypocalcemia due to hypoalbuminemia is asymptomatic (ionized calcium concentration unaffected) |
|     **Associated signs and symptoms** | Primarily neuromuscular (e.g., fatigue, depression, memory loss, hallucinations, seizures, tetany) | More severe with acute onset |
| **After insult, time to . . .** | | |
|     **Initial elevation or positive result** | Hours to years, depending on chronicity | The faster the change, the more dangerous the consequences |
|     **Peak values** | Hours to years, depending on chronicity | |
|     **Normalization** | Days, if renal function is normal | Faster with appropriate treatment |
| **Drugs often monitored with test** | Loop diuretics, calcitonin, vitamin D, calcium supplements, phosphate binders | |
| **Causes of spurious results** | Hypoalbuminemia | Ionized calcium concentration usually unaffected |

**QuickView—Phosphate**

| Parameter | Description | Comments |
|---|---|---|
| **Common reference ranges** | | |
|     **Adults** | 2.6–4.5 mg/dL (0.84–1.45 mmol/L) | |
|     **Pediatrics** | 4–7.1 mg/dL (1.3–2.3 mmol/L) | |
| **Critical value** | >8 or <1 mg/dL (>2.6 or <0.3 mmol/L) | Acute changes more dangerous than chronic abnormalities |
| **Natural substance?** | Yes | Most abundant intracellular anion |
| **Inherent activity?** | Yes | Bone and tooth integrity, cellular membrane integrity, phospholipid synthesis, acid–base balance, calcium homeostasis, enzyme activation, formation of high-energy bonds |
| **Location** | | |
|     **Storage** | Extracellular fluid, cell membrane structure, intracellular fluid, collagen, bone | 85% in bone |
|     **Secretion/excretion** | Filtration by kidneys | Mostly reabsorbed |

## QuickView—Phosphate *continued*

| Parameter | Description | Comments |
|---|---|---|
| **Major causes of . . .** | | |
| **High results** | Decreased renal excretion<br>Extracellular shifting<br>Increased intake of phosphate or vitamin D | Renal failure the most common cause |
| **Associated signs and symptoms** | Due primarily to hypocalcemia and hyperparathyroidism | QuickView for calcium (hypocalcemia) |
| **Low results** | Increased renal excretion<br>Intracellular shifting<br>Decreased intake of phosphate or vitamin D | Also can occur in renal failure |
| **Associated signs and symptoms** | Bone pain, weakness, malaise, hypocalcemia, cardiac failure, respiratory failure | Usually due to diminished intracellular ATP and erythrocyte 2,3-DPG concentrations |
| **After insult, time to . . .** | | |
| **Initial elevation or positive result** | Usually over months to years | |
| **Peak values** | Usually over months to years | |
| **Normalization** | Over days with renal transplantation | |
| **Drugs often monitored with test** | Calcium-containing antacids, vitamin D, phosphate binders | |
| **Causes of spurious results** | Hemolyzed samples (falsely elevated) and methotrexate (falsely elevated) | |

## QuickView—Copper

| Parameter | Description | Comments |
|---|---|---|
| **Common reference ranges** | | |
| **Adults** | 75–150 µg/dL (11.8–23.6 µmol/L) | |
| **Pediatrics** | 20–70 µg/dL (3.1–11 µmol/L)<br>90–190 µg/dL (14.2–29.9 µmol/L)<br>80–160 µg/dL (12.6–25.2 µmol/L) | 0–6 months<br>6 years<br>12 years |
| **Critical value** | Not applicable | |
| **Natural substance?** | Yes | |
| **Inherent activity?** | Yes | Companion to iron, enzyme cofactor, Hgb synthesis, collagen and elastin synthesis, metabolism of many neurotransmitters, energy generation, regulation of plasma lipid levels, cell protection against oxidative damage |
| **Location** | | |
| **Storage** | One-third in liver and brain; one-third in muscles; the rest in heart, spleen, kidneys, and blood (erythrocytes and neutrophils) | 95% of circulating copper is protein bound as ceruloplasmin |
| **Secretion/excretion** | Mainly by biliary excretion; only 0.5–3% of daily intake found in urine | |

*continued*

## QuickView—Copper *continued*

| Parameter | Description | Comments |
|---|---|---|
| **Major causes of . . .** | | |
| High results | Deliberate ingestion of large amounts (>15 mg of elemental copper) Wilson's disease | Uncommon in humans |
| Associated signs and symptoms | Nausea, vomiting, intestinal cramps, diarrhea | Larger ingestions lead to shock, hepatic necrosis, intravascular hemolysis, renal impairment, coma, and death |
| Low results | Infants with chronic diarrhea Malabsorption syndromes Decreased intake over months Menkes' syndrome | |
| Associated signs and symptoms | Neutropenia, iron-deficiency anemia, abnormal glucose tolerance, arrhythmias, hypercholesterolemia, atherosclerosis, depressed immune function, defective connective tissue formation, demineralization of bones | Can affect any system or organ whose enzymes require copper for proper functioning |
| **Drugs often monitored with test** | Copper supplements and hyperalimentation solutions | Serum copper concentrations not routinely monitored |

## QuickView—Zinc

| Parameter | Description | Comments |
|---|---|---|
| **Common reference ranges** | | |
| Adults and pediatrics | 70–130 µg/dL (10.7–19.9 µmol/L) | |
| **Critical value** | <70 µg/dL (<10.7 µmol/L) | Increased risk for developing symptomatic zinc deficiency |
| **Natural substance?** | Yes | |
| **Inherent activity?** | Yes | Enzyme constituent and cofactor; carbohydrate, protein, lipid, and nucleic acid metabolism; tissue growth; tissue repair; cell membrane stabilization; bone collagenase activity and collagen turnover; immune response; food intake control; spermatogenesis and gonadal maturation; normal testicular function |
| **Location** | | |
| Storage | Liver, pancreas, spleen, lungs, eyes (retina, iris, cornea, lens), prostate, skeletal muscle, bone, erythrocytes, neutrophils | 60–62% in skeletal muscle, 20–28% in bone, 2–4% in liver |
| Secretion/excretion | Primarily in pancreatic and intestinal secretions; also lost dermally through sweat, hair and nail growth, and skin shedding | Except in certain disease states, only 2% lost in urine |

## QuickView—Zinc *continued*

| Parameter | Description | Comments |
|---|---|---|
| **Major causes of . . .** | | |
| **High results** | Large intake | Uncommon in humans |
| **Associated signs and symptoms** | Drowsiness, lethargy, nausea, vomiting, diarrhea, increases in serum lipase and amylase concentrations | |
| **Low results** | Low intake (infants) Decreased absorption (acrodermatitis enteropathica) Increased utilization (rapidly growing adolescents and menstruating, lactating, or pregnant women) Increased loss (hyperzincuria) | Rare from inadequate dietary intake |
| **Associated signs and symptoms** | Manifests in numerous organs and physiological systems | Table 1 |
| **Drugs often monitored with test** | Zinc supplements and hyperalimentation solutions | Serum zinc concentrations not routinely monitored |
| **Causes of spurious results** | Hemolyzed samples; 24-hr intrapatient variability | High zinc content in erythrocytes and neutrophils |

## QuickView—Manganese

| Parameter | Description | Comments |
|---|---|---|
| **Common reference ranges** | | |
| **Adults** | 2–3 µg/L (36–55 µmol/L) | |
| **Pediatrics** | 2.4–9.6 µg/L (44–175 µmol/L) 0.8–2.1 µg/L (15–38 µmol/L) | Newborn 2–18 years |
| **Critical value** | Not applicable | |
| **Natural substance?** | Yes | |
| **Inherent activity?** | Yes | Enzyme cofactor; carbohydrate, protein, and lipid metabolism; protection of cells from free radicals; steroid biosynthesis; metabolism of biogenic amines; normal brain function Magnesium may substitute for manganese in most instances |
| **Location** | | |
| **Storage** | Bone, liver, pancreas, pituitary gland | Circulating manganese loosely bound to transmanganin |
| **Secretion/excretion** | Primarily in biliary and pancreatic juices; little lost in urine | Other GI routes also may be used in manganese overload |
| **Major causes of . . .** | | |
| **High results** | Primarily through inhalation of manganese compounds, such as in manganese mines | One of least toxic trace elements |
| **Associated signs and symptoms** | Encephalopathy and profound neurological disturbances mimicking Parkinson disease | Accumulates in liver and brain |
| **Low results** | After several months of deliberate omission from diet | Rare from inadequate dietary intake |
| **Associated signs and symptoms** | Weight loss, slow hair and nail growth, hair color change, transient dermatitis, hypocholesterolemia, hypotriglyceridemia | Seen mostly in experimental subjects |

*continued*

## QuickView—Manganese *continued*

| Parameter | Description | Comments |
|---|---|---|
| **Drugs often monitored with test** | Manganese supplements and hyperalimentation solutions | Serum manganese concentration not routinely monitored |

## QuickView—Chromium

| Parameter | Description | Comments |
|---|---|---|
| **Common reference ranges** | | |
| Adults | 1–5 µg/L (18–92 nmol/L) | Analysis of chromium in biological fluids and tissues is difficult |
| Pediatrics | Unknown | Analysis of chromium in biological fluids and tissues is difficult |
| **Critical value** | Unknown | |
| **Natural substance?** | Yes | |
| **Inherent activity?** | Yes | Cofactor for insulin and metabolism of glucose, cholesterol, and triglycerides |
| **Location** | | |
| Storage | Hair, kidneys, skeleton, liver, spleen, lungs, testes, large intestines | Chromium circulates as free $Cr^{3+}$, bound to transferrin and other proteins, and as organic complex |
| Secretion/excretion | Excretion in urine | Circulating insulin controls daily loss |
| **Major causes of . . .** | | |
| Low results | Decreased intake | |
| Associated signs and symptoms | Glucose intolerance; hyperinsulinemia; hypercholesterolemia; possibly, cardiovascular disease | Mainly due to its role as insulin cofactor |
| **Drugs often monitored with test** | Chromium supplement and hyperalimentation solution | Serum chromium concentration not routinely monitored |

# Chapter 7

# The Kidneys

*Scott L. Traub*

The kidneys play a vital role in the body's homeostasis with their ability to excrete and reabsorb various endogenous and exogenous substances selectively. This chapter describes the physiology of the kidneys, tests that measure their ability to eliminate or conserve substances, and interpretation of urinalysis.

Renal physiology as it relates to control of *serum* electrolytes was discussed in Chapter 6. Therefore, this chapter emphasizes *urine* electrolytes. Methods of estimating renal function without collecting urine also are described. Finally, the role of urinary urea nitrogen in nutritional monitoring is discussed.

## OBJECTIVES

Upon completion of this chapter, the reader should be able to

1. Describe the normal physiology of the kidneys.
2. Describe clinical situations where blood urea nitrogen (BUN) and/or serum creatinine (SCr) is elevated.
3. Cite clinical situations where BUN and SCr are and are not reliable indicators of renal function and explain why.
4. Given a case study, determine the most likely type and extent of renal dysfunction based on a BUN and SCr drawn at the same time.
5. Determine creatinine clearance (CrCl) given a patient's 24-hr urine creatinine (UCr) excretion and SCr.
6. Estimate CrCl given a patient's height, weight, sex, age, and SCr.
7. Discuss the various components assessed by macroscopic and microscopic urine analyses.
8. Identify possible medical problems given a patient's urinalysis results as part of a case study.
9. Describe situations where urinary electrolyte determinations and the fractional excretion of sodium ($FE_{Na}$) test are useful diagnostically and therapeutically.
10. Describe the uses as well as the limitations of urine urea nitrogen in monitoring nutritional status.

## RENAL PHYSIOLOGY

The functional unit of cells in the kidneys is the nephron (Figure 1), and each of the two kidneys contains about 1 million nephrons. Each nephron can be divided into the glomerulus, proximal tubule, loop of Henle, distal tubule, and collecting duct. The glomerulus is the filtering section of the nephron. Acting as microfilters, the pores of glomerular capillaries allow substances with a molecular weight of up to 40,000 to pass through them. This weight limit prevents passage of plasma proteins and red blood cells (RBCs) but not most drugs, unless they are protein bound.

The proximal tubule avidly reabsorbs large quantities of water along with glucose, amino acids, uric acid, sodium, chloride, bicarbonate, and other electrolytes. Sodium and water are further reabsorbed in the loop of Henle. The distal tubule controls the amounts of sodium, potassium, bicarbonate, phosphate, and hydrogen that ultimately are excreted, and the collecting duct regulates the amount of water in the urine.[1]

As shown in Figure 1, substances can enter the nephron from the peritubular blood (secretion) or interstitial space. Substances also are reabsorbed back into the blood via the peritubular vasculature. Creatinine enters the tubule mostly by filtration through the glomerulus; however, a small amount of creatinine is secreted directly into the tubules.

The kidneys filter about 180 L of fluid each day; of this amount, they excrete only 1.5 L as urine. Thus, more than 99% of the glomerular filtrate is absorbed back into the bloodstream. Many solutes that are not reabsorbed are concentrated in the urine, including

➢ Endogenous substances such as creatinine and urea.
➢ Exogenous substances such as drugs.

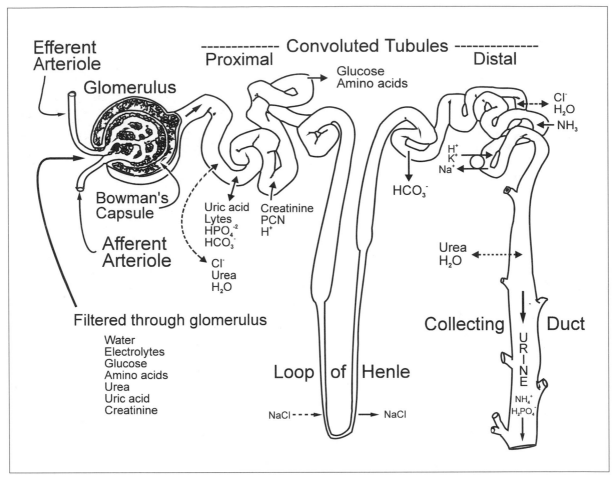

**FIGURE 1.** The nephron. Arrows pointing toward the nephron represent substances entering from the peritubular blood or interstitial space. Arrows heading away represent reabsorption. Solid arrows represent an active (energy-requiring) process, and dashed arrows represent a passive process. PCN = penicillin.

Although beta-lactam antibiotics (e.g., penicillins and cephalosporins) are filtered through the glomerulus, a large percentage enters the nephron via tubular secretion. If a renally eliminated drug or substance is filtered but not secreted from the blood into the tubule and not reabsorbed once in the tubule, its clearance is equal to the glomerular filtration rate (GFR).[1]

The GFR is the volume of water filtered or "cleared" out of the plasma per minute through the surrounding capillary walls into Bowman's spaces. Some water (urine) ultimately reaches the renal tubules, collecting ducts, and bladder. To measure the actual GFR, probes would have to be placed within Bowman's spaces. Since this procedure is not practical, clinicians order tests that measure the clearance of marker substances. These marker substances are filtered through the glomerulus and minimally (if at all) excreted into, or reabsorbed from, the tubules.

## TESTS TO ESTIMATE GLOMERULAR FILTRATION RATE

Tests that estimate the GFR use endogenous markers such

as urea and creatinine and exogenous markers such as inulin and radioactive substances [e.g., ethylenediamine tetraacetic acid ($^{51}$Cr-EDTA), diethylenetriamine pentaacetic acid ($^{99m}$Tc-DTPA), and meglumine iothalamate]. Tests for endogenous marker clearance correlate roughly with the GFR, whereas tests for exogenous marker clearance provide much closer correlations. (Since urea clearance is no longer used in clinical practice, it is not discussed here.)

Clinicians should determine whether the actual GFR (inulin clearance) or a surrogate clearance (of any substance except inulin) would give the most useful or accurate information, depending on the intended use. For example, although the GFR as measured by inulin clearance is the "gold standard" for determining renal function, CrCl may yield better results for pharmacokinetic dosing since most kinetic studies use it (as a surrogate marker) to estimate drug clearance and to develop dosing strategies. BUN and SCr also are widely used, but they provide only rough estimates of GFR-based renal function.

The following is a ranking of tests with respect to accuracy in estimating the GFR (with inulin clearance being the best estimation):

inulin clearance > $^{51}$Cr-EDTA clearance =
$^{99m}$Tc-DTPA clearance > meglumine iothalamate clearance >
CrCl > SCr > BUN

## Inulin and Related Marker Substances

Inulin, an inert carbohydrate, is filtered through the glomerulus but is not metabolized, secreted, or reabsorbed. During the inulin clearance test, the patient receives inulin as a constant infusion to achieve a steady blood concentration. The quantity in the plasma and the amount excreted in the urine are measured, and the clearance is calculated.

Although the inulin clearance test has ideal pharmacokinetics and nonradioactivity, it is mainly used in nephrological research because of its complexity. Furthermore, as mentioned, pharmacokinetic studies in patients with renal dysfunction usually relate drug clearance to CrCl as opposed to the true GFR. Therefore, dosing adjustments should (and more practically can) be based on CrCl.

Other procedures that measure the GFR include the clearance of $^{51}$Cr-EDTA, $^{99m}$Tc-DTPA, or meglumine iothalamate. Although some authorities feel that these tests are more suitable for clinical use than inulin is, they still require the injection of a foreign substance (some radioactive) into the patient's bloodstream as well as repeated blood sampling and/or timed urine collections. Therefore, these methods are not widely accepted in the clinical arena and they are not discussed further in this chapter. Alternatively, measurement of the two endogenous substances, BUN and SCr, is widely used in clinical practice.

## Blood Urea Nitrogen
*Normal range: 8–20 mg/dL or 2.9–7.1 mmol/L*

BUN is actually the concentration of nitrogen (within urea) in the *serum* and not in RBCs (blood) as the name implies. Although BUN can be a reflection of the GFR, it does not meet the requirements for an ideal GFR marker (i.e., a substance that is filtered but not secreted from the blood into the tubule and not reabsorbed once in the tubule). Its serum concentration depends on urea production (which occurs in the liver) and tubular reabsorption in addition to glomerular filtration. Therefore, clinicians must consider factors other than filtration when interpreting changes in BUN.

When viewed with other laboratory and clinical data, BUN can be used to assess or monitor hydrational status, renal function, protein tolerance, and catabolism in numerous clinical settings (Table 1). It also is used to predict the risk of uremic syndrome (Glossary) in patients with severe renal failure.[2] Concentrations above 100 mg/dL (35.7 mmol/L) are associated with this risk.

**TABLE 1.** Common Causes of True BUN Elevations (Azotemia)

| |
|---|
| **Prerenal causes** |
| *Decreased renal perfusion*: dehydration, blood loss, shock, severe heart failure |
| *Increased protein breakdown or antianabolism (urea appearance)*: gastrointestinal bleed, crush injury, burn, fever, corticosteroids, tetracyclines, excessive amino acid or protein intake |
| **Intrarenal (intrinsic) causes** |
| *Acute renal failure*: nephrotoxic drugs (Table 3), severe hypertension, glomerulonephritis, tubular necrosis |
| *Chronic renal dysfunction*: pyelonephritis, diabetes, glomerulonephritis, renal tubular disease, amyloidosis, arteriosclerosis, collagen vascular disease, polycystic kidney, chronic analgesic overuse |
| **Postrenal causes** |
| Obstruction of ureter, bladder neck, or urethra |

### *Elevated Blood Urea Nitrogen*

BUN production is increased by

- A high-protein diet (including amino acid infusions).
- Upper gastrointestinal (GI) bleeding (blood is digested as dietary protein).
- Administration of corticosteroids, tetracyclines, or any other drug with antianabolic effects.

Usually, about 50% of the filtered urea is reabsorbed, but this amount is inversely related to the rate of urine flow in the tubules. In other words, the slower the urine flows, the more time the urea has to leave the tubule and reenter surrounding capillaries (reabsorption). Urea reabsorption tends to change in parallel with sodium chloride and water reabsorption. Since severely dehydrated patients avidly reabsorb sodium chloride and water, larger amounts of urea also are absorbed.

Urine flow, in turn, is affected by fluid balance and blood pressure (BP). For example, dehydrated patients have low urine flow and develop high concentrations of urea nitrogen in the blood. Likewise, a patient with a pathologically low BP develops diminished urine flow secondary to decreased renal blood flow with a subsequently diminished GFR. Causes of abnormally high BUN (also called azotemia) are listed in Table 1.

Chloral hydrate may interfere with some assays and cause *falsely* high BUN values. Fortunately, SCr and BUN are routinely measured together in most laboratories because of predetermined automatic analyzer setups.[3] Simultaneous assays that assess the same organ may help to identify interferences when results are discordant (Chapter 3).

### *Decreased Blood Urea Nitrogen*

In and of itself, a low BUN does not have pathophysiological consequences. BUN may be truly low in patients who are malnourished or have profound liver damage (due to inability to synthesize urea). Fluid overload may initially dilute BUN (causing low concentrations), but eventually many overload causes [e.g., congestive heart failure (CHF), renal failure, and nephrotic syndrome] result in *increased* BUN when its accumulation becomes faster than that of fluid.

Chloramphenicol and streptomycin interference with some assays may also cause BUN to appear low. Likewise, assays based on urease reactions may yield falsely low BUN values (depressed up to 25%) if blood is collected in tubes containing sodium fluoride (gray-top tube), sometimes used for glucose preservation.[3]

## Creatinine
### Assays for Creatinine

The measurement of creatinine to assess the urinary excretion rate was first suggested by Folin in 1904.[1] His assay quantified creatinine by forming creatinine picrate in an alkaline environment. The picrate salt appears as varying intensities of an orange-red color. Many laboratories still use a modification (Jaffé) of this assay but read the color more accurately (±2%) with spectrophotometry. This assay is only fairly specific because noncreatinine chromogens are measured as creatinine (Causes of False Serum Creatinine Results section).

Some laboratories now use an automated enzymatic method to determine true creatinine—it does not measure noncreatinine chromogens.[4] These practitioners argue that CrCls measured using a true creatinine assay correlate better with those determined using inulin.[5] However, this automated assay is time consuming and disrupts the counterbalancing of creatinine secretion (discussed later) when the GFR is estimated from CrCl. Laboratories using true creatinine assays should report a lower normal range (0.4–1.0 mg/dL or 35–88 μmol/L).

### Serum Creatinine
*Normal range: 0.7–1.5 mg/dL or 62–133 μmol/L for adults; 0.2–0.7 mg/dL or 18–62 μmol/L for young children*

Creatinine and its precursor creatine are nonprotein, nitrogenous biochemicals of the blood. After synthesis in the liver, creatine diffuses into the bloodstream. Creatine then is taken up by muscle cells, where some of it is stored in a high-energy form, creatine phosphate. Creatine phosphate acts as a readily available source of phosphorus for regeneration of adenosine triphosphate (ATP) and is required for transforming chemical energy to muscle action.[6]

Creatinine is a spontaneous decomposition product of creatine and creatine phosphate. The daily production of creatinine is about 2% of total body creatine, which remains constant if muscle mass is not significantly changed. In normal patients at steady state, the rate of

creatinine production equals its excretion. Therefore, creatinine concentrations in the serum (SCr) vary little from day to day in patients with healthy kidneys.

For children with *normal* renal function, the expected SCr can be estimated in milligrams per deciliter by multiplying the child's height in inches by 0.01.[7] For International System (SI) units (micromoles per liter), the equation becomes height in centimeters times 0.35. These formulas are not surprising since the relationship between height and muscle mass is known. Although only rough estimates are obtained, they may be useful for children who cannot or will not tolerate venipuncture. Extensive reference range tables have been generated for infants and children[8] and are summarized in the SCr QuickView.

After an acute insult to nephrons, the amount of time needed to reach a new steady-state SCr depends on the half-life of creatinine at that time. Interpretation based on a pre-steady-state SCr concentration (if rising) leads to overestimation of the GFR. The half-life of creatinine in a 70-kg person with a CrCl of 120 mL/min is 3.5 hr. Although half-life and other physiokinetic data would predict faster accumulation rates, in general the typical maximal daily increase in SCr is 1–2 mg/dL (88–177 μmol/L). Higher rates (especially without decreased urine output) suggest an assay interference. Some evidence (albeit controversial), however, indicates that SCr may increase faster than 2 mg/dL/day (177 μmol/L/day) in rhabdomyolysis-induced renal failure.[9]

The time required to reach 95% of steady state in patients with 50, 25, and 10% of normal kidney function (120 mL/min) is about 1, 2, and 4 days, respectively. Therefore, if renal function suddenly declines to 10% of normal, SCr would not fully reflect the functional disability until 4 days later.

*Causes of true changes in serum creatinine.* A rise in SCr almost always indicates worsening renal function. Diseases and substances that adversely affect the kidney's ability to filter and excrete metabolic end-products (e.g., creatinine) and drugs (e.g., digoxin) disrupt the steady state, causing these chemicals to accumulate in the blood (Tables 2 and 3).

In addition, drugs such as cimetidine, triamterene, amiloride, spironolactone, trimethoprim,[10] probenecid, aspirin,[11] and pyrimethamine[12] inhibit tubular secretion of creatinine. Although they may cause true increases in SCr, these increases are not from a decreased GFR.[13] Pa-

**TABLE 2.** Nondrug Causes of SCr Elevations

| Hemoconcentration | Increased production |
|---|---|
| Dehydration | Excess catabolism |
| **Decreased excretion** | Excess exercise |
| Renal dysfunction | Hyperpyrexia |
| Urinary tract obstruction | Hyperthyroidism |
| | Muscular dystrophy |
| | Myasthenia gravis |

**TABLE 3.** Drugs Reported to Cause True SCr Elevations (via Nephrotoxicity)[a]

| | |
|---|---|
| Aminoglycosides | Lithium |
| Amphotericin B | Methicillin |
| Cisplatin | Methotrexate |
| Colistin | Methoxyflurane |
| Cyclosporine | Nitrofurantoin[b] |
| Dextran | Pentamidine |
| Gallium | Plicamycin |
| Hydroxyurea | Streptozocin |

[a]*BUN also would be increased from nephrotoxicity induced by these drugs.*
[b]*May accompany pulmonary reactions.*

tients on these drugs may have falsely suppressed urinary excretion of creatinine; therefore, their renal function, as estimated by CrCl, may be incorrectly assessed to be worse than it really is. Some investigators have exploited this property and used cimetidine to improve the accuracy of CrCl as an estimate of the true GFR (cimetidine inhibits most nonglomerular excretion).[14,15]

Unlike BUN, SCr is not influenced much by usual changes in diet or urine flow. A large intake of roasted meats, however, may temporarily increase SCr due to its actual ingestion. Likewise, there is a strong relationship between the amount of protein in the diet and creatinine *excretion* but not SCr.[16]

Since SCr is a by-product of muscle metabolism, severely decreased muscle mass (cachexia) or activity may be reflected by low SCr. Thus, patients with spinal cord injuries and muscle inactivity have decreased creatinine production.[17] For similar reasons, patients who have been in a coma or on neuromuscular blocking agents for a prolonged time tend to have decreased creatinine excretion rates with normal or low SCr. Conversely, very muscular patients occasionally have slightly elevated SCr with elevated creatinine excretion and normal CrCl and GFR. As expected, vigorous exercise may temporarily increase SCr (by an average of 0.5 mg/dL or 44 µmol/L), but normal exercise does not.[18]

Clinicians should rightfully surmise, therefore, that as long as no abnormalities exist in muscle mass, an increased SCr almost always reflects a decreased GFR. The converse is not always true, however; a normal SCr does not necessarily imply a normal GFR. As part of the aging process, both muscle mass and renal function diminish. Therefore, SCr remains in the normal range because as the kidneys become less capable of filtering and excreting creatinine, they also are presented with decreasing amounts. Thus, practitioners should not rely solely on SCr as an index of renal function. They should also obtain or estimate CrCl (discussed later).

Besides aging, some pathophysiological changes can affect the relationship between SCr and CrCl. For example, renal dysfunction is underestimated on the basis of SCr alone in cirrhotic patients.[19] Their low SCr is in part due to a decreased hepatic synthesis of creatine, the precursor of creatinine. In cirrhotic patients, it is prudent to calculate CrCl from SCr *and* UCr (Calculating Creatinine Clearance from Urinary Creatinine section). If the patient also has hyperbilirubinemia, assay interference by elevated bilirubin also may contribute to the low SCr.

*Causes of false serum creatinine results.* Unusually large amounts of noncreatinine chromogens (uric acid, glucose, fructose, acetone, acetoacetate, pyruvic acid, ascorbic acid, etc.) in the serum, as measured by the Jaffé (alkaline picrate) assay, commonly lead to falsely increased SCr concentrations.[20] For example, an increase in glucose of 100 mg/dL (5.6 mmol/L) is likely to elevate SCr falsely by 0.5 mg/dL (44 µmol/L) in some assays. Likewise, serum ketones high enough to spill into the urine may falsely increase SCr[21,22] and UCr. This false effect is important because diabetic patients are prone to nephropathy and are likely to undergo unnecessary evaluation for renal failure when presenting with ketoacidosis. Like ketones, acetoacetate may be elevated enough to cause falsely elevated SCr after a 48-hr fast or in diabetic ketoacidosis.

With some automated analyzers, turbid or chylous samples (occurring in patients with hyperlipidemias) may produce erratic results. Patients receiving intravenous (IV) fat emulsions may have this potential under certain circumstances. Fortunately, when astute technologists observe turbidity, they remove chylomicrons to circumvent the interference.

Another endogenous substance, bilirubin, may falsely lower results (by 0.4–0.8 mg/dL or 35–70 µmol/L) if concentrations are greater than 10 mg/dL (171 µmol/L) with both the alkaline picrate and enzymatic assays.[23] Patients with bilirubin this high are easily identified because of their jaundice (Chapter 11).

Unlike most other interferents, flucytosine affects only the enzymatic assays.[24] This interference is especially important because patients may concomitantly receive two antifungal agents, flucytosine and the nephrotoxic agent amphotericin B. An increase in SCr may be attributed to amphotericin B-induced nephrotoxicity when it is actually from an assay interference.

Potential interferences with common SCr assays are listed in Table 4 (next page)—most of the substances cause concentration-dependent alterations. Therefore, drawing serum (for SCr) far apart from anticipated peak concentrations of the listed substances should minimize interferences. Reference 34 provides more information on drug-induced alterations in SCr. Minicase 1 (pages 137 and 138) demonstrates how drugs can falsely elevate SCr.

## Concomitant Blood Urea Nitrogen and Serum Creatinine

Simultaneous BUN and SCr determinations can furnish valuable information. Examples include

**TABLE 4.** Drugs and Other Susbtances that May Interfere Chemically with SCr Assays[a]

| Substance | Interference[b] with | |
|---|---|---|
| | **Jaffé Assay** | **Enzymatic Assay** |
| Acetoacetic acid | ↑ or ↓ | – |
| Acetone | ↑ | – |
| Ascorbic acid (high doses) | ↑ | ↓ |
| Bilirubin (>10 mg/dL)[c] | ↓ | ↓ |
| Cefoxitin | ↑ | – |
| Cephalothin | ↑ | – |
| Dopamine | ↑ | ↓ |
| Flucytosine | – | ↑ |
| Fructose | ↑ | – |
| Glucose (>250 mg/dL) | ↑ | – |
| Ketones | ↑ | – |
| Levodopa | ↑ | – |
| Lidocaine[d] | – | ↑ |
| Lipid emulsions | – | ↓ |
| Methyldopa | ↑ | – |

[a]Compiled from References 3 and 25–33. These substances also may interfere with measurement of UCr if excreted in the urine mostly unmetabolized.
[b]↑ = false elevation of results; ↓ = false suppression of results; – = no significant effect.
[c]SI: 171 μmol/L total bilirubin.
[d]Interferes with the EKTA enzymatic assay.

> Acute renal failure with suspected altered hydration.
> GI bleeding during renal insufficiency.
> End-stage renal failure (SCr >7 mg/dL).

In acute renal failure with suspected dehydration, BUN and SCr are elevated. However, the BUN:SCr ratio is often 20:1 or higher (SI: 0.08:1 or higher). Similarly, in patients with GI bleeding and renal insufficiency, both BUN and SCr are elevated with a high BUN:SCr ratio due to digestion of blood and lowered effective blood volume. One study found that a BUN:SCr ratio of at least 36 suggests upper GI bleeding, whereas a ratio of less than 36 (SI: <0.144) does not help locate the source of bleeding.[35]

Usually, BUN:SCr ratios greater than 20:1 suggest prerenal causes (Table 1, Minicase 1); ratios from 10:1 to 20:1 (SI: from 0.04:1 to 0.08:1) suggest intrinsic renal damage. However, as previously noted, both types may occur simultaneously, confounding typical interpretations. Furthermore, a ratio greater than 20:1 is not clinically important if both SCr and BUN are within normal lim-

its (e.g., SCr = 0.8 mg/dL and BUN = 20 mg/dL). These interpretations are illustrated in Minicase 1.

## Creatinine Clearance
*Normal range: 90–140 mL/min/1.73 m²; QuickView shows pediatric values*

From a practical clinical perspective, determination of CrCl provides the best approximation of the GFR. Creatinine is close to the ideal natural substance for this estimation because it is eliminated almost entirely by glomerular filtration until SCr exceeds 5–10 mg/dL (442–884 μmol/L). At that point, tubular secretion significantly adds to creatinine's elimination. Creatinine also may be eliminated by gut flora, an important mechanism primarily in patients with chronic renal failure.[38,39]

Despite some nonglomerular elimination (mostly secretion), CrCl accurately estimates the GFR because substances that contribute to the color of the common Jaffé assay reaction (noncreatinine chromogens) are read as creatinine throughout the range of normal to moderately decreased GFRs. The noncreatinine chromogens (uric acid, glucose, fructose, acetone, pyruvic acid, acetoacetate, ascorbic acid, etc.) affect the serum assay much more than the measurement of creatinine in urine. The overestimation of SCr increases the denominator of the clearance equation. The impact of overestimation is canceled out by the comparable effect (in the opposite direction) of creatinine elimination by secretion (nonfiltration), which increases the numerator.

At very low GFRs, however, creatinine secretion overtakes the balancing effects of measuring noncreatinine chromogens, causing an overestimation of GFRs by as much as 50%.[5,20] In other words, CrCl (in milliliters per minute) is much greater than the GFR (in milliliters per minute). This effect has been seen particularly in patients with nephrotic syndrome.

### Using Age-Adjusted Standards and Reference Ranges

The relationship of age, sex, and SCr with CrCl is shown in Figure 2. CrCl declines with age at any given SCr. Even with a "normal" SCr of 1.5 mg/dL (133 μmol/L), an 80-year-old female has a CrCl of only 35 mL/min/70 kg. For drugs such as gentamicin, manufacturers' "usual" dosage regimens assume that the patient has a CrCl of 100 mL/min or higher.

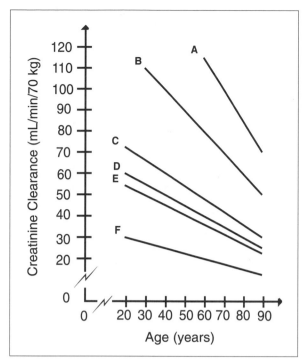

**FIGURE 2.** CrCl as it relates to SCr and age in a 70-kg person. A: male, SCr = 0.7 mg/dL (62 μmol/L). B: male, SCr = 1.0 mg/dL (88 μmol/L). C: female, SCr = 1.5 mg/dL (133 μmol/L). D: male, SCr = 2.0 mg/dL (177 μmol/L). E: female, SCr = 2.0 mg/dL. F: male, SCr = 4.0 mg/dL (354 μmol/L).

One way to estimate age-adjusted normal values of CrCl in males is with CrCl = 133 − (0.64 × age), where CrCl is in milliliters per minute per 1.73 m² and age is in years. In females, the CrCl is 93% of that value.[40] Thus, with a SCr of 1.0 mg/dL (88 μmol/L), a 30-year-old male should have a CrCl of 114 mL/min/1.73 m² and an 80-year-old female should have a CrCl of 76 mL/min/1.73 m².

In children, the CrCl (in milliliters per minute per 1.73 m²) approaches that of adults sometime between the ages of 1 and 2 years (CrCl QuickView).

### Interpreting Creatinine Clearance Values with Other Renal Parameters

As alluded to previously, the most common clinical uses for CrCl and SCr include

➤ Assessing kidney function in patients with acute or chronic renal failure.

➤ Monitoring patients on nephrotoxic drugs.

➤ Determining dosage adjustments for renally eliminated drugs.

Because the relationship between SCr and CrCl is inverse and geometric as opposed to linear, significant declines in CrCl may occur before SCr rises above the normal range. For example, as CrCl slows, SCr rises very little

## Minicase 1

A 43-year-old female, Judith C., with a long history of Crohn's disease (regional enteritis), was admitted to Community Hospital with exacerbation described as bloody, pusy, diarrhea; abdominal pain; anorexia; weight loss (5 lb); and weakness; all had worsened over the past 2 weeks.

A physical examination revealed an emaciated (5 ft 9 in; 40 kg; BSA of 1.3 m²), but mildly Cushingoid, woman with moderate abdominal distress and dehydration, tachycardia (heart rate of 100), oral temperature of 101.5 °F (38.6 °C), BP of 100/50 mm Hg, macerated anal area, pallor, and mild finger clubbing. Judith C. had been taking prednisone, 10 mg/day, for the past year and until now had experienced no serious flareups of her disease. On admission, prednisone was replaced with IV methylprednisolone 40 mg twice a day.

Laboratory work included

- Sodium, 130 mEq/L (136–145 mEq/L).
- Potassium, 3.2 mEq/L (3.5–5.0 mEq/L).
- Chloride, 96 mEq/L (96–106 mEq/L).
- Carbon dioxide, 20 mEq/L (24–30 mEq/L).
- Glucose, 185 mg/dL (70–110 mg/dL).
- Phosphorus, 2.5 mg/dL (2.6–4.5 mg/dL).
- Hemoglobin (Hgb), 9 g/dL (12–16 g/dL).
- White blood cell (WBC) count, 15,000 cells/mm³ (4800–10,800 cells/mm³) with 80% neutrophils.
- BUN, 33 mg/dL (8–20 mg/dL).
- SCr, 0.8 mg/dL (0.7–1.5 mg/dL).

Over the next 3 days, Judith C. received fluid and electrolyte replacement and 2 U of packed RBCs. On day 3, her test results were

- Sodium, 140 mEq/L.
- Potassium, 3.6 mEq/L.
- Chloride, 102 mEq/L.
- Carbon dioxide, 25 mEq/L.
- Glucose, 130 mg/dL.
- Phosphorus, 3.5 mg/dL.
- Hgb, 9.5 g/dL.
- WBC count, 18,000 cells/mm³ with 85% neutrophils.
- BUN, 25 mg/dL.
- SCr, 0.6 mg/dL.

On day 4, because Judith C.'s Hgb did not improve much, her oral nutritional intake was inadequate, and bowel rest was desired, she was given another 2 U of blood and started on total parenteral nutrition (TPN). TPN was comprised of appropriate vitamins and minerals, amino acids 3 g/kg/day, and 30 nonprotein kcal/kg/day including fat emulsion 500 mL every day. Because she was still febrile (spiking temperatures to 103 °F or 39.4 °C) with leukocytosis (WBC count of 16,000 cells/mm³) and abdominal rigidity, an intra-abdominal infection was suspected. Therefore, cefoxitin 2 g every 6 hr was started.

By day 6, Judith C. defervesced and her Hgb was 11 g/dL. However, her BUN was 40 mg/dL and her SCr was 2.2 mg/dL (serum was not turbid). Her urinalysis was normal with no ketones, glucose, muddy brown (granular) casts, or tubular epithelial cells; her

*continued*

serum glucose was 150 mg/dL. Judith C.'s urine output was difficult to determine because of loss during diarrhea.

Because her SCr was elevated, a 24-hr urine collection for creatinine was started 6 hr later, after insertion of a Foley catheter. Judith C. also was switched to cefotetan 2 g every 12 hr. At the same time, a repeat BUN and SCr were 39 and 0.8 mg/dL, respectively. On the next day, the 24-hr UCr was 700 mg in a volume of 1900 mL and SCr was 0.7 mg/dL.

*What type of renal dysfunction was Judith C. experiencing? What were the likely causes of her elevated BUN and SCr? How often should BUN and SCr be determined?*

**Discussion:** This case is rather complex because many factors might affect SCr and BUN at various times. One fairly certain interpretation is that, on day 6, cefoxitin caused the SCr to be falsely elevated to 2.2 mg/dL. The argument for this conclusion is strong because

1. SCr rarely would decline by 1.4 mg/dL in only 6–12 hr in patients not being hemodialyzed.
2. Other SCr measurements were all around 0.7–0.8 mg/dL.
3. Cefoxitin interference with common creatinine assays is well documented.[28,29,34]

Because Judith C.'s SCr was elevated to 2.2 mg/dL and because renal hypoperfusion (BP of 100/50 mm Hg) might have led to kidney damage and her urine output was unknown, a CrCl test was done to try to clarify SCr. Her CrCl was 93 mL/min/1.73 m², which would be expected if her renal function were normal. The clinician should keep in mind, however, that renal function, as determined by CrCl, may be overestimated in malnourished patients[36] like Judith C.

Although it did not seem to happen with Judith C., the measurement of UCr also would be falsely elevated if the cefoxitin washout period were inadequate and this antibiotic were still in her urine. In this case, the measured CrCl would be exaggerated. More evidence of normal renal function was that catheter-collected urine showed good output (1900 mL; almost 2 mL/kg/hr) and urinalysis revealed no significant casts (discussed later).

There are several possible reasons why Judith C.'s BUN values were elevated. On admission, dehydration could have hemoconcentrated the BUN. In fact, after rehydration, her BUN decreased to 25 mg/dL. Although her SCr also declined (albeit slightly), if hemoconcentration contributed to the initial azotemia, at first glance one would

expect other serum constituents to *decline.* The opposite occurred. There is no paradox, however, since Judith C. probably received many of these substances parenterally during the first 3 days.

Severe dehydration also may have increased her BUN secondary to diminished renal blood flow (prerenal cause). A BUN:SCr ratio of greater than 20:1 is consistent with prerenal azotemia. Judith C.'s ratio was 40:1. The patient's relatively low SCr, which may have been a reflection of little muscle mass, increased this ratio "artificially." Finally, the fact that Judith C. was on chronic steroids may have contributed to her elevated BUN.

On day 6, Judith C.'s BUN was 40 mg/dL despite rehydration. A SCr of 2.2 mg/dL and a BUN:SCr ratio of 10:1–20:1 are consistent with acute renal failure, and it is not uncommon for prerenal problems to lead to acute renal failure.[37] Fortunately, as mentioned, her SCr was spuriously elevated.

On day 6, three causes of the high BUN are possible:

1. Judith C.'s steroid dose had been increased substantially. As mentioned, steroids can lead to an elevated BUN by their antianabolic properties (a by-product of increased gluconeogenesis from cellular proteins).
2. Judith C. was receiving excessive amino acids and relatively inadequate calories. Although increasing BUN from parenteral nutrition usually occurs only with diminished renal function, it can occur in this scenario.
3. Stress from exacerbation of Crohn's disease and her infection also may have contributed to Judith C.'s elevated BUN values due to increased protein catabolism.

There is no consensus about the optimal frequency for determining SCr or CrCl. With this patient, the BUN and SCr tests were ordered whenever the clinician needed to assess therapy, renal function, or state of hydration. A CrCl was ordered only after other results appeared discrepant.

In patients in the initial phases of acute renal failure, SCr tests are done almost every day; in chronic renal failure, every 4–6 months usually suffices. While patients are on drugs such as aminoglycosides, determinations are customarily conducted every 3 days. The frequency of taking SCr levels depends on the disease or drug being monitored as well as the patient's history. In general, CrCl is tested only if renal function cannot be reliably assessed by SCr and BUN alone.

until more than 50% of the nephrons are gone. Therefore, SCr alone is not a sensitive indicator of early kidney dysfunction.

Although BUN is a more sensitive indicator of early failure, too many factors besides the GFR influence BUN, making it less specific and less useful. Practitioners should remember that anything causing a real or artifactual rise in SCr also causes a real or artifactual underestimation of CrCl. This relationship is apparent in Minicase 1, which includes integrative interpretation of CrCl, BUN, SCr, and related parameters.

### Calculating Creatinine Clearance from Urinary Creatinine

Although shorter collection periods (8 hr) appear to be adequate, CrCl is routinely calculated using a 12- or 24-hr UCr excretion result and SCr. Creatinine excretion is normally 20–28 mg/kg/24 hr in men or 15–21 mg/kg/24 hr in women. In children, normal excretion (milligrams per kilogram per 24 hr) should be around 15 + (0.5 × age), where age is in years.

Because its excretion remains relatively consistent

within these ranges, UCr is often used as a check for complete urine collection when creatinine or other substances (e.g., amylase, urea, protein, hormones, and catecholamines) are being measured. In adults, some clinicians discount a urine sample if it contains less than 10 mg of creatinine/kg/24 hr; they assume that the collection was incomplete. However, 8.5 mg/kg/day might be a better cutoff, especially in critically ill elderly patients.[41] UCr assays are affected by most of the same substances that affect SCr. To interfere significantly, however, the substance must appear in the urine in concentrations at least equal to those found in the blood.

Endogenous CrCl is calculated with the formula

$$CrCl = \frac{UV}{P} \times \frac{1.73}{BSA} \qquad (1)$$

where CrCl is in milliliters per minute per 1.73 m$^2$, U is the creatinine concentration in the urine (milligrams per milliliter), V is the urine volume (milliliters per minute), P is the creatinine concentration in the plasma or serum (milligrams per milliliter), and BSA is the patient's body surface area (square meters). It should be noted that P (essentially the same as SCr) is in milligrams per milliliter, not per deciliter as reported by most laboratories, and that V is in milliliters per minute. SI units also can be used for U and P. To adjust V to a 24-hr period, one must multiply by 1440 min.

BSA can be estimated using standard nomograms (available in *American Hospital Formulary Service Drug Information* published by the American Society of Health-System Pharmacists), derived primarily from data of Dubois and Dubois.[42] BSA also can be estimated using the following equation:[43]

$$BSA \left(m^2\right) = \sqrt{\frac{height \ (in) \times weight \ (lb)}{3131}} \qquad (2a)$$

or

$$BSA \left(m^2\right) = \sqrt{\frac{height \ (cm) \times weight \ (kg)}{3615}} \qquad (2b)$$

Adjustment of CrCl to a standard BSA (1.73 m$^2$) allows direct comparison with lists of normal CrCl ranges since such tables are in units of milliliters per minute per 1.73 m$^2$. In essence, the CrCl value adjusted for BSA is the number of milliliters cleared per minute for each 1.73 m$^2$ of the patient's BSA. Therefore, such adjustment in a large person (>1.73 m$^2$) reduces the original nonadjusted clearance value since the assumption is that clearance would be lower if the patient were smaller (only 1.73 m$^2$). In practice, it is only important to adjust CrCl for BSA in patients who are much smaller (e.g., children) or larger (e.g., tall weight-lifters) than 1.73 m$^2$.

If a full 24-hr collection period is used, the equation simplifies to the following:

$$CrCl \ (mL/min/1.73 \ m^2) = \frac{UCr \times 0.12}{SCr \times BSA} \qquad (3)$$

where UCr is in milligrams per 24 hr and SCr is in milligrams per deciliter, both in units reported by most U.S. laboratories. The same equation holds for SI units if milliliter per minute per 1.73 m$^2$ is desired. For a 12-hr urine collection, UCr is multiplied by 0.24 instead of 0.12. Thus, the mnemonic for "opposite values" is helpful: 0.24 for 12 hr and 0.12 for 24 hr.

When unadjusted for BSA and using a 24-hr collection, the formula is

$$CrCl \ (mL/min) = \frac{UCr \times 0.07}{SCr} \qquad (4)$$

### *Estimating Creatinine Clearance without Urine Collection*

An accurate 24-hr urine collection is labor intensive, expensive, time consuming, and cumbersome. The most common problem is that all excreted urine is not collected. In addition, therapy or other diagnostic studies may have to be delayed until after the collection period. Therefore, clinicians have sought methods of roughly estimating CrCl. Although results from estimations are probably not as accurate as test results from measuring UCr, they can be obtained quickly and easily. Most methods use demographic data (height, weight, age, and sex) and SCr.[44,45]

Several methods can be used, depending on the clinical situation. Methods 1–3 are for adults. Method 1 can be used despite a changing SCr (i.e., SCr is not at steady state), although it assumes that creatinine excretion is at steady state. For Methods 2 and 3, SCr and creatinine excretion should be at steady state.

The equations in Method 1 for determining the 24-hr UCr excretion (Step 2) are derived from data used to design the nomogram in Method 2; therefore, these two methods should generate similar results if SCr is relatively constant. With Method 4, which is used in children, SCr also must be relatively constant. None of these methods is valid in a patient being hemodialyzed since dialysis contributes to creatinine elimination.

For *Method 1* (modified from Reference 46), Steps 1–6 are followed.

1. *Estimate patient's ideal body mass (IBM) from height in inches:*

    $$IBM \ (lb) = 130 + 3 \ (height - 60) \ in \ males \qquad (5)$$

    $$IBM \ (lb) = 120 + 3 \ (height - 60) \ in \ females \qquad (6)$$

    For example, a 70-in-tall woman has an ideal body mass of 150 lb. These formulas were derived from Metropolitan Life Insurance Company "Desirable Weight for Height Tables."[47] If the patient's actual weight is less than the estimated ideal body mass, the actual weight should be used. Pounds are converted to kilograms (divided by 2.2) for Step 2.

2. *Estimate steady-state (unadjusted) UCr:*

$$UCr = IBM [29.3 - (0.20 \times age)] \text{ in males} \quad (7)$$

$$UCr = IBM [25.3 - (0.18 \times age)] \text{ in females} \quad (8)$$

where UCr is in milligrams per 24 hr, ideal body mass is in kilograms, and age is in years.

3. *Correct UCr for nonrenal elimination using a correction factor (CF):*

$$CF = 1.035 - 0.034(SCr) \quad (9)$$

An average SCr can be used if more than one has been run. Then:

$$UCr' = UCr \times CF \quad (10)$$

where UCr′ is creatinine excretion corrected for nonrenal (mostly GI) elimination. Step 3 can be omitted unless SCr is greater than 2.5 mg/dL; at that point, it begins to affect UCr′ more drastically.

4. *Estimate daily accumulation (or loss) of creatinine (Cr⁻):*

$$Cr^- = \frac{4(IBM)(SCr_2 - SCr_1)}{T} \quad (11)$$

where $SCr_2$ is the current SCr and $SCr_1$ is the SCr T days ago. If there has been no upward or downward trend in SCr (i.e., it is stable), creatinine approaches zero and this adjustment is not needed.

5. *Adjust UCr for daily accumulation or loss:*

$$UCr_\Delta = UCr' - Cr^- \quad (12)$$

where $UCr_\Delta$ is the estimated UCr excretion adjusted for nonrenal elimination and *changing* renal function.

6. *Calculate CrCl:*

$$CrCl \text{ (mL/min/1.73 m}^2) = \frac{UCr_\Delta \times 0.12}{SCr \times BSA} \quad (13)$$

The question of which SCr to use is controversial. If one suspects that CrCl will continue to fall or rise, the most recent value, $SCr_2$, probably should be used. Otherwise, the average of $SCr_2$ and $SCr_1$ should be used.

Although Method 1 is rather complex, it is the *only* valid method for patients whose SCr is rising or falling. The following methods are not suitable for such cases.

For *Method 2*,[48] the nomogram in Figure 3 is used. It is based on the same data that generated the equations described in Step 2 of Method 1, but no adjustment is made for rising or falling SCr. Furthermore, CrCl is in milliliters per minute and is not adjusted for BSA.

For *Method 3*, the following equation is used:

$$CrCl \text{ (mL/min)} = \frac{IBM \times (140 - age)}{72 \times SCr} \quad (14)$$

where IBM is in kilograms and age is in years.[49] When SI units (micromoles per liter) are used for SCr, the equation becomes

$$CrCl \text{ (mL/min)} = \frac{IBM \times (140 - age)}{0.8 \times SCr} \quad (15)$$

In females, the result has traditionally been multiplied by 0.85 (85%). The work of Rowe et al.,[40] however, indicated that 93% should be used for this adjustment. Therefore, 90% is suggested as a compromise.

In unusually small or large somatotypes, Equations 14 and 15 should be adjusted for BSA by multiplying the result by 1.73/patient's BSA. This adjustment generates results in milliliters per minute per 1.73 m². Some clinicians, however, prefer to adjust the milliliters per minute value to a 72-kg person (as opposed to BSA). The formula then is simplified to

$$CrCl \text{ (mL/min/72 kg)} = \frac{140 - age}{SCr} \quad (16)$$

where SCr is in milligrams per deciliter and age is in years.

*Method 4* was developed for children (1–18 years) with *stable* SCr.[45] Height can be in centimeters or inches, and SCr is in milligrams per deciliter. A nomogram (Figure 4, page 142) also was designed for quick calculations. Since adjustment for BSA is required for most children, it was built into this method:

$$CrCl \text{ (mL/min/1.73 m}^2) = 0.48 \times \frac{height \text{ (cm)}}{SCr} \quad (17)$$

$$= 1.22 \times \frac{height \text{ (in)}}{SCr} \quad (18)$$

This equation suggests that a rough bedside estimate of CrCl in children can be made by either

➤ Taking half of the height (0.5 instead of 0.48) in *centimeters* and dividing it by the SCr.

➤ Adding another approximately 25% to the height (1.25 instead of 1.22) in *inches* and dividing by SCr.

For example, a 40-in child with a SCr of 1 mg/dL has a CrCl of approximately 40 + 10 or 50 mL/min/1.73 m². If SCr is 0.5 mg/dL (as is more common in children this size), CrCl would be 100 mL/min/1.73 m². Using SI units for SCr, the equation becomes

$$CrCl \text{ (mL/min/1.73 m}^2) = \frac{42.2 \times height \text{ (cm)}}{SCr} \quad (19)$$

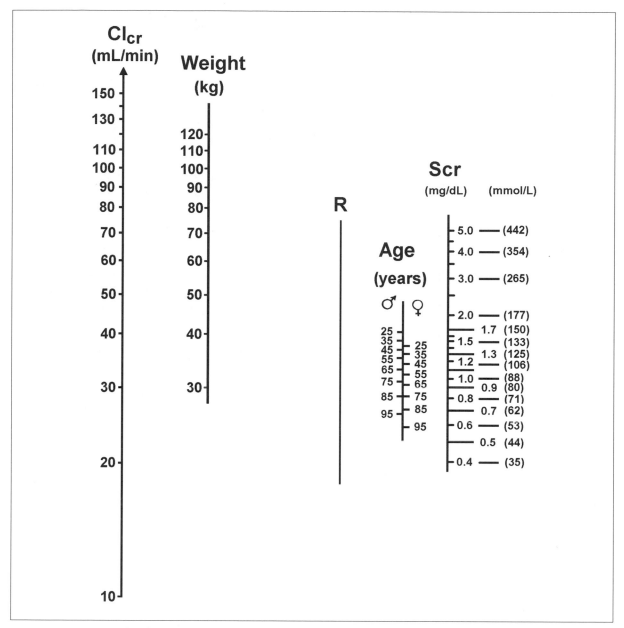

**FIGURE 3.** Nomogram for estimating CrCl (in milliliters per minute) for adults with steady-state SCr. The patient's weight and age are connected with a ruler, using the appropriate scale for sex. Then the point of intersection is marked on the center line (R). Next, R is connected with the patient's SCr, and CrCl is read where the ruler intersects the line on the far left. (Adapted, with permission, from Reference 48.)

where SCr is in micromoles per liter.

Equations 17 and 18 and similar ones[50,51] may not be accurate in all pediatric populations. For example, when a constant of 0.55 was used in Equation 17, renal function was underestimated in children with insulin-dependent diabetes mellitus;[52] a constant of 0.7 gave better predictions. However, that study used $^{99m}$Tc-DTPA to measure GFRs in contrast to original studies that used inulin or creatinine. Furthermore, the equation with 0.48 as the constant generates CrCl (the parameter used in most pharmacokinetic dosing methods) and not the actual GFR, as was measured in the diabetic children.[52]

## URINALYSIS

Urinalysis is another tool that clinicians can use to search for or evaluate renal and nonrenal problems (endocrine, metabolic, genetic, etc.). A routine urinalysis, as the name implies, is done as a screening test during many hospital admissions and initial physician visits. It also is performed periodically in patients in nursing homes and other settings. Since many different methods can assay the components of a urinalysis, only the common ones are discussed here.

Accurate interpretations can be made only if the urine

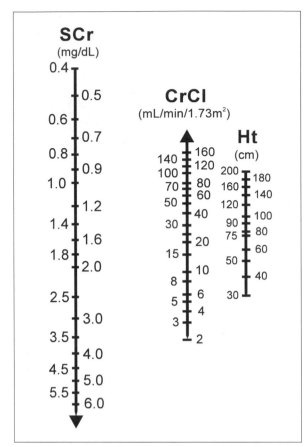

**FIGURE 4.** Nomogram for estimating CrCl (in milliliters per minute per 1.73 m²) for children 1–18 years old with steady-state SCr.[45] The patient's height (centimeters) and SCr (milligrams per deciliter) are connected with a ruler, and CrCl is read from the center line. (Derived with assays that measure noncreatinine chromogens. Adapted from Reference 45.)

is properly collected as well as handled. Techniques are mainly standardized and they aim to avoid contamination (the urine should be sterile) by normal flora of external mucous membranes of the vagina or penis (uncircumcised) or by microorganisms on the hands. Therefore, these areas are cleansed and physically kept away from the urine flow. During menses or heavy vaginal secretions, a fresh tampon should be inserted before cleansing. Midstream urine alone (one cup) is customarily used as the specimen; however, first-voided (two-cup) and even three-cup urines may provide information about the prostate in males.

Once voided, the urine should be brought to the laboratory as soon as possible to prevent its deterioration. If the sample is not refrigerated, the bacteria multiply; they use glucose (if any) as a food source. Glucose concentrations fall and ketones may evaporate with prolonged standing. Another problem is that formed elements (Microscopic Analysis section) begin decomposing within 2 hr. With excessive exposure to light, bilirubin and urobilinogen are oxidized. Unlike other substances, however,

### Minicase 2

Pam D., a 78-year-old, 5-ft 5-in, 125-lb female, was admitted to the hospital 2 days ago for pneumonia in her left lower lobe and postprandial epigastric pain. She had a history of chronic obstructive pulmonary disease requiring oral steroids two or three times a year and many previous admissions for pneumonia. She had developed worsening shortness of breath and fever over the past few days.

Pam D. also had a history of chronic renal failure secondary to diabetes and hypertension. Her SCr typically ran around 3 mg/dL, and her BUN was around 50 mg/dL. A stain of sputum revealed many Gram-negative rods, and cultures grew *Pseudomonas aeruginosa* susceptible only to ceftazidime and imipenem. Her SCr concentrations on the previous 2 days were 3.2 and 3.0 mg/dL, and her BUNs were 50 and 55 mg/dL. Her urine output averaged 1200 mL/day with an intake of about 1800 mL during the past 2 days. A Hemocult test (for blood in stools) was positive on two occasions.

Pam D. was empirically started on ceftriaxone on admission. However, the pharmacist wanted to change her antibiotic to imipenem (the attending physician usually used 500 mg every 6 hr for this type of infection) and start nizatidine. Both drugs need dosage adjustment in patients with renal dysfunction.

*How should Pam D.'s renal function be estimated? How should her drug dosages be adjusted?*

**Discussion:** Because Pam D.'s SCr values did not change significantly from her usual poor baseline, her CrCl can be estimated using either Method 2 or 3. With a SCr of 3.0 mg/dL, the nomogram gives an estimate of about 17 mL/min; Method 3 yields a CrCl of 16.3 mL/min. Equation 2a yields a BSA of 1.61 m². To adjust the CrCl for BSA, 16.3 is multiplied by 1.73/BSA to get a CrCl of 17.5 mL/min/1.73 m². This adjustment affects the CrCl insignificantly because Pam D. did not have a very large or small body size.

Because of possible active GI bleeding, the nizatidine dose is usually 150 mg twice a day. However, at a CrCl of 20–50 mL/min, the manufacturer recommends a dose of 150 mg every day; at a CrCl of less than 20 mL, 150 mg every other day is suggested. Because Pam D.'s CrCl was stable at about 17 mL/min, nizatidine should be started at 150 mg every other day but changed to every day if epigastric pain or bleeding persists.

In patients with normal renal function, imipenem 500 mg is often given every 6 hr. Occasionally, doses as high as 1000 mg every 8 hr are given for this type of infection. The manufacturer suggests using 500 mg every 6 hr if the CrCl is 31–70 mL/min, 500 mg every 8 hr if it is 21–30 mL/min, and 500 mg every 12 hr if it is 6–20 mL/min. Since Pam D.'s CrCl was 17 mL/min, she should be given 500 mg every 12 hr.

protein is hardly affected by prolonged standing.[53]

After the urine sample is collected, it may undergo three types of testing: macroscopic, microscopic, and chemical.

## Macroscopic Analysis (General Appearance)

The color of normal urine varies greatly—from totally clear to dark yellow or amber—depending on the concentration of solutes. Color comes primarily from the pigments urochrome and urobilin. Fresh normal urine is not cloudy or hazy, but urine may become cloudy if urates (in an acid environment) or phosphates (in an alkaline environment) crystallize or precipitate out of solution. These salts become less soluble as the urine cools from body temperature.

Turbidity also may occur when large numbers of RBCs or WBCs are present. An unusual amount of foam may be from protein or bile acids. Table 5 lists causes of different urine colors. Drugs that cause or exacerbate any of the medical problems listed in Table 5 also can be considered indirect causes.

## Microscopic Analysis (Formed Elements)

Microscopic analysis typically involves

1. Centrifuging the urine at 2000 revolutions per minute for 5 min.
2. Pouring off all "loose" supernatant.
3. Mixing the sediment with the residual supernatant.
4. Examining the resulting suspension under 400–455× magnification (also described as high-power field).

This segment of the urinalysis is the most time consuming and costly. Therefore, many authorities have suggested that dipstick chemical screening (described later) be used to determine whether the urine sediment should be examined microscopically.[55] Some practitioners found that when the urine was negative for protein, blood, and leukocytes, omitting microscopy missed potentially significant findings in only 1.5–3% of specimens. Whether microscopic analysis is done routinely or selectively, one should look for the three "Cs"—cells, casts, and crystals.

### Cells

Theoretically, no cells should be seen during microscopic examination of urine. In practice, however, an occasional cell or two is found. These cells include microorganisms, RBCs, WBCs, and tubular epithelial cells.

*Microorganisms (normal range: zero to trace).* Although urine is sterile normally, fungi, bacteria, and other single-cell organisms can be seen in patients with a urinary tract infection or colonization. Even if ordered, some laboratories do not perform urine cultures unless there is sig-

**TABLE 5.** Causes of Various Urine Coloring[a]

| Color | Cause | Possible Underlying Etiologies |
|---|---|---|
| Red to orange | Myoglobin | Crush injuries, electric shock, seizures, cocaine-induced muscle damage |
| | Hgb | Hemolysis (malaria, drugs, strenuous exercise) |
| | Porphyrins | Porphyria, lead poisoning, liver disease |
| | Drugs/chemicals | Drugs/chemicals causing above diseases. As dyes: rifampin, phenazopyridine, danthron,[b] emodin,[c] daunorubicin, doxorubicin, phenolphthalein,[b] phenothiazines, senna,[b] chlorzoxazone |
| | Food | Beets, rhubarb, blackberries, cold drink dyes, carrots |
| Blue to green | Biliverdin | Oxidation of bilirubin (poorly preserved specimen)[d] |
| | Bacteria | *Pseudomonas* or *Proteus* in urinary tract infections (rare), particularly in urine drainage bags |
| | Drugs/chemicals | As dyes: amitriptyline, azuresin, methylene blue, Clorets abuse, Clinitest ingestion, mitoxantrone, triamterene, resorcinol |
| Brown to black | Myoglobin | Crush injuries, electric shock, seizures, cocaine-induced muscle damage |
| | Bile pigments | Hemolysis, bleed into tissues, liver disease |
| | Melanin | Melanoma (prolonged exposure to air)[d] |
| | Methemoglobin | Methemoglobinemia from drugs, dyes, etc. |
| | Porphyrins | Porphyria and sickle cell crisis |
| | Drugs/chemicals | As dyes: cascara,[b] chloroquine, clofazimine, emodin,[b] senna,[b] ferrous salts, methocarbamol, metronidazole, nitrofurantoin, sulfonamides |

[a]Adapted from References 3, 53, and 54 and various anecdotal reports.
[b]In acidic urine.
[c]In basic (alkaline) urine.
[d]After prolonged standing or exposure to air.

nificant bacteriuria. *Significant bacteriuria* may be defined as an initial positive dipstick screen for leukocyte esterase and/or nitrites (Chemical Analysis section). Likewise, some laboratories do not process cultures further (identification, quantification, and susceptibility) if more than one or two different bacterial species is seen on initial plating.

Additionally, some labs do not perform susceptibility testing if more than one organism (some more than two) is isolated or if less than 100,000 (some use 50,000 as the cutoff) colony-forming units (cfu) per milliliter per organism is measured with a midstream, clean-catch sample. The common cutoff for urine obtained through a catheter is less than 10,000. The rationale is that the chance of isolating pathogens is low with low colony counts. In the case of multiple bacteria, contamination by vaginal, rectal, hand, or other flora is assumed. (Chapter 16 covers infectious disease tests in more detail.)

Most laboratories use unspun urine for microbiological screening. However, investigators using *centrifuged*, stained sediment found the highest sensitivity (98%) and specificity (89%) when the criterion for significant bacteriuria was one or more bacteria per oil-immersion field.[56] Microscopic findings were compared with the "gold standard," quantitative urine culture, where the isolate is deemed to be a pathogen if seen in quantities of 100,000 cfu or more per milliliter. Unfortunately, studies on this topic are difficult to compare because of slight differences in technical methods and varying ideas about what constitutes significant bacteriuria.

*Red blood cells (normal range: one to three per high-power field).* A few RBCs occasionally are found in a healthy patient's urine, particularly after exertion, trauma, or fever. If persistent, however, even small numbers may reflect urinary tract pathology. RBCs are seen in glomerulonephritis, infection (pyelonephritis), renal infarction or papillary necrosis, tumors, stones, and coagulopathies. In some of these disorders, hematuria may turn the urine pink or red (gross hematuria).

If the specimen is not collected properly, vaginal blood may contaminate the urine. Many squamous epithelial cells also appear in this case, suggesting that the erythrocytes did not originate from the urinary tract but probably from the vaginal walls.

*White blood cells (normal range: zero to two per high-power field).* Potentially significant pyuria has been defined as three or more WBCs per high-power field of centrifuged urine sediment. Alone, this finding is not specific for a particular disease and may even occur in the absence of pathology. Pyuria is usually associated with a bacterial urinary tract infection; however, inflammation in the tract also may lead to this finding.

Urethritis provides an interesting example of how integration of pyuria with other urinalysis findings can provide diagnostic information. In women complaining of dysuria, pus in the urine without microscopic bacteria is highly suggestive of chlamydial urethritis. Negative hematuria and proteinuria strengthen this diagnosis.

*Tubular epithelial cells (normal range: zero or one per high-power field).* One epithelial cell per high-power field is often found in normal subjects. Cells originating from the renal tubules are small, round, and mononuclear. Their quantity increases dramatically when the tubules are damaged (e.g., acute tubular necrosis) or heavy proteinuria (nephrotic syndrome) occurs.

Numerous flat, irregular, vaginal epithelial cells with small nuclei suggest contamination.

### Casts

Casts are cylindrical masses of glycoproteins (e.g., Tamm-Horsfall mucoprotein) that form in the tubules. As shown in Figure 5, casts have relatively smooth and regular margins (as opposed to clumps of cells) because they conform to the shape of the tubular lumen. To oversimplify, their production is similar to the pouring of wax into a tubular mold to make (usually short) candles.

Under certain conditions, casts are released into the urine (called cylinduria). Even normal urine can contain a few clear casts. These formed elements are fragile and dissolve more quickly in warm, alkaline urine. Types include hyaline, cellular, granular, waxy, and broad; their causes are listed in Table 6.

*Hyaline casts.* Being clear, hyaline casts are difficult to observe under a microscope. They are seen with exercise, fever, and proteinuria. They are not indicative of intrinsic renal disease but of a small volume of concentrated urine or a prerenal problem (CHF, dehydration, etc., as seen in Minicase 2, page 142).

*Cellular casts.* In contrast to hyaline casts, cellular casts are seen with intrinsic renal disease. They form when leukocytes, RBCs, or renal tubular epithelial cells become entrapped in the gelatinous matrix forming in the tubule. Their clinical significance is the same as that of the cells themselves; unlike free cells, however, cells in casts originate from within the kidneys. In other words, WBC casts suggest *intra*renal inflammation and/or upper urinary tract infection, usually pyelonephritis. Epithelial cell casts indicate definite tubular destruction, while RBC casts are seen in glomerulonephritis or ischemic injury to the kidneys.

*Granular and waxy casts.* Granular and waxy casts are older, degenerated forms of the other types. Granular (also called muddy brown) casts are most typical of acute tubular necrosis and, therefore, are seen in renal damage secondary to ischemic or toxic insults (e.g., shock, sepsis, liver failure with increased bilirubin, aminoglycoside toxicity,

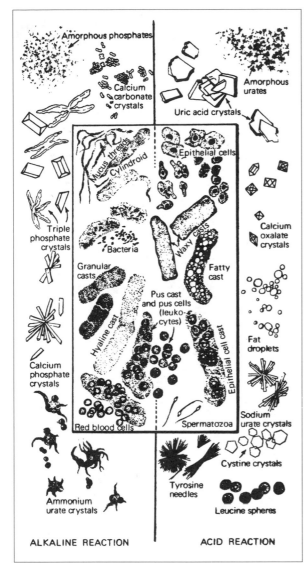

FIGURE 5. Possible microscopic (100–200×) findings (mostly abnormal) in urine sediment. Elements on the left are more likely to be seen in an alkaline urine; those on the right are more likely in an acid urine. (Reproduced, with permission, from Krupp MA, Sweet NJ, Jawetz E, et al. Physician's handbook, 19th ed. Norwalk, CT: Lange Medical Publications; 1979.)

and contrast media toxicity). Since waxy casts occur in many diseases, they do not offer much diagnostic information.

*Broad casts.* As the name implies, broad casts are much wider in diameter than other casts but can be of any type. They may be larger because they form in the collecting ducts as opposed to the narrower tubules. They probably form only when the urine flow rate is very low, as in severe acute or chronic renal failure, and are therefore called "renal failure casts."

### Crystals

Crystaluria, if differentiated by type, can help to identify

**TABLE 6.** Causes of Various Types of Casts in Urine[a]

| Cast | Cause |
| --- | --- |
| Red cell | Acute glomerulonephritis, renal infarct, subacute bacterial endocarditis, Goodpasture's syndrome, lupus nephritis, vasculitis |
| White cell | Acute pyelonephritis or interstitial nephritis |
| Epithelial cell | Toxicity from salicylates and heavy metals, tubular necrosis, cytomegalovirus infection |
| Hyaline | Prerenal azotemia (from CHF, dehydration, etc.) or strenuous exercise |
| Granular | Acute tubular necrosis; less often in severe pyelonephritis and glomerulonephritis |
| Waxy | Renal failure or severe tubular atrophy |
| Broad | May be any of above types, but larger width reflects diameter of their origin (collecting ducts); seen in acute and chronic renal failure |

[a]Adapted from Reference 53.

patients with certain local and systemic diseases. Urate crystals are found in acid urine and dissolve on warming; phosphate crystals form in alkaline urine and dissolve with acidification. The former occur in patients with uric acid uropathy; the latter occur in patients with urinary infections caused by urea-splitting bacteria (e.g., *Proteus*) and in patients with persistently alkaline urine for other reasons. Both crystals also may be found in normal urine.

## Chemical Analysis (Semiquantitative Tests)

For this discussion, biochemical analysis of urine includes protein; pH; specific gravity; bilirubin, bile, and urobilinogen; blood and Hgb; leukocyte esterase; nitrite; and glucose and ketones. All of these semiquantitative tests can be performed quickly using modern dipsticks containing one or more reagent-impregnated pads. When using these strips, the clinician must carefully apply the urine to the pads as instructed and wait the designated time before comparing pad colors to the color chart. Possible results associated with various colors are displayed in Table 7 (next page).

A few tests (protein, pH, and specific gravity) are still performed in the clinical laboratory using more traditional test tube methods.

### Protein
*Normal range: 0–1+ or <150 mg/day or <0.2 mg/mg UCr*

The more common causes of proteinuria are listed in Table

**TABLE 7.** Examples of Tests Available and Possible Results from Multitest Urine Dipstick[a]

| Test | Results | | | | | | |
|------|---------|---|---|---|---|---|---|
| Leukocyte esterase | Negative | Trace | Small + | Moderate ++ | Large +++ | | |
| Nitrite | Negative | Positive | | | | | |
| Urobilinogen | Normal 0.2 mg/dL | Normal 1 mg/dL | 2 mg/dL | 4 mg/dL | 8 mg/dL | | |
| Protein | Negative | Trace | 30 mg/dL + | 100 mg/dL ++ | 300 mg/dL +++ | ≥2000 mg/dL ++++ | |
| pH | 5 | 6 | 6.5 | 7 | 7.5 | 8 | 8.5 |
| Blood (Hgb) | Negative | Nonhemolyzed Trace | Hemolyzed Trace | Small + | Moderate ++ | Large +++ | |
| Specific gravity | 1.000 | 1.005 | 1.010 | 1.015 | 1.020 | 1.025 | 1.030 |
| Ketones | Negative | Trace 5 mg/dL | Small 15 mg/dL | Moderate 40 mg/dL | Large 80 mg/dL | Large 160 mg/dL | |
| Bilirubin | Negative | Small + | Moderate ++ | Large +++ | | | |
| Glucose | Negative | 1/10 g/dL (trace) 100 mg/dL | 1/4 g/dL 250 mg/dL | 1/2 g/dL 500 mg/dL | 1 g/dL 1000 mg/dL | ≥2 g/dL ≥2000 mg/dL | |

[a]*Multistix 10 SG, Bayer.*

8. Even the persistent presence of as little as 150 mg of protein in the urine per day is abnormal. Most protein that passes into the urine is either albumin or globulins.

Abnormal permeability of the glomerular-limiting membrane, prototypically seen with the nephrotic syndrome, allows large quantities of albumin to enter the urine. Even trace amounts in patients with noninsulin-dependent diabetes (type II) are associated with increased mortality.[57] Large quantities of globulins (e.g., Bence Jones proteins) in the urine suggest multiple myeloma. Furthermore, small to moderate amounts of protein may be seen in the urine of patients with dysfunctioning renal tubules since they cannot reabsorb the small amounts of proteins that are normally filtered.

The color indicator test strips used to detect and measure protein in the urine contain a buffer mixed with a dye (usually tetrabromphenol blue). In the absence of albumin, the buffer holds the pH at 3, maintaining a yellow color. If present, albumin reduces the activity coefficient of hydrogen ions (the pH rises), producing a blue color. However, urine containing globulins, including 50% of Bence Jones proteins, is misread as negative. Improper interpretation also may result if the buffer is neutralized by very alkaline urine or is washed off by excessive urine ("drenching"). A newer semiquantitative test uses tablets impregnated with reagents similar to those in the strips. This test, for professional use only, detects albumin concentrations as low as 4 mg/dL.

The more traditional acetic acid and sulfosalicylic

acid methods, being less specific, detect globulins and Bence Jones proteins as well as albumin. These methods are based on the denaturing of protein to produce turbidity. Although they are sensitive to more proteins, they are not specific for proteins. For example, penicillins, especially those administered in large doses (e.g., penicillin G and nafcillin), caused false positives with the acid meth-

**TABLE 8.** Causes of Proteins in Urine

**Little proteinuria (<0.5 g/day)**
  Hemoglobinuria (hemolysis)
  High BP
  Lower urinary tract infection
  Fever
  Renal tubular damage
  Exercise

**Moderate proteinuria (0.5–3 g/day)**
  CHF (severe)
  Chronic glomerulonephritis
  Acute glomerulonephritis (sometimes major)
  Diabetic nephropathy
  Pyelonephritis
  Multiple myeloma
  Preeclampsia of pregnancy

**Major proteinuria (>3 g/day)**
  Amyloid disorders
  Chronic glomerulonephritis (severe)
  Diabetic nephropathy (severe)
  Lipoid nephrosis
  Lupus nephritis
  Focal glomerulosclerosis (AIDS or heroin abuse)

ods in some studies. Discordantly, one study suggested that beta-lactam antibiotics, including penicillin G, ampicillin, methicillin, and cefazolin, do not interfere with the acid tests for urine protein.[58]

Information regarding interferences with specific tests for detecting proteinuria is included in Table 9. When the dipstick method shows negative proteinuria in a patient suspected with this problem (cloudy or foamy urine), the sulfosalicylic or acetic acid method should be used to confirm the result. Conversely, when drug interference is suspected with an acid assay, the dipstick test should be done.

### pH
*Normal range: 4.5–8.0*

Sulfuric acid, resulting from the metabolism of sulfur-containing amino acids, is the primary acid generated by the daily ingestion of food. Normally, the kidneys can eliminate the acid load by excreting acid itself and sodium hydroxide ions. In fact, healthy persons can acidify the urine to pH 4.5, although the average pH is around 6. Any pH close to the reference range can be interpreted as normal as long as it reflects the kidneys' attempts at regulating blood pH. Conversely, a pH within the reference range may be considered abnormal if it is the opposite of what normal homeostasis should produce.

In general, an acidic (versus neutral) urine deters bacterial colonization. An alkaline urine may be seen with either

> Urinary tract infections caused by urea-splitting bacteria such as *Proteus mirabilis* (via ammonia production).
> Tubular defects causing decreased net tubular hydrogen ion secretion, as in renal tubular acidosis.

By their intended or unintended pharmacological actions, drugs also can cause true pH changes; they do not interfere with the reagents used to estimate urine pH.

Drugs that induce diseases associated with pH changes are indirect causes. These and other causes of acidic and alkaline urine are listed in Table 10 (next page). Persistent pHs greater than 7.0 are associated with calcium carbonate, calcium phosphate, and magnesium–ammonium phosphate stones; pHs below 5.5 are associated with cystine and uric acid stones.

pH is usually estimated (in 0.5 increments) by use of test strips containing methyl red and bromthymol blue indicators. These strips undergo a series of color changes from orange to blue over a pH range of 5.0–8.5. In addition, pH can be precisely measured with electronic pH meters.

### Specific Gravity
*Normal range: 1.010–1.025*

The kidneys are responsible for maintaining the blood's osmolality within a narrow range (285–300 mOsm/kg). To do so, however, the kidneys must vary the osmolality of the urine over a wider range. Although osmolality is the best measure of the kidneys' concentrating ability, determining osmolality is difficult. Fortunately, it correlates well with specific gravity when the urine contains normal constituents. Because specific gravity is related to the weight (and not the number) of particles in solution, particles with a weight different from that of sodium chloride (the solute usually in the highest concentration there) can widen the disparity.

Sodium is normally the main contributor to the specific gravity of urine. Nevertheless, other endogenous substances (e.g., glucose, urea, and protein) also can affect it. If the urine contains protein or glucose, the specific gravity is greater at a fixed osmolality than in normal urine. In diabetics, for example, each increase of 270 mg/dL glucose raises the specific gravity by 0.001. This increase would not usually confound matters until the urine reached 2 g/dL, which would account for about 0.010 of the specific gravity (a 50–100% rise from baseline).

Proteinuria affects the specific gravity even less; heavy

**TABLE 9.** Interferences with Tests for Protein in Urine[a]

| Type of Test | Proteins Detected | False Positives | False Negatives |
|---|---|---|---|
| Reagent strip (dipstick) | Albumin (5–10 mg/dL) | Skin disinfectants<br>Sodium bicarbonate<br>Acetazolamide | Very dilute urine<br>High salt concentration |
| Heat and acetic acid | Albumin (5–10 mg/dL)<br>Globulins<br>Bence Jones | Phosphates and urates confusing interpretation<br>Tolbutamide, sulfonamides, penicillins (high dose), tolmetin | Highly buffered alkaline urine |
| Sulfosalicylic acid | Albumin (0.25 mg/dL)<br>Globulins<br>Bence Jones<br>Glycoproteins | Same as for heat and acetic acid, plus cephalothin and chlorpromazine | Highly buffered alkaline urine |

*[a]Adapted from Reference 53.*

**TABLE 10.** Factors Affecting Urine pH[a]

| Urine pH and Factor | Causes and Comments |
|---|---|
| **Alkaline urine** | |
| Drugs | Acetazolamide, bicarbonate salts, thiazides, citrate and acetate salts |
| Postprandial | Specimens voided shortly after meals |
| Vegetarianism | Vegetables do not produce fixed acid residues |
| Metabolic alkalosis | Hyperventilation (initial respiratory alkalosis), severe vomiting, excessive hydrochloric acid loss from GI suctioning |
| Urinary tract infection | Some bacteria (e.g., *Proteus*) split urea to ammonia, which is alkalinizing |
| Renal tubular acidosis | Impaired tubular acidification of urine and low bicarbonate and pH in blood |
| **Acidic urine** | |
| Drugs | Ammonium chloride, ascorbic acid (high dose), acetic acid (bladder irrigation) |
| Food | Cranberries, prunes, plums |
| Ketoacidosis | Diabetes, starvation, high fever |
| Metabolic acidosis | Increased ammonium excretion and cellular hypoxia with lactic acid production (shock) |
| Sleep | |

[a]*Adapted from Reference 53.*

proteinuria (0.4 g/dL) raises it by only 0.001. On the other hand, if the urine contains unusual amounts of urea (a less dense molecule), the specific gravity could be lowered and then interpreted as a sign of the kidneys having lower than actual concentrating ability.

Exogenous substances (e.g., drugs) that concentrate in the urine can increase the specific gravity. For example, after a radiologic study of the kidneys, the iodinated contrast material that appears in the urine may raise the specific gravity to 1.040. Dextran also may cause increases in this parameter. Furthermore, penicillins that are dosed in large quantities can increase the urine's specific gravity according to the following formula:

$$\text{true SG} = \text{lab SG} - \left[ 6 \times \frac{0.8 \times \text{carbenicillin (g/day)}}{24 \text{ hr urine volume (mL)}} \right] \quad (20)$$

where SG is specific gravity.[59] For penicillin G, 4.7 would be used instead of 6. Dehydrated patients typically concentrate urine to a specific gravity of 1.020–1.030. A specific gravity greater than 1.030 is likely to be caused by drugs such as carbenicillin.

Several diseases usually affect specific gravity. In chronic renal failure, the kidneys first lose their ability to concentrate and then their ability to produce dilute urine. When about 80% of the nephron mass is destroyed, the specific gravity hovers around 1.010, the specific gravity of plasma. The urine of patients with diabetes insipidus (Chapter 12) has low values (<1.005), whereas high values are found in patients with inappropriate secretion of antidiuretic hormone (ADH). In general, *urinary* specific gravity should be considered abnormal if it is the "opposite" (high versus low and vice versa) of what normal physiology should produce based on the concurrent *plasma* specific gravity.

Specific gravity is routinely measured with a urinometer or refractometer. The urinometer is akin to a graduated buoy; it requires sufficient urine volume to float freely.

The reading is adjusted according to the urine temperature. The refractometer uses the refractive index as a basis and needs only a few milliliters of urine and no temperature adjustment.

### *Bilirubin, Bile, and Urobilinogen*
*Normal range: zero to trace*

A dark yellow or brown color generally suggests bilirubin in the urine. Most test strips and some tablets (Ictotest) rely on bilirubin's reaction with a diazotized organic dye to yield a distinct color. Patients on ethoxazene, phenazopyridine, and some phenothiazines may have false-positive results. Truly positive results are found in patients with liver disease (jaundice) or internal bleeding.

Urobilinogen (formed by bacterial conversion of conjugated bilirubin in the intestine) increases in the urine when the turnover of heme pigments is abnormally rapid, as in hemolytic anemia, CHF with liver congestion, cirrhosis, viral hepatitis, and drug-induced hepatotoxicity. Elevated urobilinogen may be premonitory of early hepatocellular injury, such as hepatitis, because it is affected before serum bilirubin. Alkaline urine also has increased urobilinogen concentrations (excretion).

Urobilinogen may decrease (if previously elevated) in patients started on antibiotics (e.g., neomycin, chloramphenicol, and tetracycline) that reduce the intestinal flora producing this substance. Urobilinogen is usually absent in total biliary obstruction, since the substance cannot be formed. Increased urobilinogen in the absence of bile in the urine suggests a hemolytic process. Finally, both substances degrade in specimens exposed for prolonged periods to bright fluorescent light or room temperature.

### *Blood and Hemoglobin*
*Normal range: zero to trace*

Lysed RBCs and, therefore, Hgb may be present in the

urine when the urinary tract is damaged. In addition, after intravascular hemolysis and saturation of serum haptoglobin, free Hgb may spill into the urine. This hemoglobinuria occurs within a few hours of severe hemolysis and lasts less than a day. Hemolysis may occur with hereditary diseases (e.g., sickle cell anemia, spherocytosis, and glucose-6-phosphate dehydrogenase deficiency) or paroxysmal nocturnal hemoglobinuria and may be induced by many drugs (Chapter 15).

Hgb acts as a peroxidase and catalyzes the oxidation of *o*-tolidine by peroxide, producing a blue color. When urine is tested for occult blood with common dipsticks, povidone-iodine can cause positive readings in the absence of Hgb. Since this antiseptic is often used to prepare the urethral meatus before urine collection for cultures and the same urine also may be used for Hgb testing, this fact is clinically relevant.

Because of its structural similarity with Hgb, myoglobin in the urine (which may appear after muscle trauma, infarction, or infection) also leads to a positive test despite the absence of hematuria. Conversely, high doses of vitamin C may cause a false negative by inhibiting the reaction rate.

### Leukocyte Esterase
*Normal range: zero to trace*

Many dipsticks can detect leukocyte esterase and give a semiquantitative estimate of pyuria. WBC esterases differ enough from esterases of serum, urine, and kidney tissue to yield reliable results. Specificity and sensitivity are around 96 and 85%, respectively.

Some clinicians think that reading the strip at 5 min (as opposed to the indicated 2 min) decreases false negatives. In fact, the sensitivity of the WBC esterase test (based on more than three WBCs per high-power field in sediment of spun urine) approaches 100% if the strip is read after 5 min. As is often the case, however, increased sensitivity is at the expense of specificity. In one study, the false-positive rate increased from 4.5 to 22% with the 5-min read time.[55] Based on these findings, the WBC pad on the strip should be read at 1–2 min and, if negative, again at 5 min. If the test is positive only at the second reading, a significant—but low—number of WBCs are probably in the urine.

One example of how this test may be applied in an office or clinic involves a woman suspected of having a lower urinary tract infection (dysuria, frequency, and urgency). If she has significant pyuria (2+ or greater leukocyte esterase), she could be started immediately on empiric therapy. In the absence of pyuria, however, therapy could be withheld pending full urinalysis and culture results.[60]

Vitamin C and phenazopyridine interfere with the leukocyte esterase test. Phenazopyridine causes either false-negative or unreadable results.[61]

### Nitrite
*Normal range: none*

Nitrite may be present in the urine as a result of Gram-negative bacterial metabolism of dietary nitrates to nitrites. In this assay, an aromatic amine reacts with any nitrite to produce a colored azo dye. If bacteria that are incapable of this metabolism are causing the infection (Gram-positive bacteria), the test falsely indicates that no bacteria are present. Recent antibacterial therapy and high doses of ascorbic acid also may cause false-negative results.

A positive nitrite test usually corresponds with a positive leukocyte esterase test. However, a positive WBC test may occur with inflammation, whereas the nitrite test pad is only positive when bacteria are present.

### Glucose and Ketones
*Normal range: none*

Glucose in the urine is suggestive of diabetes mellitus. Ketones in the urine are also suggestive of diabetes mellitus, especially when glucose is present. Aspirin has been reported to cause a false-negative ketone test, whereas levodopa and phenazopyridine may cause false-positive ketone results. (These tests are discussed in detail in Chapter 12.)

## URINARY ELECTROLYTES AND FE$_{Na}$ TEST

Like most laboratory tests, urinary electrolytes are rarely definitive for any diagnosis. They can confirm suspicions of a particular medical problem from the history, physical examination, and other laboratory data. They also can assist in determining whether the kidneys are retaining these electrolytes. Along with the results of a urinalysis and serum electrolytes, urinary electrolyte tests allow the practitioner to rule possible diseases in or out of the differential diagnosis.

Because normal values per se have not been firmly established, these tests can be properly interpreted only in the context of the clinical situation and dietary intake. In general, however, because the kidneys play a major role in maintaining the balance of these electrolytes, any concentration in the urine is *normal* if it favors a normal fluid and serum electrolyte status. A related test, the FE$_{Na}$, can assist with common diagnostic dilemmas involving the kidneys' ability to regulate electrolytes. (Chapter 6 covers serum electrolytes.)

### Urinary Sodium, Potassium, and Chloride

The electrolyte that is most commonly measured in the urine is sodium. Occasionally, it also is useful to measure potassium and chloride. Interpretation of urinary sodium, potassium, and chloride is summarized in Table 11 (next page). For these electrolytes, there is no conversion to SI

**TABLE 11.** Interpretation of Urinary Sodium, Potassium, and Chloride[a,b]

| Medical Problem | Electrolyte Value | Likely Diagnosis |
| --- | --- | --- |
| | **Sodium** | |
| Volume depletion | 0–10 mEq/L | Extrarenal sodium loss |
| | >10 mEq/L | Renal sodium wasting or adrenal insufficiency |
| Acute oliguria | 0–10 mEq/L | Prerenal azotemia |
| | >30 mEq/L | Acute tubular necrosis, except contrast-media-induced failure |
| Hyponatremia | 0–10 mEq/L | Volume depletion or edematous diseases |
| | Greater than diet intake | Inappropriate ADH secretion or adrenal insufficiency |
| | **Potassium** | |
| Hypokalemia | 0–10 mEq/L | Nonrenal potassium loss |
| | >10 mEq/L | Renal potassium loss |
| | **Chloride** | |
| Metabolic alkalosis | 0–10 mEq/L | Chloride-responsive alkalosis |
| | Same as diet intake | Chloride-resistant alkalosis |

[a]Adapted from References 62 and 63.
[b]Random samples, assuming no drug therapy that will influence excretion. See exceptions in text.

units since milliequivalents per liter is equivalent to millimoles per liter.

### Sodium
*Normal range: varies widely*

The major diagnostic use of random urinary sodium concentrations is in patients with simultaneous volume depletion, acute oliguria, and hyponatremia.[62] In the volume-depleted patient, urinary sodium may help to determine the underlying cause of the sodium loss (Minicase 2, page 142). When the amount of sodium in the urine is negligible, volume depletion is probably caused by GI or other nonrenal sodium or fluid losses. On the other hand, the presence of sodium suggests renal or adrenal insufficiency if drug-induced and osmotic diuresis can be excluded.

The underlying cause of a sudden stoppage or sharp drop in urine output (acute oliguria) must be quickly assessed. Most often, it is related to either prerenal azotemia or acute tubular necrosis. Patients with pure prerenal oliguria should have markedly diminished urinary sodium concentrations (<5–10 mEq/L). Conversely, in acute tubular necrosis, the values are commonly greater than 30–40 mEq/L. Exceptions are patients with burns, cirrhosis (hepatorenal syndrome), and contrast-media-induced renal failure.[63] An $FE_{Na}$ determination or microscopic examination of the urine (showing granular casts) may firm up a diagnosis of acute tubular necrosis.

Hyponatremia associated with urinary sodium excretion that equals or exceeds dietary intake is often seen with inappropriate ADH secretion or adrenal insufficiency. Low serum sodium with very low urinary sodium (regardless of diet) is consistent with enhanced tubular reabsorption. Depletion of extracellular volume or development (or worsening) of edematous diseases (e.g., CHF, cirrhosis, and nephrotic syndrome) is the usual underlying cause. Furthermore, patients receiving therapeutic doses of heparin for more than a few days may not retain sodium properly because of impaired aldosterone activity.

In addition, clinicians responsible for monitoring drug therapy have another use for this test: assessing a patient's compliance with a diuretic regimen. Compliant patients should have moderate to high concentrations (>10–20 mEq/L) of sodium in their urine.

### Potassium
*Normal range: varies widely*

For patients with unexplained hypokalemia, urinary potassium may provide useful information. Concentrations greater than 10 mEq/L in a hypokalemic patient usually mean that the kidneys are responsible for the loss. This scenario may occur with potassium-wasting diuretics, high-dose penicillin therapy (e.g., ticarcillin), metabolic acidosis or alkalosis, and a few intrinsic renal disorders. Concomitant hypokalemia and low urinary potassium (<10 mEq/L) suggest GI loss (including chronic laxative abuse) as the cause of low serum potassium.

### Chloride
*Normal range: varies*

If metabolic alkalosis is persistent, urinary chloride determination may be of value. Since this disorder is commonly from GI losses of hydrochloric acid or is diuretic induced, urinary chloride levels are not needed.

Usually, urinary sodium and chloride concentrations parallel each other: if sodium is high, chloride is high and vice versa. The direction of change, however, may diverge if the need for urinary electroneutrality is overpowering. For example, if there is heavy excretion of cations other than sodium ($K^+$, $NH_4^+$, $Ca^{++}$, and $H^+$), more chloride than sodium would have to be excreted. Therefore, in a dehydrated patient, where typically both urinary sodium and chloride are low, this situation would lead to the appearance of only a low urine sodium. For similar reasons, the opposite divergence (only a low urinary chloride) may be seen in the dehydrated patient who is excreting large amounts of anions other than chloride [bicarbonate; high-dose penicillins such as ticarcillin and piperacillin (PCN-COO$^-$)].

Elevated urinary chloride without elevated urinary sodium generally occurs when the kidneys respond to metabolic acidosis and attempt to eliminate excess acid as ammonium chloride. Therefore, the urinary anion gap (a concept similar to the serum anion gap discussed in Chapter 8), calculated as $(U_{Na} + U_K) - U_{Cl}$, becomes negative. This calculation can be used to distinguish the normal anion gap acidosis caused by diarrhea (or other GI alkali loss) from that caused by distal renal tubular acidosis. In both disorders, serum potassium is usually low. In patients with renal tubular acidosis, however, urinary pH is always greater than 5.3.

Usually, excretion of urinary hydrogen ions during diarrhea acidifies the urine; however, hypokalemia leads to enhanced ammonia synthesis by the proximal tubular cells. Despite acidemia, the excess urinary ammonia ($NH_3$) accepts a hydrogen ion to become ammonium ($NH_4^+$), which increases the urine pH in some patients with diarrhea. The ammonium picks up chlorine ions and is excreted in the urine, creating a negative urinary anion gap. Hence, the urinary anion gap should be negative in the patient with diarrhea, regardless of the urine pH.

In contrast, although hypokalemia may result in enhanced proximal tubular ammonia synthesis in *distal* renal tubular acidosis, the inability to secrete hydrogen ions into the collecting tubule in this condition limits ammonium chloride formation and excretion. Therefore, the urinary anion gap is positive in distal renal tubular acidosis.

## FE$_{Na}$ Test

In distinguishing prerenal from intrarenal causes (e.g., acute tubular necrosis) of sudden oliguria or azotemia, the FE$_{Na}$ test has a diagnostic discrimination far better (96–100%) than urinary sodium determinations. The better discrimination is because the overlap with urinary sodium is great, the ranges being 5–40 and 10–80 mEq/L for prerenal and intrarenal diseases, respectively.[63,64]

Only a "spot" or random (versus 12–24-hr) urine collection is required, along with a concomitant serum sample. The laboratory should measure sodium and creatinine in the urine and serum. The calculation is

$$FE_{Na} (\%) = \frac{U_{Na}}{S_{Na}} \div \frac{UCr}{SCr} \times 100 \qquad (21)$$

where $U_{Na}$ and $S_{Na}$ are urine and serum sodium in milliequivalents per liter or millimoles per liter, and UCr and SCr are in milligrams per deciliter or micromoles per liter.

**TABLE 12.** FE$_{Na}$ Test Results in Various Conditions[65,a]

| Low (<1%) | High (>1%) |
|---|---|
| Prerenal azotemia | Acute tubular necrosis |
| Acute glomerulonephritis | Urinary obstruction |
| Hepatorenal syndrome | Chronic uremia |
| Renal transplant rejection | Diuretics |

$^a$See exceptions in text.

In a normal subject with a GFR of 120 mL/min and a daily sodium excretion of 120 mEq, FE$_{Na}$ is 0.5%. If the result is between 0.5 and 1%, the cause of the oliguria is probably prerenal (e.g., dehydration, volume depletion, or CHF), as in Minicase 2; if FE$_{Na}$ is 2–5% (or greater), the patient probably has acute tubular necrosis.[64] Table 12 lists FE$_{Na}$ values in various disorders.

In a few situations, however, FE$_{Na}$ may not conform to the usual patterns. It may be 1% or less despite the absence of prerenal azotemia (i.e., in the presence of nonoliguric acute renal failure) in patients with diseases causing sodium-avid states (e.g., ascites of liver disease, CHF, hepatorenal syndrome, nephrotic syndrome, and burns).[66] Moreover, with acute tubular necrosis caused by radiocontrast media, FE$_{Na}$ is often less than 1%.[67]

## URINE UREA NITROGEN AND NITROGEN BALANCE

Urine urea nitrogen is used primarily to determine the nitrogen balance in patients receiving extraordinary nutritional support (e.g., parenteral nutrition). Urine usually is collected for 24 hr, and the amount of nitrogen in urea is measured by various assays. The typical amounts found in practice are 5–25 g/day. The total nitrogen content of the urine is actually sought, and nitrogen within urea is a surrogate measure. Although clinicians assume that the urea nitrogen accounts for 80–90% of the total nitrogen content, the percentage is variable and decreases in certain diseases (e.g., liver disease).[68]

Not all assays produce the same result on the same specimen. Some laboratories use instruments that convert urea to ammonia and then quantitate nitrogen from ammonia (no correction for preexisting ammonia in the specimen). This technique generates results that are 5–10% higher than assays that do not convert urea.[69] Chloramphenicol and sulfonamides may cause falsely low results due to assay interference with most commercially available kits.

### Estimating Total Nitrogen Elimination

The formula:

$$\text{total nitrogen loss (g)} = (UUN \times 1.25) + 2 \qquad (22)$$

where UUN is urine urea nitrogen, is often used to esti-

---

**Minicase 3**

Olivia P., a 34-year-old, 120-lb, 5-ft (BSA of 1.5 m²) female, was brought into the emergency room by her father. She had passed out next to her toilet, where she had been vomiting. Her vomiting started 1 day before admission after she consumed excessive amounts of oil-of-primrose pills (and possibly some other "health foods") purchased in a health food store. Olivia P. had been told that these pills help people feel younger longer. To prevent dehydration, she had drunk lots of apple juice, but her father was not sure how much of it had stayed down. She had been in excellent health previously.

Olivia P.'s vital signs were temperature, 99 °F (37.2 °C); BP, 100/60 mm Hg supine and 70 mm Hg/not detectable sitting up; pulse, 120 and regular; and respiratory rate, 26. Olivia P. was disoriented to place and time. She had a tender abdomen, poor skin turgor, and dry mucous membranes. Laboratory work included

- Sodium, 122 mEq/L (136–145 mEq/L).
- Potassium, 3.2 mEq/L (3.5–5.0 mEq/L).
- Chloride, 80 mEq/L (96–106 mEq/L).
- Carbon dioxide, 30 mEq/L (24–30 mEq/L).
- BUN, 60 mg/dL (8–20 mg/dL).
- SCr, 3 mg/dL (0.7–1.5 mg/dL).
- Glucose, 105 mg/dL (70–110 mg/dL).

Olivia P.'s urine output was only 20 mL in the first 2 hr in the emergency room. Because she was hemodynamically unstable and disoriented, she was admitted to the intensive care unit with normal saline running at 150 mL/hr.

Over the next 3 hr with fluid replacement, Olivia P.'s urine output was only 50 mL. Spot urine sodium was 18 mEq/L, and UCr was 60 mg/dL. Urinalysis revealed frequent hyaline casts; no muddy brown casts; no crystals; rare renal tubular cells; 1+ proteinuria; urobilinogen of 1 mg/dL; negative bilirubin; trace blood, leukocyte esterase and protein; small ketones; no glucose or nitrite; a specific gravity of 1.030; and a pH of 5.

Over the next 24 hr (day 2), despite administration of normal saline, Olivia P. had to receive dopamine at 20 μg/kg/hr to maintain a systolic BP of 90 mm Hg. Because of her low output, she was becoming fluid overloaded; several doses of IV furosemide produced some short-lived increases in output. Two days (day 4) later, her urine output had improved but she was still oliguric (450 mL/24 hr). Her urinalysis revealed many muddy brown (granular) casts, renal tubular cells (loose and in casts), 2+ proteinuria, and few leukocytes and erythrocytes.

After being off diuretics for 24 hr (day 5), Olivia P.'s test results were

- BUN, 50 mg/dL (17.9 mmol/L).
- SCr, 4 mg/dL (354 μmol/L).
- UCr, 50 mg/dL (4420 μmol/L).
- Serum sodium, 138 mEq/L.
- Urine sodium, 85 mEq/L.

A 24-hr urine was collected, resulting in 750 mg creatinine in 500 mL total volume.

*What are Olivia P.'s calculated FE_Na values on days 1 and 4–5? What renal disorder was probably responsible for the oliguria at each time point? What is Olivia P.'s calculated CrCl (in milliliters per minute per 1.73 m²) from the urine collected between days 4 and 5? Also, what is her estimated CrCl from her age, sex, weight, and SCr (days 4–5) using the correct formulas? What clinical signs and symptoms and other test results are consistent or inconsistent with the underlying kidney disease at the various time points?*

**Discussion:** Olivia P.'s kidneys were hypoperfused ("shocked") from severe hypotension, secondary to her intravascular volume depletion from excessive vomiting. The initial BUN:SCr ratio of 60/3 or 20:1 is the upper limit associated with intrinsic renal disease (e.g., acute tubular necrosis) but is also consistent with prerenal azotemia. Prerenal azotemia is a probable cause of her decreased urine output given her dehydration and BP.

The $FE_{Na}$ test done in the emergency room was (18/122) ÷ (60/3) × 100 = 0.7%, typical of oliguria caused by prerenal causes (e.g., intravascular fluid deficit). Urinalysis at this time was not consistent with acute tubular necrosis given the lack of muddy brown casts and rare renal tubular cells. In retrospect, however, acute tubular necrosis probably was evolving.

A few days later (days 4–5), Olivia P.'s urine output had not improved much. Furthermore, evidence indicated that the prerenal disease had evolved into intrarenal disease, namely acute tubular necrosis with persistent oliguria. She had an elevated BUN and SCr, a BUN:SCr ratio of about 12:1 (50/4), $FE_{Na}$ of 4.9% [(85/138) ÷ (50/4) × 100], and muddy brown and renal tubular casts. Her CrCl is calculated as (UCr × 0.12)/(SCr × BSA) or (750 × 0.12)/(4 × 1.5) = 15 mL/min/1.73 m². If Olivia P.'s CrCl were estimated using Method 3, it would be (140 − age) IBM/(72 × SCr) multiplied by 0.9 for females, or [(140 − 34)54.5/(72 × 4)]0.9 = 18 mL/min or 20.8 mL/min/1.73 m². Although Method 3 is not valid here since SCr is not at steady state, the result is still close to the measured value. Method 1 (which is valid with changing SCr values) generates a CrCl of 18.5 mL/min/1.73 m².

---

mate total *body* nitrogen losses (in grams). Then this amount is compared to the amount of nitrogen intake in the form of amino acids for estimation of the nitrogen balance. The 1.25 adjusts the urine urea nitrogen to the total nitrogen content; it is assumed that only 80% of the total nitrogen content is in the form of urea (most of the rest is in ammonia). The 2 in this formula represents the amount of nitrogen (in grams) lost via nonrenal routes, primarily the stool. Some investigators, however, have proposed that urine urea nitrogen plus an actual measurement of urinary ammonia more accurately approximates the urine's total nitrogen content.[70]

## Estimating Nitrogen Balance

A positive nitrogen balance (more nitrogen in than out) is an important therapeutic goal for malnourished patients receiving parenteral and enteral nutrition. Clinicians should strive for at least a nitrogen equilibrium (in equals out).

The amount of amino acids (same as proteins) taken in by a patient can be converted to the approximate amount of incoming nitrogen (in grams) by dividing amino acids by 6.25, since 16% (1/6.25) of the average amino acid's weight is from nitrogen atoms. The amount of nitrogen going out is represented by Equation 22 or (UUN × 1.25) + 2. Therefore, a positive nitrogen balance is represented by

$$\frac{\text{amino acid intake}}{6.25} - (1.25\ \text{UUN} + 2) > 0 \qquad (23)$$

where amino acid intake and urine urea nitrogen are in grams over 24 hr. In malnourished patients, a balance of zero is not adequate. Clinicians typically strive for an excess of at least 4 g of incoming nitrogen per day. Drugs (steroids) and diseases that cause the BUN to rise due to catabolic or antianabolic activity also can cause the urine urea nitrogen to rise.

## SUMMARY

The kidneys play a major role in the regulation of fluids, electrolytes, and the acid–base balance. Kidney function is affected by the cardiovascular, pulmonary, endocrine, and central nervous systems. Therefore, abnormalities in these systems may be reflected in renal or urine tests. The urinalysis is useful as a mirror for organ systems that generate substances (e.g., blood/biliary system and urobilinogen) ultimately eliminated in the urine. A urinalysis allows indirect examination without invasive procedures.

A rise in BUN without a simultaneous rise in SCr is not specific for intrinsic renal disease; however, concomitant elevations in BUN and SCr almost always reflect intrinsic kidney damage. If there is doubt, the practitioner should collect a 12- or 24-hr UCr for CrCl and perform a urinalysis or determine $FE_{Na}$. CrCl can also be estimated—without urine collection—with various formulas and nomograms. Clinicians responsible for dosing and monitoring renally eliminated drugs rely heavily on these tests.

Urine urea nitrogen, the amount of urea nitrogen excreted in the urine per time period (usually 24 hr), is used almost exclusively for determining a patient's nitrogen balance. A positive nitrogen balance in a malnourished patient who is being fed IV or orally (especially if it occurs with a nonfluid weight gain) suggests that the patient is generating new muscular and circulating proteins.

## REFERENCES

1. Sullivan LP, Grantham JJ. Physiology of the kidney, 2nd ed. Philadelphia, PA: Lea & Febiger; 1982.
2. Beck LH, Kassirer JP. Serum electrolytes, serum osmolality, blood urea nitrogen, and serum creatinine. In: Sox HC Jr, ed. Common diagnostic tests: use and interpretation. Philadelphia, PA: American College of Physicians; 1987.
3. Young DS. Effects of drugs on clinical laboratory tests, 3rd ed. Washington, DC: American Association for Clinical Chemistry Press; 1990.
4. Fossati P, Prencipe L, Berti G. Enzymic creatinine assay: a new colorimetric method based on hydrogen peroxide measurement. *Clin Chem*. 1983; 29:1494–6.
5. Bauer JH, Brook CS, Byrch RN. Clinical appraisal of creatinine clearance as a measurement of glomerular filtration rate. *Am J Kidney Dis*. 1982; 2:337–46.
6. Jackson S. Creatinine in urine as an index of urinary excretion rate. *Health Phys*. 1966; 12:843–50.
7. Rubin MI, Barratt TM, eds. Pediatric nephrology. Baltimore, MD: Williams & Wilkins; 1975:21.
8. Savory DJ. Reference ranges for serum creatinine in infants, children and adolescents. *Ann Clin Biochem*. 1990; 27:99–101.
9. Oh MS. Does serum creatinine rise faster in rhabdomyolysis? *Nephron*. 1993; 63:255–7.
10. Muther RS. Drug interference with renal function tests. *Am J Kidney Dis*. 1983; 3:118–20.
11. Bennett WM, Porter GA. Aspirin and renal function. *N Engl J Med*. 1977; 296:1168. Letter.
12. Opravil M, Keusch G, Lüthy R. Pyrimethamine inhibits renal secretion of creatinine. *Antimicrob Agents Chemother*. 1993; 37:1056–60.
13. Perrone R, Madias N, Levey A. Serum creatinine as an index of renal function: new insights into old concepts. *Clin Chem*. 1992; 38:1933–53.
14. Hilbrands LB, Artz MA, Wetzels JFM, et al. Cimetidine improves the reliability of creatinine as a marker of glomerular filtration. *Kidney Int*. 1991; 40:1171–6.
15. Hellerstein S, Alon U, Blowey D, et al. Use of serum creatinine concentration for estimation of glomerular filtration rate. *Am J Dis Child*. 1993; 147:719–20.
16. Lew SQ, Bosch JP. Effect of diet on creatinine clearance and excretion in young and elderly healthy subjects and in patients with renal disease. *J Am Soc Nephrol*. 1991; 2:856–65.
17. Kaji D, Strauss I, Kahn T. Serum creatinine in patients with spinal cord injury. *Mt Sinai J Med*. 1990; 57:160–4.
18. Rama R, Ibáñez J, Pagés T, et al. Plasma and red cell magnesium levels and plasma creatinine after a 100 km race. *Rev Esp Fisiol*. 1993; 49:43–8.
19. Caregaro L, Menon F, Angeli P, et al. Limitations of serum creatinine level and creatinine clearance as filtration markers in cirrhosis. *Arch Intern Med*. 1994; 154:201–5.
20. Kampmann JP, Hansen JM. Glomerular filtration rate and creatinine clearance. *Br J Clin Pharmacol*. 1981; 12:7–14.
21. Lebel RR, Gutmann FD, Mazumdar DC, et al. Creatinine determination in ketosis. *N Engl J Med*. 1984; 310:1671. Letter.
22. Watts GF, Pillay D. Effects of ketones and glucose on the estimation of urinary creatinine: implications for microalbuminuria screening. *Diabetic Med*. 1990; 7:263–5.
23. Delanghe JR, Louagie HK, De Buyzere ML, et al. Glomerular filtration rate and creatinine production in adult icteric patients. *Clin Chim Acta*. 1994; 224:33–44.
24. Mitchell EK. Flucytosine and false elevation of serum creatinine level. *Ann Intern Med*. 1984; 101:278.
25. Blass KG, Ng DSK. Reactivity of acetoacetate with alkaline picrate: an interference of the Jaffé reaction. *Clin Biochem*. 1988; 21:39–47.
26. Kenny D. A study of interferences in routine methods for creatinine measurement. *Scand J Clin Lab Invest*. 1993; 212(53 Suppl):43–7.
27. Halstead AC, Nanji AA. Artifactual lowering of serum cre-

atinine levels in the presence of hyperbilirubinemia. *JAMA.* 1984; 251:38–9. Letter.

28. Piveral K, Miller SC, Baird DR, et al. Apparently raised serum creatinine levels due to cephalosporins. *JAMA.* 1986; 255:323–4. Letter.
29. Nanji AA, Poon R, Hinberg I. Interference by cephalosporins with creatinine measurement by desk-top analyzers. *Eur J Clin Pharmacol.* 1987; 33:427–9.
30. Weber JA, van Zanten AP. Interferences in current methods for measurements of creatinine. *Clin Chem.* 1991; 37:695–700.
31. Santeiro ML, Thompson DF, Sagraves R. Flucytosine interference with serum creatinine determinations. *Drug Intell Clin Pharm.* 1988; 22:879–80.
32. Viraraghavan S, Blass KG. Effect of glucose upon alkaline picrate: a Jaffé interference. *J Clin Chem Clin Biochem.* 1990; 28:95–105.
33. Nanji AA, Whitlow KJ. Spurious increase in serum creatinine associated with intravenous methyldopa therapy. *Drug Intell Clin Pharm.* 1984; 18:896–7.
34. Ducharme MP, Smythe M, Strohs G. Drug-induced alterations in serum creatinine concentrations. *Ann Pharmacother.* 1993; 27:622–33.
35. Richards RJ, Donica MB, Grayer D. Can the blood urea nitrogen/creatinine ratio distinguish upper from lower gastrointestinal bleeding? *J Clin Gastroenterol.* 1990; 12:500–4.
36. Lau AH, Berk SI, Prosser T, et al. Estimation of creatinine clearance in malnourished patients. *Clin Pharm.* 1988; 7:62–5.
37. Badr KF, Ichikawa I. Prerenal failure: a deleterious shift from renal compensation to decompensation. *N Engl J Med.* 1988; 319:623–9.
38. Jones JD, Burnett PC. Creatinine metabolism in humans with decreased renal function: creatinine deficit. *Clin Chem.* 1974; 20:1204–12.
39. Mitch WE, Mackenzie W. A proposed mechanism for reduced creatinine excretion in severe chronic renal failure. *Nephron.* 1978; 21:248–54.
40. Rowe JW, Andres R, Tobin JD, et al. Age-adjusted standards for creatinine clearance. *Ann Intern Med.* 1976; 84:567–9.
41. Pesola GR, Akhavan I, Carlon GC. Urinary creatinine excretion in the ICU: low excretion does not mean inadequate collection. *Am J Crit Care.* 1993; 2:462–6.
42. Dubois D, Dubois EF. Clinical calorimetry: X. Formula to estimate the approximate surface area if height and weight be known. *Arch Intern Med.* 1916; 17:863–71.
43. Mosteller RD. Simplified calculation of body-surface area. *N Engl J Med.* 1987; 317:1098.
44. Traub SL. Creatinine and creatinine clearance. *Hosp Pharm.* 1978; 13:715–22.
45. Traub SL, Johnson CE. Comparison of methods of estimating creatinine clearance in children. *Am J Hosp Pharm.* 1980; 37:195–201.
46. Jelliffe RW, Jelliffe SM. A computer program for estimation of creatinine clearance from unstable serum creatinine concentration. *Math Biosci.* 1972; 14:17–24.
47. Traub SL. Pharmacokinetics and apparent distribution mass. *Clin Pharmacokinet Newsl.* 1985; 2:1–4.
48. Siersback-Nielsen K, Hansen JM, Kampmann J, et al. Rapid evaluation of creatinine clearance. *Lancet.* 1971; 1:1133–4.
49. Cockcroft DW, Gault MH. Prediction of creatinine clearance from serum creatinine. *Nephron.* 1976; 16:31–41.
50. Schwartz GJ, Brion LP, Spitzer A. The use of plasma creatinine concentration for estimating glomerular filtration rate in infants, children and adolescents. *Pediatr Clin North Am.* 1987; 34:571–90.
51. Springate JE, Christensen SL, Feld LG. Serum creatinine level and renal function in children. *Am J Dis Child.* 1992; 146:1232–5.
52. Waz WR, Quattrin T, Feld LG. Serum creatinine, height, and weight do not predict glomerular filtration rate in children with IDDM. *Diabetes Care.* 1993; 16:1067–70.
53. Widmann FK. Clinical interpretation of laboratory tests, 9th ed. Philadelphia, PA: F. A. Davis; 1983.
54. Wallach J. Interpretation of diagnostic tests, 3rd ed. Boston, MA: Little, Brown; 1982:537–9.
55. Shaw ST Jr, Poon SY, Wong ET. Routine urinalysis: is the dipstick enough? *JAMA.* 1985; 253:1596–1600.
56. Jenkins RD, Fenn JP, Matsen JM. Review of urine microscopy for bacteriuria. *JAMA.* 1986; 255:3397–403.
57. Mogensen CE. Microalbuminemia predicts clinical proteinuria and early mortality in maturity-onset diabetes. *N Engl J Med.* 1984; 310:356–60.
58. Yosselson-Superstine S, Sinai Y. Drug interference with urine protein determination. *J Clin Chem Clin Biochem.* 1986; 24:103–6.
59. Zwelling LA, Balow JE. Hypersthenuria in high-dose carbenicillin therapy. *Ann Intern Med.* 1978; 89:225–6.
60. Komaroff AL. Urinalysis and urine culture in women with dysuria. *Ann Intern Med.* 1986; 104:212–8.
61. Kerr JE, Magee-Nolan C, Schuster BL. Interference with phenazopyridine with the leukocyte esterase dipstik. *JAMA.* 1986; 256:38–9.
62. Harrington JT, Cohen JJ. Measurement of urinary electrolytes: indications and limitations. *N Engl J Med.* 1975; 293:1241–3.
63. Sherman RA, Eisinger RP. The use and misuse of urinary sodium and chloride measurements. *JAMA.* 1982; 247:3121–4.
64. Espinel CH. The $FE_{Na}$ test: use in the differential diagnosis of acute renal failure. *JAMA.* 1976; 236:579–81.
65. Espinel CH. Diagnosis of acute and chronic renal failure. *Clin Lab Med.* 1993; 13:89–102.
66. Diamond JR, Yoburn DC. Nonoliguric acute renal failure associated with a low fractional excretion of sodium. *Ann Intern Med.* 1982; 96:597–600.
67. Fang LST, Sirota RA, Ebert TH, et al. Low fractional excretion of sodium with contrast media-induced acute renal failure. *Arch Intern Med.* 1980; 140:531–3.
68. Loder PB, Kee AJ, Horsburgh R, et al. Validity of urinary urea nitrogen as a measure of total urinary nitrogen in adult patients requiring parenteral nutrition. *Crit Care Med.* 1989; 17:309–12.
69. Boehm KA, Helms RA, Storm MC. Assessing the validity of adjusted urinary urea nitrogen as an estimate of total urinary nitrogen in three pediatric populations. *J Parenter Enter Nutr.* 1994; 18:172–6.
70. Burge JC, Choban P, McKnight T, et al. Urinary ammonia plus urinary urea nitrogen as an estimate of total urinary nitrogen in patients receiving parenteral nutrition support. *J Parenter Enter Nutr.* 1993; 17:529–31.

## QuickView—BUN

| Parameter | Description | Comments |
|---|---|---|
| **Common reference ranges** | | |
| Adults | 8–20 mg/dL | |
| | 2.9–7.1 mmol/L | |
| Pediatrics | 4–20 mg/dL | <1 year old |
| **Critical value** | >40 mg/dL | Unexpected; no dehydration |
| | >100 mg/dL | Risk of uremia |
| | Increasing >20 mg/dL in 24 hr | Consistent with new renal failure |
| **Natural substance?** | Yes | Nitrogenous end-product of protein metabolism |
| **Inherent activity?** | No | No normal physiological activity |
| **Location** | | |
| Production | Liver | From ammonia and carbon dioxide |
| Storage | Not stored | |
| Secretion/excretion | Excreted unchanged via glomerular filtration | Some secretion and reabsorption |
| **Major causes of . . .** | | |
| High results | Renal dysfunction | Table 1 |
| | Dehydration and high-protein diet | |
| Associated signs and symptoms | Signs and symptoms of renal failure and uremic syndrome | Decreasing urine output, etc. |
| Low results | Hepatic failure | Also overhydration |
| | Cachexia | |
| Associated signs and symptoms | Signs and symptoms of underlying disorder | Does not cause signs and symptoms directly |
| **After insult, time to . . .** | | |
| Initial elevation | 6–12 hr | Depends on cause |
| Peak values | 6 hr–6 days | Assumes insult not removed |
| Normalization | 6 hr–6 days | Assumes insult removed and no permanent damage |
| **Drugs often monitored with test** | Aminoglycosides, amphotericin B, gallium, lithium, diuretics | Table 3 |
| **Causes of spurious results** | | |
| Falsely elevated | Chloral hydrate | Assay dependent |
| Falsely lowered | Chloramphenicol and streptomycin | Assay dependent |
| | | Sodium fluoride in collection tube depresses results of urease assays |

## QuickView—SCr

| Parameter | Description | Comments |
|---|---|---|
| **Common reference ranges** | | |
| Adults | 0.7–1.5 mg/dL | |
| | 62–133 µmol/L | |
| Pediatrics | 0.2–0.7 mg/dL | SCr (mg/dL) = height (in) × 0.01 |
| | 18–62 µmol/L | |
| **Critical value** | >2 mg/dL or sudden increase >1 mg/dL | |

                    *continued*

## QuickView—SCr *continued*

| Parameter | Description | Comments |
|---|---|---|
| **Natural substance?** | Yes | Waste product of muscle metabolism |
| **Inherent activity?** | No | No physiological activity |
| **Location** | | |
|    Production | Muscle | From creatine and creatine phosphate |
|    Storage | Not stored | |
|    Secretion/excretion | Excreted unchanged via glomerular filtration | Some secretion |
| **Major causes of . . .** | | |
|    High results | Renal dysfunction | Tables 2–4 |
|      Associated signs and symptoms | Signs and symptoms of renal failure | Decreased urine output, acid–base imbalances, anemia |
|    Low results | Abnormally low muscle mass | Cachexia and chronic neuromuscular disease |
|      Associated signs and symptoms | Causes of low muscle mass | Does not cause signs and symptoms directly |
| **After insult, time to . . .** | | |
|    Initial elevation | 6–24 hr | Usual maximum increase of 1–2 mg/dL/day |
|    Peak values | 3–6 days | Assumes insult not removed |
|    Normalization | 3–6 days | Assumes insult removed and no permanent damage |
| **Drugs often monitored with test** | Aminoglycosides, amphotericin B, gallium, lithium | Table 3 |
| **Causes of spurious results** | Table 4 | Assay dependent |

## QuickView—CrCl

| Parameter | Description | Comments |
|---|---|---|
| **Common reference ranges** | | |
|    Adults | 90–140 mL/min/1.73 m$^2$<br>Based on age and sex | Males: CrCl = 133 − (0.64 × age in years)<br>Females: CrCl = 123 − (0.64 × age in years) |
|    Pediatrics | 5–7 days: 45–55 mL/min/1.73 m$^2$<br>1–2 months: 60–70 mL/min/1.73 m$^2$<br>3–4 months: 80–90 mL/min/1.73 m$^2$<br>5–12 months: 75–100 mL/min/1.73 m$^2$ | Approximates adult values after 12 months (adjusted for 1.73 m$^2$ BSA) |
| **Critical value** | Sudden decrease >20–30% | More critical at lower CrCl |
| **Major causes of . . .** | | |
|    High results | Not clinically important | High CrCl usually desirable |
|      Associated signs and symptoms | None | |
|    Low results | Decreasing renal function | Renally eliminated drugs may accumulate |
|      Associated signs and symptoms | Decreasing urine output and signs and symptoms of uremia | Toxicity from drug accumulation |

## QuickView—CrCl *continued*

| Parameter | Description | Comments |
|---|---|---|
| **After insult, time to . . .** | | |
| **Initial decline** | 6–12 hr | |
| **Nadir values** | 3–6 days | Assumes insult not removed |
| **Normalization** | 3–6 days | Assumes insult removed and no permanent damage |
| **Drugs often monitored with test** | Aminoglycosides, amphotericin B, gallium, lithium | Table 3 |
| **Causes of spurious results** | Table 4 | Assay dependent |

# Chapter 8

# Arterial Blood Gases and Acid–Base Balance

*Thomas G. Hall*

Maintenance of normal pH in the body is required for normal health. Cellular metabolism produces acidic substances that must be excreted to prevent acid accumulation. The lungs, kidneys, and a complex system of buffers allow the body to maintain acid–base homeostasis. Arterial blood gases (ABGs) include the pH, arterial partial pressures of oxygen ($PaO_2$) and carbon dioxide ($PaCO_2$), and the bicarbonate ($HCO_3^-$) concentration. By evaluating the ABGs, the clinician can assess a patient's acid–base status. The serum anion gap and lactate concentration provide additional information to classify and evaluate acid–base disorders further.

This chapter reviews acid–base physiology and control, discusses laboratory tests to assess these substances, and provides a method to evaluate a patient's acid–base status. This chapter also reviews the use of ABGs to evaluate the oxygenation and ventilation function of the lungs.

## OBJECTIVES

Upon completion of this chapter, the reader should be able to

1. Discuss the normal physiology of acid–base balance, including the importance of normal pH and usual compensatory mechanisms.
2. Describe the role of the kidneys in maintaining acid–base balance.
3. Describe the role of the lungs in gas exchange and maintenance of acid–base balance.
4. Explain the importance of the carbonic acid/bicarbonate buffer system and the roles of the various buffer system components.
5. List the four simple acid–base disorders, their important causes, and accompanying laboratory test results.
6. Evaluate a patient's acid–base status, given the clinical presentation and laboratory data.
7. In a case study, use the results of ABGs and se-

rum bicarbonate concentration to assess acid–base disorders, ventilation, and oxygenation.
8. In a case study, use the results of the anion gap and serum lactate concentration to interpret acid–base disorders.

## ACID–BASE PHYSIOLOGY

The pH of arterial blood is normally maintained within the narrow range of 7.36–7.44.[1,2] Values of arterial pH 7.35 and lower are termed *acidemia,* and values of arterial pH 7.45 and higher are termed *alkalemia.* A disorder that lowers pH is an *acidosis,* and a disorder that raises pH is an *alkalosis.* The distinction between these terms is often blurred; however, the concept underlying them is important because the arterial pH may be normal in mixed acid–base disorders (e.g., respiratory acidosis plus metabolic alkalosis).

Generally, acid–base homeostasis is maintained by the lungs and kidneys. Acid–base disorders are categorized according to the primary abnormality, the underlying pathophysiological event that disturbs the pH. When the primary abnormality is impaired excretion of carbon dioxide ($CO_2$) by the lungs, the disorder is termed *respiratory acidosis;* excessive lung excretion of carbon dioxide is termed *respiratory alkalosis.* When the primary abnormality is a deficit of bicarbonate (handled by the kidneys), the disorder is termed *metabolic acidosis;* an excess of bicarbonate is termed *metabolic alkalosis.* Laboratory assessment of acid–base status is usually performed on samples of arterial blood, which accurately reflect acid–base status in the body under most conditions.

## Acid–Base Balance

Metabolism of glucose, fats, and protein as an energy source results in the daily production of 15,000 mmol of carbon dioxide, which acts as an acid in the body, and 50–100 mEq of nonvolatile acids (e.g., sulfuric acid).[3]

This continual load of acidic substances must be buffered initially to prevent acute acidosis and then excreted to prevent exceeding the body's buffer capacity.

The principal buffer in the body is the carbonic acid/bicarbonate system. Other buffers, including proteins, phosphate, and hemoglobin (Hgb), also contribute to maintenance of normal pH. However, the carbonic acid/bicarbonate system is particularly important in understanding acid–base physiology for two reasons:

1.  The components of this system are routinely measured in clinical laboratories and used to estimate the overall acid–base status of the body. Because all buffer systems exist in equilibrium in the body, any change in acid–base status is reflected in each system.
2.  The lungs and kidneys closely regulate the concentrations of this system's components, allowing rapid and precise control over acid–base equilibrium.

## Carbonic Acid/Bicarbonate Buffer System

Carbonic acid ($H_2CO_3$), a weak acid, and its conjugate base, bicarbonate ($HCO_3^-$), exist in equilibrium with hydrogen ions ($H^+$):

$$HCO_3^- + H^+ \leftrightarrows H_2CO_3$$

If hydrogen ions are added to the body or released as a result of cellular metabolism, the $H^+$ concentration rises and is reflected by a fall in pH. However, a large portion of the hydrogen ions combines with bicarbonate to form carbonic acid, lessening the effect on pH. The effect of the acid is buffered; the pH remains at or near normal.

In aqueous solutions, carbonic acid reversibly dehydrates to form water and carbon dioxide. This reaction is catalyzed by the enzyme carbonic anhydrase (CA), which is present throughout the body:

$$HCO_3^- + H^+ \leftrightarrows H_2CO_3 \overset{CA}{\leftrightarrows} CO_2 + H_2O$$

Nearly all carbonic acid in the body exists as carbon dioxide gas. Therefore, carbon dioxide is the acid form of the carbonic acid/bicarbonate buffer system. When hydrogen ions are released, the concentration of bicarbonate falls and the concentration of carbon dioxide gas rises.

The Henderson–Hasselbalch equation for the carbonic acid/bicarbonate buffer system describes the mathematical relationship among pH, bicarbonate concentration in milliequivalents per liter, and partial pressure of carbon dioxide $PaCO_2$ (often depicted as $pCO_2$), a measure of the concentration of carbon dioxide gas in fluid) in millimeters of mercury:

$$pH = 6.1 + \log \frac{HCO_3^-}{0.03 \times PaCO_2}$$

This equation demonstrates an important point: *the ratio of the bicarbonate and carbon dioxide concentrations, not the absolute values, determines pH.* The concentration of bicarbonate or carbon dioxide can change dramatically; but if the other value changes proportionately in the same direction, pH remains unchanged.

For arterial blood, the most commonly sampled medium, the normal ratio of bicarbonate (in milliequivalents per liter) to $PaCO_2$ (in millimeters of mercury) is 0.6:1. This ratio results in a pH of 7.40 when the bicarbonate concentration is normal (24 mEq/L $\pm$ 2 or 24 mmol/L $\pm$ 2) and the $PaCO_2$ is normal (40 mm Hg $\pm$ 4 or 5.3 kPa $\pm$ 0.5). It is impossible to predict the pH accurately or to assess a patient's acid–base status from either the bicarbonate concentration or $PaCO_2$ alone. If both are known, however, the pH can be calculated from this equation. In fact, when clinical laboratories evaluate ABGs, only the pH and $PaCO_2$ are measured. The bicarbonate concentration is then calculated from this equation.

## Role of Kidneys and Lungs

The kidneys regulate the concentration of bicarbonate in extracellular fluid, and the lungs regulate the $PaCO_2$. An understanding of the functions of these organs is necessary to evaluate ABGs and acid–base status.

### Kidneys

The principal role of the kidneys in maintaining acid–base homeostasis is to regulate the concentration of bicarbonate in the blood. Since bicarbonate is readily filtered at the glomerulus, the kidneys reabsorb filtered bicarbonate to prevent depletion. Approximately 90% of this reabsorption takes place in the proximal tubule and is catalyzed by carbonic anhydrase (Figure 1). Filtered bicarbonate combines with hydrogen ions secreted by the

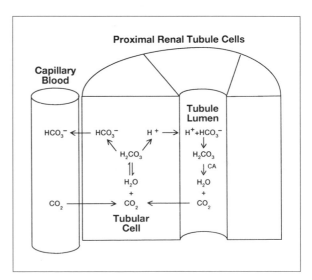

**FIGURE 1.** Reabsorption of bicarbonate from the proximal renal tubule cell.

cell to form carbonic acid. The enzyme carbonic anhydrase (located in the brush border of the tubule) catalyzes conversion of carbonic acid to carbon dioxide, which readily diffuses into the cell. Inside the cell, carbonic acid and bicarbonate are reformed, also catalyzed by carbonic anhydrase. The bicarbonate is reabsorbed into capillary blood. The net result of this process is reabsorption of sodium and bicarbonate. Drugs (e.g., acetazolamide) that are inhibitors of carbonic anhydrase can cause metabolic acidosis by inhibiting this process, causing excessive quantities of bicarbonate to be lost in the urine.

The other major role of the kidneys, as discussed previously, is to excrete the 50–100 mEq/day of nonvolatile acids that are produced by the body. This process occurs primarily in the distal tubule and also requires carbonic anhydrase. The hydrogen ions that are secreted into the tubule lumen are buffered by phosphates and ammonia, so the final urine pH is usually acidic but typically not less than 4.50.

### Lungs

The principal role of the lungs in maintaining acid–base balance is to regulate the $PaCO_2$. After blood returns from the tissues to the right side of the heart, it is pumped through the pulmonary artery to the lungs. In normal capillaries, carbon dioxide readily diffuses from the blood into the alveoli of the lungs and is excreted in exhaled air.

The rate of carbon dioxide excretion is directly proportional to the rate of air passing into and out of the lungs. Under resting conditions, normal individuals take 14–18 breaths/min. The amount of air in each breath, known as the tidal volume, is about 500 mL. Ventilation can be increased either by increasing the rate of respiration or the tidal volume.

Chemoreceptors in the arteries and the medulla in the brain are capable of rapidly increasing or decreasing ventilation in response to changes in pH, $PaO_2$, and $PaCO_2$. This ability (1) allows rapid response to changes in acid–base status and (2) is a reason that the carbonic acid/bicarbonate buffer system is physiologically important. An elevated $PaCO_2$ is usually associated with hypoventilation, and a low $PaCO_2$ is usually associated with hyperventilation.

The other major function of the lungs is to oxygenate the blood. Inspired oxygen diffuses from the alveoli into capillary blood and is bound to Hgb in red blood cells. The oxygen is carried throughout the body via the arterial system and is released to tissues for utilization. Oxygen in arterial blood is present in three forms:

- ➢ Oxygen gas (measured as $PaO_2$ or $pO_2$).
- ➢ Dissolved oxygen.
- ➢ Oxygen bound to Hgb (oxy-Hgb).

However, over 90% of the total arterial oxygen content is as oxy-Hgb. As the oxygenated blood passes through the capillaries, dissolved and gaseous oxygen are taken up by tissues, and additional oxygen rapidly dissociates from Hgb and becomes available for tissue uptake.

## COMPONENTS OF ARTERIAL BLOOD GASES

ABG evaluations include measurements of the arterial pH, $PaO_2$, and $PaCO_2$. The bicarbonate concentration is calculated from the pH and $PaCO_2$ using the equations listed previously. Proper evaluation of ABG results requires specific knowledge about each test.

### pH
*Normal range: 7.36–7.44*

The pH of arterial blood is the first value to consider when using the ABGs to assess a patient's acid–base status. As stated previously, pH values of 7.35 and lower represent acidemia, and pH values of 7.45 and higher represent alkalemia. When a patient's acid–base status is evaluated, the patient must first be classified as having normal pH, acidemia, or alkalemia.

### Arterial Partial Pressure of Carbon Dioxide
*Normal range: 36–44 mm Hg or 4.8–5.9 kPa*

Evaluation of the $PaCO_2$ (commonly seen on lab reports as $pCO_2$) provides information about the adequacy of lung function in excreting carbon dioxide, the acid form of the carbonic acid/bicarbonate buffer system. Because carbon dioxide is a small, uncharged molecule, it diffuses readily from pulmonary capillary blood into the alveoli in normal lungs. Therefore, an elevated $PaCO_2$ usually implies inadequate ventilation.

### Arterial Partial Pressure of Oxygen
*Normal range: 80–100 mm Hg or 10.7–13.3 kPa*

Evaluation of the $PaO_2$ (commonly seen on lab reports as $pO_2$) provides information about the level of oxygenation of arterial blood. If effective circulation is achieved, a normal $PaO_2$ means that oxygen delivery to tissues is adequate. $PaO_2$ commonly is reduced in conjunction with an elevated $PaCO_2$ in states associated with hypoventilation. In fact, the $PaO_2$ is more likely to be diminished because carbon dioxide is much more freely diffusible across the pulmonary capillary and alveolar membranes. Therefore, diseases that impair gas exchange in the lungs can produce hypoxemia, which stimulates increased ventilation. Hyperventilation may fail to correct the hypoxemia but may produce a low $PaCO_2$.

Figure 2 shows the sigmoid relationship between the percentage of available oxygen-binding sites on Hgb that are occupied and the $PaO_2$. The Hgb saturation remains above 90% as long as the $PaO_2$ is above 60 mm Hg (8

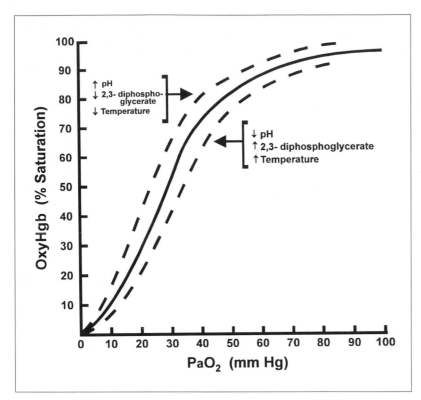

**FIGURE 2.** Oxygen–Hgb dissociation curve. (Adapted from Reference 4.)

kPa). Since most oxygen in arterial blood is present as oxy-Hgb, oxygen delivery to tissues generally remains adequate even though the $PaO_2$ drops to as low as 60 mm Hg. However, $PaO_2$ values less than 60 mm Hg are associated with rapid falls in Hgb saturation and dramatic decreases in oxygen delivery to tissues.

This relationship is important to remember because ABGs measure $PaO_2$. Even though $PaO_2$ values between 60 mm Hg (8 kPa) and normal (80–100 mm Hg or 10.7–13.3 kPa) indicate lung disease, oxygen therapy may not be urgently needed since Hgb saturation is still above 90%. However, $PaO_2$ values less than 60 mm Hg indicate that Hgb saturation is more significantly reduced, and tissue oxygen delivery may be impaired. This impairment may require rapid supplemental oxygen therapy. The atmosphere contains 21% oxygen, and increasing this concentration with supplemental oxygen therapy frequently reverses hypoxemia. Oxygen is administered by increasing the fraction of inspired oxygen ($FiO_2$) to 24–100%.

Several conditions can alter oxygen–Hgb dissociation. Acidosis, fever, and increased concentrations of 2,3-diphosphoglycerate (2,3-DPG) shift the curve in Figure 2 to the right, making oxygen more readily available for delivery to tissues. Alkalosis and decreased 2,3-DPG concentrations shift the curve to the left, increasing oxygen binding to Hgb and potentially reducing oxygen delivery to tissues.

As an alternative to $PaO_2$ values obtained with ABGs, the level of oxygenation can also be assessed by indirectly measuring the oxygen–Hgb saturation with oximetry. In oximetry, a noninvasive method of measurement, a probe is placed on the finger or earlobe and light absorption is quantified. The relative amount of absorption is proportional to the oxygen saturation, which is normally 90–100%. This method is commonly used when frequent monitoring of oxygenation is needed [e.g., for patients receiving intravenous (IV) midazolam or opiates to provide conscious sedation for invasive procedures]. Oximetry provides a continuous estimate of oxygenation without frequent arterial blood sampling.

### Serum Bicarbonate
*Normal range: 24–30 mEq/L or 24–30 mmol/L*

Once the $PaCO_2$ and pH are measured, the bicarbonate concentration is calculated and reported with the ABG results. Either the bicarbonate from the ABG determination or the total carbon dioxide content of serum (discussed below) can be used to assess acid–base disorders.

## OTHER TESTS TO ASSESS ACID–BASE STATUS

### Total Carbon Dioxide (Serum Bicarbonate)
*Normal range: 24–30 mEq/L or 24–30 mmol/L*

The total carbon dioxide concentration is determined by acidifying serum to convert all of the bicarbonate present to carbon dioxide. The total carbon dioxide content is then determined. However, since 95% of total serum carbon dioxide consists of converted bicarbonate, this value is actually a measure of the bicarbonate concentration. Therefore, the term "serum bicarbonate" is often used to describe the results of this test, even though clinical laboratories may report the test as the total carbon dioxide content. It is important to recognize that *this test represents bicarbonate, the base form of the carbonic acid/bicarbonate buffer system, even though the name "total carbon dioxide" implies that it is a measure of acid.*

### Anion Gap
*Normal range: 3–11 mEq/L or 3–11 mmol/L*

The anion gap is a calculated value that is helpful in categorizing and evaluating possible causes of metabolic acidosis.[4] For the body to remain electrically neutral, the numbers of all positively and negatively charged ions must be equal. However, not all ions are routinely measured by clinical laboratories. Most positively charged ions (e.g., sodium, potassium, calcium, and magnesium) are measured. Sodium ($Na^+$) typically accounts for the majority of cations in extracellular fluids. Some anions (e.g., chloride, bicarbonate, and phosphate) are routinely measured, but others (e.g., sulfate, lactate, and pyruvate) are not. Serum proteins are also sources of negative charges that are difficult to quantify.

The number of *unmeasured* anions normally exceeds the number of *unmeasured* cations. When this difference is increased above the upper limit of normal, it often reflects an increase in negatively charged, weak acids. The presence of an increased anion gap in conjunction with metabolic acidosis provides the clinician with useful information about possible causes of acidosis. By convention, the anion gap is calculated using sodium to approximate the measured cations, and chloride ($Cl^-$) and bicarbonate to approximate the measured anions:

$$\text{anion gap} = Na^+ - (Cl^- + HCO_3^-)$$

In conditions that cause metabolic acidosis either by production of hydrochloric acid (HCl) or by excessive loss of bicarbonate, which the kidneys primarily replace with chloride, the anion gap remains normal. This normalcy remains because chloride anions replace bicarbonate in these disorders, and both values are included in the calculation of the anion gap. These conditions are termed *hyperchloremic* or *normal anion gap* metabolic acidosis.

In other conditions, different organic acids are formed, such as formate in methanol intoxication in which methanol is metabolized to formic acid. These anions are not measured in routine electrolyte panels or included in the calculation of the anion gap. Therefore, they produce acidemia, a decrease in serum bicarbonate as this buffer is consumed, and an increase in the calculated anion gap. These conditions are examples of *elevated anion gap* metabolic acidosis.

The normal value for the anion gap has been reduced within the last few years because of changes in clinical chemistry methodologies for measuring chloride ions.[5] This shift has resulted in an increase in the normal range for chloride and a subsequent decrease in the normal value of the anion gap. Prior to this change, the normal anion gap was 8–12 mEq/L (8–12 mmol/L). The normal value at most institutions is now 3–11 mEq/L (3–11 mmol/L); however, this range may vary due to the variability in normal ranges of the values used to calculate anion gap. Clinicians should verify the normal range for anion gap at their institutions.

Various factors can alter the anion gap, making interpretation more difficult.[6] In particular, hypoalbuminemia, hyperlipidemia, lithium intoxication, and multiple myeloma decrease the anion gap. Albumin is one principal source of unmeasured anions, so hypoalbuminemia decreases unmeasured anions and the anion gap. Hyperlipidemia reduces the anion gap both by occupying space in the plasma volume and by interfering with the laboratory assay for chloride. Lithium is a positively charged ion not included in the anion gap calculation. In cases of intoxication, it can decrease the anion gap. Furthermore, multiple myeloma produces positively charged proteins and reduces the anion gap by increasing unmeasured cations. These conditions may convert an elevated anion gap metabolic acidosis to a normal anion gap metabolic acidosis.

In contrast, administration of carbenicillin, mezlocillin, azlocillin, and piperacillin may increase the anion gap because these antibiotics (1) are given in large doses (12–24 g/day), (2) are negatively charged, and (3) increase unmeasured anions. Administration of these agents may convert a normal anion gap metabolic acidosis to an elevated anion gap metabolic acidosis.

The anion gap can also be altered by many electrolyte abnormalities. In particular, abnormalities involving ions not included in the calculation of the anion gap (e.g., potassium and calcium) can affect the anion gap. Therefore, the anion gap must always be interpreted cautiously.

### Serum Lactate
*Normal ranges: 0.5–1.5 mEq/L or 0.5–1.5 mmol/L (venous) and 0.5–2.0 mEq/L or 0.5–2.0 mmol/L (arterial)*

Lactate is a byproduct of the anaerobic metabolism of glucose as an energy source.[7] Metabolism of glucose yields pyruvate, which can be converted to lactate in a reaction catalyzed by lactate dehydrogenase (LDH) (Figure 3). Lactate is transported to the liver and converted back to pyruvate.

When tissues are normally oxygenated, pyruvate is converted to acetyl coenzyme A (acetyl CoA) and is utilized as an energy source via aerobic metabolism. In patients with inadequate tissue perfusion or increased tissue metabolic rates, anaerobic metabolism predominates. Anaerobic metabolism increases the conversion of pyru-

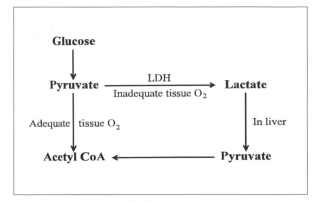

**FIGURE 3.** Lactate metabolism.

vate to lactate, increasing lactate concentrations. When inadequate tissue perfusion is present, lactate is not transported to the liver, further increasing lactate concentrations. If these processes are severe or not reversed, lactic acidosis can occur. Drugs or other conditions that impair lactate or pyruvate metabolism can also produce elevated lactate concentrations.

## BASIC PRINCIPLES IN ACID–BASE ASSESSMENT

Table 1 summarizes the expected laboratory results in the four simple acid–base disorders. For each disorder, the primary laboratory abnormality is accompanied by a compensatory change. For example, the primary abnormality in metabolic acidosis is a fall in serum bicarbonate, and the compensatory change is a fall in $PaCO_2$. These compensatory changes reflect the body's attempts to return the biocarbonate/carbon dioxide ratio and pH closer to the normal range.

An important principle in interpreting these laboratory tests is to recognize that the body never overcompensates and rarely completely compensates for an acid–base disorder. The only exception is chronic respiratory alkalosis, in which the kidneys can completely compensate. Therefore, the pH and direction of change of the $PaCO_2$ and serum bicarbonate generally can be used to classify simple acid–base disorders.

Although respiratory compensation for metabolic acid–base disorders occurs within minutes to hours because the lungs can alter carbon dioxide excretion rapidly, renal compensation for respiratory disorders is slower. Acute respiratory acidosis and alkalosis are associated with minimal compensation (Table 1). This compensation is produced by tissue buffers (e.g., protein and Hgb). Renal compensation, accomplished by altering the bicarbonate concentration, requires 6–12 hr to be initiated and is not complete for 3–5 days.

When assessing a patient's acid–base status, one should always evaluate the pH first. Once the patient is

categorized as being acidemic, alkalemic, or normal, evaluation of the $PaCO_2$ and serum bicarbonate allows categorization of the acid–base disorder. In simple disorders, either the $PaCO_2$ or the serum bicarbonate is abnormal. If compensation has occurred, the other test (serum bicarbonate or $PaCO_2$) is also altered in the same direction. The direction of change in pH, $PaCO_2$, and serum bicarbonate is usually consistent with only one form of simple acid–base disorder.

The formulas listed in Table 1 for normal levels of compensation are estimates only; variability exists in the normal response. Generally, compensatory changes within 10% of the values predicted in Table 1 are consistent with normal compensation. Changes higher than 10% from predicted values should prompt consideration of a mixed acid–base disorder, such as metabolic alkalosis plus respiratory acidosis or metabolic acidosis plus respiratory alkalosis. Changes lower than 10% from predicted values may also suggest a mixed disorder, such as a combined metabolic and respiratory acidosis or metabolic and respiratory alkalosis.

In the case of renal compensation for respiratory acid–base disorders, values intermediate between acute and chronic compensation may indicate either that a mixed disorder is present or that adequate time for compensation has not elapsed. Information from the patient's history and physical examination, including temporal relationships, must be assessed to help evaluate the laboratory data. The minicases and discussions that follow build on this overview to demonstrate evaluation of patients with acid–base disorders.

### Metabolic Acidosis

Patients with metabolic acidosis display an arterial pH less than 7.36 (acidemia) and a low serum bicarbonate concentration, determined either with ABGs or as the total carbon dioxide concentration on the serum chemistry panel. Under most circumstances, the body compensates by hyperventilating to increase carbon dioxide excretion, resulting in a low $PaCO_2$ value (Table 1).

**TABLE 1.** Laboratory Results in Simple Acid–Base Disorders[a]

| Disorder | pH | Primary Alteration | Compensatory Alteration | Normal Level of Compensation[b] |
|---|---|---|---|---|
| Metabolic acidosis | ↓ | ↓↓↓ $HCO_3^-$ | ↓↓ $PaCO_2$ | ↓ $PaCO_2 = 1.2 \times$ ↓ $HCO_3^-$ |
| Metabolic alkalosis | ↑ | ↑↑↑ $HCO_3^-$ | ↑↑ $PaCO_2$ | ↑ $PaCO_2 = 0.6 \times$ ↑ $HCO_3^-$ |
| Respiratory acidosis (acute) | ↓↓ | ↑↑↑ $PaCO_2$ | ↑ $HCO_3^-$ | ↑ $HCO_3^- = 0.1 \times$ ↑ $PaCO_2$ |
| Respiratory acidosis (chronic) | ↓ | ↑↑↑ $PaCO_2$ | ↑↑ $HCO_3^-$ | ↑ $HCO_3^- = 0.4 \times$ ↑ $PaCO_2$ |
| Respiratory alkalosis (acute) | ↑↑ | ↓↓↓ $PaCO_2$ | ↓ $HCO_3^-$ | ↓ $HCO_3^- = 0.2 \times$ ↓ $PaCO_2$ |
| Respiratory alkalosis (chronic) | ↑ | ↓↓↓ $PaCO_2$ | ↓↓ $HCO_3^-$ | ↓ $HCO_3^- = 0.4 \times$ ↓ $PaCO_2$ |

[a]Arrows signify direction and relative magnitude of change from normal values of $PaCO_2$ (40 mm Hg) and $HCO_3^-$ (24 mEq/L).
[b]Normal compensation can vary by approximately ±10% from calculated values.

**TABLE 2.** Common Causes of Metabolic Acidosis[1-4,7]

| Elevated Anion Gap | Normal Anion Gap (Hyperchloremic) |
|---|---|
| **Renal failure** | **Renal tubular acidosis** |
| **Ketoacidosis** | **Diarrhea** |
|    Diabetes mellitus | **Drugs/toxins** |
|    Starvation |    Carbonic anhydrase inhibitors (e.g., acetazolamide) |
|    Ethanol |    Amphotericin B |
| **Lactic acidosis** |    Lithium carbonate |
|    Shock—septic, cardiogenic, hypovolemic |    Lead |
|    Severe hypoxemia |    Ammonium chloride |
|    Carbon monoxide poisoning |    Arginine hydrochloride |
|    Tonic–clonic seizures | |
|    Liver disease | |
|    Biguanides (e.g., metformin and phenformin) | |
| **Intoxications** | |
|    Methanol | |
|    Ethylene glycol | |
|    Salicylates | |

Common causes of metabolic acidosis are listed in Table 2. Once metabolic acidosis is diagnosed, the next step in patient assessment is calculation of the anion gap. This step helps to determine the cause of the acidosis. As shown in Table 2, some causes of metabolic acidosis typically produce an increased anion gap, while others produce a normal gap. With a normal anion gap, the serum chloride is elevated, producing a hyperchloremic metabolic acidosis (Minicase 1).

## Metabolic Alkalosis

An elevated pH with an elevated serum bicarbonate concentration confirms the presence of metabolic alkalosis. Although some respiratory compensation occurs as a result of hypoventilation and carbon dioxide retention, compensation is relatively minor in metabolic alkalosis. The most common causes of metabolic alkalosis (Table 3, next page) are

### ✎ Minicase 1

A 27-year-old female, M. M., was brought to the emergency department in a somnolent state. Her roommate stated that M. M. was diabetic and took insulin shots several times a day. The patient complained the previous evening of a headache and fatigue. Her vital signs included heart rate (HR) 120/min with blood pressure (BP) 110/60 mm Hg supine, HR 140/min with BP 80/40 mm Hg sitting, respiration rate 28/min with deep respirations, and temperature 99.5 °F (37.5 °C). Mucous membranes were dry, and tenting of the skin was present.

M. M. responded to stimuli only by opening her eyes and mumbling; she was unable to answer questions or follow commands. Deep tendon reflexes were mildly hyporeactive. Lung, cardiac, and abdominal exams were normal. Laboratory data included sodium 132 mEq/L (136–145 mEq/L), potassium 4.0 mEq/L (3.5–5.0 mEq/L), chloride 102 mEq/L (96–106 mEq/L), total carbon dioxide 10 mEq/L (24–30 mEq/L), serum creatinine (SCr) 1.4 mg/dL (0.7–1.5 mg/dL), glucose 600 mg/dL (70–110 mg/dL), and white blood cell (WBC) count 10,000 cells/mm³ (4800–10,800 cells/mm³). ABGs on room air were pH 7.23 (7.36–7.44), $PaCO_2$ 22 mm Hg (36–44 mm Hg), $PaO_2$ 100 mm Hg (80–100 mm Hg), and serum bicarbonate 9 mEq/L (24–30 mEq/L).

*What acid–base disorder does M. M. exhibit? What is her anion gap? What is the cause of her acid–base disorder? How are the physical exam findings consistent with this acid–base disorder?*

**Discussion:** M. M.'s pH of 7.23 is clearly in the acidemic range. Further evaluation of the ABGs reveals a markedly low bicarbonate value, suggesting metabolic acidosis. The low $PaCO_2$ value, representing respiratory compensation, confirms this assessment. The level of respiratory compensation is consistent with the expected degree of compensation described in Table 1. The bicarbonate value has fallen by approximately 15 mEq/L from a normal value of 24, and the $PaCO_2$ has been reduced by 18 (1.2 × 15 mEq/L, as predicted in Table 1) to 22 mm Hg from the approximate normal of 40. These values suggest that M. M. has only metabolic acidosis and not a mixed acid–base disorder.

The importance of compensation for acid–base disorders can be appreciated by calculating the expected pH in M. M. if respiratory compensation had not occurred. If the $PaCO_2$ had stayed at 40 mm Hg with a serum bicarbonate of 9 mEq/L, the pH would be 6.98 (Henderson–Hasselbalch equation).

M. M.'s anion gap of 20 mEq/L [132 – (102 + 10)] is elevated, allowing classification of the disorder as a metabolic acidosis with elevated anion gap. The most likely cause is diabetic ketoacidosis (Table 2), as suggested by her medical history and the elevated glucose concentration. Ketoacidosis produces an elevated anion gap due to the production of the ketone bodies, β-hydroxybutyrate and acetoacetate, by-products of fat metabolism. The presence of rapid, deep respirations (Kussmaul) both (1) indicates the hyperventilation response to the acidosis and (2) represents the body's attempt to reduce the carbon dioxide concentration to maintain a more normal pH in the presence of diminished bicarbonate.

**TABLE 3.** Common Causes of Metabolic Alkalosis[1-3]

| |
|---|
| **Loss of gastric acid**[a] |
|    Vomiting |
|    Nasogastric suction |
| **Mineralocorticoid excess** |
|    Hyperaldosteronism |
|    Exogenous mineralocorticoids |
| **Hypokalemia** |
| **Alkali administration** |
|    Oral |
|    Parenteral nutrition with excessive acetate |
|    Excessive administration of bicarbonate in metabolic acidosis |
| **Diuretic therapy** |
|    Loop diuretics (e.g., furosemide) |
|    Thiazide diuretics (e.g., hydrochlorothiazide) |

[a]*May be prevented by administration of gastric acid inhibitors, including omeprazole, lansoprazole, or histamine-2 blockers (e.g., ranitidine, famotidine, and cimetidine).*

> ➤   Loss of gastric acid as a result of vomiting or nasogastric suction.
> ➤   Loss of intravascular volume and chloride ion as a result of diuretic use.

Metabolic alkalosis also occurs in hospitalized pa-

**TABLE 4.** Common Causes of Respiratory Acidosis[1-3,9]

| |
|---|
| **CNS disorders** |
|    Cerebral vascular accident |
|    Tumor |
|    Sleep apnea |
|    Drugs (e.g., opioids and sedative/hypnotics) |
| **Lung disorders** |
|    Airway obstruction |
|    Asthma |
|    Chronic obstructive pulmonary disease (e.g., chronic bronchitis) |
|    Pulmonary edema |
| **Neuromuscular disorders** |
|    Myasthenia gravis |
|    Guillain-Barré syndrome |
|    Hypokalemia |
|    Hypophosphatemia |
|    Neuromuscular blocking drugs |

tients as a result of improper anion balance in parenteral nutrition solutions or overtreatment of metabolic acidosis with bicarbonate. In parenteral nutrition solutions, anions are typically provided as acetate and chloride. Because acetate is metabolized to bicarbonate, excessive acetate and inadequate chloride delivery can produce metabolic alkalosis. In patients with metabolic acidosis due to

---

### ✎ Minicase 2

A 45-year-old male, J. C., was admitted to the general surgery service because of a constant, gnawing abdominal pain lasting 3 days. The pain was present in the left, upper abdominal quadrant and extended to his back. He came to the hospital when the pain got so severe that he was no longer able to eat or drink.

J. C. had a history of mild hypertension treated with hydrochlorothiazide 25 mg by mouth daily. He smoked one pack of cigarettes per day and admitted to consuming two or three martinis with lunch and dinner each day.

J. C.'s vital signs included HR 120/min with BP 120/70 mm Hg supine, HR 132/min with BP 100/60 mm Hg sitting, respiration rate 16/min, and temperature 98.6 °F (37 °C). His physical exam was remarkable only for marked left, upper-quadrant tenderness with guarding and dry mucous membranes. Bowel sounds were present but hypoactive, and rebound tenderness was absent.

J. C. was diagnosed with acute pancreatitis and received nothing by mouth. Intermittent nasogastric suction was initiated. Laboratory data included sodium 135 mEq/L (136–145 mEq/L), potassium 4.0 mEq/L (3.5–5.0 mEq/L), chloride 98 mEq/L (96–106 mEq/L), total carbon dioxide 32 mEq/L (24–30 mEq/L), SCr 1.4 mg/dL (0.7–1.5 mg/dL), glucose 140 mg/dL (70–110 mg/dL), calcium 9.0 g/dL (8.5–10.8 mEq/L), albumin 4.0 g/dL (3.5–5 g/dL), amylase 1100 IU/L, and lipase 840 IU/L. J. C. was given IV fluids and meperidine 75–100 mg intramuscularly every 4 hr as needed for pain.

Thirty-six hours later, his pain had improved slightly and his BP was normal, but he complained of generalized weakness. His ABGs were pH 7.53 (7.36–7.44), $PaCO_2$ 47 mm Hg (36–44 mm Hg), $PaO_2$ 100 mm Hg (80–100 mm Hg), and serum bicarbonate 38 mEq/L (24–30 mEq/L).

*What acid–base disorder is present? What is the cause? What acid–base disorder was present on admission and what was the cause?*

**Discussion:** The elevated pH of 7.53 confirms the presence of an alkalemia. The possible causes are respiratory alkalosis, which would present with a low $PaCO_2$, and metabolic alkalosis, which would present with an elevated serum bicarbonate concentration. In J. C., the elevated serum bicarbonate of 38 mEq/L and slightly elevated $PaCO_2$ are consistent with the diagnosis of metabolic alkalosis.

His degree of hypoventilation and carbon dioxide retention is consistent with the expected degree of respiratory compensation predicted in Table 1. The serum bicarbonate is elevated by 14 mEq/L from the lower of normal value of 24 mEq/L. The expected respiratory compensation for this serum bicarbonate concentration (Table 1) is approximately 8 mm Hg (0.6 × 14 mEq/L increase in bicarbonate), and the $PaCO_2$ is elevated by 7 mm Hg (from approximate normal of 40 mm Hg). Therefore, J. C. appears to have a simple compensated metabolic alkalosis. The most likely cause is the nasogastric suction, which results in removal of hydrogen ions from the stomach (Table 3).

Although definitive classification of J. C.'s acid–base status on admission is not possible since his ABGs were not done, he probably had a mild metabolic alkalosis at that time as well. The increase in bicarbonate, history of diuretic use, and evidence of intravascular volume depletion (i.e., orthostatic hypotension, dry mucous membranes, and reduced oral intake) are consistent with this conclusion.

A 63-year-old male, T. K., arrived at the Family Practice Clinic for a routine followup. He had a history of hypertension, coronary artery disease, and chronic bronchitis but had experienced no episodes of chest pain for the last month. T. K. had a chronic cough productive of approximately 2 cups of white-yellow sputum per day and shortness of breath on walking one block. These symptoms were unchanged over the past 3 months. His medications were diltiazem 240 mg oral daily, isosorbide dinitrate 40 mg oral three times a day, enteric-coated aspirin 325 mg oral daily, ipratropium bromide inhaler two puffs four times a day, albuterol inhaler two puffs as needed for shortness of breath, and nitroglycerin 0.4 mg sublingually as needed for chest pain.

T. K.'s vital signs included HR 90/min, BP 130/85 mm Hg, respiration rate 28/min, and temperature 98.6 °F (37 °C). His physical exam revealed rales and rhonchi throughout both lung fields. His laboratory data included sodium 134 mEq/L (136–145 mEq/L), potassium 3.6 mEq/L (3.5–5.0 mEq/L), chloride 92 mEq/L (96–106 mEq/L), total carbon dioxide 34 mEq/L (24–30 mEq/L), SCr 1.2 mg/dL (0.7–1.5 mg/dL), and glucose 160 mg/dL (70–110 mg/dL). ABGs on room air were pH 7.35 (7.36–7.44), $PaCO_2$ 60 mm Hg (36–44 mm Hg), $PaO_2$ 65 mm Hg (80–100 mm Hg), and serum bicarbonate 32 mEq/L (24–30 mEq/L).

*What acid–base disorder does this patient have and what is the cause? Is this disorder acute or chronic?*

**Discussion:** Inspection of the ABGs reveals that T. K. is acidemic, with a slightly low pH of 7.35. If he had a metabolic acidosis, his serum bicarbonate would be expected to be low. Instead, both the serum bicarbonate and the $PaCO_2$ are elevated. These values are consistent with a compensated respiratory acidosis. Patients with chronic bronchitis commonly exhibit chronic respiratory acidosis due to impaired ventilation (Table 4).[8] The body compensates by avidly reabsorbing bicarbonate to return the bicarbonate/carbon dioxide ratio and pH nearer to normal. The degree of renal compensation, as well as the history of chronic, stable symptoms, is consistent with a chronic disorder (Table 1). The anion gap is normal at 8 mEq/L [134 − (92 + 34)], as expected in patients with respiratory acidosis.

circulatory failure, administration of sodium bicarbonate initially returns the pH toward normal. However, after restoration of adequate circulation, excessive bicarbonate and metabolic alkalosis may be present until the kidneys return the bicarbonate concentration to normal (Minicase 2).

## Respiratory Acidosis

Respiratory acidosis is usually synonymous with hypoventilation. This condition can be a result of numerous causes (Table 4) in three general categories:

> Impaired central nervous system (CNS) respi-

ratory drive.
> Impaired gas exchange in the lungs.
> Impaired neuromuscular function affecting the diaphragm or chest wall.

Laboratory results consistent with respiratory acidosis are a low pH with an elevated $PaCO_2$, indicating inadequate excretion of carbon dioxide. Because the kidneys require 6–12 hr to initiate and 3–5 days to complete compensation, acute respiratory acidosis is associated with much greater alterations in pH than chronic respiratory acidosis. For example, the average patient with an acute rise in $PaCO_2$ to 60 mm Hg (8 kPa) will have a pH of 7.26 with a serum bicarbonate of 26 mEq/L (26 mmol/L; Table 1 and Henderson–Hasselbalch equation). If the same patient's $PaCO_2$ remains at 60 mm Hg for 3–5 days and full renal compensation occurs, the serum bicarbonate will rise to 32 mEq/L (32 mmol/L). This rise returns the arterial pH to a nearly normal value of 7.35. While acute respiratory acidosis associated with hypoxemia may be life threatening, chronic compensated respiratory acidosis usually requires no therapeutic intervention.

## Respiratory Alkalosis

Increased ventilation results in increased carbon dioxide excretion (low $PaCO_2$), elevated pH, and respiratory alkalosis. Typically, the symptoms of respiratory alkalosis are mild and consist of dizziness, lightheadedness, and paresthesias. Acute respiratory alkalosis, commonly produced by the anxiety–hyperventilation syndrome, is usually a benign disorder and reverses either spontaneously or as a result of rebreathing expired air. Chronic respira-

A 24-year-old male, B. H., was brought to the emergency department from the obstetrical floor for evaluation of syncope. He was assisting his wife in Lamaze breathing techniques when he fainted. His laboratory data included sodium 140 mEq/L (136–145 mEq/L), potassium 3.8 mEq/L (3.5–5.0 mEq/L), chloride 102 mEq/L (96–106 mEq/L), serum bicarbonate 24 mEq/L (24–30 mEq/L), SCr 0.8 mg/dL (0.7–1.5 mg/dL), and glucose 140 mg/dL (70–110 mg/dL). B. H.'s ABGs were pH 7.60 (7.36–7.44), $PaCO_2$ 25 mm Hg (36–44 mm Hg), $PaO_2$ 120 mm Hg (80–100 mm Hg), and serum bicarbonate 24 mEq/L (24–30 mEq/L).

*What acid–base disorder does this patient exhibit?*

**Discussion:** B. H.'s arterial pH is in the alkalemic range. Since the serum bicarbonate concentration is not elevated, this condition is not likely to be metabolic alkalosis. However, his $PaCO_2$ is low, consistent with respiratory alkalosis. The most likely cause is hyperventilation (Table 5). Because the alkalosis developed acutely, the kidneys did not have adequate time to compensate, and his pH rose enough to cause syncope.

A 65-year-old female, A. S., was admitted from the emergency department with a chief complaint of dysuria, fever, and back pain for the past 2 days. She had a history of glucose intolerance, obesity, and degenerative joint disease. Her vital signs included HR 100/min, BP 80/40 mm Hg, respiration rate 16/min, and temperature 102.2 °F (39 °C). She was disoriented and responded intermittently to commands. Her lungs were clear, and heart sounds were normal. She displayed costovertebral angle tenderness. Her extremities were cool and pale.

A. S.'s laboratory data included sodium 140 mEq/L (136–145 mEq/L), potassium 3.5 mEq/L (3.5–5.0 mEq/L), chloride 98 mEq/L (96–106 mEq/L), total carbon dioxide 14 mEq/L (24–30 mEq/L), SCr 1.5 mg/dL (0.7–1.5 mg/dL), glucose 200 mg/dL (70–110 mg/dL), and serum lactate 15 mEq/L (15 mmol/L). Her ABGs were pH 7.17 (7.36–7.44), $PaCO_2$ 40 mm Hg (36–44 mm Hg), $PaO_2$ 80 mm Hg (80–100 mm Hg), and serum bicarbonate 14 mEq/L (24–30 mEq/L). Her WBC count was 15,000 cells/mm³ (4800–10,800 cells/mm³) with 50% segmented neutrophils, 20% band neutrophils, 20% lymphocytes, and 10% monocytes.

Urinalysis revealed 4+ bacteria, more than 50 WBCs per high-power field, and WBC casts. A. S.'s Gram stain of urine revealed Gram-negative rods; blood and urine cultures were sent to the lab. She was admitted to the internal medicine service with a presumed diagnosis of urosepsis and started on gentamicin and ceftriaxone.

*What is the patient's acid–base status at this time? How do the other tests help to classify the acid–base disturbance and provide information regarding etiology?*

**Discussion:** The pH of 7.17 is in the acidemic range. Because her bicarbonate concentration is low and the $PaCO_2$ is normal, A. S. must have metabolic acidosis. The fact that the $PaCO_2$ is not reduced to compensate for the low bicarbonate suggests that she has a mixed acid–base disorder, with combined respiratory acidosis and metabolic acidosis. Although the $PaCO_2$ is not elevated, as is expected in respiratory acidosis, pulmonary compensation for her metabolic acidosis is absent. The mental status changes may be responsible for relative hypoventilation.

In assessing the patient's metabolic acidosis, both the anion gap and serum lactate concentration are helpful. The anion gap is elevated (28 mEq/L), as is the lactic acid concentration. These elevations help to define the most likely causes of metabolic acidosis (Table 2). In A. S., metabolic acidosis with an elevated anion gap and lactate concentration—in conjunction with a Gram-negative urinary tract infection and her clinical presentation—is most consistent with septic shock.

**Minicase 5 (continued):** Twelve hours after admission, A. S.'s mental status continued to deteriorate, and her respiratory rate dropped to 12/min. Chest film revealed diffuse pulmonary infiltrates. Repeat ABGs on room air were pH 7.07, $PaCO_2$ 50 mm Hg, $PaO_2$ 55 mm Hg, and serum bicarbonate 14 mEq/L. She was taken to the intensive care unit and placed on mechanical ventilation with 100% oxygen. This patient's repeat blood gases 60 min later were pH 7.15, $PaCO_2$ 47 mm Hg, $PaO_2$ 140 mm Hg, and serum bicarbonate 16 mEq/L.

*What acid–base disorder exists in this patient? What do these blood gases imply about A. S.'s level of oxygenation? Do the results of the second set of ABGs indicate that she needs increased or decreased mechanical ventilation?*

**Discussion (continued):** A. S. now clearly has a mixed acid–base disorder. The low pH of 7.07 is evidence of an acidemia. Evaluation of the $PaCO_2$ and bicarbonate values reveals that the $PaCO_2$ is elevated, consistent with a respiratory acidosis, and the bicarbonate is low, consistent with a metabolic acidosis. A. S. displays a mixed respiratory and metabolic acidosis due to the septic shock producing a lactic acidosis and deterioration of her mental status impairing ventilation, which superimposes a respiratory acidosis.

The blood gases also provide important information about A. S.'s level of oxygenation. The second $PaO_2$ of 55 mm Hg indicates that her blood is inadequately oxygenated. Her oxygen saturation at this level is less than 90%, in the steep portion of the Hgb–oxygen dissociation curve (Figure 2). Further decreases in $PaO_2$ will result in significant reductions in Hgb saturation and significant impairment in oxygen delivery to tissues.

After initiation of mechanical ventilation with 100% oxygen, the $PaO_2$ rises dramatically. This increase is typical when the $FiO_2$ increases from 21 (room air) to 100%. At this point, her level of oxygen saturation is more than adequate. As long as measures are taken to ensure hemodynamic stability so that proper tissue blood flow is provided, tissue oxygen delivery should also be adequate.

However, the second set of blood gases also demonstrates inadequate correction of the respiratory acidosis. The pH is still low, but correction of the metabolic acidosis may take several hours even with appropriate therapy for sepsis. However, A. S.'s $PaCO_2$ is still elevated, indicating the presence of a respiratory acidosis. The mechanical ventilation should rapidly reverse this process. Since the $PaCO_2$ is still elevated despite ample time for correction, some alteration in mechanical ventilation is needed.

Based on the ABGs, two changes are indicated in the ventilator settings. One change is a reduction in the inspired oxygen concentration, which should prevent the oxygen toxicity that occurs when $FiO_2$ exceeds 50% for prolonged periods. Oxygen toxicity is caused by production of oxygen free radicals with subsequent tissue damage in the lungs. Higher levels of $FiO_2$ and longer periods when $FiO_2$ exceeds 50% increase the risk for toxicity by depleting tissue antioxidants. Oxygen toxicity in mechanically ventilated patients is manifested by reduced lung compliance and vital capacity, followed by increased difficulty in adequate oxygenation. In this patient, the percentage of inspired oxygen should be reduced to maintain adequate saturation of Hgb (≥90%) at the minimum of inspired oxygen concentration.

Another change in ventilator settings is that the minute ventilation rate should be increased to improve carbon dioxide excretion. This change can be accomplished by increasing the ventilation rate and/or the volume of air provided with each ventilation (the tidal volume).

**TABLE 5.** Common Causes of Respiratory Alkalosis[1-3]

| |
|---|
| **Hypoxemia** |
| **Lung disease** |
|    Pneumonia |
|    Pulmonary embolism |
| **CNS–respiratory stimulation** |
|    Cerebrovascular accident |
|    Fever |
|    Liver disease |
|    Anxiety–hyperventilation syndrome |
|    Pregnancy |
|    Progesterone derivatives |
|    Salicylate intoxication |

tory alkalosis is also usually a benign disorder. Common causes of respiratory alkalosis are listed in Table 5.

## SUMMARY

This chapter reviews acid–base physiology and disorders and presents a method of evaluating a patient's acid–base status. The lungs regulate the concentration of carbon dioxide, the acid form of the carbonic acid/bicarbonate buffer system. The kidneys regulate the concentration of bicarbonate.

Evaluation of ABGs requires identification of whether the patient is acidemic or alkalemic or has a normal pH. Once this determination is made, the disorder can be categorized into a metabolic or respiratory type by examining both the $PaCO_2$ and serum bicarbonate. Assessment of the degree of compensation and comparison with expected levels of compensation, along with an evaluation of other patient information, allows detection of mixed acid–base disorders. These basic skills enable the clinician to assess a patient's acid–base status quickly and effectively.

## REFERENCES

1. Narins RG, Emmett M. Simple and mixed acid–base disorders: a practical approach. *Medicine.* 1980; 59:161–87.
2. Hall TG, Kleiman-Wexler RL. Acid–base disorders. In: Koda-Kimble MA, Young LY, eds. Applied therapeutics: the clinical use of drugs, 5th ed. Vancouver, WA: Applied Therapeutics; 1992:29-1–29-13.
3. Rose BD. Clinical physiology of acid–base and electrolyte disorders, 4th ed. New York: McGraw-Hill; 1994.
4. Rutherford KA. Principles and application of oximetry. *Crit Care Nurs Clin North Am.* 1989; 1:649–57.
5. Goodkin DA, Gollapudi GK, Narins RG. The role of the anion gap in detecting and managing mixed metabolic acid–base disorders. *Clin Endocrinol Metab.* 1984; 13:333–49.
6. Winter SD, Pearson JR, Gabow PA, et al. The fall of the serum anion gap. *Arch Intern Med.* 1990; 150:311–3.
7. Salem MM, Mujais SK. Gaps in the anion gap. *Arch Intern Med.* 1992; 152:1625–9.
8. Mizrock BA. Lactic acidosis in critical illness. *Crit Care Med.* 1992; 20:80–93.
9. Weinberger SE, Schwartzstein RM, Weiss JW. Hypercapnia. *N Engl J Med.* 1989; 321:1223–31.

## QuickView—PaO$_2$

| Parameter | Description | Comments |
|---|---|---|
| **Common reference ranges** | 80–100 mm Hg | Same in pediatrics |
| **Critical value** | <60 mm Hg | Acute changes of >10 mm Hg may require action |
| **Natural substance?** | Yes | |
| **Inherent activity?** | Yes | Essential for tissue metabolism and life |
| **Location**<br>    Production/intake<br>    Storage<br>    Secretion/excretion | <br>Not produced; inhaled by lungs<br>Stored and carried to tissues on Hgb<br>Exhaled by lungs | |
| **Major causes of . . .**<br>    High results | <br>Inhalation of oxygen-supplemented air | <br>ABG report should include indication of FiO$_2$; room air FiO$_2$ is 21% |
|         Associated signs and symptoms | None | In patients with chronic lung disease, may reduce respiratory drive and cause respiratory acidosis |
|     Low results | Cardiorespiratory arrest<br>Obstructive lung disease<br>Pneumonia<br>Pulmonary edema<br>Pulmonary embolism<br>CNS depressant drugs<br>Neuromuscular diseases | Values in normal range may still indicate disease if FiO$_2$ >21% |
|         Associated signs and symptoms | Dyspnea, tachypnea, weakness, fatigue, mental status changes, tachycardia, cyanosis | |
| **After insult, time to . . .**<br>    Initial elevation or positive result | <br>Minutes | |
|     Peak values | 1 hr | Assumes insult not removed |
|     Normalization | Minutes | Assumes insult removed or supplemental oxygen administered |
| **Drugs often monitored with test** | Not usually performed | May be used to evaluate effects of CNS respiratory depressants (e.g., barbiturates and benzodiazepines) |
| **Causes of spurious results** | Inadvertent venous sample<br>Failure to place sample on ice<br>Air in syringe | |

## QuickView—PaCO$_2$

| Parameter | Description | Comments |
|---|---|---|
| **Common reference ranges** | 36–44 mm Hg | Same in pediatrics |
| **Critical value** | >50 mm Hg | Must be interpreted in context of pH; acute changes of >5–10 mm Hg may require action |
| **Natural substance?** | Yes | |
| **Inherent activity?** | Yes | Serves as reservoir for acid form of bicarbonate buffer system |

## QuickView—PaCO$_2$ *continued*

| Parameter | Description | Comments |
|---|---|---|
| **Location** | | |
| **Production** | All tissues | By-product of glucose and fat metabolism |
| **Storage** | Stored and carried to tissues on Hgb | |
| **Secretion/excretion** | Exhaled by lungs | Excretion rate directly proportional to ventilation |
| **Major causes of . . .** | | |
| **High results** | Hypoventilation<br>Obstructive lung disease<br>Neuromuscular disease<br>Cardiorespiratory arrest | |
| **Associated signs and symptoms** | Dyspnea, headache, flushing, drowsiness | |
| **Low results** | Hyperventilation<br>CNS stimulation | Various CNS and pulmonary diseases result in inappropriate stimulation of respiratory center and increased ventilation |
| **Associated signs and symptoms** | Paresthesias, confusion, lightheadedness | |
| **After insult, time to . . .** | | |
| **Initial elevation or positive result** | Minutes | |
| **Peak values** | 1 hr | Assumes insult not removed |
| **Normalization** | 1 hr | Assumes insult removed |
| **Drugs often monitored with test** | Not usually performed | May be used to evaluate effects of CNS respiratory depressants (e.g., barbiturates and benzodiazepines) |
| **Causes of spurious results** | Inadvertent venous sample | |

## QuickView—pH (H$^+$)

| Parameter | Description | Comments |
|---|---|---|
| **Common reference ranges** | 7.36–7.44 pH units | Same in pediatrics |
| **Critical value** | <7.30 or >7.50 pH units | |
| **Natural substance?** | Yes | Negative logarithm of hydrogen ion concentration |
| **Inherent activity?** | Yes | Provides appropriate milieu for cellular metabolism |
| **Location** | | |
| **Production** | All tissues | By-product of glucose and fat metabolism |
| **Storage** | Not stored | Circulates in blood |
| **Secretion/excretion** | Excreted by kidneys or converted to carbon dioxide and excreted by lungs | In urine, ammonia and phosphate buffer excreted hydrogen ions |
| **Major causes of . . .** | | |
| **High results** | Metabolic alkalosis<br>Respiratory alkalosis | Tables 3 and 5 |
| **Associated signs and symptoms** | Paresthesias, confusion, lightheadedness | |
| **Low results** | Metabolic acidosis<br>Respiratory acidosis | Tables 2 and 4 |
| **Associated signs and symptoms** | Usually dependent on underlying cause of acidosis | |

*continued*

## QuickView—pH (H⁺) *continued*

| Parameter | Description | Comments |
|---|---|---|
| **After insult, time to . . .** | | |
| **Initial elevation or positive result** | Minutes | |
| **Peak values** | 1 hr | Assumes insult not removed |
| **Normalization** | Hours | Assumes insult removed |
| **Drugs often monitored with test** | Not usually performed | |
| **Causes of spurious results** | Inadvertent venous sample | |

## QuickView—Serum Bicarbonate

| Parameter | Description | Comments |
|---|---|---|
| **Common reference ranges** | 24–30 mEq/L | Same in pediatrics; can be determined with total carbon dioxide content in venous blood or by calculation from ABG |
| **Critical value** | <15 or >35 mEq/L | |
| **Natural substance?** | Yes | Weak base component of principal buffer system of body |
| **Inherent activity?** | Yes | Prevents excessive change in pH |
| **Location** | | |
| **Production** | All tissues | |
| **Storage** | Not stored | Circulates in blood |
| **Secretion/excretion** | Kidneys | Normally, kidneys reabsorb virtually all filtered bicarbonate |
| **Major causes of . . .** | | |
| **High results** | Metabolic alkalosis<br>Loss of gastric acid | Table 3 |
| **Associated signs and symptoms** | Paresthesias, confusion, lightheadedness, tetany, seizures | |
| **Low results** | Metabolic acidosis | Table 2 |
| **Associated signs and symptoms** | Usually dependent on underlying cause of acidosis | |
| **After insult, time to . . .** | | |
| **Initial elevation or positive result** | 1–2 hr | |
| **Peak values** | 12–24 hr | Assumes insult not removed |
| **Normalization** | Days | Assumes insult removed |
| **Drugs often monitored with test** | Not usually performed | |
| **Causes of spurious results** | Mishandling of sample | |

## QuickView—Serum Lactate

| Parameter | Description | Comments |
|---|---|---|
| **Common reference ranges** | Venous: 0.5–1.5 mEq/L<br>Arterial: 0.5–2.0 mEq/L | Same in pediatrics |
| **Critical value** | >5 mEq/L | Low values not clinically significant |
| **Natural substance?** | Yes | By-product of anaerobic metabolism of glucose. |
| **Inherent activity?** | No | |
| **Location**<br>  Production<br>  Storage<br>  Secretion/excretion | <br>All metabolically active cells<br>Not stored<br>Kidneys | <br><br>Circulates in blood<br> |
| **Major causes of . . .**<br>  **High results**<br><br>  Associated signs and symptoms<br>  **Low results** | <br>Tissue hypoxia due to shock, congestive heart failure, or cardiopulmonary arrest<br>Usually dependent on underlying cause<br>Not clinically significant | <br>Occasionally glucophage<br><br><br>Does not reflect disease |
| **After insult, time to . . .**<br>  Initial elevation or positive result<br>  **Peak values**<br>  **Normalization** | <br>Minutes<br>Hours<br>Hours to days | <br><br>Assumes insult not removed<br>Assumes insult removed or supplemental oxygen administered |
| **Drugs often monitored with test** | Not usually performed | |

## QuickView—Anion Gap

| Parameter | Description | Comments |
|---|---|---|
| **Common reference ranges** | 3–11 mEq/L | Calculated as<br>  anion gap = $Na^+ - (Cl^- + HCO_3^-)$<br>Normal value has changed recently due to alterations in chloride measurements; same in pediatrics |
| **Critical value** | Not applicable | Of value only in classifying acid–base disorders; response depends on severity and cause of disorder |
| **Major causes of . . .**<br>  **High results**<br><br><br><br>  **Low results**<br><br><br><br>  Associated signs and symptoms | <br>Metabolic acidosis due to renal failure, diabetic ketoacidosis, or lactic acidosis<br>Other causes not associated with acidosis include carbenicillin and similar penicillins<br>Hypoalbuminemia<br>Hyperlipidemia<br>Lithium intoxication<br>Multiple myeloma<br>Not applicable | <br>Table 2 lists other causes with metabolic acidosis; carbenicillin and other penicillins are negatively charged, unmeasured anions and increase anion gap when given in large doses (>12 g/day) |

 *continued*

## QuickView—Anion Gap *continued*

| Parameter | Description | Comments |
|---|---|---|
| **After insult, time to . . .** | | |
|    **Initial elevation or positive result** | Minutes | |
|    **Peak values** | 1 hr | Assumes insult not removed |
|    **Normalization** | Hours | Assumes insult removed |
| **Drugs often monitored with test** | Not usually performed | |
| **Causes of spurious results** | Exposure of blood sample to air | Any condition that causes spurious result in measurement of serum sodium, chloride, or bicarbonate causes error in calculation of anion gap |

# Chapter 9

# Pulmonary Function and Related Tests

*Gary Milavetz*

Pulmonary function tests (PFTs) are useful adjuncts in the diagnosis, evaluation, and monitoring of respiratory disease. A clear diagnosis of many pulmonary diseases is difficult without measurements of the flow or volume of air inspired and expired by the patient. Furthermore, diseases of gas exchange are also difficult to diagnose and follow without pulmonary function measurements.

The appropriate pharmacotherapeutic agents can be chosen and evaluated by using PFTs. Clinicians frequently review changes in these tests to monitor therapy for patients with asthma, cystic fibrosis (CF), emphysema, and other respiratory diseases. This chapter discusses the mechanics and interpretation of PFTs.

## OBJECTIVES

Upon completion of this chapter, the reader should be able to

1. List commonly used PFTs.
2. Describe how PFTs are performed.
3. Interpret commonly used PFTs, given clinical and other laboratory data.
4. Discuss how PFTs are used in the diagnosis of pulmonary diseases.
5. Discuss how PFTs are used in the monitoring of drug therapy.

## ANATOMY AND PHYSIOLOGY OF LUNGS

The left and right lungs are in the pleural cavity of the thorax. These two spongy, conical structures are the primary organs of respiration. The right lung has three lobes, but the left lung has only two lobes; space is thus provided for the heart.

The lungs are connected to the pharynx by the trachea. The trachea splits into the left and right main stem bronchi, and these bronchi deliver inspired air to the respective lungs. These main bronchi continue to split into smaller bronchi, bronchioles, terminal bronchioles, and finally alveoli. In the alveoli, the lungs exchange carbon dioxide for oxygen across a thin membrane separating capillary blood from inspired air.

The thoracic cavity is separated from the abdominal cavity by the diaphragm. The diaphragm—a thin sheet of dome-shaped muscles—contracts and relaxes during breathing. The lungs are contained within the rib cage but rest on the diaphragm. Between the ribs are two sets of intercostal muscles. These muscles attach to each upper and lower rib.

During inhalation, the intercostal muscles and the diaphragm contract, thereby enlarging the thoracic cavity. This action generates a negative intrathoracic pressure, allowing air to rush in through the nose and mouth down into the pharynx, trachea, and lungs. During exhalation, these muscles relax; air is then blown out by a positive intrathoracic pressure.

The purpose of the lungs is to take oxygen from the atmosphere and exchange it for carbon dioxide in the blood. The movement of air in and out of the lungs is called *ventilation*; the movement of blood through the lungs is termed *perfusion*. To have an adequate exchange of the gases, there must be a matching of ventilation (V) and perfusion (Q).

An average V:Q ratio, determined by dividing alveolar ventilation (4 L/min) by cardiac output (5 L/min), is 0.8. A mismatch may result from a cardiovascular anomaly (e.g., pulmonary embolus) that shunts blood away from normal alveoli. Ventilation in this area of the lung is "wasted," and the V:Q ratio approaches infinity. The converse occurs when there is normal perfusion to alveoli that have collapsed ("dead" space).

For the respiration process to be complete, *diffusion* must occur in the alveoli. By the diffusion mechanism, gases in the alveoli equilibrate from areas of high concentration to areas of low concentration. Hemoglobin (Hgb)

**TABLE 1.** Types of Pulmonary Disease

| Type | Pathophysiology | Example |
|------|-----------------|---------|
| Outflow obstruction | Reversible | Asthma |
| | Irreversible | Emphysema |
| Restrictive ventilation | Parenchymal infiltration | Pulmonary hemosiderosis and sarcoid |
| | Loss of lung volume | Pneumothorax, pneumonectomy, pleural effusions |
| | Extrathoracic compression | Kyphosis, morbid obesity, ascites, chest wall deformities |
| Mixed outflow obstruction and restrictive ventilation | All of the above | Chronic obstructive pulmonary disease |
| Diffusion capacity | Pulmonary fibrosis | Interstitial fibrosis |

releases carbon dioxide and adsorbs oxygen through the alveolar walls. If these walls thicken, diffusion is hampered. Membrane thickening may result from an acute or chronic inflammatory process such as

➤ Acute pulmonary edema from congestive heart failure or pneumonia.
➤ Chronic tuberculosis, silicosis, and other fibrotic conditions.

A V:Q mismatching also can decrease the pulmonary diffusing capacity.

Both the airways and lung tissue are important for an understanding of PFTs. Airway function is indicated by tests that measure airflow in or out of the lungs. Lung capacity tests mainly indicate how much air is in the lung parenchyma, even though some air is in the airways. Other specific tests may illuminate ventilation and perfusion, gas diffusion, or specific changes in airway tone or reactivity.

## CLINICAL USE OF PULMONARY FUNCTION TESTING

PFTs are useful in many clinical situations. They help to establish a baseline of respiratory function prior to surgical, medical, or radiation therapy. They also help to detect and measure lung damage caused by these therapies. Similarly, PFTs are used to evaluate the risk of exposure to environmental or occupational hazards.

Obstructive disease (e.g., asthma or chronic bronchitis) can be differentiated from restrictive disease (e.g., kyphosis or sarcoid) by using PFTs. In obstructive diseases, the underlying pathophysiology is a reversible or irreversible obstruction to airflow in the airways. In restrictive diseases, the lungs are restricted in the amount of air they can contain. Obstructive diseases usually decrease the flow of air but not its volume. On the other hand, restrictive diseases usually decrease the volume of air but not its flow (Table 1).

In brief, PFTs are performed to

➤ Evaluate respiratory symptoms.
➤ Screen for respiratory disease.
➤ Assess disease severity.
➤ Preoperatively determine the risk of thoracic or upper abdominal surgery.
➤ Monitor the course of disease.
➤ Evaluate the response to therapy.
➤ Assess the risk of pulmonary exposure to environmental toxins.

Table 2 summarizes the selected uses of PFTs.

## PROCEDURES AND EQUIPMENT
### Spirometry

During spirometry, the patient is typically seated with good posture in front of the pulmonary function equipment. Although patients may stand, they should not be supine or slumped over. Since the patient must respond to commands and have reasonably mature motor control

**TABLE 2.** Selected Uses of PFTs[a]

**Diagnosis**
Signs and symptoms of respiratory disease
Followup of historical or laboratory findings
Disease effects on pulmonary function
Drug effects on pulmonary function

**Evaluation**
Medical–legal issues
Rehabilitation

**Monitoring**
Respiratory disease progression
Prognosis
Occupational or environmental exposure to toxins
Therapeutic drug effectiveness
Drug effects on pulmonary function

[a]Adapted from Reference 1.

and coordination, children younger than about 5 years cannot perform this PFT reproducibly.

After a mouthpiece and nose clip are secured in place, the patient initially is instructed to breathe normally several times. Then the patient inhales as fully as possible and exhales rapidly, forcefully, and completely. The time of full exhalation usually takes at least 5–6 sec but may be prolonged by severe obstruction. This forced, full exhalation is a patient's *forced vital capacity* (FVC).

During this vital capacity maneuver, airflow and the total amount of air expired can be simultaneously measured by obtaining lung capacities or volumes. This maneuver generates a "flow–volume loop" on the PFT screen or a printout of the patient's results (discussed later).

The results of spirometric PFTs depend on the patient's effort. Therefore, patients are routinely asked to repeat the test until at least three efforts vary by less than 5% or 0.1 L. The experienced respiratory therapist can identify patients whose efforts may be submaximal but consistent. This consideration serves as a measure of quality control for the test results.

The physical forces of the airflow and the total amount of air exhaled are converted by transducers to electrical signals and displayed on a computer screen. Since both of these quantities used to be measured by displacement of water by a cylinder in a water bath, current spirometers are frequently called "waterless."

## Body Plethysmography

For body plethysmography, the patient is seated in a large, closed box. Inside, a mouthpiece contains a pressure transducer. It senses the intrathoracic pressure generated when the patient rapidly and forcefully puffs against the closed mouthpiece. These data are then placed into Boyle's law:

$$\frac{P_1 \times V_1}{T_1} = \frac{P_2 \times V_2}{T_2}$$

where

$P_1$ = pressure inside the box where the patient is seated (atmospheric pressure)
$V_1$ = volume of the box
$P_2$ = intrathoracic pressure generated by the patient
$V_2$ = calculated volume of the patient's thoracic cavity

Because temperature ($T_1$ and $T_2$) is constant throughout testing, it is not included in the calculations.

After these data are generated, the patient's results usually are compared to references from a presumed normal population. This comparison necessitates the generation of predicted values for that patient if he or she were completely normal and healthy. Through complex mathematical formulas, sitting and standing height, weight, age, gender, race, and altitude are factored in to give predicted values for the pulmonary functions being assessed.[2]

Instead of a patient's results being compared with set "normal values," the results are described either as a percentage of predicted values or with standard deviations (SD) from the mean from a physically matched healthy population of the same age. With few exceptions, either comparison is acceptable; some pulmonary function laboratories report both values. The exceptions are PFTs that are not normally distributed in the population.

## PULMONARY FUNCTION TESTS

PFTs measure lung volumes, lung flow, and diffusion capacity as well as airway reactivity, compliance, resistance, and conductance.

### Lung Volume Tests

Lung volume tests routinely measure the

- ➤ Tidal volume (TV).
- ➤ Inspiratory capacity (IC).
- ➤ Inspiratory reserve volume (IRV).
- ➤ Expiratory reserve volume (ERV).
- ➤ Slow vital capacity (SVC).
- ➤ Residual volume (RV).
- ➤ Functional residual capacity (FRC).
- ➤ Total lung capacity (TLC).

Lung volume tests indicate the amount of gas contained in the lungs at the various stages of inflation.[3]

RV, FRC, and TLC may be obtained by several methods, including (1) body plethysmography with application of Boyle's law and (2) gas dilution. The different methods can have small but real effects on the values reported. Gas dilution methods only measure ventilated areas, whereas body plethysmography measures both ventilated and nonventilated areas. Therefore, body plethysmography values may be larger in patients with nonventilated or poorly ventilated lung areas.[3]

### *Tidal Volume, Inspiratory Capacity, and Inspiratory and Expiratory Reserve Volumes*

The TV is the amount of air inhaled and exhaled at rest. It usually is a very small proportion of the lung volume—only 500–750 mL—and is infrequently used as a measure of respiratory disease.

The volume measured from the point of the TV where inhalation normally begins to maximal inspiration is known as the IC.

The volume measured from the "top" of the TV (i.e., initial point of normal exhalation) to maximal inspiration is known as the IRV. During exhalation, the volume from the "bottom" of the TV (i.e., initial point of normal inhalation) to maximal expiration is referred to as the ERV.

These four volumes, depicted graphically in Figure 1 (next page), are measured by spirometric PFTs.

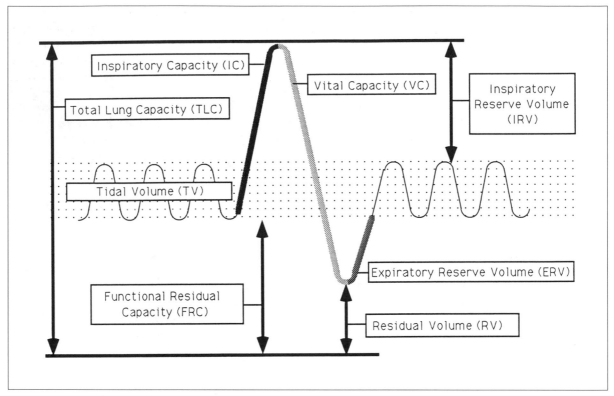

**FIGURE 1.** Lung volumes and capacities—a schematic representation of various lung compartments based on a typical spirogram. (Graphic artwork by Michele Betterton)

### Slow Vital Capacity

When the full inhalation–exhalation procedure is repeated slowly—instead of forcefully and rapidly—it is called the SVC. This value is the maximum amount of air exhaled after a full and complete inhalation.

In patients with normal airway function, SVC and FVC are usually similar. Therefore, they are shown together in Figure 1 as vital capacity. In patients with diseases, such as chronic obstructive pulmonary disease (COPD), results often show temporal divergence. During the initial stages of the disease, the FVC decreases before the SVC. The SVC remains normal because interluminal thoracic pressures are not elevated during the maneuver. Because of the forcefulness of the airflow, however, the FVC shows evidence of air trapping and airway collapse much earlier in the disease process.

### Residual Volume

Following full exhalation to the ERV, the amount of air left in the lungs is called the RV. This air volume, unmeasurable by spirometric methods, is usually obtained by body plethysmography. The RV typically approximates 1 L. Without the RV, the lungs would collapse like deflated balloons. In diseases characterized by obstructions that trap air in the lungs (e.g., asthma), the RV increases; the patient is less able to mobilize air beyond these obstructions.

### Functional Residual Capacity

The FRC is the summation of the ERV and RV. It is the volume of gas remaining in the lungs at the end of the TV. It also may be defined as a balance point between chest wall forces that increase volume and lung parenchymal forces that decrease volume.

An increased FRC represents hyperinflation of the lungs and usually indicates airway obstruction. The FRC may be decreased in diseases that affect many alveoli (e.g., pneumonia) or by restrictive changes, especially those due to fibrotic pulmonary tissue changes.

### Total Lung Capacity

The TLC is the summation of the RV and the vital capacity. It is the total amount of gas contained in the lungs. The TLC also may be referred to as thoracic gas volume.

## Lung Flow Tests

Lung flow tests routinely assess the

> ➤ Forced expiratory volume (FEV).
> ➤ Peak expiratory flow rate (PEFR).
> ➤ Forced expiratory flow (FEF).

These values and a flow–volume loop (discussed in Flow–Volume Curves section) are obtained by spirometry. The flow–volume loop is a graphic representation of inspiration and expiration.[4]

## Forced Expiratory Volume

The full, forced inhalation–exhalation procedure was already described as the FVC. Changes in this measurement from baseline reflect the degree of current airway obstruction. During this maneuver, the computer can discern the amount of air exhaled at specific time intervals of the FVC. By convention, $FEV_{0.5}$, $FEV_1$, and $FEV_3$ are the amounts of air exhaled after 0.5, 1, and 3 sec, respectively. Of these measurements, $FEV_1$ has the most clinical relevance, primarily as an indicator of large airway function. Only air contained in the large airways (oropharynx, trachea, main stem bronchi, and early, large bronchi) can be mobilized for exhalation in this short time.

The "normal range" for $FEV_1$ is 0.75–5.5 L. This range is large because of the physical variables among patients, as discussed previously. Usually, a patient's value is described either as a percentage of a predicted value or as a standard deviation from the mean of a physically matched population of the same age.

A value greater than 80% of the predicted value or within ±2 SD is considered normal. Values less than or equal to 80% or outside 2 SD are abnormal and related to airway obstruction. "Normal" values are often seen in patients with reversible airway obstruction when their disease is not "active"; during acute exacerbation, however, their $FEV_1$ values may be markedly decreased.

In both obstructive and restrictive diseases, the FEV usually shows a reduction in flow. The magnitude of change in $FEV_1$ can indicate the severity of the obstructive airway disease. Degrees of severity may be reported as mild (61–80% of predicted), moderate (41–60%), and severe (≤40%).

The ratio of $FEV_1$ to the FVC is another way to estimate the presence and amount of obstruction in the airways. This ratio indicates the amount of air mobilized in 1 sec as a percentage of the total amount of mobilizable air. Normal, healthy individuals can exhale approximately 50% of their FVC in the first 0.5 sec, about 80% in 1 sec, and about 98% in 3 sec.

Patients with obstructive disease usually show a decreased ratio, and the actual percentage reduction varies with the severity of obstruction (Minicase 1). Generally, this ratio is normal (or high) in patients with restrictive diseases, because both the FVC and $FEV_1$ are similarly reduced from normal in these disorders (Minicase 2, next page). The effects of pulmonary disease on some common PFTs are presented in Table 3 (next page).

## Peak Expiratory Flow Rate

The PEFR (or peak flow) occurs within the first milliseconds of expiratory flow and is a measure of the maximum

---

### ✎ Minicase 1

Ed W., a 22-year-old male with a 14-year history of asthma, reported increasing symptoms of coughing, wheezing, shortness of breath, and chest tightness over the past 12 hr. He came to the clinic for an evaluation of this acute exacerbation of his disease. His only treatment was two puffs of an epinephrine metered-dose inhaler, which he used every 1–2 hr with good response.

After a brief history and physical examination, pre- and postbronchodilator spirometry was performed using two puffs of isoproterenol from a metered-dose inhaler. Auscultation revealed breath sounds only on forced expiration.

The spirometry revealed the following results:

| PFT | Predicted | Prebronchodilator | | | Postbronchodilator | | % Change |
| | | Measured | % Predicted | SD | Measured | SD | |
|---|---|---|---|---|---|---|---|
| FVC (L) | 3.63 | 3.23 | 89 | –0.070 | 3.22 | –0.73 | 0 |
| $FEV_1$ (L) | 3.24 | 2.24 | 69 | –2.33 | 2.87 | –0.77 | 28 |
| $FEV_1$:FVC (%) | 89 | 69 | – | – | 89 | – | 29 |

*What would be a better treatment for Ed W.?*

**Discussion:** Isoproterenol is used because of its rapid onset, strong $\beta_2$-activity, and short duration of effect. The PFTs are obtained within 5 min of the isoproterenol dose. The predicted values are obtained from formulas that take into account the patient's age, gender, height, sitting height, weight, etc.

Although values greater than 80% of predicted are considered normal, a preferable way to evaluate PFTs is to compare the results to the population as a whole. In this manner, standard deviation is used to compare individual results to the general population. Most PFTs are normally distributed, so any value falling within ±2 SD is considered normal.

Ed W. is bronchodilator responsive, as evidenced by the reversal to normal of his $FEV_1$ and $FEV_1$: FVC values. These values are interpreted as normal because the standard deviation returns to within ±2 of the predicted percentage. Since Ed W.'s FVC is normal prebronchodilator, it cannot by definition return to normal. Auscultation of an asthmatic usually finds breath sounds on expiration. Some patients may not experience these breath sounds on expiration but exhibit them on forced expiration. In either case, this finding indicates small airway obstructions.

Because of his responsiveness, Ed W.'s therapy should include inhaled $\beta_2$-selective agonists for his acute exacerbation. Therefore, Ed W. should use an albuterol-metered dose inhaler instead of his epinephrine inhaler.

## ✎ Minicase 2

During an annual physical examination, Sandra S., a 44-year-old female with kyphosis (abnormal spinal curvature), had routine PFTs assessed. On initial review, her PFTs appeared abnormally decreased. Nevertheless, the patient had no complaints of respiratory symptoms now or in the past. Furthermore, her spinal curvature and general health had not changed.

Sandra S.'s PFTs revealed the following results:

| PFT | Predicted | Prebronchodilator | | | Postbronchodilator | | % Change |
| | | Measured | % Predicted | SD | Measured | SD | |
| --- | --- | --- | --- | --- | --- | --- | --- |
| FVC (L) | 3.05 | 0.81 | 22 | −3.73 | 0.91 | −3.57 | 12 |
| FEV$_1$ (L) | 3.05 | 0.79 | 26 | −5.12 | 0.91 | −4.96 | 15 |
| FEV$_1$:FVC (%) | 100 | 98 | – | – | 95 | – | – |
| RV:TLC (%) | 30 | – | – | – | 29 | – | – |

*Why is the FEV$_1$:FVC ratio useful in this case?*

**Discussion:** This case is an example of restrictive lung disease. Because Sandra S.'s thoracic cavity is small and deformed compared to that of a normal, healthy person of similar size and age, her PFTs appear abnormally decreased. Therefore, it is imperative to assess the FEV$_1$:FVC ratio, which is within normal limits. This result indicates that Sandra S.'s airways function normally, even though she has less than normal expansion of her lung tissue. She has an *extra*pulmonary cause for her decreased thoracic volume. An example of an important *intra*pulmonary cause for decreased thoracic volume includes neoplasm. Anything that limits (restricts) the lung's ability to expand can alter PFTs.

airflow rate. At a physician's office or a patient's home or bedside, the PEFR is easily measured with a simple hand-held device (called a peak flow meter) and is widely used as an indicator of large airway obstructions.[5]

Like FEV$_1$, the PEFR has a wide normal range. Healthy men achieve values of 400–800 L/min; healthy women achieve values of 200–600 L/min. A comparison of the current reading with a patient's best values is most useful. At the time of worsened obstruction, the patient's values are markedly decreased from the best values. Values of 50–100 L/min (or less if the flow meter is capable of lower readings) indicate severe, acute obstruction.

Usually, the peak flow is reduced in obstructive diseases but is normal in restrictive diseases. A decreased peak flow also may indicate a mechanical obstruction (e.g., foreign body aspiration). Although peak flows are both very nonspecific and effort dependent, they are commonly used as objective "at home" measurements of airway function.

Asthma is the most common disease monitored with a peak flow meter. These meters are available in community pharmacies. The National Asthma Education Program recommends peak flow monitoring in selected patients.[6] Minicase 3 demonstrates how PEFR is used to monitor asthma patients and their drug therapy.

### Forced Expiratory Flow

FEF measures airflow rate during forced expiration. While FEV measures the volume of air during expiration, FEF measures the rate of air movement. The FEF from 25 to 75% of vital capacity is known as FEF$_{25-75}$. This test specifically measures the flow rate of air in the medium and small airways (bronchioles and terminal bronchioles). Because asthma affects these airways the most, FEF$_{25-75}$ is a good indicator of obstruction.

Flow rates decrease in obstructive disease but remain normal in restrictive disease (Table 3). FEF$_{25-75}$ also gradu-

**TABLE 3.** Effects of Pulmonary Disease on PFTs

| Disease | Vital Capacity | RV | FEV$_1$:FVC |
| --- | --- | --- | --- |
| Chronic obstructive (chronic bronchitis and emphysema) | Normal or decreased | Normal or increased | Decreased |
| Reversible obstructive (asthma) | Normal or decreased | Increased | Decreased |
| Restrictive (extrapulmonary and intrapulmonary) | Decreased | Decreased | Normal |
| Combined obstructive and restrictive | Decreased | Decreased | Decreased |

The father of an 8-year-old girl with chronic asthma called the clinic pharmacy to ask if his daughter, Frances P., should begin a short course of high-dose oral corticosteroids for her increased asthmatic symptoms. Frances P. was well until 18 hr ago when she experienced increased coughing, wheezing, and chest tightness.

Frances P. used a peak flow meter twice a day, recording the best of three efforts each time. Usually, her peak flow was approximately 250 L/min. On this day, before use of her albuterol metered-dose inhaler, her peak flow was 120 L/min. After her inhaled bronchodilator, it was 170 L/min. Although Frances P.'s symptoms improved after the albuterol, they did not completely resolve.

*Should corticosteroids be used in this patient? If so, should the delivery method be oral or inhaled?*

**Discussion:** Peak flow meters are useful objective indicators of large airway function. In this case, the patient assesses her peak flow twice daily for reference. Usually, patients record the best of several efforts.

On this day, Frances P. used the meter before and after her inhaled bronchodilator to indicate whether her airway obstructions adequately responded to albuterol. Because her peak flow improved but did not return to normal, her symptoms are not fully bronchodilator responsive. Some clinicians administer a short course of high-dose oral corticosteroids at this point. Oral corticosteroids are the appropriate choice for acute exacerbation of asthma. Inhaled corticosteroids are used for maintenance therapy of chronic asthma.

ally decreases with age. The flow from 75 to 100% of vital capacity is called alveolar airflow. This parameter may markedly diminish as airways collapse with increased intrathoracic pressure. Such pressure occurs in severe acute asthma when large obstructions are present in terminal bronchioles (Minicase 4, next page).

## Diffusion Capacity Tests

Tests of gas exchange measure the ability of gases to cross (diffuse) the alveolar–capillary membrane and are useful in assessing interstitial lung disease.[7] Typically, these tests measure the per minute transfer of a gas, usually carbon monoxide, from the alveoli to the blood. The diffusion capacity may be lessened following losses in the surface area of the alveoli or thickening of the alveolar–capillary membrane. Thickening may be due to fibrotic changes.

These test results can be confounded by a loss of diffusion capacity due to poor ventilation. Poor ventilation may be related to closed or partially closed airways (as with atelectasis, pneumonia, or airway obstruction) or to a ventilation–perfusion mismatch (as with pulmonary emboli or cor pulmonale). The diffusion capacity of the lungs to carbon monoxide ($DL_{CO}$) can be measured by either a single-breath or steady-state test.

In the single-breath test, the patient deeply inhales—to vital capacity—a mixture of 0.3%, carbon monoxide, 10% helium, and air. After holding the breath for 10 sec, the patient exhales fully; the concentrations of carbon monoxide and helium are measured during the end of expiration (i.e., alveolar flow). These concentrations are compared to the inspired concentrations to determine the amount diffusing across the alveolar membrane. The mean value for carbon monoxide is about 25–30 mL/min/mm Hg.

In the steady-state test, the patient breathes a 0.1–0.2% concentration of carbon monoxide for 5–6 min. In the final 2 min, the expired gases are collected and an arterial blood gas (ABG) is obtained. The exhaled gas is

measured for total volume and concentrations of carbon monoxide, carbon dioxide, and oxygen. The ABG is analyzed for carbon dioxide. These values are used to calculate the amount of gas transferred across the alveolar membrane per unit of time—usually a minute. The usual mean value may be slightly less with the steady-state method than the single-breath method. Furthermore, females typically have slightly lower values than males, probably due in part to slightly smaller lung volumes.

These tests of diffusion capacity are useful for assessing pulmonary fibrotic changes. Diffusion capacity is decreased in diseases that cause alveolar fibrotic changes. Changes may be idiopathic, such as those seen with sarcoid or environmental or occupational disease (asbestosis), or be induced by drugs (e.g., nitrofurantoin, amiodarone, and bleomycin).[8,9] Anything that alters Hgb, decreases the red cell Hgb concentration (Chapter 14), or changes diffusion across the red cell membrane may alter the $DL_{CO}$. The $DL_{CO}$ also reflects the pulmonary capillary blood volume. An increase in this volume (pulmonary edema or asthma) increases the $DL_{CO}$.

## Flow–Volume Curves

Figure 2 (page 183) shows several flow–volume curves where the expiratory flow is plotted against the exhaled volume.[10] As explained earlier, these curves are graphic representations of inspiration and expiration. The shape of the curve indicates both the type of disease and the severity of obstruction.

Obstructive changes result in decreased airflows at lower lung volumes, revealing a characteristic concave appearance. In obstructive cases, the loop size is similar to that of a healthy individual unless there is severe, acute obstruction. Flow–volume curves are usually used with other PFTs. Minicase 5 (page 184) demonstrates other PFT values that may occur in a patient with acute obstruction producing a concave flow–volume curve.

Restrictive changes result in a shape similar to that

## Minicase 4

A 13-year-old boy, Greg A., came to a clinic complaining of increased coughing, wheezing, and chest tightness for 3 days. He had a 9-year history of asthma. His asthma usually was controlled with two puffs of a cromolyn metered-dose inhaler four times a day and two puffs of an albuterol metered-dose inhaler when needed for acute symptoms. Greg A. was currently using his albuterol four or five times a day with an incomplete response. He had had a viral upper respiratory infection for about 1 week. Chest auscultation revealed breath sounds on expiration. A chest X-ray was not obtained, nor were arterial blood gases (ABGs).

PFTs revealed the following results:

| PFT | Predicted | Prebronchodilator Measured | % Predicted | SD | Postbronchodilator Measured | SD | % Change |
|---|---|---|---|---|---|---|---|
| FVC (L) | 2.92 | 1.26 | 43 | −7.39 | 1.15 | −8.25 | −9 |
| FEV$_1$ (L) | 2.49 | 0.54 | 22 | −12.15 | 0.56 | −11.85 | 4 |
| FEV$_1$:FVC (%) | 85 | 43 | – | – | 49 | – | – |
| FEF$_{25-75}$ (L/sec) | 2.86 | 0.20 | 7 | −10.02 | 0.25 | −9.09 | 25 |

Because of the viral upper respiratory infection, subsequent increase in respiratory symptoms with increasing albuterol use, and PFT results indicating no bronchodilator response, Greg A. was placed on a short course of high-dose oral prednisone, 40 mg twice a day, until completely symptom free for 24 hr. He was told to call the clinic if he was not symptom free in 10 days. The PFTs were considered bronchodilator unresponsive because the postbronchodilator values did not normalize to within ±2 SD of the mean for that population. Greg A. called the clinic on day 11 and indicated that he had improved considerably but was not completely clear. His inhaled β$_2$-agonist use had decreased to one or two times a day with the clearing of his symptoms. He was told to continue prednisone, 40 mg twice a day, for an additional 3 days and then to return to the clinic for followup PFTs.

On day 14, Greg A.'s PFTs revealed the following results:

| PFT | Predicted | Prebronchodilator Measured | % Predicted | SD | Postbronchodilator Measured | SD | % Change |
|---|---|---|---|---|---|---|---|
| FVC (L) | 2.92 | 2.93 | 100 | 0.01 | 3.00 | 0.22 | 2 |
| FEV$_1$ (L) | 2.49 | 2.40 | 96 | −0.29 | 2.72 | 0.70 | 13 |
| FEV$_1$:FVC (%) | 85 | 82 | – | – | 91 | – | – |
| FEF$_{25-75}$ (L/sec) | 2.86 | 2.32 | 73 | −0.84 | 2.25 | 0.84 | 89 |

*Should this patient's chronic maintenance therapy be altered?*

**Discussion:** After 14 days of prednisone, the patient's asthma is back in control. The PFTs have returned to the predicted values; Greg A's coughing, wheezing, and chest tightness are resolved. Moreover, his chest is clear to auscultation.

The remaining reduced FEF$_{25-75}$ indicates residual obstructions in the patient's small airways. They would eventually be cleared up if the prednisone was continued. The oral steroid is stopped, and Greg A. started on inhaled beclomethasone, six puffs twice a day, as maintenance therapy. Because of the relatively short duration of the prednisone therapy and the beginning of inhaled beclomethasone, tapering of prednisone is not necessary.

This presentation is common for patients with viral induced asthma. They have a "cold" that lasts 10–14 days and exacerbates their asthma. The exacerbation starts with increasing asthma symptoms that may, but usually do not, respond to β-agonists. A short course of high-dose oral prednisone brings the asthma back into control.

---

of a healthy individual, but the size is considerably smaller. The flow–volume loop also reveals mixed obstructive and restrictive disease by a combination of the two patterns.

## Airway Reactivity Tests

### Bronchoprovocational Testing

Bronchoprovocational testing is usually considered a research tool. Nevertheless, it may help to confirm a diagnosis of asthma due to airway hyperreactivity when the diagnosis (based on the patient's history and traditional PFTs) is equivocal.[11] In this test, inhaled histamine or methacholine is used to provoke bronchospasms in susceptible individuals.[12] Histamine must be compounded extemporaneously, but methacholine is available commercially.[13]

Typical protocols begin by nebulizing low concentrations (0.03125 mg/mL) of either agent followed by spirometry (FEV$_1$ and/or FVC). The concentration is doubled at specific time intervals (about 5 min) until a set decrease (usually 20% from baseline) in the FEV$_1$ or FVC is attained. If the maximal concentration of the agent used is less than or equal to 8 mg/mL, the patient has increased airway reactivity. If the concentration is greater

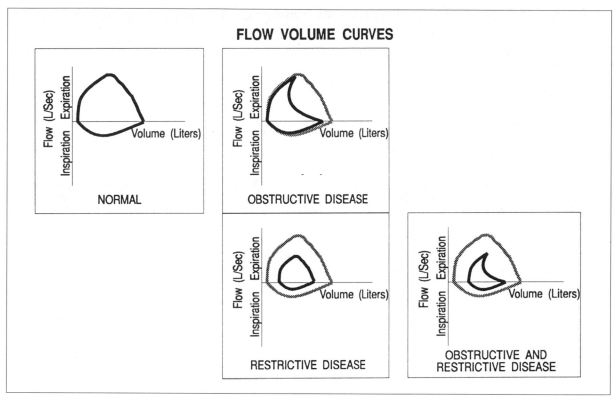

**FIGURE 2.** Flow–volume loops seen with common obstructive and restrictive pulmonary diseases. (Graphic artwork by Michele Betterton)

than 8 mg/mL, the patient has normally sensitive airways. Frequently, inhalation challenges are continued up to a concentration of 128 mg/mL, but even normal subjects usually have some bronchospasm at such high doses. The advantage of both histamine and methacholine is their short duration of effect—usually only 15–45 min.

Although increased reactivity of airways may be indicative of reversible airway disease, a diagnosis of asthma is usually not made until a careful history, physical examination, and PFTs are obtained. An attenuated response may occur in patients receiving theophylline, $\beta_2$-adrenergic agonists (e.g., albuterol), anticholinergics (e.g., ipratropium), cromolyn, or corticosteroids (e.g., prednisone or beclomethasone). The response may be intensified in patients receiving $\beta_2$-adrenergic blockers (e.g., propanolol).

*One important caution*: A patient may exhibit severe, life-threatening bronchoconstriction during the provocational challenge. Therefore, it should be performed by trained personnel only where emergency actions may be readily taken.

### Bronchodilator Studies

Bronchodilator studies are frequently used to assess a patient's response to these medications.[14] The various types of results seen with these tests are illustrated in the minicases.

The patient is asked to perform spirometry and plethysmography immediately before and after the administration of an inhaled $\beta_2$-adrenergic agonist. If the patient then has improved airflow and volume, he or she may be a candidate for bronchodilator therapy. This therapy may take the form of inhaled, $\beta_2$-adrenergic agonists (i.e., albuterol or terbutaline) or theophylline. Without a positive response, further bronchodilator therapy is unlikely to elicit significant improvement. Patients with emphysema, however, frequently show a decreased flow pattern with little PFT response to bronchodilators but still feel better after using them.

Some clinicians use anticholinergics (e.g., ipratropium or atropine) as bronchodilators instead of a $\beta_2$-adrenergic agonist, particularly for patients with COPD (e.g., chronic bronchitis or emphysema). Anticholinergics have demonstrated efficacy in treating COPD both as intervention (acute) and maintenance therapy. Efficacy is lacking in the treatment of asthma. The procedure is the same. Other medications besides $\beta_2$-adrenergic agonists, such as corticosteroids and anticholinergics, may still be necessary in controlling these respiratory diseases.

### Specialized Tests

Specialized tests may help to diagnose or evaluate respiratory response to specific agents. Exercise stress testing confirms or rules out exercise- or exertion-induced asthma (or bronchospasm). Patients are asked to maintain 60–80% of the aerobic capacity of their heart rate on a treadmill for at least 5 min. After the exercise is completed, the

### Minicase 5

A 46-year-old male, Kent N., presented to a respiratory clinic for evaluation of his persistent cough and shortness of breath. His respiratory symptoms had been consistent, neither increasing nor decreasing for several months. They had progressively worsened over the past 15–20 years. Currently, Kent N. produced a teaspoonful to a tablespoonful of sputum each 24 hr. He had no history of fever, sore throat, or rhinitis but had been smoking at least one pack of cigarettes each day for 30 years.

A brief physical exam revealed a thin adult male with breath sounds on inspiration and expiration during auscultation. His pulse was 76 beats/min with regular rate and rhythm and no murmurs heard. His blood pressure was 134/78 mm Hg, and his temperature was 98.9 °F (37.2 °C). A chest radiograph revealed increased bronchiolar markings and slight hyperinflation with barrel chest. ABGs were not obtained.

PFTs revealed the following results (postbronchodilator values were obtained after two puffs of isoproterenol from a metered-dose inhaler):

| PFT | Predicted | Prebronchodilator | | | Postbronchodilator | | |
|---|---|---|---|---|---|---|---|
| | | Measured | % Predicted | SD | Measured | SD | % Change |
| FVC (L) | 4.60 | 1.41 | 31 | −8.10 | 1.94 | −5.94 | 38 |
| FEV$_1$ (L) | 3.80 | 0.61 | 16 | −12.53 | 0.71 | −11.47 | 16 |
| FEV$_1$:FVC (%) | 83 | 43 | – | – | 37 | NA[a] | NA[a] |
| FEF$_{25-75}$ (L/sec) | 4.03 | 0.21 | 5 | −9.29 | 0.21 | −9.29 | 0 |
| SVC (L) | 4.60 | – | – | – | 2.15 | −5.22 | NA[a] |
| TLC (L) | 6.94 | – | – | – | 5.99 | NA[a] | NA[a] |
| RV (L) | 2.33 | – | – | – | 3.83 | NA[a] | NA[a] |
| RV:TLC (%) | 34 | – | – | – | 64 | NA[a] | NA[a] |

[a]NA = not applicable.

*What factors suggest a diagnosis of COPD?*

**Discussion:** The poor prebronchodilator PFT results and the lack of a postbronchodilator response support the diagnosis of COPD. Kent N.'s poor baseline PFTs indicate that he is markedly obstructed. Furthermore, his lack of response to a strong β-agonist indicates that the obstructions in his lungs are not caused primarily (if at all) by bronchospasms. The obstructions could be caused by inflammation and airway damage.

The breath sounds present during both inspiration and expiration also are compatible with a diagnosis of COPD. Breath sounds on expiration are compatible with the diagnosis of asthma, while breath sounds on inspiration are usually associated with stridor. Breath sounds occur when air rushes over and through the partial obstructions in the airways.

The chest X-ray also is compatible with long-term pulmonary changes associated with COPD. Over a long period, airway linings thicken with mucous and cellular debris. These obstructions occlude the distal airways and increase the density of pulmonary tissue to X-rays. With long-term obstructions, a patient "retains" air, increasing the RV and subsequent RV:TLC ratio. These changes result in hyperinflation on the X-ray. In addition, the patient's chest increases in thickness and becomes more rounded (barrel chested).

Although ABGs could be obtained, these tests are rarely cost effective and useful in the evaluation of a stable COPD patient. The obvious cause of Kent N.'s disease is his cigarette smoking.

patient does serial spirometry for 5–20 min. During this time period, a patient with exertion-induced asthma will have a precipitous drop of 20% or more from baseline PFTs, usually FEV$_1$.[15] For example, a patient may have an FEV$_1$ of 2.8 L while at rest; after the exercise stress, this value may be 1.91 L, a 32% decrease in pulmonary function.

Similarly, some allergists administer increasing concentrations of antigens (e.g., cat dander) to elicit an airway response.

## Compliance, Resistance, and Conductance

### Compliance

The elasticity of the lungs and/or thorax is measured by pulmonary compliance. Compliance is the change in volume divided by the change in pressure. Pulmonary compliance varies with the amount of air contained in the lungs. Therefore, compliance is often "normalized" relative to the FRC (the ratio of compliance to the FRC). This ratio is also helpful in comparing patients with normal lung function to those with disease. Pressure is related to the effort needed to expand the lungs. As the pulmonary tissue nears its maximal elastic stretch, greater pressure is needed to stretch farther.

Decreased compliance is observed in patients with decreased volume secondary to pulmonary fibrosis, edema, atelectasis, and some pneumonias. Decreased compliance also is seen when the pressure needed to expand the lungs is increased, as with the loss of surfactant (e.g., hyaline membrane disease and adult respiratory distress syndrome). Pulmonary compliance increases in conditions where less pressure is needed to inflate the lungs. Because of progressive tissue destruction and reduced tissue elasticity, patients with emphysema demonstrate increased pulmonary compliance.

### Minicase 6

Patrick E., a 14-year-old boy with CF, was admitted to a hospital for pulmonary exacerbation. He was diagnosed at age 3 after having poor growth and weight gain and a long history of respiratory symptoms. Since the diagnosis, he had required one or two hospitalizations each year to reverse his decreasing pulmonary functions and wors-

ening symptoms. Typically, his hospital treatment included intensive antibiotic therapy and chest physiotherapy.

Before therapy was started and serially every other day during this admission, PFTs were obtained with the following results:

| PFT | Predicted | Measured on Admission | | Measured on 12th Day | | Best Ever Measurements | |
|---|---|---|---|---|---|---|---|
| | | Pre[a] | Post[a] | Pre | Post | Pre | Post |
| FVC (L) | 3.61 | 2.85 | 2.78 | 3.86 | 3.85 | 3.92 | 3.92 |
| $FEV_1$ (L) | 3.18 | 1.82 | 1.90 | 2.72 | 2.75 | 2.81 | 2.91 |
| $FEF_{25-75}$ (L/sec) | 4.32 | 1.04 | 1.22 | 1.81 | 1.95 | 2.07 | 2.33 |
| SVC (L) | 3.61 | – | 3.57 | – | 3.60 | 3.63 | 3.75 |
| RV (L) | 1.37 | – | 1.62 | – | 1.62 | 1.49 | 1.41 |
| RV:TLC (%) | 29 | – | 31 | – | 31 | 30 | 30 |

[a]Pre and Post indicate before and after inhaled bronchodilator administration, respectively.

*Why monitor "best ever" values in a patient with CF?*

**Discussion:** Patrick E.'s PFTs improved until they reached the maximum possible. Since CF is a chronic, progressive disease, he probably cannot attain the predicted values. The predicted values are based on normal healthy patients, not people with a chronic progressive pulmo-

nary disease. Therefore, Patrick E.'s "best ever" results become the goals of therapy. The listed tests are usually monitored in CF patients because they represent large airway function ($FEV_1$), small airway function ($FEF_{25-75}$), trapped air (RV and RV:TLC ratio), and general lung function (FVC and SVC).

### Resistance and Conductance

When the change in pressure is divided by the change in flow, the result is airway resistance. This value may be useful in differentiating obstructive from restrictive pulmonary disease or from normal pulmonary function. In obstructive diseases, resistance related to blockage of airflow increases. The magnitude of this increase is related to the amount and severity of the obstruction. Because of airway narrowing, resistance may increase during acute asthma attacks. Increases also may be seen in emphysema and bronchitis because of obstructive changes. Decreased resistance is rarely clinically meaningful.

Some clinicians prefer to speak in terms of conductance rather than resistance. Conductance is the inverse of resistance. To compare resistance or conductance from one time or patient to another, the value is divided by the lung volume when the measurement was made. These new "normalized" values are referred to as the specific airway resistance or specific airway conductance.

### SUMMARY

This chapter discussed the importance of pulmonary function testing as it relates to the diagnosis, treatment, and monitoring of respiratory disease states. After a review of the anatomy and physiology of the lungs, the mechanics of obtaining PFTs were emphasized. By understanding these mechanics, a clinician can better understand the interpretation of PFTs. Findings from different PFTs can

help differentiate between diagnoses and therapeutic recommendations. Most PFT results need to be interpreted within the context of the other findings, both historical and laboratory results.

Common tests of airflows and lung volumes are primarily used to characterize airway functions and diseases. These measurements may indicate the need for specific pharmacotherapeutic interventions. For example, clinicians recommending a peak flow meter for home monitoring of severe asthma will find the information obtained useful when considering appropriate therapeutic interventions.

Other tests, such as diffusion capacity, indicate the ability of a gas to diffuse through lung tissues and the general "thickness" of the membranes lining the alveoli. Specialized tests, such as bronchoprovocational and bronchodilator studies, are used to clarify treatment choices. Clearly, the PFTs are an important tool to aid the clinician in decisionmaking.

### REFERENCES

1. Crapo RO. Pulmonary function testing. *N Engl J Med.* 1994; 331:25–30.
2. Clausen JL. Prediction of normal pulmonary function testing. *Clin Chest Med.* 1989; 10:135–43.
3. Walter S. Tests of pulmonary function–II. *Natl Med J India.* 1992; 5:123–8.
4. Mueller GA, Eigen H. Pediatric pulmonary function testing in asthma. *Pediatr Clin North Am.* 1992; 39:1243–58.
5. Apps MCP. A guide to lung function tests. *Br J Hosp Med.*

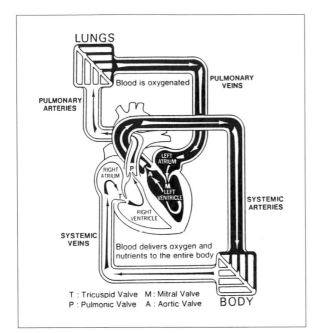

**FIGURE 1.** Structure of the heart, showing blood flow through the heart chambers. Darkened vessels carry oxygenated blood. (Reproduced, with permission, from Chung EK, ed. One heart, one life. Englewood Cliffs, NJ: Prentice-Hall; 1982.)

these cells provide a system for electrical excitation of the heart and for the rapid transmission of the electric excitatory signal throughout the heart. This electrical action potential then causes the myofibrils to contract via a linking mechanism called excitation–contraction coupling.

The normal adult human heart contracts rhythmically at approximately 70 beats/min. Each period from the end of one heart contraction to the end of the next is called a cardiac cycle. During each cycle, blood from the systemic circulation is returned to the heart via the veins; the blood empties from the superior and inferior vena cava into the right atrium. During the diastolic phase of the heart's pumping cycle, blood passively fills the right ventricle through the tricuspid valve, with an atrial contraction just prior to end-diastole.

Blood is then pumped from the right ventricle through the pulmonary artery to the lungs, where carbon dioxide is removed and the blood is oxygenated. From the lungs, blood returns to the heart via the pulmonary veins and empties into the left atrium. Again, during diastole, blood empties from the left atrium through the mitral valve into the main pumping chamber, the left ventricle. The ventricles provide the major power for circulating blood through the vascular system.

## Dysfunction

About 4–6 L/min of blood are pumped by the heart (cardiac output) when a person is at rest. This output can reach 8–12 L/min during strenuous exercise or fall to 1–

2 L/min when the heart experiences systolic dysfunction.[2] Reasons for systolic dysfunction as an etiology of heart failure include

- AMI.
- Hypertensive heart disease.
- Valvular heart disease.
- Congenital heart disease.
- Disease of the myocardium (i.e., cardiomyopathy).

Heart failure with systolic dysfunction also may occur in conjunction with volume-overload conditions (e.g., valvular regurgitation and shunts) or elevated cardiac output (high-output states such as severe anemia and pregnancy).

Moreover, there is increasing recognition that myocardial ischemia and infarction can affect the diastolic function of the heart, leading to reduced ventricular relaxation and increased ventricular stiffness. Thus, myocardial injury may frequently result in both systolic and diastolic dysfunction. Other well-described causes of diastolic dysfunction include increased myocardial stiffness from ventricular hypertrophy (e.g., hypertrophic cardiomyopathy) or infiltrative myocardial diseases (e.g., sarcoidosis) and pericardial diseases (e.g., pericarditis and pericardial effusion).

The heart muscle uses chemical energy to contract and pump. Energy is obtained mainly from aerobic metabolism of fatty acids and, to a lesser extent, metabolism of other nutrients, especially glucose and lactate. Because of this chemical energy requirement, cardiac tissues are characteristically richer in certain enzymes and isoenzymes than most other body tissues. When the heart is injured and irreversible damage occurs to cardiac cells, as during AMI, these enzymes leak through the cell membrane and enter the vascular compartment. There they can be measured in the serum with laboratory tests.

## TESTS TO EVALUATE UNSTABLE ANGINA AND MYOCARDIAL INFARCTION

The number of tests for evaluating patients with ischemic heart disease and AMI is increasing. This section discusses these tests, including diagnostic biochemical tests, electrocardiography, and noninvasive imaging techniques.

It is now well accepted that coronary artery thrombosis at the site of an atherosclerotic lesion in a major coronary artery is the most common cause of the acute ischemic events of unstable angina and AMI. Unstable angina is characterized variably by[3]

1. New onset (within 2 months of presentation) angina that is severe and occurs frequently.
2. Crescendo angina.
3. Angina occurring at rest.

In unstable angina, circumstances that result in partial coronary occlusion ensue, including fissuring of atheromatous plaques, activation of platelets, thrombus formation, and episodic embolization. New information suggesting that inflammation plays a role in unstable angina comes from histology of unstable angina plaques, evidence of thromboxane and leukotriene release, and activation of circulating leukocytes.[4]

When AMI occurs, the associated plaque rupture and thrombus formation convert a subtotal artery occlusion into a total occlusion. If the total occlusion results in a prolonged (>20–40 min) decrease in oxygen delivery to a region of cardiac muscle, permanent cell injury and ultimately cell death occur. Irreversibly damaged heart cells release several enzymes into the bloodstream over a particular period (Figure 2).

## Enzymes and Isoenzymes

The diagnosis of AMI is based on clinical judgment aided by information from the patient's history, physical examination, and specific laboratory determinations (i.e., ECG and cardiac enzyme measurements). Three enzymes assayed for diagnosis of AMI are CK (also called creatine phosphokinase or CPK), LDH (or LD), and AST (formerly called serum glutamic-oxaloacetic transaminase or SGOT). Because AST has been supplanted by the other

two enzyme tests, it is discussed only briefly in this chapter. Normal values or ranges are included for each enzyme. Nevertheless, these ranges vary from institution to institution and depend on the method of assay. Where pertinent, this information is emphasized.

Standard clinical practice is to obtain serial cardiac enzyme and isoenzyme evaluations for patients with suspected AMI. Figure 3 shows an algorithm incorporating the use of serum enzyme assays in the diagnosis of AMI.

### Creatine Kinase
*Normal range: 40–200 IU/L or 667–3334 nmol sec/L for males or 35–150 IU/L or 583–2501 nmol sec/L for females but varies with assay and laboratory*

CK is an enzyme that stimulates the transfer of high-energy phosphate groups. It is highly concentrated in the cytoplasm of tissues that require substantial amounts of energy and depend on aerobic metabolism. CK is found in greatest abundance in skeletal (striated) muscle and, to a lesser extent, in the brain and cardiac muscle. Only small amounts are found in other tissues, but injury to these tissues can increase CK.

Normal CK values vary, depending on the assay and reporting units used as well as the laboratory. In addition, the amount of CK circulating in serum is directly related to the individual's muscle mass. Therefore, males tend to have higher CK values than do females.

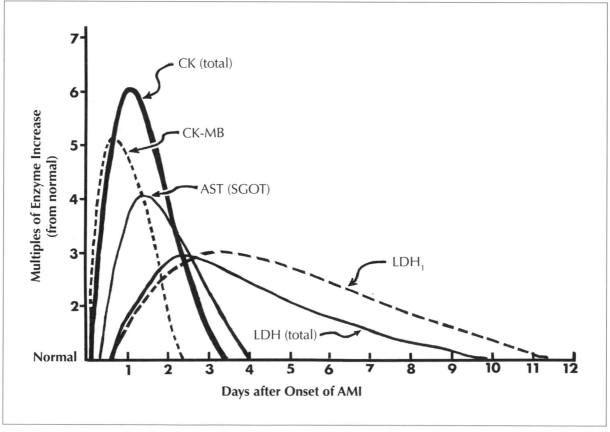

**FIGURE 2.** Time course of cardiac enzyme release following AMI. The *y*-axis is the magnitude of serum enzyme elevation.

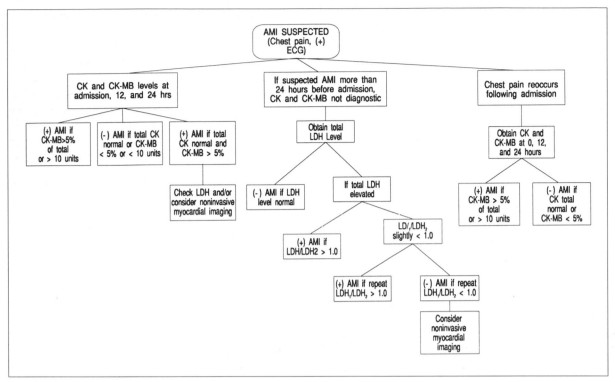

**FIGURE 3.** Algorithm for the use of serum enzyme assays in the diagnosis of AMI. Cutoff values for CK-MB represent the electrophoretic/fluorometric method used by most hospital clinical laboratories.

Serum CK concentrations rise sharply 6–8 hr after the onset of chest pain associated with AMI. Maximum CK concentrations, usually five to seven times normal values, are reached within 24 hr and return to normal in 3–4 days. Serial CK measurements following AMI provide excellent sensitivity (98%) but poor specificity (67%), as illustrated in Table 1.[5]

CK also commonly increases following trauma, intramuscular (IM) injection, surgery, vigorous exercise, convulsions, malignant hyperpyrexia, and hymenoptera (bee) stings. It also becomes elevated in patients with musculoskeletal diseases (e.g., polymyositis and muscular dystrophy) and late in the course of toxic shock syndrome. In most of these cases, the elevation is not of cardiac origin. In certain instances, however, such as after marathon running or cardiac surgery, substantial serum CK of cardiac origin may be seen.[6]

Some drugs and noxious gases also can increase total CK. These drugs include amphotericin B, clofibrate, ethanol (binge drinking), lithium, halothane and succinylcholine administered concurrently during anesthesia, barbiturate or ethchlorvynol poisoning, large doses of aminocaproic acid, and drugs administered by IM injection.[7,8] Elevations of CK from IM depo forms of drugs may be prolonged. In addition, exposure to carbon monoxide can elevate CK because of an effect on skeletal muscle.[9] Moderate to severe sample hemolysis may falsely elevate CK results.[10] Some causes of elevated CK are listed in Table 2.[11]

The major limitations of using total CK to assess AMI include

➤ The relatively short time after onset of infarction during which CK is elevated.

**TABLE 1.** Diagnostic Accuracy in AMI of ECG and Serial Assays in Patients in Critical Care Unit and Emergency Room[a]

| Test | Sensitivity[b] (%) | Specificity[c] (%) |
|---|---|---|
| ECG | 68 | 100 |
| CK-MB | 100 | 98 |
| CK | 98 | 67 |
| AST | 97 | 86 |
| LDH | 98 | 72 |
| LDH$_1$:LDH$_2$ >1 | 81 | 94 |
| LDH$_1$:LDH$_2$ >0.76 | 92 | 94 |
| LDH$_1$:total LDH >0.4 (12–24 hr after AMI) | 86 | 95 |

[a]Compiled from References 5 and 18.

[b]$Sensitivity = \dfrac{all\ patients\ with\ AMI\ and\ positive\ test}{all\ patients\ with\ AMI}$

[c]$Specificity = \dfrac{all\ patients\ without\ AMI\ and\ negative\ test}{all\ patients\ without\ AMI}$

**TABLE 2.** Some Causes of Elevated CK Levels

| | |
|---|---|
| AMI | Myocarditis |
| Cerebrovascular accident | Myxedema (hypothyroidism) |
| Dermatomyositis | Polymyositis |
| Malignant hyperthermia syndrome | Rhabdomyolysis |
| | Seizures (postictal state) |
| Muscular dystrophy | Skeletal muscle damage |
| Muscular stress | |

➤ False-positive elevations due to skeletal muscle injury (especially IM injections).

### Creatine Kinase Isoenzymes
*Normal range: CK-MB <12 IU/L or <3–6% of total CK but varies with assay*

CK enzymes exist in multiple molecular forms known as isoenzymes; they occur in different quantities in various tissues. These isoenzymes can be separated by fractionation, a process that increases the diagnostic specificity of the test for AMI.

CK is composed of two subunits, M (for muscle) and B (for brain). There are three CK isoenzymes, and their tissue sources are primarily skeletal muscle (CK-MM), heart (CK-MB), and brain (CK-BB). Although trace amounts of CK-MB appear in tissues other than the heart (including skeletal muscle), the elevated serum concentration of CK-MB is relatively specific for myocardial infarction and is currently the test of choice to confirm AMI diagnosis.

*CK-MB.* Serum CK-MB concentrations begin to rise 4–8 hr after the onset of AMI symptoms. Its peak concentration period (12–20 hr) is similar to that for total CK. Because of faster clearance from serum, however, CK-MB returns to baseline sooner than total CK (2–3 days versus 3–4 days, respectively).

Enzyme assays of both CK and CK-MB have been used to judge the size of a myocardial infarction but allow only rough, qualitative estimates because enzyme peaks can be affected by other clinical events (discussed below). For example, in myocardial infarction patients who experience either spontaneous or thrombolytic-induced early reperfusion of the infarction area, peak concentrations of these enzymes are often higher and are usually reached sooner. In these patients, total CK and CK-MB concentrations may peak as early as 8–14 hr. In addition, the total amount of enzyme released into the blood may be greater with early reperfusion than when an infarction of the same size is not reperfused or reperfuses long after the AMI. This larger amount of enzyme is believed to be secondary to the improved washout of released enzymes from the infarction area.[5] Similarly, some investigators reported that CK-MB appears in serum sooner after small non-Q-wave AMI than after Q-wave

AMI, probably reflecting early reperfusion of the infarcted region.[5]

In patients evaluated within 24 hr of onset of chest pain, serial testing of CK-MB concentrations provides near-perfect sensitivity and high specificity (Table 1). However, CK-MB levels should not be tested at the first sign of AMI symptoms because, as already noted, the serum enzyme concentrations do not begin to increase for at least 4–8 hr after onset. Single samples for CK-MB concentration drawn less than 4 hr after the onset of symptoms yield many false-negative results and are essentially worthless for the assessment of myocardial infarction.[5]

CK isoenzymes can be measured by various methods, but the ultimate goal is the determination of the quantitative amount of CK-MB in serum. Qualitative assays use column chromatography or electrophoresis to separate isoenzymes. Qualitative assays are considered positive if *any* CK-MB band is seen.

In most laboratories, electrophoretic separation is followed by fluorometric analysis of isoenzyme bands to determine the actual CK-MB concentration in international units per liter. A few laboratories use the actual CK-MB concentration determined in this fashion to define the upper limit of normal, with cutoffs ranging from 5 to 25 IU/L. More commonly, CK-MB as a percentage of the total CK concentration is determined by dividing the CK-MB concentration by the total CK concentration. The cutoff for the upper limit of normal for this value usually is 3–6%.[5] When these methods are used, for example, the diagnosis of myocardial infarction would be strongly suggested when CK-MB as a percentage of total CK was greater than 5% or when the actual CK-MB concentration was greater than 10 IU/L.

False-positive elevations of CK-MB can occur due to laboratory artifacts, and real elevations can occur due to nonischemic causes. These elevations are usually less than those seen with AMI, and the clinical presentations are different. Moreover, these conditions are less likely to cause the *acute* rise and fall in CK and CK-MB observed with myocardial infarction. The sources of these elevations can be myocardial and/or peripheral (Table 3, next page).[5]

For example, with column chromatography assays, false-positive results may be caused by carryover of elevated CK-MM isoenzyme into fractions that normally contain CK-MB. Another problem is variant isoenzymes that migrate as a band between CK-MM and CK-MB on electrophoresis; they may be interpreted as CK-MB on quantitative assays. These variants are usually due to immunoglobulin G (IgG) (Chapters 6 and 17) complexed to CK-BB or to a mitochondrial source of CK, which differs slightly from cytoplasmic CK.

An uncommon problem of qualitative electrophoretic assays is nonspecific fluorescence from other proteins (especially albumin), which may exhibit migration similar to that of other fractions. In addition, misleading eleva-

**TABLE 3.** Some Causes of Elevated CK-MB Concentrations[a]

| | |
|---|---|
| **False elevations** | **Peripheral source of CK-MB** |
|     Isoenzyme variants |     Athletic activity (e.g., marathons) |
|     Nonspecific fluorescence |     Cesarean section |
|     Spillover of CK-MM |     Gastrointestinal surgery |
| **Myocardial damage** |     Myositis |
|     Myocardial infarction |     Prostate surgery |
|     Myocardial puncture/trauma |     Rhabdomyolysis |
|     Myocarditis |     Tumors |
|     Pericarditis | **Miscellaneous** |
| **Systemic disease with cardiac involvement** |     Hypothyroidism |
|     Hyperthermia |     Renal failure |
|     Hypothermia |     Subarachnoid hemorrhage |
|     Muscular dystrophy | |
|     Reye's syndrome | |

[a]Adapted from Reference 5.

tions can be caused by decreased clearance of CK and CK-MB, as occurs with renal failure or hypothyroidism.

New CK-MB radioimmunoassay and fluorometric immunoassay methodologies use a monoclonal antibody extremely specific for the CK-MB isoenzyme. These assays measure CK-MB in nanograms per milliliter (actual concentration of CK-MB protein) rather than in units of activity per liter. According to some clinicians, if the total CK is within the normal range, no myocardial injury is suggested when CK-MB is 0–5.9 ng/mL.[12] If the total CK is above normal, then a relative index is calculated:

$$\frac{\text{concentration of CK MB}\,(ng/mL)/\text{total CK}\,(IU/L)}{100}$$

This index is useful for samples with abnormally elevated total CK to differentiate MB released from skeletal versus cardiac muscle. An index greater than 2 is suggestive of myocardial necrosis. These new monoclonal antibody immunoassay methodologies appear to be very sensitive and extremely specific. Furthermore, they do not show the interferences common to earlier immunoassay or traditional electrophoretic and chromatographic methods.[12–14]

*CK-MB subforms.* Accurate diagnosis of AMI is critical in the first 6 hr if effective therapy is to produce reperfusion and preserve the myocardium. A major limitation of CK-MB for diagnosis of AMI is that concentrations do not rise appreciably until 4–8 hr after symptoms appear. Therefore, the conventional methods of using CK-MB require at least 8–12 hr from onset of symptoms for reliable diagnostic certainty of AMI.

This delay in the rise of CK-MB to levels of diagnostic specificity also creates a dilemma in emergency rooms where patients with chest pain must be quickly triaged to a coronary care unit or to a less intensive care setting. Unfortunately, patient history and ECG can be nonspecific and a diagnostic rise in CK-MB can be delayed up to 12 hr (Minicase 1). Of patients admitted to a coronary care unit, fewer than 30% are subsequently found to have had a myocardial infarction.[15] Thus, more rapid and sensitive methods for detecting myocardial tissue damage continue to be pursued.

Recently, a method for accurately and precisely detecting subforms of CK-MB has been tested. CK-MB exists as a single form in cardiac tissue (CK-MB$_2$). When released into the blood, CK-MB$_2$ has a positively charged terminal amino acid (lysine) cleaved from its M subunit, producing a more negatively charged structure (CK-MB$_1$). In the normal state, CK-MB$_2$ and CK-MB$_1$ are present in concentrations as low as 0.5–1 U/L and at equivalent concentrations in the blood (CK-MB$_2$:CK-MB$_1$ ratio of approximately 1). AMI would be diagnosed when the CK-MB$_2$ concentration is at least 1 U/L and the ratio of CK-MB$_2$:CK-MB$_1$ is at least 1.5.[16,17]

The assay for plasma CK-MB$_2$ and CK-MB$_1$ has been automated and utilizes rapid high-voltage electrophoresis to separate the subforms in about 25 min. Experience with this assay has shown the initial plasma sample (on presentation) to be abnormal in 67% of patients, compared to 27% with the conventional CK-MB assay. Samples collected at 2–4, 4–6, and 6–8 hr after AMI showed sensitivities of 59, 92, and 100%, respectively, compared to 23, 50, and 71%, respectively, with the conventional CK-MB assay.[17]

Study of 1110 consecutive patients, evaluated in an emergency room for chest pain, revealed subform assay sensitivity to detect AMI within 6 hr after onset of symptoms to be 95.7%, compared to only 48% with the conventional CK-MB assay. Moreover, results of the subform assay were available in just over 1 hr (1.22 ± 1.17 hr).[15] Doubtless, subform assays will soon be commercially available and should limit unnecessary admission, facilitate early patient discharge, and reduce health care costs.[15]

### *Lactate Dehydrogenase*
*Normal range: 100–210 IU/L or 1667–3501 nmol sec/L*

LDH, found in the cytoplasm of almost every body cell,

## ✎ Minicase 1

William N., a 44-year-old male with no previous cardiac history, was seen by a local physician 1 day after first feeling palpitations. His physician noted a tachycardic pulse with a heart rate of about 130 beats/min. William N. was sent to the local emergency room where an ECG revealed atrial fibrillation with a ventricular rate of 200 beats/min. Adenosine 6 mg was given, resulting in transient slowing of the rate to 150 beats/min. Intravenous (IV) verapamil produced no change in either heart rate or rhythm but did drop the patient's blood pressure (BP).

Synchronized direct current cardioversion was then attempted, resulting in ventricular fibrillation. William N. was then resuscitated for approximately 90 min until normal sinus rhythm returned. During this time, he received 27 direct current cardioversions, epinephrine 12 mg, bretylium 2 g, lidocaine 550 mg, magnesium sulfate 2 g,

and 2 ampuls of sodium bicarbonate.

William N. was then transferred by emergency aircare to a university hospital and admitted to the cardiovascular intensive care unit (ICU). His ECG on admission showed a short PR interval and a wide QRS with slurred upstroke ($\delta$ wave) consistent with the Wolff-Parkinson-White syndrome. His laboratory results on admission were normal, except for an elevated leukocyte count of 23,800 cells/mm$^3$ (4800–10,800 cells/mm$^3$), serum creatinine (SCr) of 2.1 mg/dL (0.7–1.5 mg/dL), calcium of 8.2 mg/dL (8.5–10.8 mg/dL), phosphate of 6.3 mg/dL (2.6–4.5 mg/dL), uric acid of 9.9 mg/dL (3.4–7.0 mg/dL), and AST of 511 IU/L (0–37 IU/L). His glucose drawn on admission was 294 mg/dL (70–110 mg/dL). Over the ensuing 5 days, his cardiac enzymes were as follows (normal range in parentheses):

| Hospital Day | Time | CK (40–200) (IU/L) | CK-MB (0–5.9) (ng/mL) | CK-MB Index (0–1.9)[a] | LDH (100–210) (IU/L) | LDH$_1$ (20–40) (%) | LDH$_2$ (25–45) (%) |
|---|---|---|---|---|---|---|---|
| 1 | 1525 | 1843 | – | 2.6 | – | – | – |
|   | 2250 | 5062 | – | 1.1 | – | – | – |
| 2 | 0627 | 6273 | – | 0.6 | – | – | – |
|   | 1244 | 6876 | – | 0.4 | – | – | – |
|   | 1809 | 7030 | – | ND | – | – | – |
| 3 | 0611 | 7768 | – | ND | – | – | – |
| 4 | 0448 | 5478 | – | ND | – | – | – |
| 5 | 0714 | 2813 | – | 0.1 | – | – | – |
| 6 | 0755 | 1051 | – | 0.1 | – | – | – |
| 7 | 0710 | 408 | – | 0.1 | 314 | 31 | 34 |

[a]ND = not determined.

**Discussion:** In this case, the patient presented with an arrhythmia and received multiple direct current cardioversions and prolonged chest compression. He had no symptoms of AMI and no ECG changes indicative of ischemia. The CK enzymes increased to extremely high concentrations, but only the first was positive for significant MB (positive CK-MB index). This finding was not interpreted as AMI since it was the only abnormal CK-MB and probably reflected a small amount of myocardial injury due to repeated cardioversions.

The CK enzyme concentrations were increased for a prolonged period—much longer than would be expected in a usual AMI. This finding probably reflected prolonged release from traumatized tissues and slowed elimination from acute renal failure (SCr peaked at 2.1 mg/dL) that developed secondary to hypotension and reduced renal perfusion during resuscitation. Both phosphate and uric acid were elevated because of developing renal failure. The leukocyte count was elevated secondary to the stressful event and possible aspiration during resuscitation. The AST elevation most likely represented hepatic injury secondary to reduced hepatic perfusion during the code.

catalyzes the reversible reduction of pyruvate to lactate in the final step of glycolysis. High LDH concentrations occur in the skeletal muscle, liver, red blood cells (RBCs), and kidneys as well as the heart. Following AMI, LDH does not increase in serum until approximately 12 hr after the onset of chest pain. Peak concentrations are reached 2–3 days after infarction. Moreover, the magnitude of increase—usually only two to three times the upper limit of normal—is not as great as that of CK. LDH concentrations return to normal over 8–14 days (Figure 2).

The total LDH level has a high sensitivity (98%) but a relatively poor specificity (false-positive rate of about 30%). The latter is due to the high LDH concentration in tissues other than the heart, resulting in increased LDH with many diseases and conditions (Table 4, next page).[11]

In addition to the causes listed in Table 4, LDH values may increase because of assay interference and exposure to numerous drugs. Hemolysis falsely elevates LDH results. False elevations also may be caused by specimen exposure to heat, serum contact with clot, and triamterene administration.[10,11] Drugs that can truly elevate LDH include anesthetic gases, clofibrate, dicoumarol, ethanol, fluorides, imipramine, methotrexate, mithramycin, narcotic analgesics, nitrofurantoin, propoxyphene, quinidine, and sulfonamides.[10]

### Lactate Dehydrogenase Isoenzymes
*Normal ranges: LDH$_1$, 20–40%; LDH$_2$, 25–45%; LDH$_3$, 10–25%; LDH$_4$, 0–12%; LDH$_5$, 0–12%*

LDH can be differentiated into five isoenzymes (LDH$_1$–

**TABLE 4.** Some Causes of Elevated LDH Concentrations

| | |
|---|---|
| Acute pancreatitis | Inflammation |
| Central nervous system disease | Intestinal obstruction |
| | Liver disease |
| Collagen disease | Megaloblastic anemia |
| Excessive cell destruction | Muscle damage |
| Focal necrosis | Muscular dystrophy |
| Fractures | Myocardial infarction |
| Head trauma | Neoplastic states |
| Hemolytic anemia | Other lung disease |
| Hypothyroidism | Pulmonary infarction |
| Hypoxic cardiorespiratory disease | Renal infarction |
| | Shock and hypotension |
| Infectious mononucleosis | |

$LDH_5$), and most tissues contain all five. In the heart, however, $LDH_1$ and, to a lesser extent, $LDH_2$ predominate. Most assays for LDH separate the isoenzymes by electrophoresis and then estimate the ratio of $LDH_1$ to $LDH_2$. Normally, $LDH_2$ is the major isoenzyme in the blood and the serum pattern is $LDH_2$ greater than $LDH_1$. With myocardial infarction, the concentration of $LDH_1$ rises in the serum; within 14–24 hr, the ratio of $LDH_1$ to $LDH_2$ increases until a flipped pattern is seen ($LDH_1$

greater than $LDH_2$). Although a ratio of $LDH_1$:$LDH_2$ greater than 1 is used as a cutoff to support diagnoses of AMI,[5,11] some authors advocate a cutoff of 0.76, citing better detection or sensitivity (Table 1).

New methodologies may improve the clinical utility of LDH in the diagnosis of AMI. Preliminary work suggests that an $LDH_1$:total LDH ratio greater than 0.4 as early as 12 hr after symptoms has a sensitivity of 86% (nearly equal to CK-MB).[18] In addition, 24 hr after onset of symptoms, clinical sensitivity stays at 90–100% with a specificity of 95%. Although not useful in the very early detection of AMI, the $LDH_1$:total LDH ratio may be helpful in late diagnosis since the ratio persists for 2–5 days; it may be helpful even 6–15 days after symptom onset.[18] Further controlled study is needed.

The measurement of LDH isoenzymes is especially useful in patients who present more than 24 hr after the onset of chest pain (Minicase 2) and can remain diagnostic for as long as 2 weeks after the infarction.[5] The use of LDH isoenzymes is considerably more specific than total LDH levels (94 versus 72%, respectively). However, the sensitivity of LDH isoenzymes is less because other tissues, including the RBCs, kidneys, brain, stomach, and pancreas, contain $LDH_1$. Therefore, potentially misleading elevations of $LDH_1$:$LDH_2$ ratio can result from hemolysis, renal infarction, pregnancy, and myopathies.

---

### Minicase 2

Jim B., an 84-year-old male with a history of diabetes mellitus and hyperthyroidism but no previous cardiac history, was seen in the endocrinology clinic for routine followup. He complained of vague chest discomfort for the previous 24–48 hr. An ECG revealed new ST-segment elevation in leads II, III, and aVF, consistent with inferior wall myocardial ischemia.

Jim B. was admitted to the cardiovascular ICU on suspicion that he suffered or was developing an AMI. He denied any chest pain, shortness of breath, nausea, vomiting, and diaphoresis at the time of admission.

Upon admission to the cardiovascular ICU, Jim B.'s electrolytes and hematological test results were normal, except for an elevated leukocyte count of 13,000 cells/mm³ (4800–10,800 cells/mm³). His blood urea nitrogen (BUN), creatinine, and thyroid function test results were normal. However, his serum glucose, drawn 2 hr after lunch, was unusually elevated (250 mg/dL) for him. Over the next 2 days, his cardiac enzymes were as follows (normal range in parentheses):

| Hospital Day | Time | CK (40–200) (IU/L) | CK-MB (0–5.9) (ng/mL) | CK-MB Index (0–1.9) | LDH (100–210) (IU/L) | $LDH_1$ (20–40) (%) | $LDH_2$ (25–45) (%) |
|---|---|---|---|---|---|---|---|
| 1 | 1223 | 299 | – | 0.5 | 205 | 32 | 24 |
| | 1825 | 191 | 1.1 | – | 444 | 35 | 33 |
| 2 | 0025 | 168 | 0.7 | – | 416 | 35 | 33 |
| | 0635 | 163 | 1.1 | – | – | – | – |

**Discussion:** As often happens, the presentation of this patient was not classic for AMI. He was diagnosed as having a myocardial infarction despite a CK that was only slightly elevated and decreasing, a normal CK-MB, and a negative CK-MB index. The diagnosis was based on chest discomfort, ECG changes, increasing LDH (from 205 to 444), and reversal of the normal $LDH_1$:$LDH_2$ ratio (1.06). Based on history and enzyme release patterns (Figure 2), the AMI probably occurred about 2 days prior to admission. Because CK rises and declines quickly, this hall-

mark will be absent if the patient does not seek medical attention right away. Leukocytosis and hyperglycemia also were consistent with an AMI (Other Related Tests section).

As might be expected from the mild symptoms and absence of a Q wave, Jim B. did well after his AMI. He experienced no further chest discomfort and no symptoms of congestive heart failure or arrhythmia, the two most common sequelae of AMI.

### Aspartate Aminotransferase
*Normal range: 0–37 IU/L or 0–617 nmol sec/L for males or 0–31 IU/L or 0–517 nmol sec/L for females*

AST, an enzyme involved in the transfer of amino groups in amino acid synthesis, is widely distributed, with high concentrations in the liver, skeletal muscles, and heart. This distribution imparts poor specificity as an indicator of acute myocardial cell damage. Although AST was one of the first serum enzymes useful in the diagnosis of AMI, its relative nonspecificity has led to its replacement by CK and LDH enzymes. AST rises within 12 hr of infarction, peaks at about 36 hr, and returns to normal in 3–4 days.[5] (Chapter 11 discusses noncardiac AST tests.)

### Myoglobin

This biological marker, a low molecular weight heme protein, is elevated shortly (within 2 hr) after an AMI but is cleared rapidly by the kidneys. Although its diagnostic sensitivity in the early stages of AMI is superior to CK-MB, this sensitivity is lost later due to its rapid clearance. In addition, serum myoglobin measurements in the emergency room are fraught with controversy because of low specificity. Skeletal muscle injury and renal failure cause false-positive results.[19]

### Cardiac Troponins I (<1.5 ng/mL) and T (≤0.2 ng/mL)

The most recent revolution in specific labels for myocardial cell injury involves use of troponins. The calcium-mediated interaction of actin and myosin is mediated by the complex of proteins known as troponins I, C, and T.

Troponin T is found in cardiac and skeletal muscle cells. Because cardiac and skeletal muscle isoforms of troponin T are encoded by different genes, these troponins have unique amino acid sequences. This uniqueness has permitted the development of troponin-specific monoclonal antibodies with little or no cross-reactivity with the respective skeletal muscle isoforms.[19] Troponin I apparently is found only in cardiac—not skeletal—muscle.[20]

Two structurally related, but distinct, troponin C isoforms have been identified: fast skeletal (found exclusively in mammalian fast skeletal muscle) and cardiac (found in adults and usually restricted to cardiac and slow muscle). Structural similarities between the isoforms make it difficult to develop a cardiac troponin C assay without cross-reactivity with troponin C from skeletal muscle.[21]

Initial use has shown troponins I and T to possess superior specificity in situations where false-positive elevations of CK-MB are likely (e.g., perioperative AMI with skeletal muscle injury occurring during surgery). One study in patients undergoing surgery revealed a specificity of 99% for troponin I compared to 81% for CK-MB obtained perioperatively.[20] Troponin T also has prognostic value in unstable angina, detecting minor myocardial cell injury with greater sensitivity than CK-MB and, thus,

distinguishing high-risk patients.[22]

The current troponin assays require either 30 (I) or 90 (T) min to perform. However, qualitative whole blood assay kits for troponin T requiring only 10 min may soon be available.[19] Preliminary studies reveal that troponin rises within 4 hr of AMI, but improved assays may be able to detect the protein sooner. If the troponin rise can be detected within 1–2 hr after symptoms, it can be used to identify patients for thrombolysis. A new era in the diagnosis and treatment of patients with AMI would then begin.

### C-Reactive (<0.3 mg/dL) and Serum Amyloid A (<0.5 mg/dL) Proteins

As previously reviewed, recent evidence suggests that active inflammation, either in the coronary arteries or myocardium (or its microvasculature), may occur in unstable angina. Circulating inflammatory mediators (cytokines) apparently stimulate hepatic production of acute-phase reactants such as C-reactive protein and serum amyloid A.

Unstable angina patients with elevated concentrations of these proteins have a worse clinical course than patients with normal concentrations. In particular, elevated concentrations of C-reactive protein and serum amyloid A have been associated with increased frequency of recurrent angina, myocardial infarction, and coronary revascularization.[23] Thus, these acute-phase proteins may prove useful as prognostic indicators of clinical outcomes in patients with acute ischemic syndromes.[4] (More information on acute-phase reactant proteins appears in Chapter 17.)

## Electrocardiography

Cardiac cells are normally charged or polarized in their resting state (negative inside the cell compared to outside). When electrically stimulated, they "depolarize" (become internally positive) and contract. The ECG records the electrical impulses resulting from this depolarization and subsequent cardiac contraction. As the positive wave of depolarization within cardiac cells moves toward a positive electrode placed on the skin, a positive (upward) deflection is recorded on the ECG. Thus, the wave of depolarization (cells become internally positive) and repolarization (cells return to negative) appears.

The cardiac electrical impulse begins at the sinoatrial (SA) node and spreads in wave-like fashion, stimulating the atria. This electrical impulse spreads across the atria and produces a P wave on the ECG. The impulse then reaches the atrioventricular (AV) node where a $1/10$-sec pause allows blood to fill the ventricles. After this pause, the AV node is stimulated, initiating an electrical impulse that travels down the AV bundle to the bundle branches.

The QRS complex on the ECG represents the electrical impulse as it travels from the AV node to the Purkinje

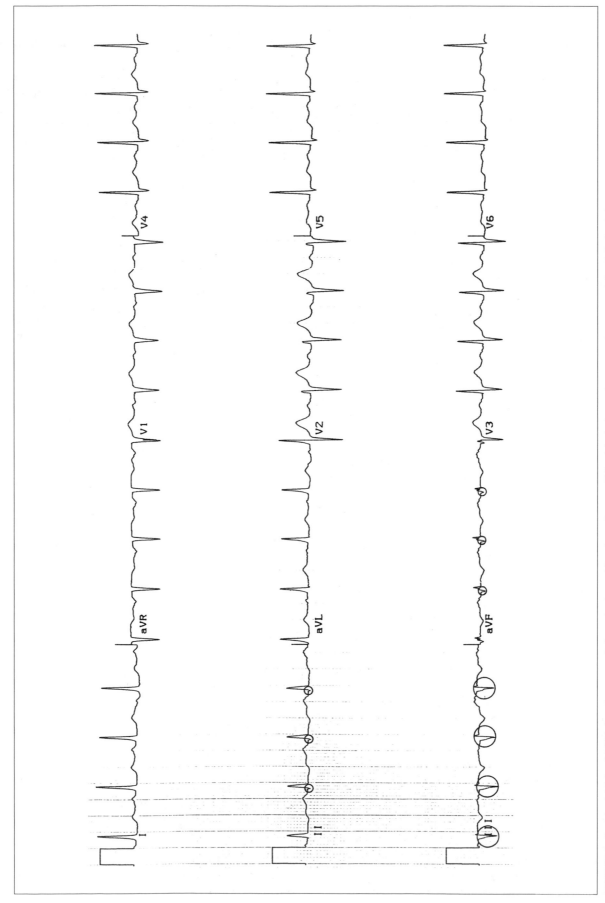

**FIGURE 4.** Standard 12-lead ECG showing normal sinus rhythm with minor abnormalities (circled areas) representing an evolving inferior infarct.

fibers and then the ventricular myocardial cells. During this time, the ventricles are simultaneously stimulated and contracted. The Q wave, the first downward stroke (often not present) of the QRS, is followed by the upward R wave. The upgoing R wave is followed by the downward S wave. This total QRS complex represents the electrical activity of ventricular contraction.

A pause occurs after the QRS complex; then a T wave (representing ventricular repolarization) appears. The atria have a very small repolarization wave, usually lost within the QRS complex and ordinarily not seen. Thus, the P (atrial contraction), QRS (ventricular contraction), and T (ventricular repolarization) waves make up the usual cardiac cycle; this cycle is repeated continuously.

The standard ECG is composed of 12 separate leads or electrodes—six limb and six chest (or precordial)—placed on the body for recording electrical activity. The limb leads are placed on the right and left arms and the left leg. Since each limb lead (I, II, III, aVR, aVL, and aVF) records from a different angle, each gives a different view of the same cardiac activity. For the six chest leads ($V_1$–$V_6$), a positive electrode is placed at six different positions across the anterior chest.

The ECG wave form looks different in the various leads because the electrical activity is monitored from different positions on the body. When a standard 12-lead ECG is recorded on paper, the six limb and six chest leads are usually grouped together in columns (Figure 4). (For a more indepth introduction to electrocardiography, the reader is referred to a programmed course.[24])

In the early diagnosis of patients with AMI symptoms (<6–10 hr after onset), the ECG is the most convenient and reliable method. ECG changes occur within seconds after acute coronary occlusion,[25,26] and about 80% of patients with infarction have abnormal recordings at presentation.[27] The overall sensitivity and specificity of serial ECGs in the diagnosis of AMI are 68–73% and 95–100%, respectively.[5,28] The classic ECG pattern of myocardial infarction is reflected by three changes[29] (Figure 5):

> ➤ T-wave inversion (or elevation).
> ➤ ST-segment elevation.
> ➤ Appearance of Q waves.

### *T-Wave Inversion*

T waves associated with myocardial ischemia have specific characteristics. In ECG leads oriented to the ischemic surface, T waves are typically inverted or upright; they are usually arrowhead in appearance, being peaked, symmetrical, and increased in magnitude. Transmural AMI (through the full thickness of the heart wall) is typically associated with an inverted T wave, which may vary from slightly flat or depressed to deeply inverted. However, inverted T waves are nonspecific and may be associated with many conditions, both normal and abnormal.[29]

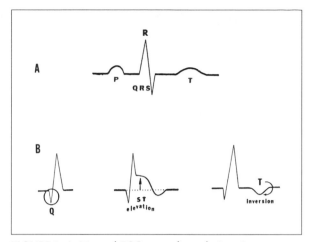

**FIGURE 5.** A. Normal ECG wave form during sinus rhythm. B. The three ECG changes characteristic of AMI: Q wave, ST elevation, and T inversion. (Adapted and reproduced, with permission, from Dubin D. Rapid interpretation of EKG's, 3rd ed. Tampa, FL: Cover Publishing; 1985.)

### *ST-Segment Elevation*

With continued occlusion of a coronary artery, a stage beyond ischemia occurs. This pattern of myocardial injury, represented by ST elevation, is still reversible. The deviated ST segments typically show an upward convexity, but they may be only slightly (0.5 mm) elevated or as much as 10 mm or more above the baseline. To be considered diagnostic of AMI, ST elevation must be at least 1 mm in at least two contiguous leads (Minicase 3, next page). Such elevation indicates that the infarction is acute.[29]

### *Q-Wave Appearance*

When occlusion of a coronary artery persists for a sufficient time (>4–6 hr from onset), irreversible structural changes occur and a pattern of necrosis appears in the ECG. This pattern evolves over hours to days. The QRS complex becomes inverted to produce a QS complex with deep and wide Q waves, the ST segment returns to the ECG baseline, and the T wave becomes upright. Q waves are considered diagnostic for infarction when they are at least 1 mm wide and/or one-third the size (height and depth) of the entire QRS complex.[29]

At one time, the appearance of Q waves was thought always to indicate a transmural infarction. An ECG without a Q wave was thought to reflect a less severe, nontransmural (subendocardial) infarction. However, relatively recent autopsy studies have shown that these beliefs are not always correct, although Q waves do occur more commonly with transmural infarction. Therefore, many authors now maintain that it is more appropriate to use the terms Q-wave and non-Q-wave infarctions (as opposed to transmural and nontransmural) when referring only to ECG abnormalities.[29]

---

### Minicase 3

Mary S., a 63-year-old female with a history of noninsulin-dependent diabetes mellitus, hypertension, and hyperlipidemia, presented to the Continuation of Care Clinic complaining of exertional chest pain over the past 2 weeks. While in the clinic, she had a similar episode of chest pain, prompting an ECG. It showed nonspecific changes.

After being given sublingual nitroglycerin, Mary S.'s systolic BP dropped from 120 to 90 mm Hg, and she developed 3-mm ST-segment elevation in leads III and aVF and ST-segment depression in leads $V_{2R}$–$V_{4R}$. When admitted to the cardiovascular ICU, she was given aspirin 325 mg, IV heparin, metoprolol 5 mg times two, and IV nitroglycerin. She then was rushed to the cardiac catheterization laboratory.

Coronary angiography showed a normal left main coronary artery, 80–90% proximal occlusion of the left anterior descending (LAD) artery, diffuse (<20%) occlu-

sion of the left circumflex, and a right coronary artery with 25% proximal, 25% mid, and 95% distal coronary occlusion. This patient then underwent percutaneous transluminal coronary angioplasty of the right coronary artery, which reduced the distal occlusion to less than 10% with brisk blood flow through the artery.

In the clinic and on admission to the cardiovascular ICU, Mary S.'s electrolytes and hematological test results were normal, except for a serum calcium of 7.8 mg/dL (8.5–10.8 mg/dL), glucose of 200 mg/dL (70–110 mg/dL), slightly low carbon dioxide at 19 mEq/L, activated partial thromboplastin time (aPTT) of longer than 150 sec (21–45 sec), prothrombin time (PT) of 22 sec (10–13 sec), and International Normalized Ratio (INR) of 3.8. These results were obtained after heparin was given. Before these tests, the patient was on warfarin for prior history of deep vein thrombosis. Her cardiac enzymes rose and fell over the next 2 days as follows (normal range in parentheses):

| Hospital Day | Time | CK (40–200) (IU/L) | CK-MB (0–5.9) (ng/mL) | CK-MB Index (0–1.9) | LDH (100–210) (IU/L) | LDH$_1$ (20–40) (%) | LDH$_2$ (25–45) (%) |
|---|---|---|---|---|---|---|---|
| 1 | 1125 | 91 | 5.6 | – | 297 | 30 | 38 |
|   | 1346 | 382 | – | 7.6 | 260 | 30 | 36 |
|   | 2109 | 668 | – | 9.9 | – | – | – |
| 2 | 0526 | 470 | – | 9.2 | – | – | – |
|   | 1343 | 331 | – | 8.5 | – | – | – |
|   | 2124 | 219 | – | 5.3 | – | – | – |
|   | 0654 | 142 | 4.2 | – | – | – | – |

**Discussion:** This case depicts ECG changes and the usual CK enzymes rise and fall associated with AMI. Mary S.'s CK apparently began to rise within 2–3 hr of her symptom onset, and CK and CK-MB peaked in approximately 9–10 hr. The early peak of CK and CK-MB may be explained by the fact that this patient probably reperfused her occluded artery early after symptom onset. This reperfusion was reflected by the fact that a stenosed, but not totally occluded, right coronary artery was observed on coronary angiography soon after her symptoms occurred.

The LDH enzymes were elevated, but the LDH$_1$:LDH$_2$ ratio had not flipped, probably because these results were

obtained before the change in enzyme ratio occurred. (This ratio was greater than 0.70, which meets criteria established by some investigators.) The glucose elevation reflected this patient's diabetes, with glucose intolerance worsening during AMI. The slight decrease in carbon dioxide is probably secondary to the patient's diabetes and some cellular hypoxia from reduced cardiac output during AMI. The PT and aPTT were prolonged because the patient presented on warfarin and then received heparin at the time of AMI. Mary S. did develop Q waves in the inferior leads of her ECG (III and aVF), further indicating myocardial damage. However, she had an uncomplicated hospital course.

---

Q waves become obscured in patients with anterior or inferior infarction if a left bundle branch block develops. The diagnosis can still be made in about two-thirds of these patients by observing evolving ST–T-wave changes on serial ECGs (Figure 4). Following an AMI, Q waves may normalize in some patients and disappear altogether.

The ECG also provides the clinician with information on the location of the myocardial infarction. Locating the site is important because prognosis depends on it. Moreover, the location also refers to the likely major coronary artery involved. This knowledge provides the clinician with early information on the likely outlook and treatment of the patient. The specific ECG leads showing

changes reflecting the infarction site are summarized in Table 5 and demonstrated in Minicase 3.

## Noninvasive Myocardial Imaging

As stated previously, the diagnosis of AMI is based primarily on the objective evidence of symptoms, ECG changes, and laboratory enzymes. However, these traditional approaches have limitations. If a reliable patient history cannot be obtained or if standard clinical and laboratory tests for AMI are equivocal, myocardial imaging may contribute to accurate diagnosis. In addition, imaging techniques may be used to identify, localize, and estimate the size of myocardial infarctions.

**TABLE 5.** Specific ECG Leads Reflecting AMI by Site and Likely Coronary Artery Involvement[a,b]

| ECG Leads Reflecting AMI (ST–T-Wave Changes or Q Waves) | Site of AMI | Likely Artery Involvement |
|---|---|---|
| $V_1$–$V_6$ | Anterior | Left main or LAD |
| II, III, aVF | Inferior | PDA |
| I, aVL, $V_6$ | Lateral | Circumflex |
| $V_1$ and $V_2$ | Posterior | RCA |
| $V_{2R}$–$V_{4R}$ and occasionally $V_1$–$V_3$ | Right ventricle | RCA |

[a]*Adapted from Reference 29.*
[b]*LAD = left anterior descending; PDA = posterior descending artery; RCA = right coronary artery; $V_{2R}$–$V_{4R}$ = special right ventricular leads of ECG.*

In the 1960s and early 1970s, radionuclide scanning techniques were shown to be capable of demonstrating areas of infarction. Techniques for imaging acute infarction areas are classified into two groups: those that image the infarct and those that image myocardial perfusion. The radiopharmaceutical currently used to image infarcts is technetium-99m (Tc-99m) pyrophosphate. The radiopharmaceuticals currently used for imaging myocardial perfusion are thallium-201 (Tl-201) and Tc-99m-labeled blood flow tracers. Antimyosin antibodies have been investigated for diagnosing myocardial necrosis (associated with ischemic heart disease) in selected trials.

### Infarct Imaging[31]

Tc-99m is an infarct-avid agent. It concentrates in necrotic myocardial tissue, presumably because it enters myocardial cells and selectively binds to calcium and calcium complexes. It also is avidly taken up by bone (the tracer used for bone scanning).

Abnormal intracellular uptake of calcium is a feature of irreversible cell death and begins as early as 12 hr after AMI and may persist for 2 weeks. Tc-99m scans may be positive as early as 4 hr after the onset of AMI symptoms. Although the peak sensitivity for the scan is between 48 and 72 hr, it generally remains positive for 1 week and becomes negative by 2 weeks. When obtained within 24–72 hr after onset of infarction, the scan has a diagnostic sensitivity of 90–95% in patients with Q-wave AMI or 38–92% in patients with non-Q-wave AMI. Tc-99m imaging has moderate specificity, with an overall range of 60–80%.

Clinical experience with this imaging technique suggests that it is usually positive when other markers (ECG and enzymes) of infarction also are positive. Because of resolution limitations that affect both sensitivity and specificity, Tc-99m is often criticized for being indeterminate when the infarct is small and subsequent enzymes and ECG findings are nondiagnostic. Since tomographic imaging can detect small infarcts, Tc-99m imaging is most useful for[31]

1. Confirming the diagnosis of AMIs at least 48 hr old (after CK-MB has normalized).
2. Testing patients with uninterpretable ECGs (e.g., obscuring conduction disturbances).
3. Detecting perioperative infarctions.
4. Diagnosing an infarction of the right ventricle.
5. Localizing and sizing infarctions.

An immunologic-based infarct-imaging technique that uses antimyosin antibody fragments has been tested. Defects in necrotic cells within the infarct allow these fragments to adhere to myosin filaments. Although this technique should allow detection of myocardial necrosis soon after coronary flow is interrupted, it cannot be performed until 24 hr after administration of the antibody. The delay allows for antibody clearance from the blood. This infarct-imaging technique has not caught on because of the delay in obtaining data and a limited clinical need.

### Myocardial Perfusion Imaging[32]

Imaging agents used to evaluate myocardial perfusion, such as Tl-201, are cations that are taken up by healthy functioning tissue in a manner similar to potassium. They are taken up at reduced rates by ischemic myocardial tissue and are not distributed to or taken up by regions of myocardial infarction. Therefore, these agents image myocardial perfusion.

*Test performance.* Imaging with Tl-201 for detection of infarction is accomplished with the patient at rest and is optimal within 6 hr of symptom onset. Thallium is injected IV, and imaging is initiated 10–20 min after injection; imaging is repeated 2–4 hr later to determine whether redistribution is present. The diagnosis of AMI must be inferred by a lack of regional myocardial uptake of the radiotracer.

If applied within the first 24 hr after symptom onset, Tl-201 imaging for a perfusion defect (i.e., probable AMI) has a sensitivity of about 90%. The sensitivity falls sharply after this period. Tl-201 imaging is not usually used clinically in the diagnosis of AMI.

*Detection of ischemia/jeopardized myocardial tissue.[33,34]*
Myocardial perfusion imaging with thallium and its analog is useful in determining if CAD is the cause of symptoms and in identifying patients at high risk of further ischemic events. Tl-201 uptake is (1) limited to viable myocardial tissue, (2) dependent on regional blood flow, and (3) taken up linearly to very high blood flow rates.

Ischemic myocardial tissue will incorporate Tl-201, but at a reduced rate; washout from these areas is also delayed. Thus, scans immediately after radionuclide injection reveal ischemic areas as areas of reduced perfusion ("cold spots"). Delayed scans (4–24 hr after injection) may show "redistribution" of Tl-201 with a reduction in defect size. The redistribution phenomenon occurs because of the delayed (compared to normal tissue) washout of Tl-201; it appears to have redistributed, with decreased contrast between normal and ischemic tissue.

The sensitivity of Tl-201 scanning in the detection of CAD is about 75% but is improved when combined with ECG or graded-exercise stress testing. Computer analysis separates the scanned images into anatomic regions and specifically localizes areas (e.g., anterior, septal, and inferior) of necrotic or ischemic myocardial tissue.

Tl-201 perfusion imaging is widely utilized in patients with atypical chest pain and nondiagnostic or false-positive stress testing to determine if CAD is the cause of symptoms and testing abnormalities. In addition, since redistribution is a marker of jeopardized but viable myocardial tissue, Tl-201 can be used to indicate the probable success of revascularization or angioplasty and for prognostic stratification of patients preoperatively. A normal Tl-201 scan indicates a benign outcome, even in patients with documented CAD. Transient defects (redistribution) indicate hemodynamically significant coronary lesions with the risk of cardiac death.

Recently, several myocardial perfusion tracers have been introduced or evaluated. They include technetium-99m sestamibi (Tc-99m MIBI), technetium-99m teboroxime, and technetium-99m tetrofosmin. These new tracers may have advantages over Tl-201 and are already changing the evaluation of regional myocardial perfusion. In many nuclear cardiology departments, Tc-99m MIBI is now being combined with Tl-201 so that rest and stress myocardial perfusion imaging studies can be performed sequentially on the same day. The patient's rest study is done first with Tl-201; imaging is started immediately after tracer injection and is completed within about 45 min. Stress testing (accomplished pharmacologically or with exercise) is begun after the rest study, and Tc-99m MIBI is injected at peak cardiac stress.

Since Tc-99m MIBI emits higher energy photons than Tl-201, its images are not subject to cross-interference from the previously administered Tl-201. Both Tl-201 and Tc-99m MIBI undergo first-pass extraction from blood by myocardial cells; both provide a "stop-frame" image of regional myocardial blood flow at the time of tracer injection. Because Tc-99m MIBI does not leak appreciably from myocardial cells, imaging can be delayed to allow blood and lung concentrations to diminish. Consequently, Tc-99m MIBI imaging can be completed between 1 and 4 hr after tracer injection without significantly reducing diagnostic reliability.

### Pharmacological Perfusion Imaging[34,35]

Pharmacological perfusion imaging with Tl-201 uses agents that "stress" the myocardium by producing a hyperemic (vasodilator or increased blood flow) response. Dipyridamole and adenosine Tl-201 have both been approved for the pharmacological diagnosis of CAD. Both agents produce coronary vasodilation.

This vasodilation is greatest in regions of a normally perfused myocardium; perfusion is reduced in areas supplied by significantly stenosed (greater than 70% luminal narrowing) coronary arteries. Therefore, the myocardium distal to coronary artery obstruction shows hypoperfusion relative to the myocardium supplied by more normal coronary arteries. This difference is evidenced by a lack of perfusion, followed by redistribution on repeat Tl-201 scanning if the myocardium is viable but jeopardized.

Similar to Tl-201 with exercise, pharmacological perfusion imaging with dipyridamole or adenosine is used to

- ➤ Detect CAD.
- ➤ Evaluate patients with known CAD.
- ➤ Assess patients after AMI.
- ➤ Indicate risk stratification prior to surgical procedures.
- ➤ Evaluate the success or status of revascularization procedures.

## Other Related Tests

Some nonspecific laboratory abnormalities may be recognized in patients with AMI. Although these abnormalities are not generally useful in establishing the diagnosis, the clinician should be aware of their coexistence with infarction to avoid misinterpretation or misdiagnosis of other disorders. Minicase 4 demonstrates results of these related tests in the presence of AMI. (These tests also are discussed in other chapters.)

### Serum Glucose
*Normal range: 70–110 mg/dL or
3.9–6.1 mmol/L when fasting*

Elevations of serum glucose, apparently related to stress, occur frequently following AMI. This elevation may be found in diabetic as well as nondiabetic patients. Several weeks may be required for glucose tolerance to return to normal.[36] Measurement of glycosylated hemoglobin may

---

George S., a 57-year-old male, previously had been in good health. On the evening of January 21, 1995, after drinking approximately eight cans of beer, he awoke with severe chest pain and diaphoresis. He was driven to the local emergency treatment center by his wife, who noted that he may have "lost consciousness a couple of times" in route.

At the emergency treatment center, George S.'s pulse was in the 30s. His ECG showed a 3° AV block in addition to acute ST-segment elevation in the inferior leads (II, III, and aVF). George S. received atropine 2 mg, aspirin 325 mg, and streptokinase 1.5 million units over 1 hr, which increased his heart rate and resolved his ST-seg-

ment elevation within approximately 30–60 min.

George S. was then transferred on IV nitroglycerin and heparin to the hospital's cardiovascular ICU. Upon admission, his ECG showed normal sinus rhythm with developing Q waves in leads II, III, and aVF. The admission laboratory showed normal electrolytes and hematological test results, except for an elevated leukocyte count of 14,800 cells/mm³ (4800–10,800 cells/mm³), aPTT of 65 sec (21–45 sec), PT of 17 sec (10–13 sec), and INR of 2.2. In addition, his AST was slightly elevated at 103 IU/L. His blood alcohol level at the local hospital was 168 mg %. Over the next 2 days, his cardiac enzymes rose rapidly as follows (normal range in parentheses):

| Hospital Day | Time | CK (40–200) (IU/L) | CK-MB (0–5.9) (ng/mL) | CK-MB Index (0–1.9) | LDH (100–210) (IU/L) | LDH₁ (20–40) (%) | LDH₂ (25–45) (%) |
|---|---|---|---|---|---|---|---|
| 1 | 0148 | 722 | – | 7.6 | 213 | 23 | 30 |
|   | 1031 | 1694 | – | 8.6 | 399 | 37 | 33 |
|   | 1836 | 1428 | – | 6.2 | 508 | 33 | 31 |
| 2 | 0710 | 276 | – | 3.5 | 415 | 43 | 36 |

**Discussion:** This patient represents a classic case of inferior wall AMI. His symptoms and ECG changes represent inferior wall location and are consistent with AMI. In addition, his initial ECG showed that he was in 3° AV block with bradycardia (about 30 beats/min), as is commonly seen with inferior AMI.

George S. received a thrombolytic agent, resulting in rapid reperfusion of his occluded artery. As a result, his CK enzymes peaked earlier than usual (within 12 hr of symptom onset) and returned to normal more rapidly (by about 24–30 hr compared to 2–3 days). His LDH enzymes

also peaked rapidly (within 24 hr), and the isoenzymes LDH₁ and LDH₂ flipped pattern within 10 hr.

In addition to these factors, the leukocytosis was consistent with AMI. George S.'s aPTT and PT were elevated because he received the thrombolytic and was on heparin. His AST was probably elevated because of chronic alcohol ingestion. Despite thrombolytic therapy, he experienced significant myocardial injury, as reflected by the enzyme rise and Q waves on his ECG 1 day after his AMI.

---

help to differentiate hyperglycemia caused by the stress of AMI from that caused by diabetes.[37,38]

### White Blood Cells (WBCs)
*Normal range: 4.8–10.8 × 10³ cells/mm³ or 4.8–10.8 × 10⁹ cells/L for adults*

WBCs frequently increase following AMI. This increase may be a response to myocardial tissue necrosis or increased secretion of adrenal glucocorticoids due to stress. WBC elevation usually develops within 2 hr of the onset of symptoms, peaks at 2–4 days, and returns to normal in 1 week. The peak WBC count ranges between 12,000 and 15,000 cells/mm³ but may reach 20,000 cells/mm³. In addition, the numbers of polymorphonuclear leukocytes may increase with a shift of the differential count to band forms.[36]

### Erythrocyte Sedimentation Rate (ESR)
*Normal range: 1–15 mm/hr for males or 1–20 mm/hr for females*

During the first 1 or 2 days after an AMI, the ESR is usually normal. It then increases to a peak on the 4th or

5th day and can remain elevated for several weeks. This increase is apparently secondary to elevated globulin and fibrinogen.[36]

## TESTS TO EVALUATE CARDIAC STRUCTURE AND FUNCTION

As explained earlier, the heart's function is to circulate blood throughout the body. The regulation of circulation depends on the structural integrity of the heart's valves and chambers as well as the complex integration of the heart, veins, and arteries. When major disease states disrupt the stability of the circulation, the heart is injured (reducing ventricular function), or its structure is altered, hemodynamics may deteriorate rapidly.

Subtle and quickly changing *clinical* findings often do not allow reliable assessment of a patient's status. However, advances in biomedical engineering and invasive monitoring techniques can provide immediate objective data on complex and dynamic cardiac functions. This section discusses the measurement and evaluation of cardiac structural integrity and function by many methods.

## Cardiovascular Hemodynamic Monitoring

Central hemodynamic monitoring via a central venous catheter inserted at the bedside provides minute-by-minute measurements to guide the selection of appropriate therapy, particularly

> ➤ Preload reducing agents (e.g., diuretics and nitrates).
> ➤ Afterload reducing agents (e.g., nitroprusside, angiotensin-converting enzyme inhibitors, and calcium antagonists).
> ➤ Inotropes (e.g., dopamine and dobutamine).

Since invasive hemodynamic monitoring has become the standard of care in the United States, clinicians in a critical care environment should be familiar with the associated equipment and concepts. Although complete discussion is beyond the scope of this chapter, it is provided by an excellent review.[39]

## Echocardiography[40,41]

Echocardiography uses ultrasound to investigate and visualize the heart's structural anatomy, to calculate the left ventricular ejection fraction (LVEF), and to assess wall thickness and motion. This simple, noninvasive test can be performed at the bedside of an unstable patient. It is the preferred procedure for valvular dysfunction, wall motion abnormalities, congenital abnormalities, pericardial effusions, and endocarditis of valves.

Echocardiography is based on the principle that different tissues present different acoustical impedance (resistance to transmitting sound). Therefore, sound waves from a transducer directed across cardiac tissues transmit back sound waves of different frequencies. After correction for underlying structures and their depth, these frequencies are displayed on an oscilloscope (the electronic monitor where the image is traced). Therefore, anatomic structures can be visualized. Great advances in technology and technique have made echocardiography a capable and sophisticated diagnostic tool.

Application of echocardiography to the diagnosis of CAD resulted with the recognition that ventricular wall motion abnormalities result from ischemia. In particular, abnormalities are seen as altered thicknesses of various segments of the heart and decreases in segmental wall movement (e.g., anterior, septal, or inferior). AMI with scar formation appears as a thinning of the myocardial wall in that area. Post-AMI echocardiography is useful for detection of ventricular aneurysms and left ventricular thrombi. Both global left ventricular function and regional function can be assessed with the calculation of LVEF.

Various echocardiographic approaches are now available including M mode (motion), two dimensional, and Doppler. In addition, echocardiography can be performed using a transthoracic approach or transesophageal echocardiography (TEE) and can be done either at rest or with stress testing (e.g., pharmacologically with dobutamine). With the latter method, echocardiography can visualize stress-induced structural or functional abnormalities (e.g., wall motion abnormality associated with ischemia).

### M Mode

M-mode echocardiography provides a one-dimensional, single-axis view of a narrow region of the heart, dependent on transducer placement. Although it can provide only static objects in a single plane, it does visualize the right ventricle, left ventricle, posterior left ventricular wall, and pericardium. Results are improved by sweeping the transducer in an arc from the cardiac apex to the base. This approach adds visualization of the valves as well as the left atrium.

### Two Dimensional

Two-dimensional echocardiography records multiple views of the heart using the same basic principle as M mode. When collected onto video tape, these views produce a "motion picture" of the heart's structures and lateral movement. Two-dimensional echocardiography provides improved visualization and more accurate determination of ventricular volume, wall thickness, and valvular stenosis.

### Doppler

Doppler echocardiography uses sound or frequency ultrasound to record the velocity and direction of blood and wall motion; it is based on the principle of bouncing ultrasound off of a moving object (e.g., RBCs). This method permits the quantification of valvular abnormalities (e.g., aortic stenosis or regurgitation and mitral regurgitation) and wall motion abnormalities, measurement of hemodynamic alterations, and visualization and quantification of congenital abnormalities.

### Transesophageal Echocardiography

TEE is a recent development. Much like endoscopy in gastroenterology, the transducer is passed into the esophagus and positioned just behind the heart. Images then can be obtained in a horizontal or vertical plane. In contrast to the transthoracic approach, there is reduced interference from ribs, lungs, and subcutaneous tissues. Furthermore, because the transducer is closer to the heart, resolution and structural detail are improved.

The improved image resolution with TEE has widened the clinical application of echocardiography. Compared to the transthoracic approach, the visualization of cardiac valves (e.g., mitral valves) is superior, permitting more accurate evaluation of both native and prosthetic valves. Moreover, identification and quantification of valvular endocarditis have improved significantly. Small vegetation on valves can be visualized, and complications such as thrombosis or valvular leaks can be identified and monitored.

TEE also is used to identify cardiac thrombi, especially in the atria. The proximity of the transducer to the atria and the increased resolution provide an improved image, including atrial enlargement and thrombi in the atria or outflow tract into the ventricles.

Intraoperative TEE during valvular surgery is another important application of this technology. TEE with Doppler can be used to plan as well as monitor surgical corrections.

## Cardiac Catheterization and Angiography[42-44]

The development of cardiac catheterization and angiography has been an important contribution to the diagnosis and evaluation of cardiovascular disease. Although this procedure has many uses, it is primarily done to

> ➤ Diagnose the presence or absence of CAD.
> ➤ Define the anatomy of coronary arteries.
> ➤ Evaluate cardiac and valvular performance by measuring cardiac chamber pressures, blood flow, and oxygenation.
> ➤ Visualize and quantitate valvular abnormalities.

This technique also is used in therapeutic procedures such as balloon angioplasty and atherectomy of coronary arteries.

Basically, cardiac catheterization involves inserting a flexible, radiopaque catheter through a peripheral vein (access to right heart, pulmonary artery, and pulmonary "wedge" position) or artery (access to left heart) and guiding it either fluoroscopically or with pressure monitoring. Pressures are recorded, blood samples are drawn, and contrast material can be injected through the catheter. Table 6 lists the general types of cardiac catheterization and their associated uses.

Cardiac catheterization with coronary angiography is the definitive method for assessing CAD and stenosis. The lower limit of lesion detection by angiography is approximately 20%. Occlusions of 70% or more are almost always easily seen. Significant narrowing is usually defined as 50% or more, although some studies use 70–75% as the critical cutoff.

Ventriculography (direct injection of contrast dye into the left ventricle) studies also are usually performed to evaluate chamber contour as well as global and seg-

**TABLE 6.** Types of Cardiac Catheterization and Associated Uses

| Type of Cardiac Catheterization | Associated Uses |
|---|---|
| Right sided | Right heart pressure readings<br>Oximetry<br>Cardiac shunt studies<br>Calculation of cardiac output<br>Angiography of right atrium, right ventricle, tricuspid and pulmonary valves, and pulmonary artery |
| Left sided | Pressure readings of aorta and left-sided chambers<br>Left ventricular function evaluations<br>Mitral and aortic valve function evaluations<br>Shunt studies<br>Angiography of coronary arteries, aortic root, and left ventricle |

mental function. Regional wall motion abnormalities can be assessed, and the presence of left ventricular thrombi can usually be identified. It is now routine to complete ventriculography studies to obtain LVEF and other information, unless these data are already available from noninvasive studies or a large contrast dye injection is contraindicated.

## Radionuclide Ventriculography (Intraventriculogram and Multiple-Gated Blood Pool Imaging)[45]

Radionuclide ventriculography or blood pool scintigraphy is used to evaluate ventricular wall motion and function as well as left ventricular volume. Human serum albumin or the patient's RBCs are tagged with Tc-99m and injected IV into the patient. A scintillation camera records the radioisotope as it passes through the ventricle. Imaging can be "gated" or linked with a simultaneous ECG recording (and thus to the systolic and diastolic events of the cardiac cycle).

The camera images the heart in at least two views, and they are combined to produce a cine film. This film permits evaluation of ventricular chamber size, wall motion, filling defects, and ventricular ejection fraction. Blood pool imaging is probably the most common method used clinically to assess ventricular ejection fraction and regional wall motion abnormalities at rest.

### High-Speed Computed Axial Tomography (Cine CT)[46,47]

Although cine CT is not used as a primary diagnostic procedure, it can help to assess cardiac function and it provides detailed images of cardiac structure. In CT, an intense, focused electron beam is swept along target rings by electromagnets. When the electron beam strikes the target ring, a fan of X-rays is produced and moves around the patient.

Until recently, CT of the heart was limited by cardiac motion and the need to couple CT scan slices with the cardiac cycle. Gating of the CT scan with a simultaneous ECG recording, as in blood pool scintigraphy, has overcome this problem. In addition, extremely fast (cine) CT scanners now allow scanning in real time without gating.

CT scanning provides precise visualization of cardiac structure from the inner endocardial wall to the epicardial surface and pericardium. The extent of ventricular wall thickening during the cardiac cycle also can be determined if the CT scan is gated. Like ventriculography and echocardiography, cine CT can provide ejection fraction and chamber dimensional data. It has been shown to be equal to other tests at identifying wall motion abnormalities and is a superior diagnostic tool for imaging cardiac masses and thrombi, pericardial disease, and possibly congenital heart defects.[46,47]

## Magnetic Resonance Imaging[47,48]

MRI (formerly nuclear magnetic resonance) is a noninvasive imaging technique with tremendous potential for cardiovascular diagnosis and research. It is capable of direct tissue characterization and blood flow measurements.

For MRI, patients are placed in a device generating a magnetic field thousands of times stronger than that of the Earth. This device aligns the protons of the body's hydrogen atoms relative to the magnetic field, much like a compass lines up with the Earth's magnetic field. Radio waves pulsed through the field force the protons to shift their orientation. When the radio waves stop, the protons return to their previous orientation, giving off energy in the form of radio waves.

These waves, detected by a scanner, are converted via computer into an image which can be examined in 0.8-mm thick sections. Since lack of motion is essential for obtaining quality MRI images, the images are physiologically gated to an ECG to improve their quality for cardiac evaluation. The patient must be able to lie completely still throughout the procedure; many patients, especially infants and children, require sedation.

To achieve the magnetic field strength required by MRI, a small internal diameter device (about 60 cm) is necessary. For some patients, the size and noise produced can be frightening and claustrophobic. Unstable patients, patients who cannot remain motionless, and patients suffering from claustrophobia are contraindicated for MRI. In addition, patients with metal prostheses (e.g., pacemakers and ferromagnetic intracerebral clips) should not undergo MRI.

At present, MRI is only available at some medical centers because of the cost, scan time, and need for specialized equipment and personnel in a suitable environment. The role of MRI in cardiovascular disease assessment is still being defined. Nevertheless, it is proving useful for evaluation of aortic abnormalities, congenital heart disease, and pericardial disorders.

## Left Ventricular Ejection Fraction Assessment

A widely used technique for assessing cardiac performance involves measurement of the LVEF. LVEF represents the fraction of end-diastolic volume of the ventricle that is ejected with each heartbeat. LVEF is considered the best single index of global left ventricular function. In addition, the ejection fraction is a major determinant of outcome after myocardial infarction.[49]

Several methods, both invasive and noninvasive, can qualitatively and quantitatively measure LVEF. As reviewed previously, they include echocardiography, cardiac angiography (ventriculography), radionuclide ventriculography, high-speed (cine) CT, and MRI. In normal subjects, the ejection fraction of the two ventricles is approximately equal and averages $0.67 \pm 0.08$ (SD).[50]

When disease produces ventricular dysfunction, the resulting degrees of depression in the LVEF can be empirically classified based on the measured resting LVEF (Table 7). A cutoff value of 40% is commonly considered indicative of systolic dysfunction and has been used extensively in clinical trials of post-AMI interventions. The global ejection fraction has been studied to define the effects of pharmacological agents on ventricular function. The goals have been to explore general mechanisms of drug action and efficacy and to guide therapy selection in a specific patient.[51] Digitalis and milrinone,[52] ß-adrenergic blockers,[53] and calcium channel antagonists, as well as antineoplastic agents (e.g., anthracyclines),[54] have been studied.

Although the end-systolic volume of the left ventricle may be an even more important index of left ventricular function than is LVEF, data are limited. Currently, LVEF is widely determined and firmly established in clinical practice as the most useful measure of impaired left ventricular function—the major predictor of mortality after AMI.[55]

## Myocardial Viability Assessment

Positron emission tomography (PET) is a nuclear imaging technique capable of measuring, qualitatively and/or quantitatively, in vivo functions (e.g., blood flow and metabolism of substrates such as fatty acids, glucose, and oxygen) of various organs, including the heart. PET technology has existed for about 25 years but has been applied clinically only recently.

**TABLE 7.** LVEF as a Measure of Ventricular Function

| Ejection Fraction (%) | Class of Left Ventricular Function |
|---|---|
| 55–80 | Normal |
| 40–54 | Mild dysfunction |
| 25–39 | Moderate dysfunction |
| <25 | Severe dysfunction |

PET uses the properties of short-lived, positron-emitting, isotope-labeled compounds coupled with mathematical models of physiological function.[56] Its most relevant clinical use for cardiovascular evaluation is detection of viable myocardium that appears irreversibly injured (necrotic) by other measures. At this time, PET is not widely available. Nevertheless, it has the potential to become a routine clinical procedure, providing information on the pathophysiology, diagnosis, treatment, and prognosis of heart disease.[57]

## COSTS OF CARDIOVASCULAR ASSESSMENT AND TESTING

The costs associated with the various laboratory tests for evaluating cardiovascular disease are unquestionably important. Practitioners should have a general idea of these costs so that they can balance the best results with the least expense.

Of the tests discussed in this chapter, those for CK, LDH, and their isoenzymes are the least costly. Catheterization and angiograms are the most expensive procedures for the patient.

## SUMMARY

The heart is a muscular pump that circulates blood first to the lungs for oxygenation and then throughout the vascular system to supply oxygen and nutrients to every cell in the body. Many diseases—the most important being coronary atherosclerosis—affect the heart's function and can result in AMI.

The classic laboratory workup for AMI includes the measurement of serum CK and its more specific isoenzymes. LDH and its isoenzymes play a limited role, and measurement of AST is no longer practical. Classic ECG changes such as T-wave inversion, ST-segment elevation, and Q-wave appearance also may be present and useful in characterizing AMI. In addition to confirming an equivocal diagnosis, imaging techniques may localize and estimate the size of myocardial infarctions. After an AMI, LVEF may be determined for prognostic information and guidance in selection of appropriate drug therapy.

The clinician must have knowledge of these and other methods used to diagnose and characterize AMI, as well as a general understanding of the techniques used to measure cardiac performance. These determinations have a significant impact on decisions regarding medical and surgical management of a patient.

## REFERENCES

1.  American Heart Association. 1987 heart facts. Dallas, TX: American Heart Association National Center; 1986.
2.  Guyton AC. Textbook of medical physiology. Philadelphia, PA: W. B. Saunders; 1986.
3.  Braunwald E, Jones RH, Mark DB, et al. Diagnosing and managing unstable angina. *Circulation*. 1994; 90:613–22.
4.  Alexander RW. Inflammation and coronary artery disease. *N Engl J Med*. 1994; 331:468–9. Editorial.
5.  Lee TH, Goldman L. Serum enzyme assays in the diagnosis of acute myocardial infarction. *Ann Intern Med*. 1986; 105:221–33.
6.  Siegel AJ, Silverman LM, Evans WJ. Elevated skeletal muscle creatine kinase MB isoenzyme levels in marathon runners. *JAMA*. 1983; 250:2835–7.
7.  Tilkian AG. Clinical implications of laboratory tests. St. Louis, MO: C. V. Mosby; 1983.
8.  Tilkian SM, Conover MB, Tilkian AG. Clinical implications of laboratory tests. St. Louis, MO: C. V. Mosby; 1987.
9.  Teitz NW. Fundamentals of clinical chemistry. Philadelphia, PA: W. B. Saunders; 1987.
10. Teitz NW. Clinical guide to laboratory tests. Philadelphia, PA: W. B. Saunders; 1983.
11. Jacobs DS, Kasten BL, DeMott WR, et al., eds. Laboratory test handbook. Cleveland, OH: Lexi-Comp/Mosby; 1988.
12. Chapelle J-P, Allaf ME. Automated quantification of creatine kinase MB isoenzyme in serum by radial partition immunoassay, with use of the stratus analyzer. *Clin Chem*. 1990; 36:99–101.
13. Panteghini M, Bonora R, Pagani F, et al. A new immunoenzymometric assay for quantification of creatine kinase MB (CK-MB) in serum evaluated. *Clin Biochem*. 1989; 22:404. Abstract.
14. Apple FS, Preese LM, Gerken K, et al. Clinical utility of a monoclonal anti-CK MB antibody-based assay on the stratus immunoassay system. *Clin Biochem*. 1989; 22:404. Abstract.
15. Puleo PR, Meyer D, Wathen C, et al. Use of a rapid assay of subforms of creatine kinase MB to diagnose or rule out acute myocardial infarction. *N Engl J Med*. 1994; 331:561–6.
16. Puleo PR, Guadagno PA, Roberts R, et al. Sensitive, rapid assay of subforms of creatine kinase MB in plasma. *Clin Chem*. 1989; 35:1452–5.
17. Puleo PR, Guadagno PA, Roberts R, et al. Early diagnosis of acute myocardial infarction based on assay of subforms of creatine kinase-MB. *Circulation*. 1990; 82:759–64.
18. Onigbinde TA, Wu AHB, Johnson M, et al. Clinical evaluation of an automated chemical inhibition assay for lactate dehydrogenase isoenzyme 1. *Clin Chem*. 1990; 36:1819–22.
19. Hamm CW. New serum markers for acute myocardial infarction. *N Engl J Med*. 1994; 331:607–8. Editorial.
20. Adams JE III, Sicard GA, Allen BT, et al. Diagnosis of perioperative myocardial infarction with measurement of cardiac troponin I. *N Engl J Med*. 1994; 330:670–4.
21. Pharmacek MS, Leider JM. Structure, function, and regulation of troponin C. *Circulation*. 1991; 84:991–1003.
22. Hamm CW, Ravkilde J, Gerhardt W, et al. The prognostic value of serum troponin T in unstable angina. *N Engl J Med*. 1992; 327:146–50.
23. Liuzzo G, Biasucci LM, Gallimore JR, et al. The prognostic value of c-reactive protein and serum amyloid A protein in severe unstable angina pectoris. *N Engl J Med*. 1994; 331:417–24.
24. Dubin D. Rapid interpretation of EKGs, 4th ed. Tampa, FL: Cover Publishing; 1989.
25. Griffin B, Timmis AD, Crick JCP, et al. The evolution of myocardial ischaemia during percutaneous transluminal coronary angioplasty. *Eur Heart J*. 1987; 8:347–53.

26. Norell MS, Lyons JP, Gershlick AH, et al. Assessment of left ventricular performance during coronary angioplasty: a study of digital subtraction ventriculography. *Br Heart J.* 1988; 59:419–28.

27. Lee TH, Rouan GW, Weisberg MC, et al. Sensitivity of routine clinical criteria for diagnosing myocardial infarction within 24 hours of hospitalization. *Ann Intern Med.* 1987; 106:181–6.

28. Lott JA, Stang JM. Differential diagnosis of patients with abnormal serum creatine kinase enzymes. *Clin Lab Med.* 1989; 9:627–42.

29. Marriott HJL (with Wagner GS). Myocardial infarction. In: Marriott HJL, ed. Practical electrocardiography, 8th ed. Baltimore, MD: Williams & Wilkins; 1988:419–50.

30. Goldschlager N. Goldman MJ. Principles of clinical electrocardiography. East Norwalk, CT: Appleton & Lange; 1989.

31. Olson HG, Lyons KP. Technetium-99m stannous pyrophosphate myocardial scintigraphy in the diagnosis of acute myocardial infarction. In: Lyons KP, ed. Cardiovascular nuclear medicine. East Norwalk, CT: Appleton & Lange; 1988:163–80.

32. Reisman SA. Myocardial perfusion imaging with thallium-201 in the detection and assessment of coronary artery disease. In: Lyons KP, ed. Cardiovascular nuclear medicine. East Norwalk, CT: Appleton & Lange; 1988:117–44.

33. Mahmarian JJ, Verani MS. Exercise thallium-201 perfusion scintigraphy in the assessment of coronary artery disease. *Am J Cardiol.* 1991; 67:2D–11D.

34. Zaret BL, Wackers FJ. Nuclear cardiology (first of two parts). *N Engl J Med.* 1993; 329:775–83.

35. Beller GA. Pharmacological stress testing. *JAMA.* 1991; 265:633–8.

36. Pasternak RC, Braunwald E, Sobel BE. Acute myocardial infarction. In: Braunwald E, ed. Heart disease: a textbook of cardiovascular medicine. Philadelphia, PA: W. B. Saunders; 1988:1222–313.

37. Soler NG, Frank S. Value of glycosylated haemoglobin measurements after acute myocardial infarction. *JAMA.* 1981; 246:1690–3.

38. Husband DJ, Alberti KGM, Julian DG. "Stress" hyperglycaemia during acute myocardial infarction: an indicator of pre-existing diabetes? *Lancet.* 1983; 1(8343):179–81.

39. Hoffman EW. Basics of cardiovascular hemodynamic monitoring. *Drug Intell Clin Pharm.* 1983; 16:657–68.

40. Feigenbaum H. Echocardiography. In: Braunwald E, ed. Heart disease: a textbook of cardiovascular medicine. Philadelphia, PA: W. B. Saunders; 1988:83–139.

41. Popp RL. Echocardiography (first and second of two parts). *N Engl J Med.* 1990; 323:101–9; 165–72.

42. Canobbio MM. Cardiovascular disorders. St. Louis, MO: C. V. Mosby; 1990.

43. Grossman W, Barry WH. Cardiac catheterization. In: Braunwald E, ed. Heart disease: a textbook of cardiovascular medicine. Philadelphia, PA: W. B. Saunders; 1988: 242–67.

44. Levin DC, Gardiner GA. Cardiac arteriography. In: Braunwald E, ed. Heart disease: a textbook of cardiovascular medicine. Philadelphia, PA: W. B. Saunders; 1988: 268–310.

45. Berger HJ, Zaret BL. Nuclear cardiology (second of two parts). *N Engl J Med.* 1993; 329:855–63.

46. Farmer D, Lipton MJ, Gould R, et al. High speed (cine) computed tomography of the heart. *Cardiovasc Clin.* 1986; 17(1):345–56.

47. Higgins CB. Newer cardiac imaging techniques: digital subtraction angiography, computerized tomography, magnetic resonance imaging. In: Braunwald E, ed. Heart disease: a textbook of cardiovascular medicine. Philadelphia, PA: W. B. Saunders; 1988:356–82.

48. Higgins CB, Byrd B III, Lipton MJ. Magnetic resonance imaging of the heart. In: Pohost GM, Higgins CB, Morganroth J, et al., eds. New concepts in cardiac imaging 1985. Boston, MA: G. K. Hall Medical Publishers; 1985:278–99.

49. Multicenter Postinfarction Research Group. Risk stratification and survival after myocardial infarction. *N Engl J Med.* 1983; 309:331–6.

50. Braunwald E. Assessment of cardiac function. In: Braunwald E, ed. Heart disease: a textbook of cardiovascular medicine. Philadelphia, PA: W. B. Saunders; 1988: 449–70.

51. Berger HJ, Zaret BL. Nuclear cardiology (second of two parts). *N Engl J Med.* 1981; 305:855–65.

52. DiBianco R, Shabetai R, Kostuk W, et al. (for Milrinone Multicenter Trial Group). A comparison of oral milrinone, digoxin, and their combination in the treatment of patients with chronic heart failure. *N Engl J Med.* 1989; 320:677–83.

53. Marshall RC, Wisenberg G, Schelbert HR, et al. Effect of oral propranolol on rest, exercise and postexercise left ventricular performance in normal subjects and patients with coronary artery disease. *Circulation.* 1981; 63:572–83.

54. Schwartz RG, McKenzie WB, Alexander J, et al. Congestive heart failure and left ventricular dysfunction complicating doxorubicin therapy: seven-year experience using serial radionuclide angiocardiography. *Am J Med.* 1987; 82:1109–18.

55. White HD, Norris RM, Brown MA, et al. Left ventricular end-systolic volume as the major determinant of survival after recovery from myocardial infarction. *Circulation.* 1987; 76:44–51.

56. Phelps ME, Mazziotta JC, Schelbert HR. Positron emission tomography and autoradiography: principles and applications for brain and heart. New York: Raven Press; 1986.

57. Grover-McKay M. Clinical applications of positron emission tomography in cardiology. In: Lyons KP, ed. Cardiovascular nuclear medicine. East Norwalk, CT: Appleton & Lange; 1988:293–318.

## QuickView—CK

| Parameter | Description | Comments |
|---|---|---|
| **Common reference ranges** | | |
| Adults | Males: 40–200 IU/L<br>Females: 35–150 IU/L | Females have lower values due to smaller muscle mass |
| Pediatrics | >6 weeks = adult value | |
| **Critical value** | 150–200 IU/L without signs and symptoms warrants further evaluation | At >70 IU/L, some laboratories automatically test for CK-MB |
| **Natural substance?** | Yes | Muscle enzyme |
| **Inherent activity?** | Yes | Catalyzes transfer of high-energy phosphate groups |
| **Location** | | |
| Production | Skeletal and cardiac muscle and brain | |
| Storage | Not stored as such | |
| Secretion/excretion | Excreted via glomerular filtration | Elimination may decrease in renal failure |
| **Major causes of . . .** | | |
| High results | Myocardial infarction | Table 2 |
| Associated signs and symptoms | AMI: chest pain, nausea, vomiting, diaphoresis<br>Signs and symptoms of underlying disorder | Decreased or increased heart rate and BP, anxiety, and confusion, depending on AMI size, location, and duration<br>High CK does not cause signs and symptoms directly |
| Low results | Abnormally low muscle mass | Cachexia and neuromuscular disease |
| Associated signs and symptoms | Causes of abnormally low muscle mass | Does not cause signs and symptoms directly |
| **After AMI, time to . . .** | | |
| Initial elevation | 6–8 hr | Sooner with non-Q-wave myocardial infarction or early use of thrombolytic agent |
| Peak values | 24 hr | Sooner with non-Q-wave myocardial infarction or early use of thrombolytic agent |
| Normalization | 3–4 days | Sooner with non-Q-wave myocardial infarction or early use of thrombolytic agent |
| **Drugs often monitored with test** | None | |
| **Causes of spurious results** | Table 2 | Assay dependent |

## QuickView—CK-MB Isoenzymes

| Parameter | Description | Comments |
|---|---|---|
| **Common reference ranges** | | |
| Adults | <12 IU/L<br><3–6% of total CK<br>0–5.9 ng/mL | Assay dependent |
| **Critical value** | ≥12 IU/L<br>>6% of total CK<br>>5.9 ng/mL | Assay dependent |
| **Natural substance?** | Yes | Muscle enzyme |

 *continued*

## QuickView—CK-MB Isoenzymes *continued*

| Parameter | Description | Comments |
|---|---|---|
| Inherent activity? | Yes | Catalyzes transfer of high-energy phosphate groups |
| **Location** Production | Primarily cardiac muscle | Release from traumatized skeletal muscle can be incorrectly interpreted as cardiac |
| Storage | Small amounts in skeletal muscle | |
| Secretion/excretion | Excreted via glomerular filtration | Eliminated at slightly faster rate than total CK |
| **Major causes of . . .** High results | Myocardial infarction | Table 3 |
| Associated signs and symptoms | AMI: chest pain, nausea, vomiting, diaphoresis | Decreased or increased heart rate and BP, anxiety, and confusion, depending on AMI size, location, and duration |
| Low results | Not significant | No lower limit for normal |
| Associated signs and symptoms | None | Does not cause signs and symptoms |
| **After AMI, time to . . .** Initial elevation | 4–8 hr | Sooner with non-Q-wave myocardial infarction or early use of thrombolytic agent |
| Peak values | 12–20 hr | Sooner with non-Q-wave myocardial infarction or early use of thrombolytic agent |
| Normalization | 2–3 days | Sooner with non-Q-wave myocardial infarction or early use of thrombolytic agent |
| Drugs often monitored with test | None | |
| Causes of spurious results | Table 3 | Assay dependent |

© 1996, American Society of Health-System Pharmacists, Inc. All rights reserved.

## QuickView—CK-MB Isoenzyme Subforms (CK-MB$_2$ and CK-MB$_1$)

| Parameter | Description | Comments |
|---|---|---|
| **Common reference ranges** Adults | 0.5–1 U/L | CK-MB$_2$ and CK-MB$_1$ in equilibrium |
| Critical value | CK-MB$_2$: ≥1 U/L CK-MB$_2$:CK-MB$_1$ ratio: ≥1.5 | CK-MB$_2$ and ratio increase soon after AMI until new equilibrium reached |
| Natural substance? | Yes | CK-MB$_2$ found in myocardial cells CK-MB$_1$ formed from CK-MB$_2$ in plasma after in vivo loss of terminal lysine |
| Inherent activity? | CK-MB$_2$: yes CK-MB$_1$: unknown | Catalyzes final step of glycolysis |
| **Location** Production | Heart and skeletal muscle | |
| Storage | Not stored | |
| Secretion/excretion | Excreted via glomerular filtration | |

© 1996, American Society of Health-System Pharmacists, Inc. All rights reserved.

## QuickView—CK-MB Isoenzyme Subforms (CK-MB$_2$ and CK-MB$_1$) *continued*

| Parameter | Description | Comments |
|---|---|---|
| **Major causes of . . .** | | |
| High results | AMI | Table 3 |
| Associated signs and symptoms | Chest pain, nausea, vomiting, diaphoresis | Decreased or increased heart rate and BP, anxiety, and confusion, depending on AMI size, location, and duration |
| Low results | Normal finding | No lower limit for normal |
| Associated signs and symptoms | None | Does not cause signs and symptoms |
| **After AMI, time to . . .** | | |
| Initial elevation | 2–4 hr | Sooner with non-Q-wave myocardial infarction or early use of thrombolytic agent |
| Peak values | 6–8 hr | Sooner with non-Q-wave myocardial infarction or early use of thrombolytic agent |
| Normalization | 10–14 days | Sooner with non-Q-wave myocardial infarction or early use of thrombolytic agent |
| **Drugs often monitored with test** | None | |
| **Causes of spurious results** | False-positive elevations likely in muscular dystrophy<br>Severe skeletal muscle damage | Table 3 |

## QuickView—LDH

| Parameter | Description | Comments |
|---|---|---|
| **Common reference ranges** | | |
| Adults and/or pediatrics | 100–210 IU/L | |
| **Critical value** | >210 IU/L | Dependent on assay and clinical setting |
| **Natural substance?** | Yes | Found in cell cytoplasm |
| **Inherent activity?** | Yes | Catalyzes final step of glycolysis |
| **Location** | | |
| Production | High concentration in skeletal muscle, liver, RBCs, kidneys, and heart | |
| Storage | Not stored | |
| Secretion/excretion | Excreted via glomerular filtration | |
| **Major causes of . . .** | | |
| High results | Inflammation<br>Myocardial infarction<br>Liver disease<br>Hemolysis | Table 4 |
| Associated signs and symptoms | Underlying causes of inflammation, myocardial infarction, liver disease, or hemolysis | Does not cause signs and symptoms |
| Low results | Normal finding | No lower limit for normal |
| Associated signs and symptoms | None | Does not cause signs and symptoms |
| **After AMI, time to . . .** | | |
| Initial elevation | 12 hr | Sooner with non-Q-wave myocardial infarction or early use of thrombolytic agent |

*continued*

**QuickView—LDH** *continued*

| Parameter | Description | Comments |
|---|---|---|
| Peak values | 2–3 days | Sooner with non-Q-wave myocardial infarction or early use of thrombolytic agent |
| Normalization | 8–14 days | Sooner with non-Q-wave myocardial infarction or early use of thrombolytic agent |
| Drugs often monitored with test | None | Can be used to rule out drug-induced liver disease or hemolysis |
| Causes of spurious results | Table 4 | |

## QuickView—LDH Isoenzymes (LDH$_1$)

| Parameter | Description | Comments |
|---|---|---|
| **Common reference ranges** Adults | 20–40% total LDH | |
| **Critical value** | LDH$_1$:LDH$_2$ ratio: >1 | >0.76 used in some laboratories |
| **Location** | High concentration in heart and RBCs Smaller amounts in kidneys, brain, stomach, and pancreas | |
| **Major causes of . . .** High results | AMI | Table 4 |
| Associated signs and symptoms | Chest pain, nausea, vomiting, diaphoresis | Decreased or increased heart rate and BP, anxiety, and confusion, depending on AMI size, location, and duration |
| Low results | Normal finding | No lower limit for normal |
| Associated signs and symptoms | None | Does not cause signs and symptoms |
| **After AMI, time to . . .** Initial elevation | 12 hr | Sooner with non-Q-wave myocardial infarction or early use of thrombolytic agent |
| Peak values | 3–4 days | Sooner with non-Q-wave myocardial infarction or early use of thrombolytic agent |
| Normalization | 10–14 days | Sooner with non-Q-wave myocardial infarction or early use of thrombolytic agent |
| **Drugs often monitored with test** | None | |
| **Causes of spurious results** | Potentially misleading elevations of ratio from hemolysis, renal infarction, pregnancy, and myopathies | Table 4 |

## QuickView—Troponins I and T

| Parameter | Description | Comments |
|---|---|---|
| Common reference ranges | Troponin I: <1.5 ng/mL<br>Troponin T: ≤0.2 ng/mL | |
| Critical value | Troponin I: >1.5 ng/mL<br>Troponin T: >0.2 ng/mL | |
| Natural substance? | Yes | Regulatory proteins found in muscle cells |
| Inherent activity? | Yes | Regulates calcium-mediated interaction of actin and myosin |
| Location | Troponin I: cardiac muscle<br>Troponin T: cardiac and skeletal muscle | Cardiac troponin T and skeletal muscle troponin T have different amino acid sequences |
| **Major causes of . . .**<br>High results | Myocardial infarction<br>Unstable angina | |
| Associated signs and symptoms | Chest pain, nausea, vomiting, diaphoresis | Decreased or increased heart rate and BP, anxiety, and confusion, depending on AMI size, location, and duration |
| Low results | Normal finding | No lower limit for normal |
| Associated signs and symptoms | None | Does not cause signs and symptoms |
| **After AMI, time to . . .**<br>Initial elevation or positive result | 4 hr | Time course studies of release needed |
| Peak values | Biphasic pattern: 14 hr and 3–5 days | |
| Normalization | 5–7 days | |
| Drugs often monitored with test | None | |
| Causes of spurious results | None known | |

# Chapter 11

# Liver and Gastroenterology Tests

*Paul Farkas and Douglas Hyde*

Hepatic and other gastrointestinal (GI) diseases are fascinating areas of human physiology and medicine, and several major medical advances recently occurred in this field. This chapter covers the common liver function studies and their relationship to various hepatic and nonhepatic problems. The tests are divided into those associated with (1) general liver function, (2) cholestasis, (3) hepatocellular injury, (4) bilirubin metabolism, (5) ammonia, and (6) viral hepatitis.

This classification is not exact because many interclass relationships exist. In addition, except for serological tests for hepatitis, these tests are often nonspecific; accurate diagnosis of liver disease is possible only with a complete history and physical examination. Furthermore, diagnosis usually requires additional radiographic testing or, ultimately, a biopsy of the liver.

This chapter also describes several nonhepatic tests such as assays for the causative agent of most peptic ulcer disease, tests for pseudomembranous colitis, and tests used to diagnose and assess pancreatitis.

## OBJECTIVES

Upon completion of this chapter, the reader should be able to

1. Discuss how the anatomy and physiology of the liver and pancreas affect interpretation of pertinent laboratory test results.
2. Discuss and interpret tests associated with the liver's synthetic ability.
3. Compare and contrast tests that facilitate assessment of cholestatic and hepatocellular diseases.
4. Explain how hepatic and other diseases, as well as drugs and analytical interferences, cause abnormal laboratory test results for bilirubin.
5. List diseases that may alter laboratory test results for ammonia.
6. Given a case study, describe important patterns of results from multiple tests used in diagnosing and monitoring hepatobiliary disorders.

7. Discuss temporal relationships of the appearance and magnitude of hepatitis markers.
8. Discuss the role of *Helicobacter pylori* in peptic ulcer disease and the tests used to diagnose it.
9. Discuss tests and procedures that are used to evaluate pseudomembranous and similar forms of colitis.
10. Given a case study, interpret laboratory test results for assessing the pancreas.

## ANATOMY AND PHYSIOLOGY OF LIVER AND PANCREAS

### Liver

The liver is the largest solid organ in the human body. Weighing between 1200 and 1500 g, it is located in the right upper quadrant of the abdomen.[1] The liver has two sources of blood supply:

- ➤ The hepatic artery, from the aorta, supplies arterial blood rich in oxygen.
- ➤ Portal veins shunt the venous outflow of the intestines and spleen—blood with less oxygen but rich in nutrients—to the liver.

The liver is divided into thousands of lobules (Figure 1, next page). Each lobule is composed of plates of hepatocytes (liver cells) that radiate from the central vein much like spokes in a wheel. Between the plates of liver cells are small bile canaliculi. The hepatocytes continually form and secrete bile into these canaliculi, which empty into terminal bile ducts. Subsequently, like tiny streams forming a river, these bile ducts empty into larger and larger ducts until they ultimately merge into the common duct. Bile then drains into either the gallbladder or the duodenum.

The liver is an extremely complex organ with many functions.[1] It produces bilirubin, a product of hemoglobin (Hgb) breakdown. Bilirubin is excreted via the bile ducts into the intestinal tract, where it plays a crucial role

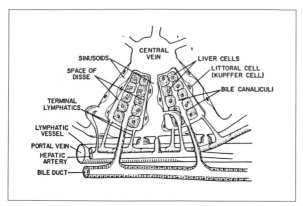

**FIGURE 1.** Basic structure of a liver lobule including the lymph flow system comprised of the spaces of Disse and interlobular lymphatics. (Reproduced, with permission, from Guyton AC. Medical physiology, 5th ed. Philadelphia, PA: W. B. Saunders; 1976.)

in digestion. Salts of bilirubin aid in making ingested fats more soluble to facilitate their absorption. The liver also plays a major role in amino acid and carbohydrate metabolism. It produces many crucial proteins, including coagulation factors and albumin. The liver breaks down some amino acids to yield urea, which is then excreted by the kidneys.

Most lipid and lipoprotein metabolism, including cholesterol synthesis, occurs in the liver. Hepatocytes synthesize cholesterol, which is then excreted into the bile. Therefore, cholesterol may be high in patients with cholestatic disorders and low in patients with cirrhosis or liver failure.

The liver is the primary location for most drug and hormone metabolism including barbiturates, certain tranquilizers, sex hormones, $H_2$-blockers, and many narcotics. Thus, in patients with liver failure, standard dosing of some medications can lead to dangerously high serum concentrations and toxicity.

With its double blood supply, large size, and critical role in regulating body metabolic pathways, the liver is affected by many systemic diseases. In addition, numerous illnesses affect primarily the liver. Fortunately, it has a tremendous reserve capacity and often can maintain its function in spite of significant disease. Furthermore, the liver is one of the few human organs capable of regeneration.

## Pancreas

The pancreas is an elongated gland located in the retroperitoneum. Its head lies in close proximity to the duodenum, and the pancreatic ducts empty into the duodenum. The pancreas has both exocrine glands, which secrete into the ducts, and endocrine glands, which secrete into the circulation.

The pancreatic exocrine glands produce primarily enzymes or proenzymes (enzymes requiring further break-

down in the duodenum) that aid in digestion. These enzymes include trypsin, chymotrypsin, lipase, and amylase. Insufficient enzyme production (i.e., pancreatic insufficiency) is associated with malabsorption of nutrients, leading to progressive weight loss and severe diarrhea.

The pancreatic endocrine glands produce many hormones including insulin and glucagon. Insufficient insulin production leads to diabetes mellitus (Chapter 12). Thus, the pancreas plays an important role in digestion and absorption of food as well as metabolism of sugar. Like the liver, the pancreas has a tremendous reserve capacity; over 90% glandular destruction is required before diabetes or pancreatic insufficiency develops.

Pancreatitis—inflammation of the pancreas—is the most common disease of this gland. Although the clinical presentation is often the same, pancreatitis can have many causes: gallstones, hypercalcemia, hyperlipidemia, medications, alcoholism, trauma, collagen vascular diseases, and penetrating duodenal ulcers.

## TESTS OF LIVER SYNTHETIC CAPABILITIES

The term *liver function test* (LFT) is overused. Most so-called LFTs really measure hepatic or biliary inflammation. Hepatic synthetic reserves are such that, even with massive inflammation, the liver may be able to perform its synthetic functions normally.

To determine the actual functional capabilities of the liver, its synthetic products must be measured. The human liver produces albumin, fibrinogen, prothrombin, haptoglobin, transferrin, and other proteins. The two factors most often used to assess liver function are albumin and prothrombin time (PT). Occasionally, total protein and globulin are measured with albumin. Additionally, an elevated ammonia may indicate liver failure, but the value of this test is controversial.

### Albumin
*Normal range: 3.5–5 g/dL or 35–50 g/L*

The liver synthesizes albumin using amino acids derived from either the gut or the breakdown of proteins. Albumin is responsible for maintaining plasma oncotic pressure, and it binds numerous hormones, anions, drugs, and fatty acids.[2] Normally, the liver synthesizes about 12 g of albumin daily, although it can double its albumin production if needed.

The normal serum half-life of albumin is about 20 days,[3] but this time can be shortened in hypermetabolic states. Because of albumin's long lifespan, serum albumin measurements are slow to fall after the onset of hepatic dysfunction. Complete cessation of albumin production results in only a 25% decrease in serum concentrations after 8 days.[1]

Because albumin reflects the liver's synthetic ability, its concentration may remain normal in many liver diseases when liver function is preserved. However, as the liver is progressively damaged and its synthetic capabilities are impaired (e.g., patients with severe hepatitis or cirrhosis), the albumin concentration progressively declines. Low concentrations (<2.5 g/dL) in liver disease are associated with a poor prognosis.

Some nonhepatic causes of hypoalbuminemia include malnutrition, malabsorption, overhydration, nephrotic syndrome (albumin is lost in the urine), protein-losing enteropathy (protein is lost through the gut), pregnancy, burns, and chronic illness. Thus, isolated hypoalbuminemia may not be caused by liver disease; clinicians must always consider other possibilities.

Hypoalbuminemia usually is not associated with specific symptoms or findings until concentrations become quite low. At very low concentrations (2–2.5 g/dL), patients can develop peripheral edema, ascites, or pulmonary edema. Low serum albumin allows hydrostatic pressure (e.g., blood pressure) to overcome oncotic pressure (pressure that holds fluid in the vasculature). Subsequently, fluid leaks from the intravascular to the interstitial spaces of subcutaneous tissues or to body cavities. Finally, low albumin concentrations affect the interpretation of total serum calcium and concentrations of drugs that are highly protein bound (e.g., phenytoin and salicylates) (Chapters 5 and 6).

Hyperalbuminemia is seen in patients with marked dehydration and is associated with concurrent elevations of blood urea nitrogen (BUN) and hematocrit (Hct). Patients taking anabolic steroids may demonstrate truly increased albumin concentrations, but those on heparin or ampicillin may have falsely elevated results with some assays. Hyperalbuminemia does not cause any symptoms or findings.

Depending on the assay methods used, albumin concentrations can be lowered in supine patients (≤0.15 g/dL), icteric patients, or patients on penicillin.[4]

## Prealbumin
*Normal range: 16–40 mg/dL*

Like albumin, prealbumin is also a protein synthesized by the liver. Although it is not often used to assess the liver's synthetic capability, it is quite useful for assessing a patient's nutritional status. Because prealbumin binds thyroxine ($T_4$), it is sometimes referred to as *thyroxine-binding prealbumin* or *transthyretin*. These terms are misleading, however, since most (75%) $T_4$ is bound to globulin (Chapter 12) and prealbumin is usually not an important factor in thyroid function. Prealbumin also binds to retinol-binding protein; then the dual carrier protein complexes with vitamin A, allowing the fat-soluble vitamin to circulate in the bloodstream.

Prealbumin has a much shorter half-life than albumin (2 versus 20 days), an attribute that makes it a sensitive marker of *acute* liver disease as well as of acute changes in nutritional status. It is routinely used to monitor patients receiving parenteral nutrition.[5] When malnourished patients are fed, prealbumin concentrations rise before albumin concentrations do. Optimal refeeding leads to increases of greater than 1 mg/dL/day. After maintenance rates of parenteral nutrition (or therapeutic enteral feedings) are reached, a goal for prealbumin concentrations in malnourished, hospitalized patients might be an increase of at least 3–5 mg/dL/week until 20 mg/dL is achieved along with a nonfluid weight gain of at least 1 kg/week. Concentrations of less than 10.7 mg/dL are associated with severe malnutrition; those between 10.7 and 16 mg/dL are associated with moderate malnutrition.

This test also is used in head trauma patients. Prealbumin is normally 2–7% of the protein found in cerebrospinal fluid (CSF), while albumin makes up 56–76% of CSF protein. The absolute prealbumin concentration in CSF is equal to that in serum. However, due to the relatively low concentrations of other proteins in CSF, prealbumin makes up a larger percentage of the protein there (12 times higher in CSF than in serum). In head trauma patients where one might question a CSF leak into the nasal passages, detection of prealbumin in nasal discharge is consistent with CSF rather than common nasal fluid.

In addition to malnutrition and acute liver disease, prealbumin is decreased in thyrotoxicosis, postsurgery, parturition, severe illness, and trauma. Finally, a variant form (one amino acid different) of prealbumin (commonly referred to as *transthyretin*) is one of the proteins that deposits in the extracellular spaces and causes certain forms of amyloidosis.[6]

## Globulin
*Normal range: 2–3 g/dL or 20–30 g/L*

Globulin refers to the total measurement of immunoglobulins in serum. Immunoglobulins are synthesized by B-cell lymphocytes located throughout the body. There are five immunoglobulin classes (IgA, IgD, IgE, IgG, and IgM), also referred to as antibodies.

Low globulin concentrations result from many causes including immunodeficiency syndromes, malabsorption, and protein-losing enteropathy. Because globulins are produced elsewhere in addition to the liver, hepatocellular dysfunction does not lower globulin concentrations unless associated with malabsorption or malnutrition.

Elevation of globulin concentrations is a sign of inflammation and may be present in hepatitis, especially in chronic viral or autoimmune hepatitis. Patients with chronic hepatitis may have a lower albumin concentration in association with elevated immunoglobulin. IgM concentrations may be elevated in primary biliary cirrhosis, and alcoholic patients can have markedly elevated IgA concentrations.

Nonhepatic causes of elevated globulin concentra-

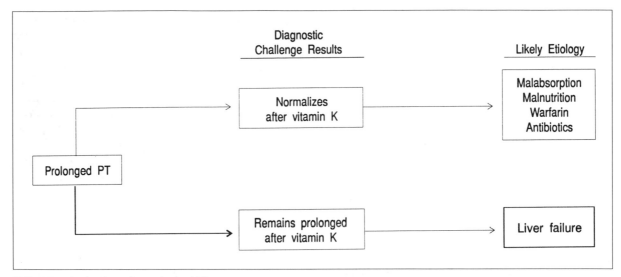

**FIGURE 2.** Evaluation of a prolonged PT.

tions include chronic infections, chronic inflammatory states, and some blood dyscrasias, including multiple myeloma. In these situations, globulin concentrations may exceed albumin concentrations; thus the albumin–globulin ratio is elevated to more than 1 (normally about 0.6).

(Detailed discussion of globulins is beyond the scope of this chapter, but Chapters 15 and 16 provide further information.)

## Total Protein
*Normal range: 5.5–9 g/dL or 55–90 g/L*

Total protein refers primarily to the sum of albumin and globulin, although many other important serum proteins exist. Any syndrome causing elevation of either albumin or globulin also increases total protein. The converse is also true. The value of obtaining a total protein concentration is limited if albumin and globulin results are already known.

(Discussion of all aspects of serum protein electrophoresis—the process that breaks down total protein into its various components—is not in this chapter.)

## Prothrombin Time
*Normal range: 10–13 sec*

The liver synthesizes six coagulation factors: I, II (prothrombin), V, VII, IX, and X. Because all of these factors are produced in excess of need and because the liver has tremendous synthetic reserves, only substantial hepatic impairment leads to decreased synthesis of these factors and subsequent clotting abnormalities.

Abnormalities of these clotting factors can be assessed either directly by their individual measurement or by tests (e.g., PT) involving the interrelationship of these factors. The activated partial thromboplastin time (aPTT) also may become prolonged in patients with severe liver dysfunction. (Chapter 15 contains a detailed discussion of

tests for blood coagulation.)

The prolongation of PT is not specific for liver disease. It can be seen in many situations including

> Inadequate vitamin K in the diet.
> Poor fat absorption (vitamin K is a fat-soluble vitamin).
> Poor or inadequate nutrition.
> Use of drugs such as warfarin, salicylates (high dose), and certain antibiotics (e.g., tetracyclines, moxalactam, cefoperazone, and cefamandole).

In these cases, the underlying cause of the PT elevation is not the liver's inadequate synthetic capability but rather a vitamin K deficiency; vitamin K catalyzes the synthesis of clotting factors II, VII, IX, and X. The prolonged PT with warfarin is due to its interference with vitamin K rather than insufficient intake or absorption. Tetracyclines may kill vitamin K-producing flora in the gut, and beta-lactam antibiotics (by virtue of their *N*-methylthiotetrazole side chain) may inhibit the enzymatic reactions that require vitamin K in the activation of clotting factor precursors to prothrombin. A prolonged PT also can be seen in certain diseases, usually collagen vascular [e.g., systemic lupus erythematosus (SLE) (Chapter 16)], where anticoagulants are circulating.

Clinically, the approach to an elevated PT of uncertain etiology is to provide vitamin K (10 mg) subcutaneously, intramuscularly (IM), or intravenously (IV) (Figure 2). When the PT is prolonged due to malabsorption, warfarin, or a lack of vitamin K, it usually returns to normal within 24 hr. Paradoxically, large doses of vitamin K (50 mg) may be associated with a PT prolongation, but the mechanism is not understood. If the PT remains prolonged despite parenteral vitamin K, it is considered a sign of substantial hepatic dysfunction and, as with hypoalbuminemia, of extensive liver damage with a poor

## Minicase 1

A 50-year-old woman, J. M., presented to her physician complaining of increasing fatigue and a 20-lb weight loss over the past 4 months. Initial evaluation showed an albumin of 2 g/dL (3.5–5 g/dL) and a PT of 18 sec (10–13 sec). J. M. was referred for evaluation of possible cirrhosis. On further questioning, she denied any history of hepatitis, exposure to hepatotoxins, alcohol use, family history of liver disease, and liver disease.

The patient's physical examination did not suggest liver disease; there was no evidence of ascites, palmar erythema, asterixis, hepatomegaly, splenomegaly, or spider angiomata. It was noted that she had pedal edema. Liver function studies were otherwise normal: alanine aminotransferase (ALT), 12 IU/L (3–30 IU/L); aspartate aminotransferase (AST), 20 IU/L (8–42 IU/L); total bilirubin, 1 mg/dL (0.3–1.0 mg/dL); and alkaline phosphatase (ALP), 56 IU/L.

An IM dose of vitamin K 10 mg corrected the PT (12 sec) within 48 hr. Workup showed that J. M. had malabsorption due to sprue, a disease of the small bowel. With proper dietary management, her symptoms resolved and she gained weight. At a followup visit 3 weeks later, her albumin concentration was 3.7 g/dL and her edema had resolved.

*Why did this patient develop a low albumin and a prolonged PT? What caused her pedal edema?*

**Discussion:** This case demonstrates that while low albumin and a prolonged PT suggest advanced liver disease, other causes need to be considered. Administration of vitamin K promptly corrected J. M.'s PT, suggesting malabsorption of vitamin K. If she had had cirrhosis, her PT would not have corrected with the vitamin K. Similarly, her hypoalbuminemia was not due to her liver's inability to synthesize albumin but to the malabsorptive disorder that was interfering with protein absorption. Therefore, J. M. had a low albumin and elevated PT in the absence of liver disease. Her pedal edema was due to hypoalbuminemia secondary to malabsorption.

prognosis.[2] Moreover, administration of parenteral vitamin K 10 mg does not correct a prolonged PT caused by severe liver dysfunction.

In the management of hepatic dysfunction, the PT also allows assessment of the patient's tendency to bleed before surgical or diagnostic procedures. Bleeding is a dramatic complication of hepatic failure. When the PT is elevated, bleeding may be controlled or at least diminished by fresh frozen plasma, which contains the needed clotting factors and often corrects the PT temporarily.

A prolonged PT in a patient with hepatic failure who is not bleeding generally does not require treatment with fresh frozen plasma. Instead, it is reasonable to try vitamin K in the hope that malnutrition may be a contributing factor (Minicase 1).

## TESTS TO ASSESS CHOLESTATIC DISEASE AND HEPATOCELLULAR INJURY

Liver diseases tend to fall into two broad categories: cholestatic and hepatocellular. In cholestatic diseases, there is primary interference with the metabolism or secretion of bilirubin, anywhere from its initial production in the hepatocytes to its secretion into the duodenum. Therefore, cholestasis is defined as the failure of normal amounts of bile to reach the duodenum.

In hepatocellular diseases, the hepatocytes are inflamed or damaged. Examples include viral and drug-induced hepatitis. However, these two categories often overlap. For example, patients with cirrhosis can have elements of both hepatocellular and cholestatic processes.

### Cholestatic Liver Disease

Clinically, in cholestatic liver disease, there is an accumulation of substances normally excreted by the liver into the bile. This accumulation can result in jaundice (from bilirubin), pruritis (from bile salts), or xanthomas (from lipid deposits in skin). Weight loss can be caused by anorexia and difficulty with intestinal absorption of nutrients (predominantly fat and the fat-soluble vitamins A, D, E, and K), partly due to a lack of bile salts. Other manifestations include (1) osteomalacia secondary to failure to absorb vitamin D and (2) PT elevation due to either intrinsic liver disease or failure to absorb vitamin K.

Cholestatic syndromes may be subclassified as either[7]

> ➤ Intrahepatic—the problem is in the liver cells or the bile ducts *within* the liver.
> ➤ Extrahepatic—the obstruction is in the major bile ducts *outside* the liver.

### *Intrahepatic Cholestasis*

Intrahepatic cholestasis can be seen in patients with viral hepatitis (especially type A), alcoholic hepatitis, or acquired immunodeficiency syndrome (AIDS). Certain drugs can cause cholestatic jaundice (Table 1). Cholestasis also occurs in patients with severe bacterial infections or those receiving parenteral hyperalimentation. Other causes are liver diseases such as primary biliary cirrhosis, sclerosing cholangitis, cholangiocarcinoma, benign recurrent cholestasis, and cholestasis of pregnancy. Cirrhosis also can present with a cholestatic picture.

**TABLE 1.** Drugs that May Cause Intrahepatic Cholestasis

| | |
| --- | --- |
| Chlorpropamide | Niacin |
| Erythromycin | Penicillamine |
| Estrogens | Phenothiazines |
| Gold salts | Sulfa drugs |
| Methyltestosterone | |

### *Extrahepatic Cholestasis*

Extrahepatic cholestasis involves obstruction of the large bile ducts outside of the liver, a situation previously only remediable with surgery. Causes include obstruction by strictures (after surgery), stones, or tumors (of pancreas, ampulla of Vater, duodenum, or bile ducts). Other causes include sclerosing cholangitis, a disease causing diffuse inflammation of the bile ducts, often both intrahepatic and extrahepatic. Although previously referred to as "surgical cholestasis," extrahepatic cholestasis can now often be treated (or at least palliated) using endoscopic means (e.g., dilation of strictures).

## Tests Associated with Cholestasis

Laboratory tests do not distinguish between intra- and extrahepatic cholestasis. This distinction is usually made clinically (assessment of a history of drug use, hepatitis exposure, etc.) or radiographically. In most instances of extrahepatic cholestasis, a "damming" effect on the bile ducts above the obstruction causes their progressive dilation. This condition can be demonstrated with either computed tomography (CT) scanning or ultrasound. Occasionally, contrast dye is injected into the ducts to demonstrate the dilation and to determine the etiology of the obstruction. This dye can be injected either through the liver, as with a percutaneous cholangiogram, or through the bile ducts, as with an endoscopic retrograde cholangiogram.

The laboratory tests most often used to diagnose and monitor cholestatic diseases include alkaline phosphatase (ALP), 5′-nucleotidase, and γ-glutamyl transpeptidase (GGTP). Other tests that may be abnormal in this situation but will not be reviewed here include serum cholesterol (Chapter 13), bile acid levels, leucine aminopeptidase, and hepatic copper levels.

### *Alkaline Phosphatase*
*Normal range: varies with assay*

ALP refers to a group of enzymes whose exact function remains unknown. These enzymes are found in many body tissues including the liver, bone, small intestine, kidneys, placenta, and leukocytes. In adults, most serum ALP activity comes from liver and bone. The serum half-life

of ALP is 7 days.[7] Normal values are not listed because each different assay—about seven—has its own range. Normal ranges should be obtained from the laboratory performing the test.

Normal ALP concentrations vary primarily with age. In children and adolescents, an elevated ALP concentration results from osteoblasts of developing bone. Similarly, the increase during late pregnancy is related to placental ALP.[8,9] In the third trimester, concentrations can double, making interpretation problematic. Additionally, concentrations can be elevated for 3 weeks postpartum. In adults younger than 50 years, ALP tends to be higher in males than females, but this difference evens out between 60 and 70 (Chapter 1).

In patients with liver disease, the mechanism of ALP elevation is not yet clear. ALP is a component of the cell cannicular membrane, and bile retention appears to induce hepatocyte synthesis of it.[10] With biliary obstruction, ALP is regurgitated into the serum rather than excreted into the bile. ALP concentrations persist until the obstruction is removed and then, consistent with a serum half-life of 7 days, they return to normal within 2–4 weeks.

Clinically, ALP elevation is associated with cholestatic disorders and, as mentioned previously, does not help to distinguish between intra- and extrahepatic disorders. Approximately 75% of patients with primarily cholestatic disorders have ALP concentrations more than four times normal (Table 2). ALP elevations are typical in any infiltrative process involving the liver including granulomatous diseases, amyloidosis, neoplasia, and abscesses. Concentrations of three times normal or less are nonspecific and can occur in all types of liver disease. Even at the highest concentrations seen in the serum, ALP has no toxicological activity. Therefore, elevated concentrations per se do not *cause* symptoms—they only reflect tissue damage.

When faced with an elevated ALP concentration, a clinician must determine whether it is coming from the liver. One approach is to fractionate the ALP isoenzymes, but this method is expensive and often time consuming. Two other tests can serve the same purpose. If ALP is elevated, an elevated 5′-nucleotidase or GGTP indicates that the source is primarily hepatic (e.g., intra- or extrahepatic cholestatic syndromes). With normal 5′-nucle-

**TABLE 2.** Initial Evaluation of Elevated ALP Concentrations in Context of Other Test Results

| ALP | GGTP | Aminotransferases (ALT and AST) | Differential Diagnosis |
|---|---|---|---|
| Mildly elevated | Within normal limits | Within normal limits | Pregnancy; nonhepatic causes (Table 3) |
| Moderately elevated[a] | Markedly elevated | Within normal limits or minimally elevated | Cholestatic syndromes |
| Mildly elevated[b] | Mildly elevated | Markedly elevated | Hepatocellular disease |

[a]Usually greater than four times normal limits.
[b]Usually less than four times normal limits.

**TABLE 3.** Some Nonhepatic Causes of Elevated ALP

| Bone Disorders | Other Disorders and Drugs |
| --- | --- |
| Healing fractures | Acromegaly |
| Osteomalacia | Anticonvulsant drugs (e.g., phenytoin and phenobarbital) |
| Paget's disease | |
| Rickets | Hyperthyroidism |
| Tumors | Lithium (bone isoenzymes) |
| | Neoplasia |
| | Oral contraceptives |
| | Sepsis |

otidase or GGTP, one must search for a nonhepatic cause.

Some nonhepatic causes of an elevated ALP are listed in Table 3 and discussed in Minicase 2. Mild elevations (usually <1.5 times normal) can be seen in "normal" patients. Some families have inherited elevated concentrations (two to four times normal), usually as an autosomal dominant trait.[11] Markedly elevated concentrations (greater than four times normal) are generally seen only in cholestasis or Paget's disease.

ALP concentrations can be lowered by vitamin D intoxication, scurvy, hypothyroidism, milk-alkali syndrome, and hypophosphatasia. ALP concentrations can be falsely elevated in patients whose blood is drawn 2–4 hr after a fatty meal, due to a rise in intestinal ALP, or with prolonged (>1 day) storage of serum at room temperature.

### 5'-Nucleotidase
*Normal range: varies*

Although 5'-nucleotidase is found in many tissues, including liver, brain, heart, and blood vessels, serum 5'-nucleotidase is elevated only in hepatic diseases. Because 5'-nucleotidase is not elevated in bone disorders, it is useful when distinguishing between hepatic and skeletal causes of an elevated ALP. Usually, an elevated ALP with a normal 5'-nucleotidase is not associated with liver disease.

### γ-Glutamyl Transpeptidase
*Normal range: varies*

Like 5'-nucleotidase, GGTP, a biliary excretory enzyme, can help sort out the etiology of an elevated ALP. Because GGTP has no origin in bone or placenta, it is not elevated in disorders of these tissues. An elevated ALP associated with a normal GGTP points to a nonhepatic etiology (Table 2). As mentioned previously, ALP concentrations may be normally elevated in pregnant or young patients, especially during growth spurts. An elevated GGTP (or 5'-nucleotidase) in such patients may point to underlying hepatobiliary disease.

GGTP concentrations are usually markedly elevated in patients with alcoholic liver disease, whether or not they are drinking when tested. Therefore, this test is po-

tentially useful in screening for this disease. A GGTP/ALP ratio greater than 2.5 may be highly indicative of alcohol abuse.[12] With abstinence, GGTP concentrations often decrease by 50% within 2 weeks. GGTP also can be elevated in pancreatic diseases, myocardial infarction, severe chronic obstructive pulmonary diseases, some renal diseases, and diabetes. In these situations, elevations are usually mild and ALP tends to be normal. GGTP elevations also have been reported in patients with SLE.

GGTP can be confoundingly elevated in patients on phenytoin, phenobarbital, carbamazepine, tricyclic antidepressants, benzodiazepines, warfarin, or other enzyme inducers; these drugs increase production of GGTP and other "liver" enzymes. In such situations, therefore, elevation of GGTP does not necessarily imply liver injury when 5'-nucleotidase is normal. Another drug, acetaminophen, has been reported to increase GGTP; however, this increase occurs only at toxic concentrations and reflects real liver injury.

### Minicase 2

When presenting for a routine school physical, A. S., a 16-year-old girl, was found by her pediatrician to be slightly jaundiced. She denied any history of liver disease, abdominal pain, alcohol use, and abdominal trauma. Lab evaluation showed a moderately elevated bilirubin of 2.3 mg/dL (0.3–1.0 mg/dL) along with ALP and GGTP concentrations of about four times normal. Her AST was 23 IU/L (8–42 IU/L).

A. S. denied being on any medications (except for vitamins), taking illicit drugs, and being exposed to toxins. Nothing suggested the possibility of a neoplastic or infectious process [temperature of 98.9 °F (37.2 °C) and white blood cell (WBC) count of 7.5 × 10³ cells/mm³ (4.8–10.8 × 10³ cells/mm³)]. Ultrasound of the liver and biliary system was normal, with no evidence of biliary dilation.

The patient's parents then took her to a pediatric hepatologist. After much discussion (and threat of a liver biopsy), A. S. tearfully revealed that she had gone to a local family planning clinic and was using birth control pills.

*How might oral contraceptives cause a cholestatic picture? What was the importance of the ultrasound? What is the usual outcome of patients who develop jaundice while taking oral contraceptives?*

**Discussion:** This case demonstrates that oral contraceptives, primarily because of their estrogen content, can cause alterations in cholestatic test results (manifested by an elevated bilirubin, GGTP, and ALP) with relatively normal aminotransferases. The ultrasound helped to distinguish between intra- and extrahepatic cholestasis. The absence of biliary dilation suggested intrahepatic cholestasis. The normal AST suggested that jaundice was not due to hepatitis.

Cholestasis from oral contraceptives is generally benign and reverses promptly when the medication is withdrawn. Patients often omit mentioning their use of birth control pills.

## Hepatocellular Injury

The aminotransferases and lactate dehydrogenase (LDH) are used to assess hepatocellular inflammation or injury (hepatitis). Although elevations of these enzymes usually lead to a diagnosis of hepatitis, they do not reliably correlate with the degree of inflammation, type of hepatitis, or prognosis. In most forms of hepatic injury, the prognosis is best related to albumin concentrations and PT.

There are multiple causes of hepatitis. One common type is viral hepatitis, which is classified A, B, C, D (delta hepatitis), or E, based on the causative virus. These viruses, and the tests for them, are discussed in detail in the Viral Hepatitis section. Other forms of viral hepatitis may be caused by the Epstein-Barr virus as well as cytomegalovirus.

Hepatitis also may be caused by various medications, and such drug-induced hepatitis can be either acute or chronic.[13] Some drugs commonly implicated in cellular hepatotoxicity are listed in Table 4. In addition, elevation of aminotransferases has been reported in patients receiving heparin.[14] ALT is elevated in up to 60% of these patients, with a mean maximal value of 3.6 times the baseline. However, virtually every drug can potentially cause hepatic injury. Moreover, drugs extensively metabolized by the liver are particularly likely to cause these problems. Although numerous drugs may result in aminotransferase elevations, such elevations are usually minor, not associated with any symptoms, transient, and of no clinical consequence.[15]

Some other causes of hepatic inflammation are listed in Table 5.

It is often difficult to determine the exact etiology of hepatic inflammation (hepatitis). A careful history, especially for exposure to drugs, alcohol, or toxins, and a detailed physical examination are crucial. Additional laboratory studies are usually necessary to distinguish one form of hepatitis from another. Radiological testing or liver biopsy may be indicated.

Aminotransferases and LDH, therefore, serve prin-

**TABLE 4.** Drugs Noted for Causing Hepatocellular Injury[a]

| | |
|---|---|
| Acetaminophen | Ketoconazole |
| Allopurinol | Lovastatin |
| Amiodarone | Methotrexate |
| Cisplatin | Methyldopa |
| Dapsone | NSAIDs[b] |
| Ethionamide | Phenothiazines |
| Etretinate | Plicamycin |
| Halothane | Valproic acid |
| Isoniazid | |

[a]*Hepatocellular injury is reflected by increased ALT, AST, and LDH. In severe cases, jaundice and hepatic failure may ensue.*
[b]*NSAIDs = nonsteroidal anti-inflammatory drugs. Diclofenac has the highest incidence (4%) of significant elevations.*

**TABLE 5.** Some Nondrug Causes of Hepatic Inflammation

| |
|---|
| Alcoholic liver disease |
| Congestive heart failure |
| Hypotension |
| Iron overload—hemochromatosis |
| Liver infections |
| Wilson's disease |

cipally as an indication of hepatic inflammation, although they may be somewhat elevated in patients with cholestatic syndromes (Table 2). These tests do not indicate the etiology or severity of the inflammation. Since these enzymes do not have any inherent toxicological activity, they do not cause signs or symptoms. Their increased serum concentrations only reflect a prior insult to tissue where they reside. Figure 3 is an algorithm for the differential diagnosis of suspected hepatitis.

## Tests Associated with Hepatocellular Injury

### Aminotransferases (AST and ALT)

The aminotransferases, formerly called transaminases, are the most frequently measured indicators of hepatic disease. Both AST (also called SGOT) and ALT (also called SGPT) are very sensitive indicators of hepatic inflammation and necrosis. Damage to liver cells, with subsequent disruption of their plasma membranes, allows these enzymes to "leak" into the systemic circulation.[16]

Markedly elevated concentrations (>1000 IU/L) are usually associated with acute viral hepatitis, severe drug or toxic reactions, or ischemic hepatitis. Very high concentrations, however, may or may not indicate a greater level of necrosis. Furthermore, high concentrations do not correlate with a poor prognosis, nor do low concentrations necessarily correlate with a good one. In some patients on drugs such as methotrexate, complete hepatic failure can develop despite minimally elevated aminotransferase concentrations.

These tests are primarily elevated in hepatocellular liver disease; in cholestatic syndromes (Tests Associated with Cholestasis section), they may be normal or minimally elevated. Additionally, unexplained false positives often occur. In one study, an isolated aminotransferase concentration found on a screening chemistry profile had an 84% chance of being falsely elevated since repeat studies showed normal concentrations.[17]

Generally, prior to a workup for mildly elevated aminotransferases, a practitioner should see either elevation of more than one test (i.e., both AST and ALT) or repeated elevations of a single test. Serum concentrations of aminotransferases follow a diurnal pattern, with the peak at around 4 p.m. and the valley at around 8 a.m. The magnitude of this variation, however, is only about 10–15% from the daily mean.[18]

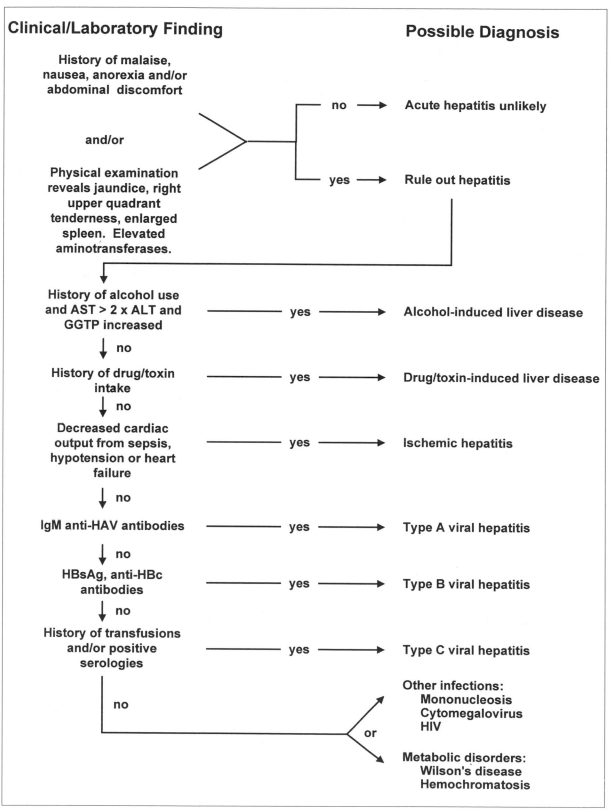

**FIGURE 3.** Algorithm for differential diagnosis of suspected hepatitis.

*Aspartate aminotransferase (normal range: 8–42 IU/L for adults but varies with assay)*. AST, an intracellular enzyme, is found primarily in the liver, cardiac muscle, kidneys, brain, pancreas, and lungs. Concentrations may be elevated in myocardial infarction (usually peaking after about 24 hr; Chapter 10), musculoskeletal diseases (including muscular dystrophy, dermatomyositis, trichinosis, and gangrene), intestinal injury, hypothyroidism, hemolysis, pericarditis, renal infarction, pulmonary embolus, and necrotic tumors.

Patients on levodopa, methyldopa, tolbutamide, *p*-aminosalicylic acid,[19] or erythromycin may have falsely elevated concentrations of AST because these drugs interfere with some assays.[4] These false elevations also may be seen in patients with diabetic ketoacidosis when the automated chemistry profile SMA 12/60 is used.

Furthermore, calcium dust in the air (caused by construction) can interfere with laboratory assays for this enzyme. Hyperlipidemia and hemolysis also can interfere in vitro. AST concentrations can be suppressed in patients with uremia.[20] Metronidazole and trifluoperazine can lower AST in vivo, as can vitamin $B_6$ deficiency.[4]

*Alanine aminotransferase (normal range: 3–30 IU/L for adults but varies with assay)*. High concentrations of ALT, another intracellular enzyme, are found primarily in the liver. Therefore, ALT is much more specific for hepatocellular disease than is AST. However, ALT can be elevated in patients with muscular disease, myocardial injury, and renal infarction; it can be falsely elevated by hemolyzed serum.

The ratio of AST to ALT is of value in diagnosing alcoholic liver disease. Both numbers are usually under 300, but AST generally is at least twice the amount of ALT in alcoholic liver disease.[21] This condition is also suggested by elevated GGTP and mean cell volume (MCV) values in the absence of folic acid or vitamin $B_{12}$ deficiency (Chapter 14) (Minicase 3). There are no important causes of a low ALT, although concentrations can be suppressed in patients deficient in vitamin $B_6$.

### Lactate Dehydrogenase
*Normal range: 100–225 IU/L for adults but varies with assay*

LDH is found in most human tissues but primarily in myocardium, liver, skeletal muscle, brain, kidneys, and red blood cells (RBCs). An elevated LDH can be seen in a patient with myocardial infarction (Chapter 10), myocarditis, hemolysis (including in vitro), renal infarction, untreated pernicious anemia, malignancy, muscle disease, burns, trauma, or pulmonary embolus. Markedly elevated LDH concentrations also occur in patients who are reabsorbing extravasated blood (e.g., after trauma). Therefore, an elevated LDH is not a very specific finding. Fortunately, however, LDH has five isoenzymes; type 5 ($LDH_5$) corresponds with liver disease (Table 6).

Although $LDH_5$ is less sensitive to liver disease than the aminotransferases, elevated concentrations occur in patients with hepatitis, biliary obstruction, metastatic liver disease, or exacerbation of cirrhosis. In some situations, $LDH_5$ can be elevated when total LDH is normal. According to some clinicians, an $LDH_5$ concentration significantly greater than $LDH_4$ is suggestive of primary or secondary liver disease.

There are no important causes of a truly low LDH; however, vitamin C at therapeutically attainable concentrations may falsely lower LDH concentrations in vitro.

(LDH is discussed from the cardiac perspective in Chapter 10.)

---

### ✎ Minicase 3

A 36-year-old executive, D. D., was referred to a prominent medical center for a second opinion. Her physician had found an elevated AST of 180 IU/L (8–42 IU/L) on a routine screening exam. D. D. had no symptoms; her physical examination had been normal, without any signs of liver disease or hepatomegaly.

Additional studies showed an ALT of 60 IU/L (3–30 IU/L), a markedly elevated GGTP of 380 IU/L (<60 IU/L), and a minimally elevated ALP of 91 IU/L (26–88 IU/L). The patient's WBC count was elevated at $20 \times 10^3$ cells/$mm^3$ ($4.8$–$10.8 \times 10^3$ cells/$mm^3$). After much discussion, she revealed that she was drinking 1 pint of vodka a day.

D. D. then enrolled in Alcoholics Anonymous and stopped drinking. Three months later, all of her tests were normal: ALT, 28 IU/L; GGTP, 54 IU/L; and ALP, 54 IU/L.

*What findings suggested alcoholic liver disease? Why did all of D. D.'s numbers return to normal? What else might have happened in this situation?*

**Discussion:** This case demonstrates several aspects of alcoholic liver disease. The diagnosis was suggested by an elevated AST out of proportion to the ALT, as well as by a markedly elevated GGTP with a normal (or virtually so) ALP. An elevated MCV, if present, also would have supported this diagnosis. Patients with alcoholic liver disease may have markedly elevated WBC counts.

Alcoholic liver disease tends to have several different stages. The earliest manifestation may be just a "fatty liver," which is generally reversible with cessation of alcohol intake. Alcoholic hepatitis and cirrhosis can follow with excessive alcohol intake. Unfortunately, alcoholic cirrhosis can develop without any warning signs. If D. D. had alcoholic cirrhosis, stopping alcohol consumption probably would not have significantly altered her abnormal test results.

Clinicians should remember that a patient does not need to be a "skid row" alcoholic to develop alcoholic cirrhosis. Women are more susceptible to the hepatotoxic effects of alcohol than are men, and as few as two or three drinks a day can cause significant liver disease in susceptible persons.

**TABLE 6.** Isoenzymes of LDH

| Isoenzyme | Tissue with Increased Amount of Enzyme[a] | Typical Percentage of Total LDH in Adult | Typical Reference Range (IU/L) |
|---|---|---|---|
| LDH$_1$ | Heart, brain, RBCs | 33 | 22–85 |
| LDH$_2$ | Heart, brain, RBCs | 45 | 30–100 |
| LDH$_3$ | Brain, kidneys, lungs | 18 | 15–65 |
| LDH$_4$ | Liver, muscle, kidneys | 3 | 5–25 |
| LDH$_5$ | Liver, muscle, ileum | 1 | 2–25 |

[a]*These tissues are richest in the indicated enzymes. However, significant amounts of LDH$_1$ also are found in the renal cortex; LDH$_3$ also is found in the lymphocytes, spleen, and pancreas.*

## BILIRUBIN METABOLISM

Upon reaching senescence, RBCs are taken up and destroyed primarily in the spleen. Every day, about 1% of the circulating RBCs (about 50 mL of blood) is destroyed in this fashion. The Hgb released from these cells is ultimately broken down to bilirubin. Approximately 6 g of Hgb is broken down daily,[22] and 250 mg of bilirubin is formed. This conversion occurs primarily at the site of the RBC destruction and yields unconjugated bilirubin (water insoluble). This bilirubin is bound to albumin while being transported to the liver. Unconjugated bilirubin is taken up by the liver and conjugated with glucuronic acid.

Conjugated bilirubin (water soluble) is excreted into the bile and, ultimately, the gut. There it is broken down to urobilinogen, and some is reabsorbed and excreted again by the liver into the gut or excreted by the kidneys. The remaining conjugated bilirubin is excreted in feces. With liver damage, urinary urobilinogen may increase; with obstruction, it is usually absent or reduced.[23]

### Total Bilirubin
*Normal range: 0.3–1.0 mg/dL or 5–17 µmol/L but varies with assay and age*

The sum of conjugated and unconjugated bilirubin equals total bilirubin. Unconjugated and conjugated bilirubin are also referred to as *indirect* and *direct* bilirubin, respectively. These terms are based on the original van den Bergh reaction. This test is still used in many clinical chemistry laboratories to determine serum bilirubin concentrations. As mentioned, direct bilirubin gives an approximate estimate of conjugated or water-soluble bilirubin. Indirect bilirubin gives an estimate of unconjugated or water-insoluble bilirubin.

The van den Bergh method does not accurately reflect the true values of direct and indirect bilirubin, especially at low total serum bilirubin concentrations. It tends to overestimate the conjugated bilirubin actually in serum. More accurate concentrations require liquid chromatography, which shows that almost 100% of serum bilirubin is unconjugated in normal individuals.

An elevated total serum bilirubin concentration is not a sensitive indicator of the hepatic dysfunction or prognosis. Furthermore, an elevated bilirubin can be seen in conditions other than liver disease (e.g., hemolysis and ineffective RBC production). Concentrations may double with anorexia or fasting for 36 hr or more. In addition, biliary obstruction is associated with increases in bilirubin and ALP out of proportion to, and greater than, the aminotransferases.

In vitro elevations also can occur. In chronic renal failure without dialysis, a propranolol metabolite accumulates and spuriously elevates bilirubin by up to 2–3 mg/dL in two automated methods.[24] False elevations also occur with certain automated methods in some patients taking levodopa, phenelzine, methyldopa, nitrofurantoin, or ascorbic acid.[4] Likewise, some bilirubin assays generate spuriously high or low results in patients receiving IV methotrexate.[4] Finally, if specimens are exposed to bright daylight, bilirubin may decrease by as much as 30%/hr.[4]

The hallmark of hyperbilirubinemia is jaundice, icterus, or a yellowish skin color. Although quinine derivatives (e.g., quinacrine) and carotenes can cause a similar skin discoloration, the sclerae of the eyes remain their normal white color; in jaundice, the sclerae may also turn yellow.

Jaundice usually becomes visible when the total bilirubin concentration is 2–4 mg/dL. Low concentrations are often missed in clinical settings with artificial light because they are best observed in natural light. Urine may turn quite dark, almost brown, as excess conjugated bilirubin is excreted by the kidneys. Elevated bilirubin concentrations (generally >15 mg/dL) may be associated with intense itching, probably related to the elevation in bile salts seen in the same conditions.

In infants, elevated concentrations of unconjugated bilirubin (often >20 mg/dL) can lead to bilirubin encephalopathy or kernicterus. Kernicterus can present as lethargy and low grade fevers but progress to spasticity, seizures, and death if untreated. Survivors may develop mental retardation and spastic paraplegia. In adults, bilirubin has no known inherent physiological or toxicological activity.

## Unconjugated/Indirect Bilirubin

*Normal range: 0.2–0.7 mg/dL or 3.4–12 μmol/L*

Because there are no important causes of low unconjugated bilirubin concentrations, further discussion concerns hyperbilirubinemia. Patients with primarily (>85%) unconjugated hyperbilirubinemia often have no signs or symptoms of liver disease and have normal aminotransaminase concentrations. These patients have one of four conditions, as discussed below.

### Hemolysis

Hemolysis results in increased destruction of RBCs with a consequent increase in bilirubin production, occasionally exceeding the liver's ability to conjugate it. Generally, bilirubin is 85% unconjugated in pure hemolysis. For example, total bilirubin could be 2.8 mg/dL with an indirect bilirubin of 2.5 mg/dL and a direct bilirubin of 0.3 mg/dL. Bilirubin rarely exceeds 4 mg/dL in hemolysis.

Patients with large hematomas or transfusions of old blood may have similar values. Additionally, a picture similar to hemolysis can be seen in patients with pernicious anemia or other conditions of ineffective erythropoiesis such as myelofibrosis and metastatic replacement of bone marrow. (Chapter 14 presents more information on the evaluation of hemolysis.)

### Gilbert's Syndrome

This syndrome is an inherited, entirely benign trait that may be present in 5% of the population. It involves intermittent (increased with fasting, stress, or illness) elevation of unconjugated bilirubin (rarely >4 mg/dL) (Minicase 4).

### Crigler–Najjar Syndrome

This syndrome is a rare congenital disease—conjugating enzymes are missing or markedly deficient. Infants with this disease rapidly develop a deep jaundice (bilirubin >20 mg/dL) and can suffer brain damage (kernicterus). Some patients can be treated with phenobarbital; it dramatically lowers bilirubin concentrations, probably due to induction of the enzyme glucuronyl transferase.

### Neonatal Jaundice

The onset of jaundice, usually 2–5 days after birth, is both common and generally benign. It is associated with a temporary lack of liver enzymes (glucuronyl transferase) that conjugate bilirubin. In some instances, neonatal jaundice requires phototherapy to reduce bilirubin concentrations. As discussed previously, elevated concentrations of unconjugated bilirubin in neonates can lead to kernicterus.

## Conjugated/Direct Bilirubin

*Normal range: 0.1–0.3 mg/dL or 1.7–5 μmol/L*

Although rare congenital disorders can present with primarily conjugated hyperbilirubinemia (Dubin–Johnson and Rotor's syndromes), conjugated hyperbilirubinemia is generally associated with elevation in other hepatic enzymes and, as such, reflects underlying hepatic disease. The level of bilirubin elevation has no value in discriminating intrahepatic cholestasis from extrahepatic obstruction. Therefore, the practitioner must always also evaluate the concentrations of ALT, AST, ALP, and GGTP to decide whether the problem is mostly hepatocellular or cholestatic.

Hyperbilirubinemia associated primarily with aminotransferase elevation is generally due to hepatitis or cirrhosis. Hyperbilirubinemia associated with marked elevation in ALP and GGTP suggests a cholestatic disorder (Table 7). Unlike the benign causes of hyperbilirubinemia already described, bilirubin concentrations can exceed 20 mg/dL in these disorders. Generally, the degree of bilirubin elevation does not correlate with the prognosis. The exceptions (when it does correlate with ultimate outcome) include alcoholic liver disease, primary biliary cirrhosis, and halothane toxicity.

**TABLE 7.** Evaluation of Elevated Bilirubin Concentrations in Context of Other Test Results

| Total Bilirubin | Direct Bilirubin | Indirect Bilirubin | ALT, AST, GGTP | Differential Diagnosis |
|---|---|---|---|---|
| Moderately elevated | Within normal limits or low | Moderately elevated | Within normal limits | Hemolysis,[a] Gilbert's syndrome,[a] Crigler–Najjar syndrome,[b] neonatal jaundice |
| Moderately elevated | Moderately elevated | Within normal limits | Within normal limits | Cogenital syndrome:[c] Dubin–Johnson[d] Rotor's |
| Mildly elevated | Mildly elevated | Moderately elevated | Moderately elevated | Liver disease |

[a]*Usually indirect bilirubin is less than 4 mg/dL but may increase to 18 mg/dL.*
[b]*Usually indirect bilirubin is greater than 12 mg/dL and may go as high as 45 mg/dL.*
[c]*These syndromes are distinguished in the laboratory by liver biopsy.*
[d]*Usually direct bilirubin is 3–10 mg/dL.*

---

**✎ Minicase 4**

A 19-year-old college student, J. N., anxiously reported to the infirmary when his girlfriend noticed that he was becoming yellow. He felt well and had a normal physical examination. On discussion, he indicated that he had recently embarked on a rigorous crash diet in anticipation of winter break in Florida.

Evaluation showed an elevated total bilirubin of 4.8 mg/dL (0.3–1.0 mg/dL), of which 90% was unconjugated (4.3 mg/dL). The absence of hemolysis was established by microscopic examination of a blood smear, normal reticulocyte count, and LDH, which was 112 IU/L (100–225 IU/L). J. N.'s other LFTs were normal: ALT, 21 IU/L (3–30 IU/L); and ALP, 76 IU/L (21–91 IU/L).

*What was the most likely cause of this young man's signs and symptoms? How should his condition be managed? What is his prognosis?*

**Discussion:** Elevated bilirubin concentrations do not necessarily indicate severe liver disease. The normal ALT and ALP ruled out hepatocellular and cholestatic liver diseases. AST, if done, would have been normal. The normal LDH, RBC microscopic exam, and reticulocyte count ruled out hemolysis (Chapter 14) as a cause of the elevated bilirubin. The normal LDH was also consistent with a lack of intrinsic liver disease.

J. N. should be reassured that he has Gilbert's syndrome and might become somewhat jaundiced with fasting or acute or chronic illness. Gilbert's disease is not associated with any symptoms, is totally benign, and requires no treatment. When a patient has an elevated bilirubin, a practitioner should always obtain LFTs before either providing a diagnosis or performing unnecessary tests.

---

## AMMONIA

*Normal range: 30–70 µg/dL or 17–41 µmol/L
but varies with assay*

Protein (whether from food or blood) in the large intestine is digested by bacteria, and ammonia is then released. Normally, this ammonia is absorbed into the bloodstream. It is metabolized by the liver, usually with the production of urea, and is then excreted by the kidneys.

In patients with cirrhosis, ammonia concentrations in serum or CSF may increase. Serum ammonia concentrations are best measured with arterial blood samples because venous serum concentrations may be falsely elevated by muscular exercise, seizures, or prolonged tourniquet placement. Generally, however, venous concentrations are used because they are the easiest to obtain and practitioners hesitate to do arterial sampling in patients who may have underlying coagulopathy from liver disease. Since blood ammonia increases rapidly at room temperature, all test specimens must be placed on ice immediately.

Ammonia levels are used primarily to evaluate patients with hepatic encephalopathy or coma. Patients with severe liver disease can progressively deteriorate in mental

---

**✎ Minicase 5**

A 47-year-old alcoholic, S. F., was admitted after being found on a park bench surrounded by empty beer bottles. Known to have cirrhosis, S. F. was thought to be showing signs of hepatic encephalopathy as he slowly lapsed into a deep coma over the first 4 days of hospitalization. His physical examination was significant in that he had hepatomegaly and splenomegaly.

Lab evaluation showed a normal urine drug screen for central nervous system (CNS) depressants with glucose normal at 120 mg/dL. All serum electrolytes also were normal: sodium, 140 mEq/L; potassium, 4 mEq/L; chloride, 98 mEq/L; carbon dioxide, 25 mEq/L; and magnesium, 1.5 mEq/L. S. F.'s blood alcohol concentration on admission was 150 (normal: 0). His serum GGTP was 321 IU/L (<60 IU/L), and his AST was 87 IU/L (8–42 IU/L).

Unfortunately, efforts at treating hepatic encephalopathy did not reverse the patient's coma. When it was noted that his ammonia concentration was normal at 48 µg/dL (30–70 µg/dL), further examination and testing were undertaken. A large bruise was then noticed on the side of S. F.'s head, and a CT scan revealed a large subdural hematoma. With surgical treatment of the hematoma, he promptly awoke and began asking for more beer.

*How does one establish the diagnosis of hepatic encephalopathy for this patient? What is the role of the serum ammonia concentration in the diagnosis?*

**Discussion:** This case demonstrates that the diagnosis of hepatic encephalopathy is not always straightforward. Hepatic encephalopathy is only one cause of altered mental function in patients with advanced liver disease. Other causes may include drug accumulation, head trauma, hypoglycemia, delirium tremens, and electrolyte imbalance. The diagnosis of hepatic encephalopathy is suggested by

- Elevated ammonia concentrations.
- Presence (in early stages) of asterixis or a flapping tremor of the hands.
- Absence of other causative factors.
- Characteristic electroencephalographic findings (rarely used).

The response to therapy (usually correction of electrolyte imbalances, rehydration, and lactulose or neomycin) further supports this diagnosis.

Serum ammonia concentrations, therefore, are just one piece of this puzzle. An elevated concentration suggests, but does not establish, this diagnosis. Furthermore, although normal ammonia concentrations may cause one to question the diagnosis of hepatic encephalopathy, they can occur in this condition.

functioning—from subtle personality changes to complete coma. The exact cause of this deterioration, referred to as hepatic encephalopathy, remains unclear. The disease seems to be toxin related, however, because the encephalopathy rapidly clears with improved liver function or after liver transplantation. Ammonia is not the only postulated toxin;[25] in certain studies, infusing ammonia into patients with cirrhosis did not worsen the encephalopathy. Furthermore, a given ammonia concentration is not predictive of an encephalopathy level, because different patients with the same ammonia concentration can be awake or comatose.[26]

Nonetheless, ammonia concentrations are commonly used to diagnose hepatic encephalopathy. For a particular patient, improvement or deterioration can be followed by tracing serial ammonia concentrations. Their greatest value is in the evaluation of the altered mental status of a patient with liver disease. In such patients, a normal concentration may suggest other causes (e.g., head trauma, drugs, and infection) while an elevated concentration may indicate hepatic encephalopathy.

Ammonia concentrations can be elevated in patients

> With inborn disorders of the urea cycle.
> With Reye's syndrome.
> On very high protein diets.
> On valproic acid.

Ammonia also can be elevated in infants receiving large amounts of parenteral nutrition. Urinary infections may be caused by bacteria that break down the urea in urine to ammonia (urea-splitting organisms such as *Proteus*); patients with urinary diversions may be susceptible to developing very high concentrations of ammonia and even encephalopathy.[27] Therapy of the infections reverses the encephalopathy, usually within 24–36 hr. Ammonia concentrations decline with proper therapy for hepatic encephalopathy (e.g., lactulose or neomycin); the concentrations, along with mental status, are used as a guide to drug therapy.

# VIRAL HEPATITIS

The onset of *acute* viral hepatitis may be quite dramatic and present as an overwhelming infection, or it may be entirely subclinical and not be noticed by the patient. In the usual prodromal period, the patient has a nonspecific illness that may include nausea, vomiting, fatigue, malaise, or a flu-like syndrome. This period may be followed by clinical hepatitis with jaundice. During this time, the most abnormal laboratory studies are usually the aminotransferases, which can be in the thousands (normally <50 IU/L). Bilirubin may be quite elevated, but ALP only mildly so.

The major types of viral hepatitis are reviewed here, but it is often clinically impossible to distinguish one type from another without serological studies. (Serological testing is also discussed from different perspectives in Chapters 2, 16, and 17.) *Chronic* hepatitis can develop after infection from hepatitis B or C viruses. Because of the mild symptoms seen with acute infection, most patients with chronic viral hepatitis are detected at blood bank screenings or during general physical examinations. Table 8 lists groups at high risk of contracting infection by the various hepatitis viruses.

## Type A Hepatitis

Type A hepatitis, also known as infectious hepatitis, is caused by a ribonucleic acid (RNA) virus. This virus, spread primarily by a fecal–oral route (i.e., contaminated food or water), has an incubation period of 3–5 weeks

**TABLE 8.** Groups at High Risk of Infection by Various Hepatitis Viruses

| Hepatitis A Virus | Hepatitis B Virus | Hepatitis C Virus | Hepatitis D Virus[a] | Hepatitis E Virus |
|---|---|---|---|---|
| Contacts with infected persons | Family of infected persons | Dialysis and transplant patients | Health care professionals | Contacts of infected persons |
| Daycare workers and attendees | Health care professionals | Health care professionals | Institutionalized persons | Travelers to Latin America, Egypt, India, and Pakistan |
| Institutionalized persons | Hemodialysis patients | IV drug users | IV drug users | |
| International travelers | Homosexual men | Multipartner heterosexuals | Multiply transfused patients | |
| Military personnel | IV drug users | Multiply transfused patients | | |
| | Morticians | Tatooed persons | | |
| | Multipartner heterosexuals | | | |
| | Newborns of HBsAg-carrier mothers | | | |
| | Sexual partners of HBsAg carriers | | | |
| | Tatooed persons | | | |

[a]Requires presence of HBsAg.

with a several-day prodrome before the onset of jaundice and malaise. Many patients who get type A hepatitis never become clinically ill.

Unlike the B and C hepatitis viruses, the hepatitis A virus (HAV) does not cause a chronic disease. Perhaps 10% of all patients become symptomatic, and only 10% of these patients become jaundiced. This small percentage may explain the serological evidence of remote infection in a large percentage of the population, most of whom do not recall ever having had hepatitis.[28]

There is no direct serum test for the virus itself. Presently, the only tests measure antibodies to the hepatitis A virus. These antibodies are either IgM or IgG types. Acute hepatitis A is suggested by the detection of IgM antihepatitis A antigen antibodies (anti-HAV IgM) in the serum. These antibodies are present at the onset of jaundice and usually resolve over 2–3 months. IgG antihepatitis A antibodies indicate previous infection and lasting immunity; they can be present in up to 75% of certain populations. Figure 4 illustrates temporal relationships of serologies with the onset of jaundice and infectious status.

Therefore, the diagnosis of acute hepatitis type A is made by the finding of IgM antibodies. The finding of antibodies to hepatitis A virus thus mandates fraction-

ation to IgG versus IgM antibodies, a process that many clinical laboratories do automatically.

## Type B Hepatitis

Hepatitis B virus (HBV) is a complex deoxyribonucleic acid (DNA) virus. It is spread by bodily fluids, most commonly via contaminated needles, blood products, or sexual intercourse. The incubation period of hepatitis B from initial exposure to development of clinical disease varies from 2 to 4 months, much longer than that of hepatitis A.

The clinical illness can be quite severe. Unfortunately, up to 20% of the patients develop a chronic illness that is often mild but can be devastating as it progresses to cirrhosis and liver failure. Fortunately, a safe vaccine is available.

### Antigenic Components and Their Antibodies

The hepatitis B virus is surrounded by a protein coat called the surface antigen (HBsAg) (Figure 5, next page). Inside this coat, a core (HBcAg) protein coat surrounds the DNA and DNA polymerase. Another protein that seems to be in this virus is the e antigen (HBeAg). Detection of HBeAg

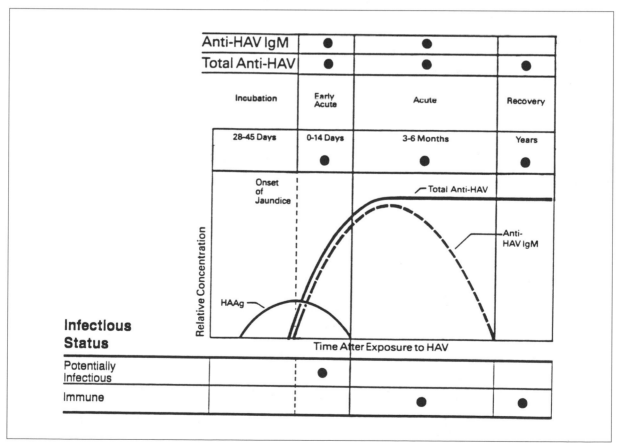

**FIGURE 4.** Temporal relationships of serologies for hepatitis A with onset of jaundice and infectious status. Anti-HAV IgM is the IgM antibody against the hepatitis A virus. HAAg is the hepatitis A antigen (virus). Total anti-HAV is primarily IgG antibodies (and some IgM in acute phase) against hepatitis A virus. (Adapted, with permission, from educational material of Abbott Laboratories, North Chicago, IL.)

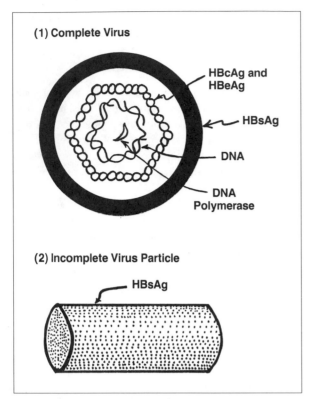

**FIGURE 5.** Hepatitis B virus and its antigenic components. The complete and infectious virus (1), originally known as the Dane particle, is composed of the outer layer (HBsAg) and inner nucleocapsid core. The inner core is comprised of HBcAg intermeshed with HBeAg and encapsulates the viral DNA. HBeAg may be an internal component or degradation product of the nucleocapsid core. An incomplete and noninfectious form (2) is composed exclusively of HBsAg and is cylindrical in shape.

indicates large amounts of circulating hepatitis B virus; these persons are five to 10 times more likely to transmit this virus than are HBeAg-negative persons.[29] The infected liver produces a great excess of surface antigen that is found in the serum in a tubular or cylindrical form and is not infectious (Figure 5). Of the antigens, HBsAg and HBeAg can be detected in clinical laboratories but HBcAg cannot.

In response to infection with hepatitis B virus, the body produces antibodies to the antigens: antisurface antigen (anti-HBs), anticore antigen (anti-HBc), and anti-e antigen (anti-HBe). All of these antibodies can be detected in clinical laboratories.

Discussion of all permutations and combinations of the antigens and antibodies is beyond the scope of this chapter. However, Table 9 should be useful when interpreting the most common serological patterns.

### Acute Hepatitis B

HBsAg titers usually develop within 4–12 weeks of infection. Consequently, they can be seen even before elevation in aminotransferases or clinical symptoms. The development of HBsAg is followed rapidly by the development of anti-HBc titers, which persist after resolution of symptoms. Anti-HBs titers often develop while symptoms are resolving and may persist for some time. The development of this antibody indicates resolution of the acute symptomatic phase of the type B infection. Figure 6 illustrates typical temporal patterns of serological tests, infectious status, and symptoms of acute hepatitis B (Minicase 6, page 230).

### Chronic Hepatitis B

Up to 20% of patients who develop type B hepatitis fail to develop anti-HBs and do not resolve their infections. These patients may develop chronic hepatitis, varying from a very mild syndrome requiring no intervention (10%) to a devastating course ultimately progressing to liver failure and death (10%). Another sequela of chronic infection is hepatocellular carcinoma. Chronic disease develops in 90% of neonates with acute infection.

The development of chronic hepatitis is suggested by persistence of elevated LFTs (generally aminotransferases) and is supported by persistence of HBsAg and anti-HBc markers (Figures 6 and 7). Chronic hepatitis B carriers do not clear HBsAg from their blood within 3 months of the acute infection. Some patients do not seroconvert; they do not develop antibodies against the e antigen of the hepatitis B virus (anti-HBe). Others do not produce anti-HBe until well after the acute infection phase is over (late seroconversion). In patients who do not develop chronic hepatitis, anti-HBe can be detected as early as 3 months and is usually present by 6 months.

### Hepatitis B Vaccine

The hepatitis vaccine consists of just the spherical HBsAg particles that are not infectious. Initially, this vaccine was produced by separating these particles from the blood of

**TABLE 9.** Interpretation of Common Hepatitis B Serological Test Results

| HBsAg | Anti-HBs | Anti-HBc | Interpretation |
|---|---|---|---|
| Positive | Negative | Positive | Acute infection or chronic hepatitis B |
| Negative | Positive | Positive | Resolving hepatitis B or previous infection |
| Negative | Positive | Negative | Resolving or recovered hepatitis B or patient after vaccination |

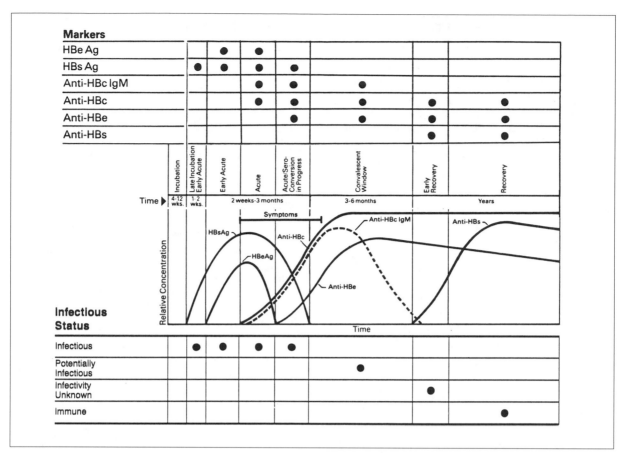

**FIGURE 6.** Serological profile, including temporal relationships integrated with infectious status and symptoms, in 75–85% of patients with *acute* type B hepatitis. (Adapted, with permission, from educational material of Abbott Laboratories, North Chicago, IL.)

patients infected with type B hepatitis. Because of growing concerns over AIDS (although never demonstrated to be a problem in vaccine production), a recombinant vaccine is now produced by genetically manipulated yeast.

Although HBsAg is not infectious, it stimulates the

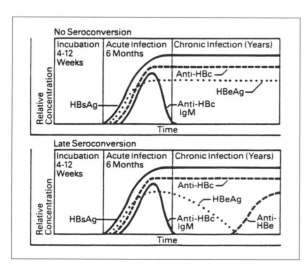

**FIGURE 7.** Serological profiles of patients who chronically carry hepatitis B virus. (Reproduced, with permission, from Abbott Laboratories, North Chicago, IL.)

production of antibodies (HBsAb) that protect patients from the disease. Thus, 90–95% of patients who receive the vaccine should have detectable HBsAb titers as early as 1 month later; these titers are present for at least 5 years.

## Type C Hepatitis

Before the late 1980s, up to 1% of patients receiving multiple transfusions developed hepatitis that tested negatively for antibodies to type A or B hepatitis and cytomegalovirus. It was referred to as "non-A/non-B" hepatitis. Then an RNA virus was identified as being responsible for 90% of these cases.[30] This virus, now referred to as type C hepatitis (HCV), is probably responsible for 20–40% of the viral hepatitis cases in this country. With the advent of testing for type C hepatitis, the risk of developing hepatitis after multiple blood transfusions is down to 0.03%.[31]

Although type C hepatitis can be spread parenterally, no clear route of exposure can be determined in many cases. Hepatitis C is prevalent in multiply transfused patients, transplant recipients, dialysis patients, and drug abusers (Table 8). There is some evidence that hepatitis C virus may be a main pathogenic factor in porphyria cutanea tarda.[32]

---

M. C., a 45-year-old executive, presented to his physician after noticing that he was turning yellow. Other than increased fatigue, he felt well. His physical examination was normal except for his jaundice and tenderness over a slightly swollen liver. Initial laboratory studies showed elevations of the aminotransferases with an ALT of 1235 IU/L (3–30 IU/L) and an AST of 2345 IU/L (8–42 IU/L). His total bilirubin was 18.6 mg/dL (0.3–1.0 mg/dL).

The tentative diagnosis was acute hepatitis. However, M. C. had not had any transfusions, used parenteral drugs, or had recent dental work. No exposure to medications or occupational exposure accounted for the disease, and there was no family history of liver disease. Careful review of the patient's history offered no explanation for his development of hepatitis.

Ultimately, serologies showed a positive HBsAg and anti-HBc antibody. A diagnosis of acute type B hepatitis was established. After much questioning, M. C. revealed that he had a "brief encounter" with a prostitute on a recent business trip. His wife was treated with the vaccine and hepatitis B immunoglobulin, a γ-globulin with high concentrations of antibodies to HBsAg. Although M. C.'s wife did not develop hepatitis, she did divorce the patient after learning that his secretary developed type B hepatitis about 3 months later.

*How was this diagnosis established? How should this patient be followed and what is the likely outcome?*

**Discussion:** This case demonstrates why a determination of the etiology of hepatitis is often difficult. The practitioner must obtain a detailed history of exposures to medicines, drugs, alcohol, infected people, family members with similar illness, and ongoing medical illness. In this case, the exposure to the prostitute put M. C. at risk for hepatitis B, C, and D and for human immunodeficiency virus (HIV). The diagnosis was established by the serologies. Had just the anti-HBc antibody been present, this patient could have

- ◆ Been in the "window" phase of the acute disease where this antibody is positive and HBsAg is negative.
- ◆ Previously recovered from hepatitis B.
- ◆ Been a chronic carrier.

Although the additional presence of HBsAg helped to secure the diagnosis, the clinical picture still had to be considered; both of these tests also can be positive in patients with chronic hepatitis B (Table 9). Determination of the type of hepatitis has prognostic value and, in this case, made it possible to administer prophylactic medications to people who might have been exposed.

There is no generally accepted drug therapy for acute viral hepatitis. M. C. should have repeated examinations and LFTs (specifically albumin, PT, AST, ALT, and bilirubin). There is a less than 1% chance that he will develop fulminant hepatitis and die. Most likely, he will recover completely, with his LFTs normalizing over 1–2 months. However, there is a 10–20% chance that he will develop either chronic persistent hepatitis, generally considered benign, or chronic active hepatitis, which could lead to cirrhosis.

The prostitute probably had chronic active hepatitis, but her HIV status was unknown. Unfortunately, even after this case was reported to the public health department, nothing could be done to prevent the prostitute from spreading these diseases to other contacts.

---

The mean incubation period of type C hepatitis is 6–12 weeks, between those of types A and B. Usually, the acute course is mild and asymptomatic. However, more than 50% of patients with acute C hepatitis develop chronic disease. Given the mildness of the acute attack and the tendency to develop into chronic hepatitis, it is understandable why many patients with this disease first present with cirrhosis or (more commonly) chronic elevations in aminotransferases.

Chronic hepatitis is defined as persistently elevated LFTs for 6 months. In chronic hepatitis C, the LFTs are usually minimally elevated, with ALT and AST values commonly in the 60–100-IU/L range. These values can fluctuate and occasionally return to normal, only to be elevated when next checked. Chronic active hepatitis C can be confirmed by a liver biopsy and treated with interferon.

Antibodies against hepatitis C virus are used to diagnose infection (acute or chronic) and thus probable infectivity. The "first-generation" test, the enzyme-linked immunosorbent assay (ELISA), was designed to detect antibodies to hepatitis C (anti-HCV). However, this assay gives many false-positive and false-negative results. False-negative results tend to occur in early infections, immunosuppressed patients (e.g., with HIV or transplants), and patients with different strains of hepatitis C (viral heterogeneity). False positives occur in patients with hypergammaglobulinemia due to connective-tissue disorders, autoimmune hepatitis, primary biliary cirrhosis, and in patients receiving IV IgG therapy.

The recombinant immunoblot assay (RIBA), the "second-generation" test for hepatitis C, also can be affected by viral heterogeneity and hypergammaglobulinemia. A newer RIBA (RIBA-3) may overcome some of these difficulties.

The present "state of the art" confirmatory test involves the detection of RNA from the hepatitis C virus. This test uses a cDNA-polymerase chain reaction to show hepatitis C viral sequences (HCV RNA) in liver and sera. This test is positive within 1–2 weeks of exposure, while the other tests may not be positive until 9–20 weeks after exposure. All anti-HCV-positive test results should be validated by a confirmatory test such as RIBA or HCV RNA (Minicase 7).[33,34]

## Type D Hepatitis

Hepatitis D, or delta hepatitis, is caused by a fascinating RNA virus (HDV) that requires the presence of hepatitis

### ✎ Minicase 7

Approximately 2 weeks after donating blood, a 48-year-old woman, K. M., received a notice that her blood could not be used because her aminotransferases were elevated and a test for hepatitis C was positive. She was referred to a specialist who found that her ALT was 87 IU/L (3–30 IU/L) and her AST was 103 IU/L (8–42 IU/L). Her bilirubin was 0.8 mg/dL (0.3–1.0 mg/dL).

A liver biopsy demonstrated chronic active hepatitis. After considerable discussion, K. M. was placed on interferon. Even after 3 months of therapy, however, her aminotransferases were not responding and she was referred for a second opinion.

Type C hepatitis was excluded when the patient's RIBA and RNA polymerase studies were negative. Additional history then was obtained. K. M. had been reluctant to tell her local family physician that, about 6 months previously, she had a positive skin test for tuberculosis (TB) after discovering that her partner was HIV positive. Being embarrassed, she had sought treatment in a nearby city and been placed on isoniazid. Although she had finished the prescriptions, she had never returned to the clinic.

*What are the roles of the second- and third-generation tests in the diagnosis of hepatitis C? What other nonviral forms of hepatitis can present as chronic hepatitis?*

**Discussion:** This case demonstrates several points. Many patients with chronic active hepatitis remain totally asymptomatic, their disease first being detected during routine blood work or when symptoms of cirrhosis or liver failure develop. Now that all blood donors are checked for hepatitis C and abnormal aminotransferases, many patients with chronic liver disease are detected before symptoms are present. Unfortunately, however, the blood banks tend to use the less expensive and less accurate ELISA test for hepatitis C, which (as in this case) gives many false-positive results. Before starting interferon therapy or establishing a diagnosis of type C hepatitis, a practitioner should confirm the diagnosis with either a RIBA or RNA polymerase.

There are many nonviral causes of chronic hepatitis including medications such as isoniazid, methyldopa, furantoins, and dantroline. A similar picture also may be seen in autoimmune hepatitis, Wilson's disease, α-antitrypsin deficiency, and hemochromatosis. Isoniazid, a common medication for TB, can cause serious liver damage that may be clinically and histologically indistinguishable from viral chronic active hepatitis. Therefore, aminotransferases need to be carefully monitored in patients on this drug. This problem tends to occur in patients over the age of 50, particularly women.

The aminotransferases may be only minimally elevated, as in this patient. Generally, hepatitis develops after about 2–3 months of drug therapy. With withdrawal of the medication, the numbers usually return to normal over an additional 1–2 months. When the diagnosis of chronic active hepatitis is considered, a patient's medications must be very carefully reviewed.

B surface antigen (HBsAg) to cause infection. Therefore, for people to contract type D hepatitis, they must have type B hepatitis. When hepatitis D occurs at the same time as hepatitis B (co-infection), the ensuing hepatitis may be particularly severe.

Hepatitis D also can occur in patients with chronic hepatitis B (superinfection). In this setting, the clinical picture is that of a patient, with known or unknown chronic hepatitis, who suddenly develops an acute flare, often with worsening jaundice, debilitating fatigue, anorexia, and deterioration of liver function. Occasionally, the patient may develop ascites, hepatic encephalopathy, or coagulopathy with subsequent variceal bleeding. Acute co-infection is usually self-limited, with rare development of chronic hepatitis. In contrast, superinfection becomes chronic in more than 75% of cases.

Transmission of hepatitis D in North America is generally by parenteral routes, although no obvious cause can be determined in some cases. Hepatitis D can lead to either a chronic infection or fulminant hepatitis (Figure 8) and may be responsive to interferon therapy.

The diagnosis is made serologically by titers of IgG and IgM anti-HDV. These titers generally become positive 2 months after exposure. Assays of serum for hepati-

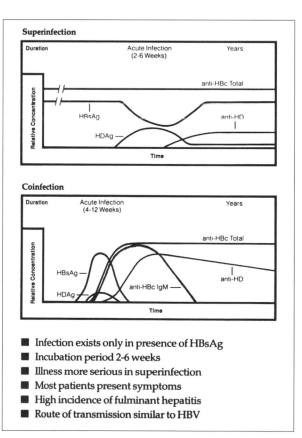

■ Infection exists only in presence of HBsAg
■ Incubation period 2-6 weeks
■ Illness more serious in superinfection
■ Most patients present symptoms
■ High incidence of fulminant hepatitis
■ Route of transmission similar to HBV

**FIGURE 8.** Two serological profiles of patients infected with the hepatitis D virus. HDAg = hepatitis D antigen (the virus); anti-HD = antibodies against hepatitis D virus. (Reproduced, with permission, from Abbott Laboratories, North Chicago, IL.)

tis D virus RNA also should be positive.[35]

## Type E Hepatitis

Like the hepatitis A virus, the hepatitis E virus (HEV) causes an enteric form of hepatitis, generally spread by contamination of food or water supplies. Clinically, this disease resembles type A and is characterized by a mild course without development of chronic disease. Fulminant hepatitis has occurred in women in their third trimester of pregnancy, occasionally in large outbreaks. The disease is rare in the United States.

Although tests are not commercially available, antibodies to hepatitis E can be measured. When these tests are available, it will be important to remember that the e antigen found in type B hepatitis has nothing to do with type E hepatitis.

## TESTS TO ASSESS THE PANCREAS

The tests discussed in this section, amylase and lipase, are primarily used to diagnose pancreatitis. Pancreatitis, or inflammation of the pancreas, can be acute or chronic. It generally presents with severe midepigastric abdominal pain, often radiating to the back. The pain tends to be continuous and can last for several days.

This condition is often associated with nausea and vomiting; in severe cases, fever, ileus, and hypotension can occur. Ultimately, there can be progressive anemia, hypocalcemia, hypoglycemia, hypoxia, renal failure, and death. The clinician faces the challenge of establishing this diagnosis, because many conditions (e.g., ulcers, biliary diseases, myocardial infarctions, and intestinal ischemia) can present in a similar manner.

Gallstones and alcohol abuse are causative factors in 60–80% of pancreatitis cases.[36] Often, however, it is impossible to determine a definite cause of a patient's attack.

## Amylase

*Normal range: 44–128 IU/L but varies with assay*

Amylase, an enzyme, helps break starch into its individual glucose molecules. It is secreted by the pancreas and salivary glands to aid in digestion. The serum amylase concentration is balanced by its entry into the circulation and its rate of clearance. This enzyme's most frequent clinical use is in the diagnosis of acute pancreatitis. However, increased release from some nonpancreatic sources or decreased plasma clearance also may elevate concentrations.

Most circulating amylase originates from the pancreas and salivary glands; much smaller amounts are released from the lungs, fallopian tubes, thyroid, tonsils, and some neoplasms. Approximately 40% of total serum amylase originates from pancreatic sources, while the other 60% is of salivary origin.

The kidneys are responsible for about 50% of the metabolic clearance, but remaining extrarenal mechanisms are poorly understood. The serum half-life is between 1 and 2 hr.[37,38] Although there is no amylase activity in neonates and only small amounts at 2–3 months of age, concentrations increase to the normal adult range by 1 year.

In the diagnosis of acute pancreatitis, serum amylase is clearly the single most useful biochemical test. Concentrations rise within 2–6 hr after the onset of symptoms and peak after 12–30 hr if the underlying inflammation has not reflared. In uncomplicated disease, these concentrations frequently return to normal within 3–5 days. More prolonged, mild elevations occur in up to 10% of patients with pancreatitis and may indicate ongoing pancreatic inflammation or associated complications (e.g., pancreatic pseudocyst).

Although serum amylase concentrations may increase up to 25 times the upper limit of normal in acute pancreatitis, the peak does not correlate with disease severity or prognosis. In contrast, elevations from opiate-induced spasms of the sphincter of Oddi are two to 10 times normal. Unfortunately, the magnitude of enzyme elevation can overlap in these situations; ranges are not very specific.

Drugs that may cause pancreatitis are listed in Table 10. In addition, hypercalcemia and hypertriglyceridemia can cause *actual* pancreatitis, which manifests with increased serum amylase.[39]

Urine amylase concentrations (normal range: <32 IU for 2-hr collection or <384 IU for 24-hr collection) usually peak later than serum concentrations, and elevations may persist for 7–10 days. If a patient does not arrive at the hospital before some acute symptoms have subsided, urine levels may be helpful. In patients with end-stage renal disease, serum amylase may be elevated without pancreatic or salivary disease due to diminished urinary clearance of the enzyme. Although amylase exhibits enzyme activity in the serum and urine, markedly elevated concentrations do not cause any pathology; they merely reflect a source tissue injury.

As shown in Table 11, numerous conditions are associated with elevated serum amylase concentrations. In some settings, fractionating amylase into its pancreatic and salivary components may be helpful (Minicase 8).

**TABLE 10.** Drugs that May Cause Pancreatitis

| | |
|---|---|
| Asparaginase | Nitrofurantoin |
| Azathioprine | Pentamidine |
| Cimetidine | Ranitidine |
| Didanosine | Steroids |
| Estrogens | Sulfonamides |
| Furosemide | Sulindac |
| Mercaptopurine | Tetracycline |
| Methyldopa | Thiazides |
| Metronidazole | Valproic acid |

**TABLE 11.** Other Causes of Elevated Serum Amylase Concentrations

| | |
|---|---|
| Alcoholism | Infections |
| Drugs (Table 10) | Penetrating ulcers |
| Gallstones | Pregnancy |
| Hypercalcemia | Trauma |
| Hypertriglyceridemia | Vasculitis |

However, if diseases or conditions are difficult to distinguish from acute pancreatitis, the elevated concentrations also may be due to an increased pancreatic component. In these cases, other clinical and radiographic information may establish a definitive diagnosis. Amylase fractionation may be especially helpful if the enzyme is chronically elevated but symptoms are nonspecific.

Macroamylasemia is a benign condition where amylase molecules are bound to abnormal proteins and form large complex molecules. Since these molecules can be between 150,000 and 1 million daltons, they are too large to be filtered by the kidneys. This condition, present in 1–2% of the population, results in serum concentrations up to 10 times the normal limit.[40] Macroamylasemia can be detected by fractionating serum amylase or by checking urine for amylase concentrations.

In marked hypertriglyceridemia, serum amylase measurements greater than 2000 mg/dL may be artificially normal in acute pancreatitis. This finding is clinically relevant since hypertriglyceridemia (>800 mg/dL) is a potential cause of acute pancreatitis. Fortunately, urinary amylase or serum lipase would typically be abnormal.

## Lipase
*Normal range: <1.5 U/mL but varies with assay*

Lipase, an enzyme, helps to digest fat by breaking triglycerides into diglycerides and fatty acids. Although mostly excreted by the pancreas, lipase can be found in the stomach, tongue, and liver. Serum lipase, however, tends to be mostly of pancreatic origin.[41]

After the onset of acute pancreatitis, lipase concentrations parallel amylase concentrations: initial elevation at 2–6 hr, peak at 12–30 hr, and fall to baseline in 2–4 days without further injury. As with amylase, peak lipase concentrations typically range from three to five times the upper limit of the reference range. At a concentration three times normal, serum lipase has a sensitivity and specificity of virtually 100% in the detection of acute alcoholic pancreatitis.[41]

Serum lipase, in general, is less sensitive but more specific than total serum amylase in pancreatitis. A serum lipase concentration that is greater than three times the upper limit of normal has a better diagnostic accuracy than serum amylase in differentiating nonpancreatic abdominal pain from acute pancreatitis.[42] Lipase is elevated in approximately 85% of patients with acute pancreati-

---

### ✎ Minicase 8

A 24-year-old male, B. W., was admitted to the hospital with a 5-day history of excruciating midepigastric pain radiating to the back and associated nausea and vomiting. He described a long history of recurring pancreatitis of undetermined etiology with similar symptomatology as his acute complaints. On admission, he had stable vital signs but appeared very uncomfortable. His physical examination was unremarkable except for fairly impressive tenderness in his epigastrium.

All of the patient's admission blood work was normal:

- WBC count of 10,000 cells/mm³ (4800–10,800 cells/mm³) with normal differential.
- AST of 20 IU/L (8–42 IU/L).
- ALT of 25 IU/L (3–30 IU/L).
- ALP of 80 IU/L (26–88 IU/L).
- Bilirubin of 1 mg/dL (0.3–1.0 mg/dL).
- Glucose of 80 mg/dL (70–110 mg/dL fasting).
- Calcium of 9 mg/dL (8.5–10.8 mg/dL).
- Serum amylase of 95 IU/L (44–128 IU/L).
- Lipase of 1.3 U/mL (<1.5 U/mL).

However, urinary amylase concentrations were markedly elevated, with over 1000 IU/2-hr specimen (<32 IU) on two determinations.

Radiographic workup, including abdominal ultrasound and computer-assisted tomography, was normal. Nevertheless, B. W. continued to require large amounts of narcotics to control his pain. One night, a nurse observed him expectorating into his urine specimen. A fractionation of the urinary amylase showed that the elevated amylase concentrations in the urine specimen were of salivary origin. When his narcotics were withdrawn, he signed out against medical advice to begin his search for the next gullible physician.

*What symptoms of B. W.'s were consistent with the diagnosis of pancreatitis? Which were not? What was the source of this patient's hyperamylasuria?*

**Discussion:** This patient, clearly seeking narcotics, knew the signs and symptoms of acute pancreatitis. His symptom of epigastric pain radiating to the back was consistent with the diagnosis he suggested (led the doctors to believe) when giving a history of previous pancreatitis attacks. The elevated urinary concentrations of amylase further supported this diagnosis.

The diagnosis of pancreatitis, however, was not supported by the normal serum concentrations of amylase and lipase, lack of a fever, normal WBC count, and normal radiographic tests. After the nurse made her observation, it became clear that the amylase elevation in the urine was salivary amylase due to B. W. deliberately expectorating into the specimen cup. Saliva, as the patient no doubt had learned, has a very large amount of amylase.

tis, but it is usually normal when serum amylase is falsely elevated. An elevated amylase with a normal lipase suggests that the amylase is of salivary origin or represents macroamylasemia.

Lipase concentrations may be elevated in patients with nonpancreatic abdominal pain such as a ruptured abdominal aortic aneurysm, cholelithiasis, small bowel obstruction, small bowel ischemia, or nephrolithiasis. In these situations, elevations tend to be less than three times normal. In the condition of macrolipasemia, macromolecular complexes of lipase to IgA lead to falsely elevated serum concentrations of lipase.[43]

## Other Test Results in Pancreatitis

In severe cases of acute pancreatitis, occasionally several days after the insult, organic soaps may form in fat necrosis and bind calcium. Serum calcium concentrations then decrease (low albumin may contribute also), sometimes enough to cause tetany. When pancreatitis is of biliary tract origin, typical elevations in ALP, bilirubin, AST, and ALT are seen. Some researchers believe that an increase of ALT to three times baseline or higher is relatively specific for gallstone-induced pancreatitis.[44]

Pancreatitis also may be associated with hemoconcentration and subsequent elevations of the BUN or Hct. Depending on the severity of the attack, lactic acidosis, azotemia, anemia, hyperglycemia, hypoalbuminemia, and hypoxemia also may occur.

Other lab tests are available to diagnose pancreatitis, including serum trypsin, serum elastase, and phospholipase A. They are not commonly used in practice but were recently reviewed.[42]

## ULCER DISEASE

Up to 10% of the U.S. population will develop ulcers at some point in life. In 1975, about 4 million Americans had ulcer disease for a total cost of 3.2 billion dollars.[45] Until recently, ulcers were believed to be primarily due to acid. Traditional therapy with antacids, $H_2$-blockers, and even proton pump inhibitors has been effective in treating ulcers but not in preventing recurrences.

### Helicobacter pylori

Only in the past decade were bacteria identified as a possible cause of ulcer disease. A curved Gram-negative rod, first called *Campylobacter pylori* and subsequently renamed *Helicobacter pylori*, was indicated as the probable causative organism. This bacterium inhabits the protective mucus layer coating the surface of gastric epithelial cells. It is best grown under microaerophilic conditions at pH 6–7 on selective media containing vancomycin, polymyxin, and trimethoprim.[46]

*H. pylori* seems to be transmitted by a fecal–oral route,

and its prevalence increases with age. In the United States, about 50% of the people have these bacteria in their stomachs by age 50. The incidence of infection is even higher in underdeveloped countries, where about 90% are infected by age 20. However, most people with *H. pylori* do not get ulcers. What role traditional "hyperacidity" plays in the development of peptic ulcers is now unclear. Nevertheless, 90–100% of patients with duodenal ulcers are infected by this bacteria, and 70% of people with gastric ulcers also have *H. pylori*. Furthermore, the bacteria are associated with the development of antral gastritis, gastric cancer, and certain types of gastric lymphoma.[47,48]

## Diagnosis

These bacteria break down urea to release ammonia and carbon dioxide. In a breath test, 13C- or 14C-labeled urea is given by mouth. If the bacteria are present, the radiolabeled urea is broken to radiolabeled carbon dioxide, which is readily measured in exhaled air. However, this test is not commonly used.

A serological test for *H. pylori* detects IgG antibody against an outer membrane protein of the bacteria. Since this test measures antibodies, it is positive (with positive titers) during the acute infection with the organism and remains positive for months after therapy. Normal values vary with the reporting lab, but titers greater than 1 generally are considered positive. A continual drop, with a 50% reduction, in antibody titers in two samples taken 3 and 6 months after therapy is good evidence of successful eradication. The absence of a fall in titer or the gradual rise in a previously declining titer indicates reinfection or recrudescence of an inadequately treated infection.[49] The infection itself probably does not result in symptoms; any symptoms are secondary to ulcer disease, gastritis, or tumors.

Many ulcer disease and gastritis cases are diagnosed during an upper endoscopy when stomach biopsies can be obtained easily. These biopsies can be cultured or examined for the bacteria. The bacteria usually grow in 3–4 days but may take as long as 7 days.

In a new test, the rapid urease or CLO test, a gastric biopsy is placed in a special medium containing urea and a pH indicator. The urease in the bacteria produces ammonia, which then changes the pH of the medium. This pH change is reflected by a color change from yellow to orange. This test is 98% specific and 90–95% sensitive.[50]

*H. pylori* is probably responsible for virtually all duodenal ulcers not related to nonsteroidal anti-inflammatory drugs (NSAIDs) or steroid use. Many practitioners now recommend empiric therapy in these cases without testing for *H. pylori*. Since gastric ulcers can be malignant, they require further investigation, generally with endoscopy. Similarly, there are many potential causes of gastritis; in most cases, confirmation of *H. pylori* is useful prior to therapy.

# PSEUDOMEMBRANOUS COLITIS

Colitis—acute inflammation of the colon—often presents quite dramatically with profound diarrhea, urgency, and abdominal cramping. It is generally distinguished from other causes of diarrhea by

➤ WBCs in stools.
➤ A positive Hemoccult test.
➤ An elevated WBC count in the blood.

There are many causes of colitis. Infectious colitis is caused by invasive organisms including *Campylobacter jejuni, Shigella, Salmonella*, and invasive *Escherichia coli*. Ameba can present in this manner, as can certain complications of AIDS (cytomegalovirus infection). Noninfectious colitis includes ischemic colitis (blood flow to the colon is insufficient), drug-induced colitis (as with gold salts), NSAID colitis, inflammatory bowel disease (Crohn's or ulcerative colitis), and radiation injury.

## *Clostridium difficile*

Pseudomembranous colitis is almost always caused by a bacterium, *Clostridium difficile*. It proliferates after the use of certain antibiotics (Table 12) and alters the gut's normal bacterial flora. Pathogenic strains of *C. difficile* produce a toxin that causes colitis, but 25% of *C. difficile* isolates neither produce toxins nor cause disease. Most hospital inpatients who grow *C. difficile* from the stool are asymptomatic. Fewer than 1% of healthy adults are carriers, but about 25% of antibiotic-treated persons are colonized with this bacterium.

This anaerobic, Gram-positive bacillus is readily cultured on an agar medium containing cycloserine and cefoxitin. Colonies have a flat, yellow, ground-glass appearance with a surrounding yellow halo.[52] Colitis patients usually have at least $10^4$ colony-forming units/g of *C. difficile*, while healthy carriers have many fewer bacteria.[53]

Pseudomembranous colitis can occur spontaneously and without antibiotic usage, but it commonly follows the use of antibiotics. Although clinical manifestations

(e.g., diarrhea) can start while the person is on the causative drug, signs and symptoms may not appear until weeks after the regimen is completed. Surprisingly, even one antibiotic dose may cause this condition. Furthermore, pseudomembranous colitis has been reported in patients with flares of inflammatory bowel disease who had not been on antibiotics.[54] Antineoplastic agents with antimicrobial activity (e.g., methotrexate) also can induce this disease.

Infection results from ingestion of *C. difficile* spores—they are heat resistant and can remain viable for months or years. They survive the acid environment of the stomach and transform into vegetative forms in the colon. However, cleaning with hypochlorous acid destroys these spores. Infection is usually acquired nosocomially. Although neonates are commonly colonized with the bacteria, pediatric patients develop infections only after the first year of life.[51]

## Diagnosis

It is quite difficult to culture *C. difficile* (hence its name). Stool cultures, while of value in excluding infectious forms of diarrhea, have little value in making this particular diagnosis. Although sigmoidoscopy may demonstrate characteristic pseudomembranes, it may be falsely negative if the disease is mainly proximal. In one study, up to one-third of the patients only had lesions in the right colon.[55]

Two toxins of *C. difficile* have been identified and are almost always present together:

➤ Toxin A (enterotoxin).
➤ Toxin B (cytotoxin).

The "gold standard" test has been the detection of toxin B in stool samples by demonstration of its cytopathic effect in cell cultures. This test is cumbersome, expensive, and time consuming. Moreover, there are false positives since healthy infants can have this toxin.[53] Additionally, this toxin can be inactivated during storage and transport. Nevertheless, this assay has both high sensitivity (94–100%) and specificity (99%).[56]

ELISA tests can detect *both* toxins in stool samples

**TABLE 12.** Antimicrobials Causing *C. difficile*-Associated Diarrhea and Colitis[a]

| Frequent Induction[b] | Infrequent Induction | Rare or No Induction |
|---|---|---|
| Amoxicillin | Chloramphenicol | Aminoglycosides (IV/IM) |
| Ampicillin | Erythromycin | Bacitracin |
| Cephalosporins[c] | Fluoroquinolones | Metronidazole |
| Clindamycin | Sulfonamides | Vancomycin |
| | Tetracyclines | |
| | Trimethoprim | |

[a]Adapted from Reference 51.
[b]Frequency may be due to prevalence of clinical usage as well as spectrum.
[c]Especially those with broad-spectrum activity against enteric bacteria.

---

### ✎ Minicase 9

J. T. presented to her physician after several days of crampy abdominal pain, diarrhea, fevers up to 102.5 °F (39.2 °C), and chills. On physical examination, she was noted to be well hydrated. Her abdomen was soft and nontender. Stools were sent for pathogenic bacterium cultures including *Shigella, Salmonella, Campylobacter*, entero-invasive *E. coli*, and *Yersinia*; meanwhile, J. T. was given a prescription for diphenoxylate.

Twenty-four hours later, the patient presented to the emergency room doubled over with severe abdominal pain. Her abdomen was distended and tender with diffuse rigidity and guarding. Clinically, she was dehydrated. Her WBC count was elevated at 23,000 cells/mm³ (4800–10,800 cells/mm³), and her BUN was 34 mg/dL (8–20 mg/dL). Abdominal X-rays showed a dilated colon (toxic megacolon) and an ileus. The emergency room physician then learned that, about 6 weeks earlier, J. T. had taken two or three of her sister's amoxicillin pills because she had thought she was developing a urinary tract infection.

Although pseudomembranous colitis was tentatively diagnosed, J. T. could not take oral medication because of her ileus. Therefore, IV metronidazole was started. This patient continued to get sicker, however; early the next day, her colon was removed and an ileostomy was created.

*What is the time course of pseudomembranous colitis? Did the use of diphenoxylate influence the outcome?*

**Discussion:** Pseudomembranous colitis can occur even after only one or two doses of a systemic antibiotic or after topical antibiotic use. Moreover, it can occur up to 6 weeks later. A complete history of antibiotic use is critical when dealing with diarrhea patients.

Diphenoxylate or loperamide use in the face of colitis is associated with a risk, although small, of toxic megacolon. In this medical emergency, the colon has no peristalsis; together with the inflammation in the colon wall (colitis), this condition leads to progressive distention. If untreated, perforation and death ensue. The development of a megacolon or ileus in this patient is especially worrisome because the best treatment—oral antibiotics—would be of little benefit. However, IV metronidazole is excreted into the bile in adequate bactericidal levels to eradicate the bacteria.

---

and are rapid and inexpensive. Although they have a high specificity, their sensitivity is variable (69–87%). Results of toxin assays are reported as either positive or negative since no clinical correlation is apparent between stool concentrations and disease severity. Therefore, the cytotoxicity assay remains the best method for diagnosing *C. difficile* diarrhea, even though results are not obtained for 48–96 hr.[51]

Susceptibility testing has not been useful in predicting treatment outcomes. After treatment, repeat cultures or cytotoxin assays for "test of cure" may be positive in up to 40% of asymptomatic patients.[53]

## SUMMARY

Solving the etiology of a given liver or other GI disease is much like putting together a puzzle. A detailed patient history and physical examination are two important pieces. Perhaps even more important is the appropriate use of laboratory studies.

The extent of liver injury or synthetic ability can best be evaluated by measuring the products of the liver, including albumin, prealbumin, and PT (an indirect assay of liver production of coagulation factors). Serum bilirubin is also useful as a marker of liver function since it reflects liver uptake, conjugation, and excretion. Although bilirubin can be elevated in some congenital diseases and hemolysis, it may indicate the degree of liver inflammation.

The degree of hepatocellular inflammation is best evaluated with the aminotransferases (ALT and AST), which leak into the blood after damage to liver (and other)

cells. Concentrations greater than eight to 10 times normal are characteristic of viral hepatitis or drug- or toxin-induced hepatic necrosis. The presence of cholestasis is best detected with ALP, 5'-nucleotidase, and GGTP, although they are not totally specific for liver disease. Elevations in serum ammonia may indicate severe liver disease as well as explain altered mental status in patients with cirrhosis. Various serological tests are available to help distinguish among the many forms of viral hepatitis.

This chapter also reviewed some recent developments in gastroenterology. Elevated amylase and lipase tests are used to diagnose acute pancreatitis. Most ulcer disease is believed to be related to the bacterium *H. pylori*. Diagnosis with serological and biopsy tests can aid in curing and preventing relapse of this disease. Antibiotics play a role in causing colitis, and tests for pseudomembranous colitis can confirm this diagnosis.

## REFERENCES

1. Sherlock S, Dooley J. Diseases of the liver and biliary system, 9th ed. London, England: Blackwell Scientific; 1993.
2. Johnson PJ, McFarlane IG. The laboratory investigation of liver disease. London, England: Bailliere Tindall; 1989.
3. Chopra S, Griffin PH. Laboratory tests and diagnostic procedures in evaluation of liver disease. *Am J Med*. 1985; 79:221–30.
4. Young DS. Effects of drugs on clinical laboratory tests, 3rd ed. Washington, DC: American Association for Clinical Chemistry Press; 1990.
5. Spiekerman AM. Proteins used in nutritional assessment. *Clin Lab Med*. 1993; 13:353–69.
6. Ghiso J, Wisniewski T, Frangione B. Unifying features of systemic and cerebral amyloidosis. *Mol Neurobiol*. 1994;

8:49–64.

7. Knapp AB, Farkas PS. Diagnostic diagrams: gastroenterology. Baltimore, MD: Williams & Wilkins; 1985.

8. Reichling JJ, Kaplan MM. Clinical use of serum enzymes in liver disease. *Dig Dis Sci.* 1988; 33:1601–14.

9. Birkett DJ, Done J, Neale FC, et al. Serum alkaline phosphatase in pregnancy: an immunologic study. *Br Med J.* 1966; 1:1210–2.

10. Bakerman S, Bakerman P, Strausbauch P. ABC's of interpretive laboratory data, 3rd ed. Myrtle Beach, SC: Interpretive Laboratory Data; 1994.

11. Wilson JW. Inherited elevation of alkaline phosphatase activity in the absence of disease. *N Engl J Med.* 1979; 301:983–4.

12. Kaplan MM, Matloff DS, Selinger MJ, et al. Biochemical basis for serum enzyme abnormalities in alcoholic liver disease. In: Chang NC, Chan NM, eds. Early identification of alcohol abuse. NIAAAA research monograph 17. Rockville, MD: U.S. Department of Health and Human Services; 1985:186–98.

13. Ockner RK. Drug induced liver disease. In: Zakim D, Boyer TD, eds. Hepatology: a textbook. Philadelphia, PA: W. B. Saunders; 1982:691–723.

14. Dukes GE, Sanders SW, Russo J, et al. Transaminase elevations in patients receiving bovine or porcine heparin. *Ann Intern Med.* 1984; 100:646–50.

15. Jick H. Drug-associated asymptomatic elevations of transaminase in drug safety assessments. *Pharmacotherapy.* 1995; 15(1):23–5.

16. Fregia A, Jensen D. Evaluation of abnormal liver tests. *Compr Ther.* 1994; 20(1):50–4.

17. Flora KD, Keefe EB. Significance of mildly elevated liver test in screening biochemical profiles. *J Insur Med.* 1990; 22:206–10.

18. Rivera-Coll A, Fuentes-Arderiu X, Diez-Noguera A. Circadian rhythms of serum concentrations of 12 enzymes of clinical interest. *Chronobiol Int.* 1993; 10:190–200.

19. Glynn KP, Cefaro AF, Fowler CW, et al. False elevations of serum glutamic oxaloacetic transaminase due to para-aminosalicylic acid. *Ann Intern Med.* 1970; 72:525–7.

20. Cohen GA, Goffinet JA, Donabedian RK, et al. Observations on decreased serum glutamic oxaloacetic transaminase (SGOT) activity in azotemic patients. *Ann Intern Med.* 1976; 84:275–80.

21. Cohen GA, Kaplan MM. The SGOT/SGPT ratio an indicator of alcoholic liver disease. *Dig Dis Sci.* 1979; 11:835–8.

22. Scharschmidt BF, Goldberg HI, Schmidt R. Current concepts in diagnosis: approach to the patient with cholestatic jaundice. *N Engl J Med.* 1983; 308:1515–9.

23. Rosalki SB, Dooley JS. Liver function profiles and their interpretation. *Br J Hosp Med.* 1994; 51:181–6.

24. Belsey R, Mueggler P, Swanson JR. Propranolol and spurious hyperbilirubinemia. *JAMA.* 1984; 251:38. Letter.

25. Gammal SH, Jones EA. Hepatic encephalopathy. *Med Clin North Am.* 1989; 73:793–813.

26. Zieve L. The mechanism of hepatic coma. *Hepatology.* 1981; 1:360–5.

27. Kaveggia FF, Thompson JS, Schafer EC, et al. Hyperammonemic encephalopathy in urinary diversion with urea-splitting urinary tract infection. *Arch Intern Med.* 1990; 150:2389–92.

28. Lemon SM. Type A viral hepatitis: new developments in an old disease. *N Engl J Med.* 1985; 313:1059–67.

29. Alter HJ. Transmission of hepatitis C virus—route, dose, and titer. *N Engl J Med.* 1994; 330:784–6.

30. Schiff ER. The patient with chronic hepatitis C. *Hosp Pract.* 1993; 28(8):25–33.

31. Donahue JG, Munoz A, Ness PM, et al. The declining risk of post transfusion hepatitis C virus infection. *N Engl J Med.* 1992; 327:369–73.

32. Fargion S, Piperno A, Cappellini M. Hepatitis C virus and porphyria cutanea tarda: evidence of a strong association. *Hepatology.* 1992; 16:1322–6.

33. Gross JB Jr, Persing DH. Hepatitis C: advances in diagnosis. *Mayo Clin Proc.* 1995; 70:296–7.

34. Alter HJ. Descartes before the horse: I clone, therefore I am: the hepatitis C virus in current perspective. *Ann Intern Med.* 1991; 8:644–9.

35. Dusheiko GM. Rolling review—the pathogenesis, diagnosis, and management of viral hepatitis. *Aliment Pharmacol Ther.* 1994; 8:229–53.

36. Gregory PB. Diseases of pancreas. *Sci Am Med.* 1994; 4(V):1–15.

37. Soergel K. Acute pancreatitis. In: Sleisenger MH, Fordtran JS, eds. Gastrointestinal disease, 5th ed. Philadelphia, PA: W. B. Saunders; 1993:1638–9.

38. Pieper-Bigelow C, Strocchi A, Levitt MD. Where does serum amylase come from and where does it go? *Gastroenterol Clin North Am.* 1990; 19:793–810.

39. Steinberg W, Tenner SM. Acute pancreatitis. *N Engl J Med.* 1994; 330:1198–1210.

40. Gumaste VV. Diagnostic tests for acute pancreatitis. *Gastroenterologist.* 1994; 2:119–30.

41. Gumaste VV, Dave P, Sereny G. Serum lipase: a better test to diagnose acute alcoholic pancreatitis. *Am J Med.* 1992; 92:239–42.

42. Gumaste VV, Roditis N, Mehta D, et al. Serum lipase levels in nonpancreatic abdominal pain versus acute pancreatitis. *Am J Gastroenterol.* 1993; 88:2051–5.

43. Bode C, Riederer J, Brauner B, et al. Macrolipasemia: a rare cause of persistently elevated serum lipase. *Am J Gastroenterol.* 1990; 85:412–6.

44. Ros E, Navarro S, Bru C, et al. Occult microlithiasis in "idiopathic" acute pancreatitis: prevention of relapses by cholecystectomy or ursodeoxycholic acid therapy. *Gastroenterology.* 1991; 101:1701–9.

45. Von Haunalter G, Chandler W. Cost of ulcer disease in the United States. Stanford Research Institute Project 5894. In: Sleisenger MH, Fordtran JS, eds. Gastrointestinal disease, 4th ed. Philadelphia, PA: W. B. Saunders; 1989:814–78.

46. Levine TS, Price AB. Helicobacter pylori: enough to give anyone an ulcer! *Br J Clin Pract.* 1994; 47:328–32.

47. Nomura A, Stemmermann GN, Chyou PH, et al. Helicobacter pylori infection and gastric carcinoma among Japanese Americans in Hawaii. *N Engl J Med.* 1991; 325:1132–6.

48. Parsonnet J, Friedman GD, Vandersteen DP, et al. Helicobacter pylori infection and the risk of gastric carcinoma. *N Engl J Med.* 1991; 325:1127–31.

49. Kendall BJ, Marshall BJ. Helicobacter pylori. *Contemp Intern Med.* 1993; 5:49–66.

50. Marshall BJ, Warren JR, Francis GJ, et al. Rapid urease test in the management of Campylobacter pyloridis associated gastritis. *Am J Gastroenterol.* 1987; 82:200.

51. Barbut F, Kajzer C, Planas N, et al. Comparison of three enzyme immunoassays, a cytotoxicity assay, and toxigenic culture for diagnosis of Clostridium difficile associated diarrhea. *J Clin Microbiol.* 1993; 31:963–7.

52. Peterson LF, Kelly PJ. The role of the clinical microbiology laboratory in the management of Clostridium difficile-associated diarrhea. *Infect Dis Clin North Am.* 1993; 7:277–93.

53. Fekety R, Shah AB. Diagnosis and treatment of Clostridium difficile colitis. *JAMA*. 1993; 269:71–5.

54. Trnka YM, LaMont JT. Association of Clostridium difficile toxin with symptomatic relapse of chronic inflammatory bowel disease. *Ann Intern Med*. 1981; 80:693–9.

55. Robesin SE, Levine MS, Glick SN, et al. Pseudomembranous colitis with rectosigmoid sparing on barium studies. *Radiology*. 1989; 170:811.

56. Kelly CP, Pothoulakis C, LaMont JT. Current concepts: Clostridium difficile colitis. *N Engl J Med*. 1994; 330:257–62.

## QuickView—Albumin

| Parameter | Description | Comments |
|---|---|---|
| **Common reference ranges** | | |
| Adults | 3.5–5 g/dL | |
| Pediatrics | 2–3.6 g/dL | <1 year old |
| | 2.6–4.2 g/dL | 1–3 years old |
| **Critical value** | <2.5 g/dL | In adults |
| **Natural substance?** | Yes | Blood protein |
| **Inherent activity?** | Increases oncotic pressure of plasma; carrier protein | |
| **Location** | | |
| Production | Liver | |
| Storage | Serum | |
| Secretion/excretion | Broken down in liver | Half-life of about 20 days |
| **Major causes of . . .** | | |
| High or positive results | Dehydration | |
| | Anabolic steroids | |
| Associated signs and symptoms | Limited to underlying disorder | No toxicological activity |
| Low results | Decreased hepatic synthesis | Seen in liver disease |
| | Malnutrition or malabsorption | Substrate deficiency |
| | Protein losses | Via kidney in nephrotic syndrome or via gut in protein-losing enteropathy |
| | Pregnancy or chronic illness | |
| Associated signs and symptoms | Edema, pulmonary edema, ascites | At levels <2–2.5 g/dL |
| **After insult, time to . . .** | | |
| Initial depression or positive result | Days | |
| Lowest values | Weeks | Half-life of about 20 days |
| Normalization | Days | Assumes insult removed and no permanent damage |
| **Drugs often monitored with test** | Parenteral nutrition | Goal is increased levels |
| **Causes of spurious results** | | |
| Falsely elevated | Ampicillin and heparin | |
| Falsely lowered | Supine patients, icterus, penicillin | |

## QuickView—PT

| Parameter | Description | Comments |
|---|---|---|
| **Common reference ranges** | | |
| Adults and pediatrics | 10–13 sec | |
| **Critical value** | >15 sec | Unless on warfarin |
| **Natural substance?** | Yes | |
| **Inherent activity?** | Indirect measurement of coagulation factors | |
| **Location** | | |
| Production | Coagulation factors produced in liver | |
| Storage | Carried in bloodstream | |
| Secretion/excretion | None | |

 *continued*

## QuickView—PT *continued*

| Parameter | Description | Comments |
|---|---|---|
| **Major causes of . . .** | | |
| **Prolonged elevation** | Liver failure | Liver unable to produce coagulation factors; does not correct with vitamin K |
| | Malabsorption or malnutrition | Vitamin K aids in synthesis of coagulation factors and is not absorbed; defect corrects with parenteral vitamin K |
| | Warfarin | Corrects with vitamin K |
| | Antibiotics | Interfere with vitamin K production or metabolism |
| **Associated signs and symptoms** | Increased risk of bleeding and ecchymoses | Easy bruising |
| **Low results** | None | |
| **After insult, time to . . .** | | |
| **Initial elevation or positive result** | 6–12 hr | |
| **Peak values** | Days to weeks | Depends on etiology |
| **Normalization** | 24 hr if vitamin K responsive (due to malabsorption, maldigestion, warfarin, etc.) but 2–4 days if due to liver disease and liver disease reverses | |
| **Drugs often monitored with test** | Warfarin | |
| **Causes of spurious results** | Improper specimen collection | |

## QuickView—ALP

| Parameter | Description | Comments |
|---|---|---|
| **Common reference ranges** | | |
| **Adults** | Varies with assay | Elevated in pregnancy |
| **Pediatrics** | Varies; can be two- to threefold higher than in adults | Elevated with developing bone |
| **Natural substance?** | Yes | Metabolic enzyme (intracellular) |
| **Inherent activity?** | Elevation alone causes no symptoms | Intracellular activity only |
| **Location** | | |
| **Production** | Intracellular enzyme | |
| **Storage** | Liver, placenta, bone, small intestine, leukocytes | These tissues are rich in ALP |
| **Secretion/excretion** | None | |
| **Major causes of . . .** | | |
| **High or positive results** | Cholestasis | Hepatic; associated with elevation of GGTP |
| | Bone | Paget's disease, bone tumors, rickets, osteomalacia, healing fracture |
| | Pregnancy | Placental ALP |
| | Childhood | Related to bone formation |
| **Associated signs and symptoms** | Limited to underlying disorder | Reflects tissue or organ damage |
| **Low results** | Vitamin D intoxication | |
| | Scurvy | |
| | Hypothyroidism | |
| **Associated signs and symptoms** | Limited to underlying disorder | |

## QuickView—ALP *continued*

| Parameter | Description | Comments |
|---|---|---|
| **After insult, time to . . .** | | |
| Initial elevation or positive result | Hours | |
| Peak values | Days | |
| Normalization | Days | Assumes insult removed and no ongoing damage |
| **Drugs often monitored with test** | None | |
| **Causes of spurious results** | Blood drawn after fatty meal and prolonged serum storage | |

## QuickView—AST (SGOT)

| Parameter | Description | Comments |
|---|---|---|
| **Common reference ranges** | | |
| Adults | 8–42 IU/L | Varies with assay |
| Newborns/infants | 20–65 IU/L | Varies with assay |
| **Critical value** | >80 IU/L | Two times upper limit of normal |
| **Natural substance?** | Yes | Metabolic enzyme |
| **Inherent activity?** | None in serum | Intracellular activity only |
| **Location** | | |
| Production | Intracellular enzyme | |
| Storage | Liver, cardiac muscle, kidneys, brain, pancreas, lungs | These tissues are rich in AST |
| Secretion/excretion | None | |
| **Major causes of . . .** | | |
| High or positive results | Hepatitis | Elevated in any disease with hepatocyte inflammation (liver cells) |
| | Hemolysis | Elevated in any disease with damage to tissues rich in enzyme |
| | Muscular diseases | |
| | Myocardial infarction | |
| | Renal infarction | |
| | Pulmonary infarction | |
| | Necrotic tumors | |
| Associated signs and symptoms | Varies with underlying disease | Reflects tissue or organ damage |
| Low results | None | |
| **After insult, time to . . .** | | |
| Initial elevation or positive result | 2–6 hr | |
| Peak values | 24–48 hr (without further cell damage) | With extensive liver or cellular damage, levels can go up to thousands |
| Normalization | 24–48 hr | Assumes insult removed and no ongoing damage |
| **Drugs often monitored with test** | Isoniazid and cholesterol-lowering agents (e.g., lovastatin, allopurinol, ketoconazole, valproic acid, and methotrexate) | Monitoring frequency varies with drug |
| **Causes of spurious results** | | |
| Falsely elevated | Heparin, levodopa, methyldopa, tolbutamide, *p*-aminosalicylic acid, erythromycin, diabetic ketoacidosis | |
| Falsely lowered | Metronidazole, trifluoperazine, vitamin $B_6$ deficiency | |

## QuickView—ALT (SGPT)

| Parameter | Description | Comments |
|---|---|---|
| **Common reference ranges** | | |
| Adults | 3–30 IU/L | Varies with assay |
| Newborns | 3–60 IU/L | Decreases to adult values within a few months |
| **Critical value** | >60 IU/L | Greater than two times normal limit |
| **Natural substance?** | Yes | Metabolic enzyme |
| **Inherent activity?** | None in serum | Intracellular activity only |
| **Location** | | |
| Production | Intracellular enzyme | |
| Storage | Liver, muscle, heart, kidneys | These tissues are rich in ALT |
| Secretion/excretion | | Normally contained intracellularly but, with cell damage, serum concentrations increase |
| **Major causes of . . .** | | |
| High or positive results | Hepatitis | Elevated in any disease with hepatocyte inflammation (liver cells) |
| | Hemolysis | Elevated in any disease with damage to tissues rich in enzymes |
| | Muscular diseases | |
| | Myocardial infarction | |
| | Renal infarction | |
| Associated signs and symptoms | Varies with underlying disease | Reflects tissue or organ damage |
| Low results | Patients deficient in vitamin $B_6$ | |
| Associated signs and symptoms | None | |
| **After insult, time to . . .** | | |
| Initial elevation or positive result | 2–6 hr | |
| Peak values | 24–48 hr (without further cell damage) | With extensive liver or cellular damage, levels can go up to thousands |
| Normalization | 24–48 hr | Assumes insult removed and no ongoing damage |
| **Drugs often monitored with test** | Isoniazid and cholesterol-lowering agents (e.g., lovastatin, allopurinol, ketoconazole, valproic acid, and methotrexate) | Monitoring frequency varies with drug |
| **Causes of spurious results** | Heparin (false elevation) | |

## QuickView—Bilirubin

| Parameter | Description | Comments |
|---|---|---|
| **Common reference ranges** | | |
| Adults | 0.3–1.0 mg/dL | Varies slightly with assay |
| Pediatrics | 2–6 mg/dL | 24-hr infant |
| | 6–8 mg/dL | 48-hr infant |
| | 0.3–1.3 mg/dL | >1 month old |
| **Critical value** | >4 mg/dL | In adults |
| **Natural substance?** | Yes | By-product of Hgb metabolism |
| **Inherent activity?** | Yes | CNS irritant or toxin in high levels in newborn (not adult) |

## QuickView—Bilirubin *continued*

| Parameter | Description | Comments |
|---|---|---|
| **Location** | | |
| Production | Liver | |
| Storage | Gallbladder | Excreted into bile |
| Secretion/excretion | Stool and urine | Bilirubin and urobilinogen |
| **Major causes of . . .** | | |
| High or positive results | Liver disease, both hepatocellular and cholestatic<br>Hemolysis<br>Metabolic abnormalities (e.g., Gilbert's syndrome) | |
| Associated signs and symptoms | Jaundice | |
| Low results | No important causes | |
| **After insult, time to . . .** | | |
| Initial elevation or positive result | Hours | |
| Peak values | 3–5 days | Assumes insult not removed |
| Normalization | Days | Assumes insult removed and no evolving damage |
| **Drugs often monitored with test** | None | |
| **Causes of spurious results** | Fasting, levodopa, phenelzine, methyldopa, ascorbic acid (false elevation) | |

## QuickView—Ammonia

| Parameter | Description | Comments |
|---|---|---|
| **Common reference ranges** | | |
| Adults and pediatrics | 30–70 µg/dL | Varies with assay |
| Newborns | 90–150 µg/dL | Varies with assay |
| **Critical value** | Varies; generally 1.5 upper limit of normal | |
| **Natural substance?** | Yes | Product of bacterial metabolism of protein (in gut) |
| **Inherent activity?** | Probably | Progressive deterioration in neurologic function |
| **Location** | | |
| Production | In gut (by bacteria) | |
| Storage | None | |
| Secretion/excretion | Liver metabolizes to urea | Urea cycle; diminished in cirrhosis |
| **Major causes of . . .** | | |
| High or positive results | Liver failure<br>Reye's syndrome<br>Metabolic abnormalities (urea cycle) | |
| Associated signs and symptoms | Hepatic encephalopathy | |
| Low results | No important causes | |

*continued*

## QuickView—Ammonia *continued*

| Parameter | Description | Comments |
|---|---|---|
| **After insult, time to . . .** | | |
|     **Initial elevation or positive result** | Hours | |
|     **Peak values** | No peak value; rises progressively | |
|     **Normalization** | Days | After appropriate therapy or resolution of underlying liver disease |
| **Drugs often monitored with test** | Valproic acid | |
| **Causes of spurious results** | Sensitive test (discussed in text) | |

# Chapter 12

# Endocrine Disorders

*Scott L. Traub*

Endocrine disorders often result from a deficiency or excess of a hormone—a chemical substance produced in the body that acts on receptors in specific target tissues to trigger a biological response. Usually, negative feedback mechanisms regulate hormone concentrations. Therefore, laboratory assessment of an endocrine disorder is based on concentrations of a plasma hormone as well as on the integrity of the feedback mechanism regulating that hormone. In this chapter, the evaluation of thyroid gland function serves as an example of these concepts.

This chapter also discusses how the relationship between a hormone (insulin) and a target substrate (glucose) serves as the basis for evaluating diabetic control. The relationship between vasopressin (antidiuretic hormone) and serum and urine osmolality is used to demonstrate the basis for the water deprivation test in diagnosing diabetes insipidus. This chapter also discusses the role of the specific hormonal (estrogen and progesterone) receptor assays, although not true "endocrine" tests, in selecting hormonal treatment for breast and ovarian cancers.

## OBJECTIVES

Upon completion of this chapter, the reader should be able to

1. Describe the actions of thyroxine ($T_4$), triiodothyronine ($T_3$), and thyroid-stimulating hormone (TSH), and the feedback mechanisms regulating them.
2. List the signs and symptoms associated with abnormally high and low concentrations of thyroid hormones.
3. Given a case description including thyroid function test results, identify the type of thyroid disorder and describe how tests are used to monitor and adjust related therapy.
4. Differentiate among the various types of glucose imbalances using laboratory tests and clinical findings.

5. Identify the medications or chemicals that may induce hyperglycemia or hypoglycemia.
6. Describe the use of glycosylated hemoglobin (Hgb $A_{1c}$) as a therapeutic monitoring tool.
7. Discuss the use of estrogen and progestin receptor assays in determining therapy for patients with breast and ovarian cancers.
8. Describe the relationship between the antidiuretic hormone vasopressin and serum and urine osmolality.
9. Differentiate between central and nephrogenic diabetes insipidus based on the water deprivation test or plasma vasopressin concentrations.

## THYROID

### Anatomy and Physiology

The thyroid gland is composed of two connecting lobes that span the trachea. The thyroid produces the hormones thyroxine ($T_4$) and triiodothyronine ($T_3$). Approximately 80 and 30 µg of $T_4$ and $T_3$, respectively, are produced daily in normal adults. $T_4$ is produced solely by the thyroid gland, but only about 20–25% of $T_3$ is directly secreted by this gland. Approximately 80% of $T_3$ is formed by the hepatic and renal deiodination of $T_4$.

$T_4$ has a longer plasma half-life than $T_3$ (approximately 7 versus 1 day). At the cellular level, however, $T_3$ is three to four times more active physiologically.[1-3] When the conversion of $T_4$ to $T_3$ is impaired, a stereoisomer of $T_3$ (reverse $T_3$) is produced; it has no known biological effect.

Thyroid hormones have many biological effects, both at the molecular level and on specific organ systems. These hormones stimulate the basal metabolic rate and can affect protein, carbohydrate, and lipid metabolism. They are also essential for normal growth and development. Thyroid hormones act to

> Stimulate neural and skeletal development during fetal life.

➤ Stimulate oxygen consumption at rest.

➤ Stimulate bone turnover by increasing bone formation and resorption.

➤ Promote the conversion of carotene to vitamin A.

➤ Promote chronotropic and inotropic effects on the heart.

➤ Increase the number of catecholamine receptors in heart muscle cells.

➤ Increase basal body temperature.

➤ Increase the production of red blood cells (RBCs).

➤ Increase the metabolism and clearance of steroid hormones.

➤ Alter the metabolism of carbohydrates, fats, and protein.

➤ Control the normal hypoxic and hypercapnic respiratory drives.

The synthesis of thyroid hormones depends on iodine and the amino acid tyrosine. The thyroid gland, using an energy-requiring process, transports dietary iodide ($I^-$) from the circulation into the thyroid. Iodide is oxidized to iodine ($I_2$) and then combined with tyrosyl residues within the thyroglobulin molecule to form thyroid hormones (iodothyronines). Thus, the thyroid hormones are formed and stored within the thyroglobulin protein for release into the circulation.[1,2,4]

$T_4$ and $T_3$ circulate in human serum bound to four proteins: the majority to thyroxine-binding globulin (TBG) and the remainder to thyroxine-binding prealbumin (TBPA or transthyretin), albumin, and apolipoproteins. Only 0.02% of $T_4$ and 0.2% of $T_3$ circulate unbound,[5] free to diffuse into tissues. The "free" fraction is the metabolically active component. Total and free hormones exist in an equilibrium state in which the protein-bound fraction serves as a reservoir for making the free fraction available to tissues.[6]

Thyroid hormone secretion is regulated by a feedback mechanism involving the hypothalamus, anterior pituitary, and thyroid gland itself (Figure 1). The release of $T_4$ and $T_3$ from the thyroid gland is regulated by thyrotropin, also called TSH, which is secreted by the anterior pituitary. The intrathyroidal iodine concentration also influences the thyroid gland activity. TSH secretion primarily is regulated by a dual negative feedback mechanism:

1. Thyrotropin-releasing hormone (TRH) or protirelin is released by the hypothalamus, which stimulates the synthesis and release of TSH from the pituitary gland. Basal TSH concentrations in persons with normal thyroid function are about 0.3–5.0 mU/L. The inverse relationship between TSH and free $T_4$ is logarithmic. A 50% decrease in free $T_4$ concentrations leads to a 50-

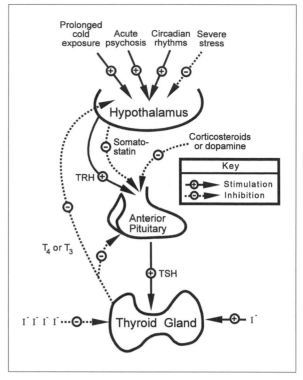

**FIGURE 1.** The hypothalamic–pituitary–thyroid axis. (Adapted, with permission, from Katzung BG, ed. Basic and clinical pharmacology, 4th ed. Norwalk, CT: Appleton & Lange; 1989.)

fold increase in TSH concentrations and vice versa.[7]

2. Unbound $T_4$ and $T_3$ (mainly the concentration of intracellular $T_3$ in the pituitary) directly inhibit pituitary TSH secretion. Consequently, increased concentrations of free thyroid hormones cause decreased TSH secretion, and decreased concentrations of $T_4$ and $T_3$ cause increased TSH secretion.[8]

Prolonged exposure to cold and acute psychosis may activate the hypothalamic–pituitary–thyroid axis, whereas severe stress may inhibit it. While TRH stimulates pituitary TSH release, somatostatin corticosteroids and dopamine inhibit it. Small amounts of iodide are needed for $T_4$ and $T_3$ production, but large amounts inhibit their production and release.

Most recent evidence based on the most sensitive assays suggests that no physiologically relevant change in serum TSH concentrations occurs in relation to age.[9]

## Thyroid Disorders

Patients with a normally functioning thyroid gland are said to be in a euthyroid state. When this state is disrupted, thyroid disease may result. It occurs four times more often in women than in men and may occur at any age, but it peaks between the third and sixth decades of life. A family history of this disease often is present, especially for the autoimmune thyroid diseases.

Diseases of the thyroid usually involve an alteration in the quantity or quality of thyroid hormone secretion and may manifest as hypothyroidism or hyperthyroidism. In addition to the signs and symptoms discussed below, thyroid disease may produce an enlargement of the thyroid gland known as goiter.

### Hypothyroidism

Hypothyroidism results from a deficiency of thyroid hormone secretion, causing a generalized slowing of the metabolism. Symptoms include lethargy; constipation; dry, coarse skin and hair; paresthesias and slowed deep tendon reflexes; facial puffiness; cold intolerance; decreased sweating; impaired memory, confusion, and dementia; slow speech and motor activity; and anemia. Interestingly, these typical signs and symptoms have been observed in as few as 25% of elderly hypothyroid patients.[9]

Hypothyroidism is usually caused by one of three mechanisms. Primary hypothyroidism is failure of the thyroid to secrete thyroid hormone, secondary hypothyroidism is failure of the anterior pituitary to secrete TSH, and tertiary hypothyroidism is failure of the hypothalamus to secrete TRH. Most patients with symptomatic primary hypothyroidism have TSH concentrations greater than 20 mU/L. Patients with mild signs or symptoms (usually not the reason for the visit to the doctor) have TSH values of 10–20 mU/L. Patients with secondary and tertiary hypothyroidism often do not have an elevated TSH, but other hormones (e.g., prolactin, cortisol, and gonadotropin) can be measured to confirm pituitary insufficiency.

Table 1 outlines the numerous etiologies of hypothyroidism.

**TABLE 1.** Classification of Hypothyroidism by Etiology[1,10,11]

| |
|---|
| **Primary** |
|     Iodide deficiency |
|     Excessive iodide intake (e.g., kelp and contrast dyes) |
|     Thyroid ablation: surgery, post [131]I treatment of thyrotoxicosis, radiation of neoplasm |
|     Hashimoto's thyroiditis |
|     Subacute thyroiditis |
|     Genetic abnormalities of thyroid hormone synthesis |
|     Drugs: propylthiouracil, methimazole, potassium perchlorate, thiocyanate, lithium, amiodarone |
|     Food: excessive intake of goiterogenic foods (e.g., cabbage and turnips) |
| **Secondary** |
|     Hypopituitarism: adenoma, ablative therapy, pituitary destruction, sarcoidosis |
| **Tertiary** |
|     Hypothalamic dysfunction |
| **Other** |
|     Abnormalities of $T_4$ receptor |

**TABLE 2.** Classification of Hyperthyroidism by Etiology[1,9–11]

| |
|---|
| **Overproduction of thyroid hormone** |
|     Graves' disease[a] |
|     TSH-secreting pituitary adenomas |
|     Hydatidiform moles/choriocarcinomas[b] |
|     Multinodular goiter |
| **"Leaking" thyroid hormone due to thyroid destruction** |
|     Lymphocytic thyroiditis |
|     Granulomatous thyroiditis |
|     Subacute thyroiditis |
|     Radiation |
| **Drugs** |
|     Thyroid-replacement drugs (excessive), amiodarone, iodinated radiocontrast agents, kelp[c] |
| **Ovarian teratomas with thyroid elements** |
| **Metastatic thyroid carcinoma** |

[a]*Most frequent cause. The mechanism is production of thyroid-stimulating antibodies; usually associated with diffuse goiter and ophthalmopathy.*
[b]*Tumor production of chorionic gonadotropin, stimulating the thyroid.*
[c]*Patients at risk of hyperthyroidism from these agents usually have some degree of thyroid autonomy.*

### Hyperthyroidism

Thyrotoxicosis results when excessive amounts of thyroid hormones are circulating and usually is due to hyperactivity of the thyroid gland (hyperthyroidism). This condition affects about 2% of women and 0.2% of men.[12] Its signs and symptoms include nervousness; fatigue; weight loss; heat intolerance; increased sweating; tachycardia or atrial fibrillation; muscle atrophy; warm, moist skin; and, in some patients, exophthalmos. These signs and symptoms occur much less frequently in the elderly, except for atrial fibrillation, which occurs three times more often.[9]

Table 2 summarizes the specific causes of hyperthyroidism.

## Nonthyroid Laboratory Tests in Patients with Thyroid Disease

Both hypo- and hyperthyroidism may cause pathophysiology outside the thyroid gland. Table 3 (next page) lists nonthyroid laboratory tests that may indicate a thyroid disorder. The influence on these tests reflects the widespread effects of thyroid hormones on peripheral tissues. Findings from these tests cannot be used alone to diagnose a thyroid disorder; however, they may support a diagnosis of thyroid dysfunction when used with specific thyroid function tests and the patient's presenting signs and symptoms.

## Thyroid Function Tests

Tests more specific for thyroid status or function can be categorized as those that (1) measure the concentration of products secreted by the thyroid gland, (2) evaluate

**TABLE 3.** Nonthyroid Laboratory Tests Consistent with Thyroid Disorders[1,4,10,11]

| Hypothyroidism | Hyperthyroidism |
|---|---|
| **Decreased** | |
| Hgb/hematocrit (Hct)[a] | Granulocytes |
| Serum glucose | Hgb/Hct |
| Serum sodium | Serum cholesterol |
| Urinary excretion of 17-hydroxysteroids | Serum triglycerides |
| Urinary excretion of 17-ketosteroids | |
| **Increased** | |
| Aspartate aminotransferase (SGOT/AST) | Alkaline phosphatase (ALP) |
| Capillary fragility | Lymphocytes |
| Cerebrospinal fluid protein | Serum ferritin |
| Lactate dehydrogenase (LDH) | Urinary calcium excretion |
| Partial pressure of carbon dioxide (pCO$_2$) | |
| Serum carotene | |
| Serum cholesterol | |
| Serum creatine phosphokinase (CPK) | |
| Serum prolactin | |
| Serum triglycerides | |

[a]Associated with normocytic and/or macrocytic anemias.

the integrity of the hypothalamic–pituitary–thyroid axis, (3) assess inherent thyroid gland function, and (4) detect antibodies to thyroid tissue.[13] Tests that directly or indirectly measure the concentrations of T$_4$ and T$_3$ include

> Free T$_4$.
> Total serum T$_4$.
> Serum T$_3$ resin uptake.
> Free T$_4$ index.
> Total serum T$_3$.

The integrity of the hypothalamic–pituitary–thyroid axis is assessed by measuring

> TSH.
> TRH.

### Free Thyroxine
*Normal range: 0.8–2.7 ng/dL or 10–35 pmol/L*

This test measures the unbound T$_4$ in the serum and is the most accurate reflection of thyrometabolic status. The low concentration of free T$_4$ in the serum (<1% of total T$_4$) makes accurate measurement a difficult and laborious process. Therefore, free T$_4$ is assayed primarily when T$_4$-binding globulin alterations or nonthyroidal illnesses confound interpretation of conventional tests (Tables 4 and 5).

Several methods can determine free T$_4$. Some methods perform well only in otherwise healthy hypo- and hyperthyroid patients and in euthyroid patients with mild abnormalities of TBG. However, in patients with severe alterations of T$_4$ binding to carrier proteins (e.g., severe nonthyroidal illness), only the direct equilibrium dialysis method maintains accuracy[14] (Table 5).

A decreased direct equilibrium dialysis free T$_4$ with

**TABLE 4.** Free T$_4$ and TSH in Thyroidal and Nonthyroidal Disorders[a]

| Diagnosis | Free T$_4$ Index or Direct Equilibrium Dialysis Free T$_4$ | TSH (mU/L) |
|---|---|---|
| **Hypothyroidism** | | |
| Primary | | |
| Normal | ↓ | ↑ |
| On dopamine or glucocorticoids | ↓ | ↓ |
| Secondary or tertiary—functional hypopituitarism | | |
| Recent thyroid withdrawal | ↓ | <0.10 |
| Recently treated hyperthyroidism | ↓ | <0.10 |
| **Hyperthyroidism** | ↑ | <0.10[b] |
| With severe nonthyroidal illness | ↓/WNL/↑[c] | <0.10[b] |
| **Euthyroid states** | WNL | WNL |
| Low total T$_4$ of nonthyroidal illness | ↓/WNL/↑[d] | WNL/↑ |
| After T$_3$ therapy | ↓ | WNL/↓ |
| After T$_4$ therapy | WNL | WNL |
| High total T$_4$ of nonthyroidal illness | ↑ | WNL/↑ |
| High total T$_4$ from amiodarone or iodinated contrast media | ↑ | ↑ |
| Decreased T$_4$-binding proteins | ↓/WNL[e] | WNL |

[a]↑ = increased; ↓ = decreased; WNL = within normal limits.
[b]Usually absent TSH response to TRH; also may be normal with hyperthyroidism from TSH-secreting tumors.
[c]Normal or low using free T$_4$ index estimation; increased using the direct equilibrium dialysis free T$_4$ assay.
[d]Decreased using free T$_4$ index estimation; normal to high using the direct equilibrium dialysis free T$_4$ assay.
[e]Decreased using free T$_4$ index estimation; normal using the direct equilibrium dialysis free T$_4$ assay.
(Adapted from Reference 3.)

**TABLE 5.** Performance and Availability of Free $T_4$ Methods

| Assay | % of Euthyroid Patients with Severe TBG Depression or Severe Nonthyroidal Illness in which Assay Underestimates Free $T_4$ | Comments |
|---|---|---|
| Free $T_4$ index[a] or single-step immunoassays | 50–80%[3] | Available in most clinical labs |
| Immunoextraction or radioimmunoassay[b] | 10–30%[3] | Available in some clinical labs |
| Direct equilibrium dialysis[c] | 0–5%[15,d] | Available in reference labs and large medical center labs; gold standard |
| Ultrafiltration[c] | 0–5%[15] | Available only in research labs |

[a]Corrects total $T_4$ values using an assessment of $T_4$-binding proteins.
[b]Uses a $T_4$ analog or two-step-back titration with solid-phase $T_4$ antibody but does not use membranes to separate free from bound hormone.
[c]Uses minimally diluted serum that separates free $T_4$ from bound $T_4$ using a semipermeable membrane.
[d]May be underestimated in about 25% of patients on dopamine.[16]

an elevated TSH is diagnostic of primary hypothyroidism, even in patients with severely depressed TBG. Conversely, an increased direct equilibrium dialysis free $T_4$ with a TSH of less than 0.01 mU/L is consistent with nonpituitary hyperthyroidism.[3] Decreased direct equilibrium dialysis free $T_4$ with normal or decreased TSH concentrations may be seen in patients on $T_3$ therapy. Although free $T_4$ assays are becoming widely available (Table 5), most clinicians initially rely on the traditional *total* serum $T_4$ measurement by radioimmunoassay (RIA).

### Total Serum Thyroxine
#### Normal range: 4–12 µg/dL or 51–154 nmol/L

Although ultrasensitive TSH and free $T_4$ assays are gradually supplanting this RIA, total serum $T_4$ still is the standard initial screening test to assess thyroid function because of its wide availability and quick turnaround time. In most patients, the total serum $T_4$ level is a sensitive test for the functional status of the thyroid gland. It is high in 90% of hyperthyroid patients and low in 85% of hypo-

thyroid patients. This test measures both bound and free $T_4$ and is, therefore, influenced by any alteration in the concentration or binding affinity of thyroid-binding protein.

Conditions that increase or decrease thyroid-binding protein result in an increased or decreased total serum $T_4$, respectively, but do not affect the amount of metabolically active free $T_4$ in the circulation. Therefore, thyrometabolic status may not always be truly represented by the results. To circumvent this problem, most clinicians concomitantly obtain the $T_3$ resin uptake test (discussed later) so they can factor out this interference. Table 6 lists factors that alter thyroid-binding protein.

*Increased total serum thyroxine.* An increased total serum $T_4$ may indicate hyperthyroidism, elevated concentrations of thyroid-binding proteins, or nonthyroid illness. Total serum $T_4$ elevations have been noted in patients, particularly the elderly, with relatively minor illnesses. These transient elevations may be due to TSH secretion stimulated

**TABLE 6.** Factors Altering Thyroid-Binding Protein[1,4,6,8,10,a]

| Factors that Increase Thyroid-Binding Protein | Factors that Decrease Thyroid-Binding Protein |
|---|---|
| Acute infectious hepatitis | Acromegaly |
| Acute intermittent porphyria | Androgen therapy |
| Chronic active hepatitis | L-Asparaginase |
| Clofibrate | Cirrhosis |
| Estrogen-containing oral contraceptives | Genetic deficiency of total binding protein |
| Estrogen-producing tumors | Glucocorticoid therapy (high dose) |
| Estrogen therapy | Hypoproteinemia |
| 5-Fluorouracil | Malnutrition |
| Genetic excess of total binding protein | Nephrotic syndrome |
| Heroin | Testosterone-producing tumors |
| Methadone | |
| Perphenazine | |
| Pregnancy | |

[a]Factors have the opposite effect on $T_3$ resin uptake (Serum Triiodothyronine Resin Uptake section).

by a low $T_3$ concentration. Similarly, up to 20% of all patients admitted to psychiatric hospitals have had transient total serum $T_4$ elevation on admission.[6,17] Thus, the differential diagnosis for a patient with this elevation must include nonthyroid illness versus hyperthyroidism if other evidence of thyroid disease is weak.

*Decreased total serum thyroxine.* A decreased total serum $T_4$ may indicate hypothyroidism, decreased concentrations of thyroid-binding proteins, or nonthyroid illness (also called "euthyroid sick syndrome"). Nonthyroid illness may lower the total serum $T_4$ concentration with no change in thyrometabolic status. Typically in this syndrome, total serum $T_4$ is decreased (or normal), total serum $T_3$ is decreased, reverse $T_3$ is increased, and TSH is normal. Neoplastic disease, diabetes mellitus, burns, trauma, liver disease, renal failure, prolonged infections, and cardiovascular disease are nonthyroid illnesses that can lower total serum $T_4$ concentrations.

Several mechanisms probably contribute to this low $T_4$ state. The concentration of serum-binding proteins may diminish hormone-binding capacity. Moreover, the conversion of $T_4$ to $T_3$ may be inhibited, causing an increase in the production of reverse $T_3$. Another theory suggests that a circulating thyroid hormone inhibitor may bind to the thyroid-binding protein.

In general, a correlation exists between the degree of total serum $T_4$ depression and the prognosis of the illness (i.e., the lower the total serum $T_4$, the poorer the disease outcome). Since severely ill patients may appear to be hypothyroid, it is important to differentiate between patients with serious nonthyroid illnesses and those who are truly hypothyroid.[6,10] The TSH concentration (Laboratory Diagnosis of Hypothalamic–Pituitary–Thyroid Axis Dysfunction section) often can be helpful in making this distinction.

*Drugs causing true alterations in total serum thyroxine.* Medications can cause a true alteration in total serum $T_4$ and a corresponding change in free $T_4$ concentrations (Table 7). In such cases, the total serum $T_4$ (and free $T_4$) result remains a true reflection of thyrometabolic status. High-dose salicylates and phenytoin also may lower total serum $T_4$ significantly via decreased binding in vivo. Phenytoin may lower free $T_4$, and salicylates may increase it.[18]

As implied in Table 7, iodides can significantly alter thyroid status. They have the potential to inhibit thyroid hormone release and to impair the organification of iodine (known as the Wolff-Chaikoff effect). In healthy individuals, this effect lasts only 1–2 weeks. However, individuals with subclinical hypothyroid disease may develop clinical hypothyroidism after treatment with iodides. Iodide-induced hypothyroidism has also been noted in patients with cystic fibrosis and emphysema.[6]

Iodides may also *increase* thyroid function. A previously euthyroid patient may develop thyrotoxicosis from exposure to increased quantities of iodine (Jodbasedow effect). The supplemental iodine causes autonomously functioning thyroid tissue to produce and secrete thyroid

**TABLE 7.** Medications that Cause a True Alteration[a] in Total Serum $T_4$ and Free $T_4$ Measurements

| Mechanism | Increase Total Serum $T_4$ and Free $T_4$ | Decrease Total Serum $T_4$ and Free $T_4$ |
|---|---|---|
| Interference in central regulation of TSH secretion at hypothalamic–pituitary level | Amphetamines | Glucocorticoids (acutely) |
| Interference with thyroid hormone synthesis and/or release from thyroid | Amiodarone[b]<br>Iodides[b] | Aminoglutethimide<br>Amiodarone[b]<br>Iodides[b]<br>Lithium carbonate<br>6-Mercaptopurine<br>Sulfonamides |
| Altered thyroid hormone metabolism | Amiodarone[a]<br>Iopanoic acid<br>Ipodate<br>Propranolol (high dose) | Phenobarbital |
| Inhibition of gastrointestinal absorption of exogenous thyroid hormone | | Antacids<br>Cholestyramine<br>Colestipol<br>Iron<br>Sodium polystyrene sulfonate<br>Soybean flour (infant formulas)<br>Sucralfate |

[a]In true alterations, the concentration change is not due to assay interference or alteration in thyroid-binding proteins.
[b]May increase or decrease total serum $T_4$ and free $T_4$.
(Compiled, in part, from References 1, 4, 6, 8, and 10.)

hormones, leading to a significant increase in $T_4$ and $T_3$ concentrations. This phenomenon commonly occurs during therapeutic iodine replacement in patients who live in areas of endemic iodine deficiency.

Similarly, patients with underlying goiter who live in iodine-sufficient areas may develop hyperthyroidism when given pharmacological doses of iodide. The heavily (37%) iodinated antiarrhythmic medication amiodarone may induce hyperthyroidism (1–5% of patients) as well as hypothyroidism (6–10% of patients).[6,19] Table 8 lists iodine-containing compounds.

Although antithyroid drugs such as propylthiouracil and methimazole are not listed in Table 7, they are used in hyperthyroid patients to decrease hormone concentrations. Both $T_4$ and $T_3$ concentrations decrease more rapidly with methimazole.[20]

### Serum Triiodothyronine Resin Uptake
*Normal range: 25–35% or 0.25–0.35*

The $T_3$ resin uptake test indirectly estimates the number of binding sites on thyroid-binding protein occupied by $T_3$. This result is also referred to as the thyroid hormone-binding ratio. The $T_3$ resin uptake usually is high when the thyroid-binding protein is low and vice versa.

In this test, radiolabeled $T_3$ is added to endogenous hormone. An aliquot of this mixture then is added to a resin that competes with endogenous thyroid-binding proteins for the free hormone. Radiolabeled $T_3$ binds to any free endogenous thyroid-binding protein; at the saturation point, the remainder binds to the resin. The amount of thyroid-binding protein can be estimated from the amount of radiolabeled $T_3$ taken up by the resin. The $T_3$ resin uptake result is expressed as a percentage of the total

**TABLE 8.** Iodine-Containing Compounds that May Influence Thyroid Status

| |
|---|
| **Oral radiopaque agents** |
| Diatrizoate |
| Iocetamic acid |
| Iopanoic acid |
| Ipodate |
| Tyropanoate |
| **Expectorants** |
| Iodinated glycerol[a] |
| Potassium iodide solution |
| SSKI (supersaturated potassium iodide) |
| **Parenteral radiopaque agents** |
| Diatrizoate meglumine |
| Iodamide meglumine |
| Iopamidol |
| Iothalamate meglumine |
| Metrizamide |
| **Miscellaneous compounds** |
| Amiodarone |
| Kelp-containing nutritional supplements |

[a]*No longer available; most products reformulated with guaifenesin.*
*(Compiled, in part, from References 6 and 10.)*

radiolabeled $T_3$ that binds to the resin. The $T_3$ resin uptake can verify the clinical significance of measured total serum $T_4$ and $T_3$ concentrations, because it is an indicator of thyroid-binding protein-induced alterations of these measurements.

Elevated $T_3$ resin uptake concentrations are consistent with hyperthyroidism, while decreased concentrations are consistent with hypothyroidism. However, this test is never used alone for diagnosis. The $T_3$ resin uptake is low in hypothyroidism because of the increased availability of binding sites on the thyroid-binding globulin. However, in nonthyroidal illnesses with a low $T_4$, the $T_3$ resin uptake is elevated. Therefore, the test may be used to differentiate between true hypothyroidism and a low $T_4$ state caused by nonthyroid illness.

All of the disease states and medications listed in Table 6 can influence thyroid-binding protein and, consequently, alter $T_3$ resin uptake results. Radioactive substances taken by the patient also will interfere with this test. In practice, the $T_3$ resin uptake test is used only to calculate the free $T_4$ index.

### Free Thyroxine Index
*Normal range: 1.2–4.2 but varies with laboratory*

The free $T_4$ index is the product of total serum $T_4$ multiplied by the percentage of $T_3$ resin uptake:

$$\text{free } T_4 \text{ index} = \text{total serum } T_4 \text{ (mg/dL)} \times T_3 \text{ resin uptake (\%)}$$

The free $T_4$ index adjusts for the effects of alterations in thyroid-binding protein on the total serum $T_4$ assay. The index is high in hyperthyroidism and low in hypothyroidism. Patients taking phenytoin or salicylates have low total serum $T_4$ and high $T_3$ resin uptake with a normal free $T_4$ index. Pregnant patients have high total serum $T_4$ and low $T_3$ resin uptake with a normal free $T_4$ index. Patients taking therapeutic doses of levothyroxine may have a high free $T_4$ index, because total serum $T_4$ and $T_3$ resin uptake are high. In addition to affecting total serum $T_4$ and free $T_4$ (Table 7), propranolol in doses greater than 200 mg/day commonly causes mild elevations in the free $T_4$ index.

### Total Serum Triiodothyronine
*Normal range: 78–195 ng/dL or 1.2–3.0 nmol/L*

This RIA measures the highly active thyroid hormone $T_3$. Like $T_4$, almost all of $T_3$ is protein bound. Therefore, any alteration in thyroid-binding protein influences this measurement. As with the total serum $T_4$ test, changes in thyroid-binding protein increase or decrease total serum $T_3$ but do not affect the metabolically active free $T_3$ in the circulation. Therefore, the patient's thyrometabolic status remains unchanged.

The total serum $T_3$ primarily is used as an indicator of hyperthyroidism. This measurement usually is made to detect $T_3$ toxicosis when $T_3$, but not $T_4$, is elevated.

Generally, the serum $T_3$ assay is not a reliable indicator of hypothyroidism because of the lack of reliability in the low to normal range.

Drugs that affect $T_4$ concentrations (Table 7) have a corresponding effect on $T_3$ concentrations. Additionally, propranolol, propylthiouracil, and glucocorticoids inhibit the peripheral conversion of $T_4$ to $T_3$ and cause a decreased $T_3$ concentration ($T_4$ usually stays normal).[21]

Total serum $T_3$ concentrations can be low in euthyroid patients with conditions (e.g., malnutrition, cirrhosis, and uremia) in which the conversion of $T_4$ to $T_3$ is suppressed. $T_3$ is low in only half of hypothyroid patients, because these patients tend to produce relatively more $T_3$ than $T_4$. A patient with a normal total serum $T_4$, a low $T_3$, and a high reverse $T_3$ has euthyroid sick syndrome.

### Thyroid-Stimulating Hormone
*Normal range: 0.3–5.0 µU/mL or mU/L; text describes interpretation of first- and second-generation assays*

Although the older, "first-generation" TSH assays have been useful in diagnosing primary hypothyroidism, they have not been useful in diagnosing hyperthyroidism. Almost all patients with symptomatic primary hypothyroidism have TSH concentrations greater than 20 mU/L; those with mild signs or symptoms have TSH values of 10–20 mU/L. TSH concentrations often become elevated before $T_4$ concentrations decline. All assays can accurately measure *high* concentrations of TSH.

The first-generation TSH assays, however, cannot distinguish low-normal from abnormally low values because their lower limit of detection is 0.5 mU/L, while the lower limit of basal TSH is 0.2–0.3 mU/L in most euthyroid persons. This distinction usually can be ascertained with the second-generation assays, which can accurately measure TSH concentrations as low as 0.05 mU/L. Occasionally, some euthyroid patients have concentrations of 0.05–0.5 mU/L. Therefore, supersensitive, third-generation assays have been developed; they can detect TSH concentrations as low as 0.005 mU/L. Concentrations below 0.05 are almost always diagnostic of primary hyperthyroidism in patients younger than 70 years.

Some clinicians feel that neither a low basal TSH concentration nor a blunted TSH response to TRH (discussed later) is a reliable predictor of hyperthyroidism in elderly patients.[22] Although third-generation assays usually are not required to make or confirm this diagnosis, they provide a wider margin of tolerance so that discrimination at 0.1 mU/L can be assured even when the assay is not performing optimally.[17]

*Use in therapy.* In patients with primary hypothyroidism, TSH concentrations also are used to adjust the dosage of levothyroxine replacement therapy. In addition to achieving a clinical euthyroid state, the goal should be to lower TSH into the midnormal range (Minicase 1, page 254).

TSH concentrations reflect long-term thyroid status, while serum $T_4$ concentrations reflect acute changes. Patients with long-standing hypothyroidism often notice an improvement in well-being 2–3 weeks after starting therapy. Significant improvements in heart rate (HR), weight, and puffiness are seen early in therapy, but hoarseness, anemia, and skin/hair changes may take many months to resolve.[23]

Unless undesirable changes in signs or symptoms occur, it is rational to wait at least 6–8 weeks after starting or changing therapy to repeat TSH and/or $T_4$ concentrations to refine dosing.[3,24] The hypothalamic–pituitary axis requires this time to respond fully to changes in circulating thyroid hormone concentrations.

This slow readjustment can be exploited elsewhere. One study[25] found that greater than 50% of TSH elevations in patients being treated with levothyroxine were attributed to noncompliance; with counseling alone, TSH normalized on subsequent visits. Noncompliant hypothyroid patients who take their levothyroxine pills only before being tested may have elevated TSH concentrations despite a normal $T_4$ concentration.[17]

Because of slow axis readjustment, patients given antithyroid drugs (e.g., methimazole) may maintain low TSH concentrations for 2–3 months after $T_4$ and $T_3$ concentrations have returned to normal. Single, daily doses of 10–20 mg of methimazole usually lead to euthyroidism within several weeks.[26] Treatment should not be adjusted too early using (low) TSH concentrations alone. However, the dose should be reduced within the first 8 weeks if TSH concentrations become elevated.

Patients with thyroid cancer often are treated with TSH suppressive therapy, usually levothyroxine. The therapeutic endpoint is a basal TSH concentration of about 0.1 mU/L.[27] Some clinicians suggest more complete suppression with TSH concentrations less than 0.005 mU/L, while others think that it leads to toxic effects of overreplacement (e.g., accelerated bone loss).[17,28]

*Potential misinterpretation and drug interference.* TSH is a glycoprotein with two subunits, alpha and beta. The alpha subunit is similar to those of other hormones secreted from the anterior pituitary: follicle-stimulating hormone, human chorionic gonadotropin (HCG), and luteinizing hormone. The beta subunit of TSH is unique and renders its specific physiological properties. Therefore, during the first trimester of pregnancy or whenever HCG concentrations are high, some TSH assays may yield falsely high results.

Most patients who have secondary or tertiary hypothyroidism have a low or normal TSH concentration. In patients with nonthyroid illness, TSH may be suppressed by factors other than thyroid hyperfunction. As mentioned previously, the TSH concentration typically is normal in patients with the euthyroid sick syndrome.

Thyroid function tests are known to be altered in

depressed patients. With the advent of the third-generation TSH assays, investigators hoped that TSH concentrations could help to determine various types of depression and response to therapies. Unfortunately, neither TSH nor its response to TRH has proven useful in this way.[29]

Because endogenous dopamine inhibits the stimulatory effects of TRH, any drug with dopaminergic activity can inhibit TSH secretion. Therefore, levodopa, glucocorticoids, bromocriptine, and dopamine are likely to lower TSH results. The converse also is true—the dopamine antagonists metoclopramide and domperidone may increase TSH concentrations.

### Thyrotropin-Releasing Hormone

TRH, a hormone secreted by the hypothalamus, regulates TSH secretion from the pituitary. The TRH test measures the ability of injected TRH to stimulate the pituitary to release TSH (and prolactin). This test has been the most reliable indicator of hyperthyroidism in patients whose other thyroid function tests are equivocal, primarily with the older, less sensitive TSH assays. With second- and third-generation TSH assays becoming more widely available, this TRH test infrequently is required. Nevertheless, it still is useful to distinguish primary from secondary hypothyroidism (Table 9).

This test is performed by drawing a baseline serum TSH concentration and then administering approximately 200–400 µg of TRH (synthetic protirelin) intravenously (IV) over 30–60 sec. TSH concentrations are drawn at 30–60 min. A normal response, indicative of the euthyroid state, is defined as a TSH rise of 5 µU/mL over baseline. A significant increase virtually rules out hyperthyroidism. A blunted or absent TSH response suggests hyperthyroidism. However, a rise of less than 5 µU/mL can be seen in euthyroid men over age 40, in depressed patients, and in patients with glucocorticoid excess. A blunted response may occur in euthyroid patients receiving adequate thyroid suppression therapy, dopamine, glucocorticoid, somatostatin, or L-dopa therapy.

Endogenous TRH secretion is enhanced by norepinephrine and serotonin. As alluded to previously, the need

for this test should decrease with the advent of the sensitive TSH immunometric assays. Patients with basal TSH concentrations less than 0.1 µU/mL typically do not have a TSH increase after a TRH challenge.

### Radioactive Iodine Uptake Test

This test is used to detect the ability of the thyroid gland to trap and concentrate iodine and, thereby, produce thyroid hormone. In other words, this test assesses the intrinsic function of the thyroid gland. This test is not very specific, and its reference range must be adjusted to the local population. Therefore, its use is declining. In patients with a normal thyroid gland, 12–20% of the radioactive iodine is absorbed by the gland after 6 hr and 5–25% is absorbed after 24 hr. The radioactive iodine uptake test is an indirect measure of thyroid gland activity and should not be used as a basic screening test of thyroid function. This test is most useful in distinguishing hyperthyroidism caused by subacute thyroiditis (with absent or reduced uptake) from Graves' disease.[11,30,31]

A high radioactive iodine uptake is noted with[11,30,31]

> Thyrotoxicosis.
> Iodine deficiency.
> Post-thyroiditis.
> Withdrawal rebound after thyroid hormone or antithyroid drug therapy.

A low test result occurs in[11,30,31]

> Acute thyroiditis.
> Euthyroid patients who ingest iodine-containing products.
> Patients on exogenous thyroid hormone therapy.
> Patients who are taking antithyroid drugs such as propylthiouracil.
> Hypothyroidism.

The radioactive iodine uptake test is affected by the body's store of iodine. Therefore, the patient should be carefully questioned about the use of iodine-containing products prior to the test. This test is contraindicated during pregnancy.

### Antithyroid Antibodies
*Normal range: varies with antibody*

Antibodies that "attack" various thyroid tissue can be detected in the serum of patients with autoimmune disorders such as Hashimoto's thyroiditis and Graves' disease. Thyroid microsomal antibody is found in 95% of patients with Hashimoto's thyroiditis, 55% of patients with Graves' disease, and 10% of adults without thyroid disease. In patients who have nodular and hard goiters, high antibody titers strongly suggest Hashimoto's thyroiditis as opposed to cancer. In Grave's disease, hyperthyroidism is caused by antibodies activating TSH receptors. In

**TABLE 9.** Differentiation of Hypothyroid Disorders Based on TSH and TRH Challenge Test Results[a]

| Dysfunctioning Tissue or Gland | TSH Before TRH Challenge | TSH After TRH Challenge |
|---|---|---|
| Thyroid | High | Exaggerated |
| Pituitary | Low/absent | No response |
| Hypothalamus | Low | Sluggish response |

[a]*Patients with hyperthyroidism have a suppressed pretest TSH and no response or a blunted response to TRH infusion.*

### ✎ Minicase 1

Amy T., an 18-year-old female, visited her physician with complaints of weakness, fatigue, weight gain, hoarseness, cold intolerance, and unusually heavy periods worsening over the past 2–3 months. Her pulse was 50, and her blood pressure (BP) was 110/70. Her physical exam was normal, except for a mildly enlarged thyroid gland, pallor, and diminished tendon reflexes. She denied taking any medications or changing her diet.

The patient's chemistry results were sodium 130 mEq/L (136–145 mEq/L), potassium 3.8 mEq/L (3.5–5.0 mEq/L), carbon dioxide 28 mEq/L (24–30 mEq/L), calcium 9.5 mg/dL (8.5–10.8 mg/dL), magnesium 2 mEq/L (1.5–2.2 mEq/L), glucose 80 mg/dL (70–110 mg/dL), blood urea nitrogen (BUN) 20 mg/dL (8–20 mg/dL), serum creatinine (SCr) 1.1 mg/dL (0.7–1.5 mg/dL), and cholesterol 235 mg/dL (<200 mg/dL). The cholesterol concentration was elevated since a screening 6 months ago. A test for mononucleosis was negative. Hematocrit (Hct) was low at 35% (37–47%)—close to her usual. Her total serum $T_4$ was 8 µg/dL (4–12 µg/dL), her $T_3$ resin uptake was 15% (25–35%), and her free $T_4$ index was 1.2 (1.2–4.2).

*How should these results be interpreted? Are confirmatory tests needed?*

**Discussion:** Clinically, all of the history and physical findings point to hypothyroidism. The pallor and weakness are also consistent with anemia, but an Hct of 35% is unlikely to cause such significant symptoms. Amy T.'s cholesterol recently became elevated, consistent with primary hypothyroidism.[33] Classically, both the total serum $T_4$ and $T_3$ resin uptake should be low in hypothyroid patients. In Amy T., only the $T_3$ resin uptake is low, and the free $T_4$ index is borderline normal, making laboratory diagnosis unclear. Confirmatory tests should prove useful.

**Minicase 1 (continued):** A few days later, Amy T. revisited her physician for additional tests. When questioned, she admitted that she has been taking oral contraceptives and would like to continue. The following day, her TSH was 25 mU/L (0.3–5.0 mU/L), her thyroid microsomal antibody was greater than 1:500, and her thyroglobulin antibody was greater than 1:1000.

*Does this information help to elucidate the diagnosis?*

**Discussion (continued):** The high titers of antibodies confirm that Amy T. has Hashimoto's thyroiditis, which has manifested as hypothyroidism. An elevated TSH confirms primary hypothyroidism. The reason for equivocal total serum $T_4$ and $T_3$ resin uptake is now apparent—the estrogens in the birth control pills. Estrogens elevate total serum $T_4$ and thyroid-binding protein and lower $T_3$ resin uptake. If Amy T. had not been taking estrogens, her total serum $T_4$ probably would have been below normal and her $T_3$ resin uptake probably would have been higher (but still below normal). The diagnosis would have been clear earlier. If oral contraceptive use had been identified at the first visit, a TSH concentration should have been performed then.

**Minicase 1 (continued):** Amy T. was started on levothyroxine 0.2 mg/day, and her TSH was 6 mU/L 3 weeks later. Clinically, she improved but was not fully back to normal. Six weeks after starting therapy, she complained of jitteriness, palpitations, and increased sweating. Her TSH was less than 0.3 mU/L. Her physician lowered the dose of levothyroxine to 0.1 mg/day, and Amy T. became asymptomatic after about 2 weeks. Eight weeks later, her TSH was 1.5 mU/L and she remained asymptomatic. Her cholesterol was 100 mg/dL, sodium was 138 mEq/L, and Hct was 40%.

*Which test(s) should be used to determine proper dosing of levothyroxine? How long after a dosage change should clinicians wait before repeating the test(s)?*

**Discussion (continued):** Although total serum $T_4$, $T_3$ resin uptake, and free $T_4$ index can be used to monitor and adjust doses of thyroid supplements in patients with a hypothyroid disorder, the highly sensitive TSH is most reliable. Chemically, the goal is to achieve a TSH in the normal range, as was ultimately achieved in Amy T. (TSH of 1.5 mU/L). Because of her continued use of birth control pills, TSH is the best test for this patient. The newer TSH assays make it possible to determine whether TSH secretion is being excessively suppressed by thyroid replacement (<0.3 mU/L).

With the increased availability of this sensitive test, TSH is becoming the standard for adjusting thyroid replacement therapy in most patients. The 0.2-mg levothyroxine dose was excessive, given the "hyperthyroid" symptoms and the fully suppressed TSH. Eight weeks later, after $T_4$ steady state was reached on the 0.1-mg/day dose and after the hypothalamic–pituitary–thyroid axis reached homeostasis, TSH was within the desired range. Amy T.'s cholesterol, sodium, and Hct also normalized as she became euthyroid.

chronic autoimmune thyroiditis, hypothyroidism may be caused by antibodies competitively binding to TSH receptors, thereby blocking TSH from eliciting a response.[32]

If a significant amount of antibodies is present in the blood, agglutination (clumping) occurs. The test for this antibody is based on hemagglutination (Glossary). Results are reported as the highest titer causing agglutination. Titers in excess of 1:100 are significant and usually can be detected even during remission.

Antibodies (>1:10) to thyroglobulin are present in 60–70% of adults with active Hashimoto's thyroiditis but typically are not detected during remission. Titers above 1:1000 are found only in Hashimoto's thyroiditis or Graves' disease (25 or 10%, respectively). Lower titers may be seen in 4% of the normal population, although the frequency increases with age in females. The thyroid microsomal antibody and thyroglobulin antibody serological tests may be elevated or positive in patients with nonthyroidal autoimmune disease.

Anti-TSH receptor antibodies are present in virtually all patients with Graves' disease, but the test usually is not necessary for diagnosis. These antibodies mostly stimulate TSH receptors but also may compete with TSH and, thus, inhibit TSH stimulation. High titers allow a confirmation of Graves' disease in asymptomatic patients, such as those whose only manifestation is exophthalmos (Minicase 1).

## Laboratory Diagnosis of Hypothalamic–Pituitary–Thyroid Axis Dysfunction

The laboratory diagnosis of primary *hypothyroidism* can be made with a low free $T_4$ index and an elevated TSH concentration. The presence of a low free $T_4$ index and a normal or low serum TSH concentration indicates secondary or tertiary hypothyroidism or nonthyroid illness. In such patients, the $T_3$ resin uptake may differentiate between hypothyroidism and a low $T_4$ state due to nonthyroid illness. An elevated reverse $T_3$ concentration also suggests nonthyroid illness. The TRH test may be used to pinpoint the thyroid axis defect (Table 9). $T_3$ is of limited usefulness in diagnosing hypothyroidism because it may be normal in up to one-third of hypothyroid patients.[11,13,30,31] With the availability of ultrasensitive TSH assays, many clinicians begin their evaluations with this test. One such approach is illustrated in Figure 2 and Minicase 2.

The newer TSH assay can also be used to diagnose *hyperthyroidism* (<0.1 mU/L). The total serum $T_4$ and free

### 📎 Minicase 2

Helen T., a 32-year-old female being assessed for infertility, was found to have a TSH concentration of 8.2 µU/mL (0.3–5.0 µU/mL) as measured by a second-generation assay. Her physical exam revealed no abnormalities, and she was clinically euthyroid. Her total serum $T_4$ was 10 µg/dL (4–12 µg/dL). She was treated with 0.125 mg/day of levothyroxine for 1 month, and a repeat TSH was 6.8 µU/mL. Her dose was increased to 0.2 mg/day.

After 2 months, Helen T.'s TSH was 8.8 µU/mL, while her total serum $T_4$ was 15 µg/dL, her total serum $T_3$ was 200 ng/dL (78–195 ng/dL), her TBG was 32 nmol/L (14–41 nmol/L), and her free $T_3$ was 4.7 pmol/L (3.2–5.1 pmol/L). She was slightly hyperthyroid. Levothyroxine therapy was stopped and, on that day, a TRH challenge (200 µg IV) evoked only minimal increases in TSH concentrations. Magnetic resonance imaging (MRI) of the hypothalamic–pituitary area was normal.

*What could have caused Helen T.'s initial elevated TSH?*

**Discussion:** TSH is classically elevated in patients with primary hypothyroidism; however, Helen T. did not have any clinical signs or symptoms of this disorder. Inappropriate elevation of TSH can be caused by a TSH-secreting pituitary tumor, thyroid hormone resistance, or assay interference. Tumor was ruled out by the normal MRI. Hormone resistance is not consistent with the patient's picture. If Helen T. had pituitary-confined resistance, persistent secretion of TSH and thyroid hormones would have led to clinical hyperthyroidism. If resistance had been general, she would have been euthyroid (as she was), but $T_4$ and $T_3$ concentrations would have been elevated along with TSH.[35]

Finally, transiently elevated TSH may be found in patients recovering from major physiological stress (e.g., intensive care illnesses and trauma), which was not the case here. Thyroid status should be evaluated after major medical problems have stabilized. The TRH challenge showed essentially no response, a finding that reflects the iatrogenic hyperthyroidism at the time. Therefore, by exclusion, Helen T.'s elevated TSH concentration most likely is an artifact, probably interfering antibodies. This condition is rare but has been described.[36]

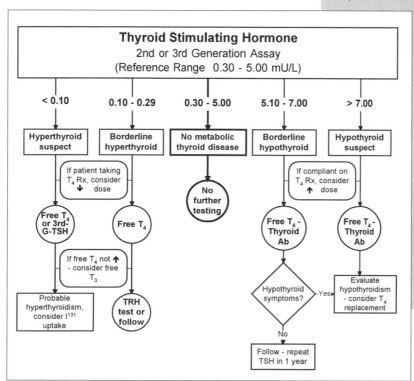

**FIGURE 2.** Algorithm for investigation of thyroid disease using second- or third-generation TSH assay as an initial test in patients without pituitary or neuropsychiatric disease. (Adapted, with permission, from Reference 17.)

$T_4$ or free $T_4$ index still are commonly used here and are increased in almost all hyperthyroid patients. Usually, both $T_3$ and $T_4$ are elevated. However, a few (<5%) hyperthyroid patients exhibit normal $T_4$ with el-

**TABLE 10.** Test Results Seen in Common Thyroid Disorders and Drug Effects on Test Results[3,13,17,33,34,a]

| Disease | Total Serum T$_4$ | Total Serum T$_3$ | T$_3$ Resin Uptake | Free T$_4$ Index | RAIU | TSH | Comment |
|---|---|---|---|---|---|---|---|
| Hypothyroidism | ↓ | ↓ | ↓ | ↓ | ↓ | ↑/↓[b] | |
| Hyperthyroidism | ↑ | ↑ | ↑ | ↑ | ↑ | ↓ | |
| T$_3$ thyrotoxicosis | No change | ↑ | No change | No change | No change/↑ | ↓ | T$_3$ resin uptake may be slightly increased |
| Euthyroid sick syndrome | No change/↓ | ↓ | ↑ | Variable | No change | No change | |
| Corticosteroids | ↓ | No change/↓ | ↑ | No change | ↓ | No change/↓ | |
| Phenytoin/aspirin | ↓ | ↓ | ↑ | No change | ↓ | No change | Large salicylate dose |
| Radiopaque media | No change/↑ | No change/↓ | No change | No change/↑ | ↓ | No change | |

[a]RAIU = radioactive iodine uptake test; ↑ = increased; ↓ = decreased.
[b]Increased TSH diagnostic of primary hypothyroidism. TSH is decreased in secondary and tertiary types.

evated T$_3$ (T$_3$ toxicosis). Second-line tests such as antithyroid antibody serologies are necessary to diagnose autoimmune thyroid disorders. Table 10 summarizes test results seen with common thyroid disorders.

# GLUCOSE

This section discusses tests that assess glucose homeostasis as it relates primarily to diabetes mellitus. Other forms of glucose imbalance (e.g., glucose intolerance and hypoglycemia), often assessed with some of the same tests, are discussed in less detail. The factors that can cause glucose concentrations to truly or spuriously rise or fall are also covered. Before considering the specific pathogeneses of diabetes mellitus and other disorders assessed by these tests, one must understand normal glucose metabolism and homeostasis.

## Glucose Homeostasis

Glucose serves as the fuel for most cellular functions and is necessary to sustain life. Glucose enters the body as dietary starch or sugar. Enzymatic reactions cleave glucose from these complex forms. The sugar is either metabolized directly for energy, with priority given to the central nervous system, or stored as glycogen in the liver or muscle for future use. The maintenance of adequate blood glucose concentrations is a function of complex regulatory mechanisms that are primarily under hormonal control.

Cells within the islets of Langerhans in the pancreas secrete at least three kinds of hormones:

➢ Glucagon.
➢ Insulin.
➢ Somatostatin.

Glucagon is secreted by the alpha cells in response to hypoglycemia, and insulin is secreted by the beta cells in response to hyperglycemia. Glucagon stimulates gluconeogenesis and the breakdown of glycogen (to glucose), fatty acids, and amino acids. Insulin stimulates their uptake, use, and storage. The third pancreatic hormone, somatostatin, is secreted by delta cells and inhibits the secretion of both glucagon and insulin as well as growth hormone from the pituitary.[37,38]

In addition to glucagon secretion, hypoglycemia leads to secretion of epinephrine, cortisol, and somatostatin. Glucagon and, to a lesser degree, epinephrine promote an immediate breakdown of glycogen and the synthesis of glucose. Cortisol and somatostatin act within hours to produce an increase in blood glucose concentrations.

Moreover, serum glucose concentrations are affected by anything that can influence glucose production or insulin production or secretion. Approximately 30–50 U of insulin normally are released into the portal vein per day. Fasting suppresses the rate of insulin secretion, and feasting generally increases insulin secretion. Other factors that may influence insulin secretion are shown in Table 11. Increased insulin secretion lowers serum glucose concentrations, and decreased secretion raises glu-

**TABLE 11.** Stimulants and Inhibitors of Insulin Secretion[37,39–41]

| Stimulants | Inhibitors |
|---|---|
| β-Adrenergic agonists | α-Adrenergic agonists |
| Amino acids | L-Asparaginase |
| Glucose | Beta-blockers |
| Sulfonylurea drugs | Diazoxide |
| Vagal stimulation | Phenytoin |
| | Somatostatin |
| | Vinblastine |

cose concentrations.

Most secreted insulin is taken up by the liver, while the remainder is metabolized by the kidneys. About 80% of glucose uptake is independent of insulin. These insulin-independent cells include nerve tissue, RBCs, liver cells, mucosal cells of the gastrointestinal (GI) tract, and exercising skeletal muscle.[42] The liver, skeletal muscle, and adipose tissue are the main tissues affected by insulin. Insulin must bind to specific cell-surface receptors to elicit a biological response.

# Hyperglycemia

Persistently elevated blood glucose concentrations suggest diabetes mellitus. If this diagnosis cannot be made in patients with elevated glucose concentrations, then the label "fasting hyperglycemia" or "glucose intolerance" may be used. Such patients may eventually develop diabetes mellitus, remain within these classifications, or return to normal glucose control. The classification, pathophysiology, and causes of diabetes mellitus and hyperglycemia are discussed here.

## Classification

The classification of diabetes mellitus is standardized. This disorder may be divided into

➤ *Insulin-dependent* diabetes mellitus (IDDM) or type I (also called ketosis prone).
➤ *Noninsulin-dependent* diabetes mellitus (NIDDM) or type II (formerly called adult onset).

IDDM is characterized by a lack of endogenous insulin, predisposition to ketoacidosis, and generally abrupt onset. Typically, this type of diabetes mellitus is diagnosed in juveniles. In contrast, patients with NIDDM are not normally dependent on exogenous insulin to sustain life and are not ketosis prone, but they usually are obese and more than 40 years old. NIDDM patients are both insulin deficient and insulin resistant.

Patients with NIDDM may present with polyuria, polydipsia, and polyphagia as well as the classical signs and symptoms of diabetes after years of subclinical glucose intolerance. Or, they may be asymptomatic so diagnosis often depends on laboratory studies. Concentrations of ketone bodies in the blood and urine typically are low or absent, even in the presence of hyperglycemia. This finding is common because the lack of insulin is not severe enough to lead to abnormalities in lypolysis and significant ketosis or acidosis.

Because of the chronicity of asymptomatic NIDDM, the long-term complications of the disease (retinopathy, nephropathy, atherosclerotic cardiovascular disease, and neuropathy) may be the first indicators. NIDDM often is identified during glucose screening sponsored by hospitals and other health care institutions.

Patients with *gestational diabetes*, a third type of glucose intolerance, develop this intolerance during pregnancy. A diabetic female who becomes pregnant is not included in this category. Glucose intolerance that develops secondary to pregnancy is associated with an increased risk of perinatal complications and an increased risk that the mother will develop overt diabetes later in life.

## Pathophysiology

In the diabetic patient, the lack of insulin action on the previously mentioned target tissues results in numerous effects. Insulin deficiency produces hyperglycemia by causing the breakdown of glycogen to glucose (glycogenolysis), causing gluconeogenesis, and decreasing the transport of glucose into cells. Cellular dehydration stimulates polydipsia. The lack of glucose as cellular fuel results in polyphagia with paradoxical weight loss. In IDDM, the glucagon response to hypoglycemia also declines.[43,44]

When liver cells are deprived of insulin, the conversion of amino acids to glucose and urea (azotemia) occurs. In addition, the breakdown and mobilization of fatty acids (lipolysis) is enhanced. These excess acids are metabolized to ketone bodies and released into the circulation. A metabolic acidosis may result (Diabetic Ketoacidosis section). In summary, insulin promotes glucose utilization and anabolism, while insulin deficiency promotes glucose intolerance and catabolism.

## Causes

Diabetes mellitus may be the result of other diseases (pancreatic and hormonal), medications, and abnormalities of the insulin receptor, or it may be due to genetic predisposition.[38] Diabetes mellitus may be due to an absolute or relative deficiency of insulin or to a resistance to its action. Deficient insulin may be the result of pancreatic beta-cell damage, impaired insulin secretion, or an abnormality in the insulin molecule itself.

NIDDM occurs when insulin's action is inadequate. This inadequacy can be caused by abnormalities of insulin-dependent cell receptors and/or a relative lack of insulin secretion. In NIDDM, lack of insulin secretion is less severe than in IDDM.

*Pancreatic cell destruction* may be related to diseases, such as cystic fibrosis, or autoimmune conditions. It can also be related to administered agents (e.g., L-asparaginase, streptozocin, and pentamidine). Similarly, hyperglycemia may result from hormonal disease in which concentrations of circulating catecholamines and glucocorticoids are increased. Such diseases include catecholamine-secreting pheochromocytoma and Cushing's disease, respectively.

*Autoimmunity* plays a major role in the pathogenesis of IDDM. Autoimmune destruction of the pancreas' beta cells is believed to be the most common etiology of

IDDM.[45] The frequent presence of the following support this hypothesis:[45,46]

> ➤ Islet cell antibodies.
> ➤ Islet cell autoantibodies.
> ➤ Antibodies to glutamic acid decarboxylase.

In fact, islet cell autoantibodies are detected in 70–80% of patients newly diagnosed with IDDM.[45] Some antibodies are directed against the beta-cell surface, and others bind to all islet cells.[47]

Various *medications or chemicals* may induce hyperglycemia and glucose intolerance. Diuretics suppress the release of insulin by inducing hypokalemia and directly inhibiting glucose transport systems. However, potassium-sparing diuretics have little or no effect on glucose. ß-Adrenergic blocking agents may impair insulin secretion in diabetic patients.

Oral contraceptives influence glucose tolerance to varying degrees, depending on the ingredients. In one study, women taking combination oral contraceptives for at least 3 months had plasma glucose concentrations 43–61% higher than controls.[48] Monophasic and triphasic combination products diminished glucose tolerance, whereas progestin-only products did not. Insulin resistance was the proposed mechanism, and fasting plasma glucose concentrations were not adversely affected. Table 12 lists medications with the potential to cause hyperglycemia.

Although 50 different substances have been listed as potential causes of methodological interference with serum glucose assays,[18] these interferences are unlikely under most laboratory and clinical situations today.

**TABLE 12.** Medications and Chemicals that May Cause Hyperglycemia[18,37–40,48–51]

| Diuretics | Steroids/hormones |
|---|---|
| Chlorthalidone | Estrogens |
| Loop diuretics[a] | Glucocorticoids |
| Metolazone | Oral contraceptives[d] |
| Thiazides | Thyroid hormones |
| **Antihypertensives** | **Miscellaneous drugs** |
| Calcium antagonists[b] | Amiodarone[b] |
| Clonidine[b] | L-Asparaginase |
| Diazoxide | Epinephrine[e] |
| **Phenothiazines**[b] | Lithium[b] |
| **Pyriminil**[c] | Nicotinic acid |
| | Pentamidine[f] |
| | Phenytoin |
| | Streptozocin |

[a]*Loop diuretics are furosemide, bumetanide, and ethacrynic acid. Torsemide has less effect on glucose concentrations.*[52]
[b]*Clinical significance is less clear.*
[c]*A rodenticide.*
[d]*Progestin-only products do not affect glucose tolerance.*
[e]*Oral sympathomimetics, such as those found in decongestants, are unlikely to be more of a cause of increased glucose than the "stress" from the illness for which they are used.*
[f]*After initial hypoglycemia, which occurs in about 4–14 (average 11) days.*

## Laboratory Tests to Assess Glucose Control

The fasting plasma glucose and 2-hr postprandial glucose tests commonly are used for evaluating glucose homeostasis. The oral glucose tolerance test mainly is used to assess equivocal results from these two tests. Hgb $A_{1c}$ and fructosamine tests are used to monitor long- and medium-term glucose control, respectively. Urine glucose monitoring in patients with diabetes mellitus gradually is being supplanted by finger-stick blood glucose tests; therefore, discussion of this test is relatively brief.

With all of these tests, proper collection and storage of the sample and performance of the procedure are important. Improper collection and storage of samples for glucose determinations can lead to false results and interpretations. Even after collection, RBCs and white blood cells (WBCs) continue to metabolize glucose in the sample tube. This process occurs unless (1) the RBCs can be separated from the serum using serum separator tubes (Appendix D) or (2) metabolism is inhibited using fluoride-containing (gray-top) tubes or refrigeration. Otherwise, glucose concentration drops by 5–10 mg/dL (0.3–0.6 mmol/L) per hour and does not reflect the patient's fasting plasma glucose at collection time. In vitro metabolic loss is hastened in samples of patients with leukocytosis or leukemia.

### Fasting Plasma Glucose and 2-Hr Postprandial Glucose
*Normal ranges: 70–110 mg/dL or 3.9–6.1 mmol/L and <150 mg/dL or 8.4 mmol/L, respectively*

A fasting plasma glucose concentration is the best indicator of glucose homeostasis. This test measures the ability of endogenous or exogenous insulin to prevent fasting hyperglycemia by regulating glucose anabolism and catabolism. Fasting plasma glucose may be used to monitor therapy in patients being treated for glucose abnormalities. For this test, the patient maintains his or her usual diet, and the assay is performed on awakening (before breakfast). This timing usually allows for an 8-hr fast.

A fasting plasma glucose greater than 140 mg/dL (>7.8 mmol/L), found on at least two occasions, is diagnostic for at least glucose intolerance. Some clinicians diagnose diabetes mellitus at this point if other signs and symptoms support it. Others confirm the diagnosis by performing a 2-hr postprandial glucose concentration; a sample is drawn 2 hr after a meal.

The diagnosis of diabetes mellitus usually can be made if the 2-hr postprandial glucose is greater than 200 mg/dL (>11.2 mmol/L), especially if previous tests reveal fasting hyperglycemia. If the results of these tests are equivocal (Diabetes Mellitus or Glucose Intolerance section), the oral glucose tolerance test should be performed.

### Oral Glucose Tolerance Test

The oral glucose tolerance test is used to assess patients

who have signs and symptoms of diabetes mellitus but who have normal or borderline fasting plasma glucose concentrations (<140 mg/dL or <7.8 mmol/L). The oral glucose tolerance test measures both the ability of the pancreas to secrete insulin following a glucose load and the body's response to insulin action. Interpretation of the test is based on the plasma glucose concentrations drawn before and during the exam. This exam may also be used in diagnosing diabetes with onset during pregnancy if the disease threatens the health of the mother and fetus. The oral glucose tolerance test is not indicated in patients who have fasting plasma glucose greater than 140 mg/dL on at least two separate occasions. Such values are already highly suggestive of diabetes mellitus. Administration of a glucose load would serve only to exacerbate hyperglycemia.

The oral glucose tolerance test is performed by giving a standard 75-g dose of an oral glucose solution over 5 min following an overnight fast. The pediatric dose is 1.75 g/kg up to a maximum of 75 g. Blood samples commonly are drawn before the test, between 0 and 2 hr, and at 2 hr. In pregnant women, the test dose is 100 g; plasma glucose concentrations are drawn before the test (fasting) and at 1-, 2-, and 3-hr intervals. The samples should be collected into tubes containing sodium fluoride, unless the assay will be performed immediately.

If the patient vomits the test dose, the exam is invalid and must be repeated. The oral glucose tolerance test is diagnostic for diabetes mellitus if the fasting plasma glucose is at least 140 mg/dL (7.8 mmol/L) or if the 2-hr plasma glucose is at least 200 mg/dL (11.2 mmol/L). The patient is considered to have impaired glucose tolerance if the fasting value is less than 140 mg/dL but the 2-hr concentration is 140–200 mg/dL (7.8–11.2 mmol/L).

The oral glucose tolerance test should not be performed on individuals who are chronically malnourished, consume inadequate carbohydrates (<150 g/day), or are bedridden. Alcohol consumption and medications that cause hyperglycemia (Table 10) should be stopped 3 days prior to the examination. Coffee and smoking are not permitted during the test.[38]

### Glycated Hemoglobin
*Normal range: 3–6% but varies*

Hgb $A_{1c}$, also referred to glycosylated or glycated Hgb $A_{1c}$, is a component of the Hgb molecule. During the 120-day lifespan of a RBC, glucose is irreversibly bound to the Hgb moieties in proportion to the average serum glucose. The process is called glycosylation. Measurement of Hgb $A_{1c}$ is, therefore, indicative of glucose control during the preceding 2–3 months. The total Hgb $A_1$ molecule—composed of $A_{1a}$, $A_{1b}$, and $A_{1c}$—is not used because subfractions $A_{1a}$ and $A_{1b}$ are more susceptible to nonglucose adducts in the blood of patients with opiate addiction, lead poisoning, uremia, and alcoholism.[53] Be-

cause the test is for Hgb, the specimen analyzed is RBCs and not serum or plasma.

Hgb $A_{1c}$ may be used to monitor diet, exercise, and drug therapy in diabetic patients. Results are not affected by daily fluctuations in the blood glucose concentration, and a fasting sample is not required. Results reflect overall patient compliance to treatment regimens. With most assays, 95% of normal individuals' Hgb is 3–6% glycated. However, patients with persistent hyperglycemia may have an Hgb $A_{1c}$ up to 20%. An Hgb $A_{1c}$ greater than 13% suggests poor glucose control.

The mean daily plasma glucose concentration can be estimated with the formula $10 \times (Hgb\ A_{1c} + 4)$.[12] Reference ranges and interpretations vary with the assay method.

A few situations confound interpretation of test results. False elevations in Hgb $A_{1c}$ may be noted with uremia, chronic alcohol intake, and hypertriglyceridemia.[54] Patients who have diseases with chronic or episodic hemolysis (e.g., sickle cell disease and thalassemia) generally have spuriously low Hgb $A_{1c}$ concentrations caused by the predominance of young RBCs (which carry less Hgb $A_{1c}$) in the circulation. In splenectomized patients and those with polycythemia, Hgb $A_{1c}$ is increased. If these disorders are stable, the test still can be used, but values must be compared with the patient's previous results rather than published normal values. Both falsely elevated and falsely lowered measurements of Hgb $A_{1c}$ may also occur during pregnancy; therefore, it should not be used to screen for gestational diabetes.

### Fructosamine
*Normal range: <285 μmol/L but varies*

Fructosamine is a general term that is applied to any glycated protein. Unlike the Hgb $A_{1c}$ test, only glycated proteins in the serum or plasma (e.g., albumin)—not erythrocytes—are measured. In nondiabetics, the unstable complex dissociates into glucose and protein. Therefore, only small quantities of fructosamine circulate. In diabetic patients, higher glucose concentrations favor the generation of more stable glycation, and higher concentrations of fructosamine are found.

Fructosamine has no known inherent toxicological activity but can be used as a marker of medium-term glucose control. Fructosamine correlates with glucose control over 2–3 weeks based on the half-lives of albumin (14–20 days) and other serum proteins (2.5–23 days). As a result, high fructosamine concentrations may alert caregivers to deteriorating glycemic control earlier than increases in Hgb $A_{1c}$.

Several limitations to this test exist. Falsely elevated results may occur when

> Serum (not whole blood) Hgb concentrations are greater than 100 mg/dL (normally <15 mg/dL).

➢ Bilirubin is greater than 4 mg/dL.

➢ Ascorbic acid is greater than 5 mg/dL.

Methyldopa and calcium dobesilate, used outside the United States to minimize myocardial damage after an acute infarction, also may cause falsely elevated results. Serum fructosamine concentrations are lower in obese diabetics compared to lean diabetic patients.[55] Some clinicians advocate the use of fructosamine concentrations as a screening test.[56]

### Urine Glucose
*Normal: negative*

Glucose "spills" into the urine when the serum glucose concentration exceeds the renal threshold for glucose reabsorption (normally 180 mg/dL). However, poor correlation exists between urine glucose and concurrent serum glucose concentrations. This poor correlation occurs because urine is "made" hours before it is tested, unless the inconvenient double-void method (urine is collected 30 min after emptying of the bladder) is used. Furthermore, the renal threshold varies among patients and tends to increase in diabetes over time, especially if renal function is declining.

Although urine testing gradually is being replaced by convenient finger-stick blood sugar testing, some patients (especially with diabetes controlled by diet and exercise alone) still use urine testing routinely to monitor glycemic control. Unfortunately, over 50% of them do not perform the procedure correctly.[57]

The presence and amount of glucose in the urine can be determined by two different techniques. Commercial products that use copper-reducing methods (e.g., Clinitest) provide the most quantitative estimate of the degree of glycosuria. Therefore, this method is preferred for patients who spill large quantities of glucose into the urine. The two-drop method can detect higher quantities of glucose (3–5%) than the five-drop method, which can quantitate only up to 2%. Generally, copper-reducing products have poor specificity for glucose (Table 11).

Contrary to popular belief, isoniazid, methyldopa, and ascorbic acid do not interfere with Clinitest. The literature is unclear on whether chloral hydrate, nitrofurantoin, probenecid, and nalidixic acid interfere with this method. Most antibacterial classes have been tested. If the substances are not listed in Table 13, they are unlikely to interfere.[58]

**TABLE 13.** Drugs Causing False-Positive Results with Clinitest[18,37,39–41,58]

| | |
|---|---|
| Aztreonam[a] | Levodopa |
| Cephalosporins[b] | Penicillins[a] |
| Imipenem[a] | Salicylates |

[a]*May also cause false-negative results.*
[b]*May also cause green-brown uninterpretable results.*

Patients should be aware that a "pass-through" phenomenon occurs with this test when more than 2% glucose is in the urine. During the test, a fleeting orange color may appear at the climax of the reaction and fade to a greenish brown when the reaction is complete. The latter color (0.75–1%) may be incorrectly used, and the glucose concentration actually may be much greater.

The second method of urine glucose testing is specific for glucose and provides a more qualitative assessment of it in the urine. Commercial products of this type (e.g., Tes-Tape, Clinistix, Diastix, and Chemstrip) consist of plastic dipsticks with paper pads that have been impregnated with glucose oxidase. These tests are sensitive to 0.1% glucose (100 mg/dL). Substances that may cause false-negative results with this type of test include ascorbic acid (high dose), salicylates (high dose), and levodopa. Interference also has been reported with phenazopyridine and X-ray contrast media, but the likelihood is less clear.[58]

### Self-Monitoring Tests

Reagent strips and stripless glucose sensors are commercially available so that patients may perform blood glucose monitoring. These strips and sensors are based on the ability of glucose oxidase to generate hydrogen peroxide. These systems are also used frequently in hospitals, where nurses rely on quick results for determining insulin requirements according to a prescribed sliding scale. The reagent strips may be used with or without a colorimeter. Manual or automatic lancet injectors are used to obtain a capillary blood sample from a fingerstick. The blood droplet is placed on a reagent strip, and the color that appears is compared to a color chart corresponding to specific blood glucose values. Use of a colorimeter eliminates the need to estimate the color match and provides the result on a digital display.

Most, if not all, hydrogen peroxide-based blood glucose monitors are not affected by ascorbic acid, Hgb, acetaminophen, SCr, bilirubin, uric acid, heparin, and high-lipid concentrations. The only exception is high-dose ascorbic acid, which may falsely suppress glucose readings with some equipment (e.g., Glucostix).[59] With some machines, swabbing the finger with iodine can falsely elevate the reading. Conversely, dopamine infusions can lead to falsely low readings. The ExacTech Pen and Companion, Pen 2, Companion 2, and Glucometer Elite use an amperometric measurement and are smaller than the other devices. These devices, except Glucometer Elite, do not require wiping of the blood from the strip before inserting it in the machine, because the end of the strip that contains the blood does not enter the meter. Most products take 0.5–1.5 min to run through the procedure and can read glucose concentrations of 20–600 mg/dL.[60]

Generally, blood glucose concentrations determined by these methods are clinically useful estimates of corresponding plasma glucose concentrations measured by the laboratory. Therefore, home blood glucose monitoring is preferred to urine testing. However, the high cost of supplies, a patient's reluctance to "stick" himself or herself, and a lack of manual dexterity may preclude the use of home blood glucose monitoring in certain patients. Furthermore, dirty machines may lead to falsely low readings at home. This problem can be identified by comparing results with a machine at the clinic or office. Nevertheless, for capable patients, home blood testing clarifies the relationship between symptomatology and blood glucose concentrations.

## Diagnosis of Hyperglycemia

The diagnosis of patients with hyperglycemia commonly falls into one of three categories: (1) diabetes mellitus or glucose intolerance, (2) diabetic ketoacidosis, and (3) hyperosmolar nonketotic hyperglycemia syndrome.

### *Diabetes Mellitus or Glucose Intolerance*

The diagnosis of diabetes mellitus may be made on the basis of any one of the following criteria:

> Any unequivocal or gross elevation of plasma glucose (>200 mg/dL or >11.2 mmol/L) in conjunction with the classic signs of diabetes (i.e., polyuria, polydipsia, and polyphagia).
> A fasting plasma glucose greater than 140 mg/dL (>7.8 mmol/L) on at least two separate occasions.
> Oral glucose tolerance test values at 2 hr and at least one other sampling during the exam greater than 200 mg/dL.

Table 14 summarizes the diagnostic indicators of glucose intolerance based on the fasting plasma glucose and the oral glucose tolerance test (Minicase 3, next page).

*Goals of therapy.* Once diabetes mellitus is diagnosed, the clinician needs to establish a therapeutic goal with respect to glucose control. The ideal goal would be to maintain

concentrations at normal physiological levels. For IDDM patients, this effort requires tight control. Tight control could include preprandial plasma glucose concentrations of 70–120 mg/dL (3.9–6.7 mmol/L) and postprandial concentrations of less than 180 mg/dL (<10 mmol/L). Control this tight requires intensive therapy and monitoring (three or more insulin injections per day and self-monitoring of glucose concentrations).

However, recent data from the Diabetes Control and Complications Trial (DCCT) suggest that the effort leads to significant health benefits.[63] Overall, the study showed that intensive therapy delays the onset and slows progression of diabetic retinopathy, nephropathy, and neuropathy in patients with IDDM. Microvascular (retinopathy and nephropathy) and neurological complications were diminished, as were macrovascular (large vessel) diseases. The difference in macrovascular complications, however, did not reach statistical significance.[63] No difference existed between the conventional and intensive therapy groups with respect to absolute risk for cardiac events. Statistical significance may not have been reached due to the short followup period (6.5 years) and the young average age (34 years). In IDDM patients, the peak frequency for development of coronary disease is age 55. Macrovascular diseases include peripheral vascular disease, stroke, and coronary heart disease. Whether these results can be extrapolated to NIDDM patients is not known.

Although tight control seems beneficial, most clinicians feel that control should not be so "tight" as to cause recurrent, overt episodes of hypoglycemia. If these episodes are severe enough, they may lead to immediate, permanent brain damage. There often is a tradeoff. For example, patients in the intensive therapy arm of the DCCT had a two- to threefold higher frequency of severe hypoglycemia.

*Impact of exogenous insulin on glucose concentrations.* Because the most common and effective means to manage IDDM is with insulin, the importance of the relationship between insulin injection and interpretation of glucose concentrations is briefly discussed. In general, 1 U

**TABLE 14.** Diagnosis of Glucose Tolerance Based on Fasting Plasma Glucose Concentration and Oral Glucose Tolerance Test (OGTT)[61,62]

| Level of Glucose Tolerance | Venous Plasma Glucose[a] (mg/dL) | | | |
| --- | --- | --- | --- | --- |
| | Fasting Plasma Glucose | OGTT Value at 30, 60, or 90 min | OGTT Value at 2 hr | OGTT Value at 3 hr |
| "Normal" | <115 | <200 | <140 | |
| Impaired glucose tolerance (age <50 years) | <140 | >200 | 140–200 | |
| Diabetes mellitus | >140 | >200 | >200 | |
| Gestational diabetes | <105 | >190 (1 hr) | >165 | >145 |

[a]Multiply number by 0.056 to convert glucose to International System (SI) units (mmol/L).

## ✎ Minicase 3

Laura O., a 5-ft 5-in, 195-lb, 58-year-old female, visited a community walk-in clinic for the first time with complaints of weakness and polyuria worsening over the past few weeks. Because she had to go to the bathroom often during the past few nights, she did not sleep much and was exhausted. She has no steady health care provider in the area. Her past medical history included hypertension (treated with hydrochlorthiazide 50 mg daily) and a 10-year history of glaucoma (treated with timolol 0.5% eyedrops). She also had taken estrogen and calcium carbonate for the past 8 years. She gained 30 lb over the past year, and a calorie estimate revealed that she took in about 2800 kcal/day.

Laura O. had no known family history of diabetes. Her physical exam was normal, except for slightly dry skin, legs cool to touch with weak pedal pulses, and slightly diminished pedal pinprick sensation. Her vital signs were BP 110/60, temperature 97.5 °F (36.4 °C), HR 60/min, and respiration rate 20/min. A dipstick of her urine was normal, except for 1+ (30 mg/dL) protein and trace (100 mg/dL) glucose. A finger-stick blood glucose was 180 mg/dL 2 hr after breakfast. Her physician told her to decrease her diuretic dose to 25 mg daily and to call back in a few days if that did not help her polyuria.

Four days later, Laura O. visited the clinic again because her symptoms were not any better even though she followed directions. Her fasting plasma glucose (no food for 8 hr) was 210 mg/dL. Her BUN and SCr from the previous visit were normal at 15 and 1.2 mg/dL, respectively, as were all other chemistries (including uric acid and lipids). Her urine glucose was 250 mg/dL with negative ketones, and she still had 1+ proteinuria. Her specific gravity was normal at 1.010.

*What type of glucose intolerance afflicts Laura O.? Is there enough evidence for a definitive diagnosis at this time? Are there any factors contributing to the hyperglycemia that may be corrected in the short term? In the long term?*

**Discussion:** Laura O. seems to have "idiopathic" NIDDM, although it could certainly be drug induced or exacerbated. Her picture is not clear based solely on the first two criteria for diagnosis of diabetes mellitus. She had classic symptoms and a blood glucose concentration of 180 mg/dL on her first visit. However, this concentration is not unequivocal, especially since it was taken only about 2 hr after her last meal. She was spilling small amounts of glucose then and slightly more on the second visit. This spilling apparently was enough to cause an osmotic diuresis and polyuria/nocturia.

Laura O. had a fasting plasma glucose greater than 140 mg/dL (>7.8 mmol/L) on only one occasion. The polyuria could have been caused by the diuretic. However, the dose had not changed for years, and a dosage reduction led to no improvement. The diuretic and estrogens could be contributing to the diabetes, as could her weight gain. The estrogen could be stopped and the diuretic changed to an angiotensin-converting enzyme inhibitor (e.g., enalapril) to see if the drugs were contributing.

The fact that Laura O. has some signs of NIDDM complications indicates that she has had a subclinical form of the disease for many years. These signs include legs cool to the touch and weak pedal pulses (evidence of macrovascular disease), slightly diminished pedal pinprick sensation (evidence of early neuropathy), and microalbuminemia (evidence of early stages of microvascular nephropathy). Although one more bona fide fasting glucose greater than 140 mg/dL or a positive glucose tolerance test would allow a definitive diagnosis, it is not needed with all of the other evidence.

Laura O.'s management should include diet and exercise control, which will lead to weight loss. Some overweight diabetics become euglycemic with weight loss. If these measures are not successful, oral hypoglycemic drugs will be needed.

---

of any type (human or pork) or form (regular or NPH) of insulin gives the same metabolic activity as another. Every 1–2-U increase in the insulin dose usually leads to a 30–50-mg/dL decrease in the glucose concentration. Although the amount of *total* activity is equal for any given number of units of any insulin, the activity is not elicited evenly over time. A clinician must know the activity-over-time profiles of various insulin types at various injection sites for various species to anticipate correctly a dose's effect on glucose concentrations at a particular time (Table 15).

Figure 3 illustrates the concentrations of insulin activity relative to meals over time after various regimens of subcutaneous insulin injections. The regimens on the left are less intensive than those on the right, which require at least three injections per day. The intensive regimens attempt to mimic those seen with normal physiological responses to meals and sleep.

In a minimal regimen (a), one mixed injection (intermediate-acting insulin and regular insulin) is administered before breakfast. Regular insulin is active in the morning, whereas the activity of intermediate-acting insulin peaks in the afternoon or evening. The patient is most prone to hypoglycemia before lunch and during the late afternoon, and fasting hyperglycemia may occur because of waning insulin activity overnight.

A mixed injection of intermediate-acting and regular insulin is administered before breakfast and dinner in an average regimen between minimal and intensive (b). In addition to the risk of hypoglycemia before lunch and in the late afternoon, the administration of intermediate-acting insulin before dinner predisposes patients to hypoglycemia from 2 to 4 a.m.

An average regimen (c) combines a mixed injection of intermediate-acting and regular insulin given before breakfast with another injection of intermediate-acting insulin given before bedtime. Intermediate-acting insulin administered at bedtime provides safer, more effective overnight glucose control. Without insulin administered before dinner, however, glucose concentrations may be-

**TABLE 15.** Relative Effects of Injection Site, Insulin Type, and Insulin Species on Absorption Rate and Duration of Activity in a Given Individual[a]

| Insulin Kinetics and Dynamics | Site of Injection | | | |
|---|---|---|---|---|
| | Abdomen | Arm | Leg | Buttock |
| Absorption rate (onset) | Fastest | Fast | Slow | Slowest |
| Duration of activity | Shortest | Short | Long | Longest |

| Insulin Kinetics and Dynamics | Insulin Type | | | |
|---|---|---|---|---|
| | Regular | NPH | Lente | Ultralente |
| Absorption rate (onset) | Fastest | Intermediate | Slow | Slowest |
| Duration of activity | Shortest | Intermediate | Long | Longest |

| Insulin Kinetics and Dynamics | Insulin Species | | | |
|---|---|---|---|---|
| | Human | Pork | Beef and Pork | Beef[b] |
| Absorption rate (onset) | Fastest | Fast | Slow | Slowest |
| Duration of activity | Shortest | Short | Long | Longest |

[a]*The rates listed are relative to each other within the same group (i.e., site, type, and species) and within a given individual. They are only semiquantitative and should be used merely as a guide in anticipating changes in glucose concentrations after changes in one of the above factors.*
[b]*Beef insulin is no longer commercially available but is included for historical comparison.*
*(Adapted from Reference 64.)*

come unacceptably high *after* dinner.

In one intensive regimen (**d**), the patient administers three injections: a mixed injection before breakfast, regular insulin before dinner, and intermediate-acting insulin before bedtime. Intensive regimens require more

frequent monitoring and are accompanied by an increased risk of hypoglycemia.

In another intensive regimen (**e**), three preprandial injections of regular insulin are combined with one injection of intermediate-acting insulin before bedtime.

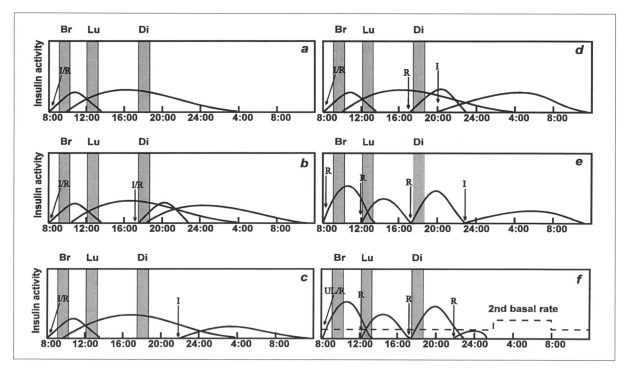

**FIGURE 3.** Insulin activity profiles of six insulin formulations and combinations of formulations. I = intermediate-acting insulin; R = rapid-acting (regular) insulin; UL = long-acting insulin (dashed line). Arrows indicate time of administration [breakfast (Br), lunch (Lu), and dinner (Di)]. (Reprinted, with permission, from Nathan DM. Metabolism. In: Dale DC, Federman DD, eds. Scientific American Medicine, vol 2. New York: Scientific American Medicine; 1995.)

Preprandial doses of regular insulin are adjusted according to glucose concentrations, meal size, and anticipated exercise.

In a third intensive regimen (f), either ultralente insulin or an insulin pump supplies the basal rate. To achieve normal fasting glucose concentrations, a second basal rate may need to be established by providing a higher rate of insulin infusion via the insulin pump (usually from 2 to 8 a.m.). This higher rate meets the rise in insulin requirements during the dawn hours (the "dawn phenomenon") and may be 1.5–2 times higher than the basal rate during the day. Regular insulin is given before meals and occasionally before bedtime.

For all regimens in Figure 3, regular insulin should be given 30–45 min before meals unless the preprandial glucose concentration is below 70 mg/dL (<3.9 mmol/L). If the concentration is less than 70 mg/dL, the patient should eat immediately. In all regimens, regular insulin doses are adjusted on the basis of self-monitored preprandial glucose concentrations. One adjustment algorithm is displayed in Table 16. Intermediate-acting insulin doses can also be adjusted on the basis of the glucose concentration pattern.

Of course, insulin alone cannot regulate glucose. Diet, exercise, and stress must always be considered.

Based on the typical effect of insulin on glucose concentrations, clinicians have designed algorithms or "sliding scales" to bring and keep glycemia under control. Although the patient's sensitivity to insulin can and should change the algorithm, a common sliding scale for patient self-adjustment of supplemental regular insulin is given in Table 16. This algorithm assumes that the patient's basic insulin dose (usually prebreakfast daily dose of NPH or Lente) has adequately controlled the prebreakfast glucose until the present, while exercise and diet have remained relatively constant.

With the advent of accurate, user-friendly blood glucose meters, sliding scales for insulin administration now are based on glucose concentrations in the blood as opposed to the urine. The algorithm applies to preprandial concentrations and regular insulin. In other words, if the prelunch concentration is higher than desired, the patient increases the prebreakfast regular insulin dose. On subsequent days, this increase in units may be added to the basic daily dose of intermediate-acting insulin (NPH or Lente) while adjusting at this time interval. If the predinner concentration is high, the patient increases the prelunch supplemental dose of regular insulin. The benefits of tighter control can be realized more easily with these protocols.

The posthypoglycemic hyperglycemia phenomenon is another concept that affects therapeutics. The clinician must appreciate it to prevent inappropriate changes in insulin dosage when responding to glucose concentrations. This event (also known as the Somogyi effect) usually occurs during the early morning after the patient administers too much insulin or eats too few calories the previous day. Counter-regulatory hormones (e.g., glucagon, cortisol, and epinephrine) increase glucose concentrations during sleep so that the patient awakes to high fasting glucose concentrations in the morning. This paradoxical situation may lead the patient to increase the insulin dose inappropriately. Low glucose concentrations taken at 3–4 a.m. help to identify this problem. Insulin regimens should be adjusted so that pharmacological activity during the early morning hours (2–4 a.m.) is decreased. Moreover, nightmares and night sweats suggest this effect.

### Diabetic Ketoacidosis

The clinical and laboratory abnormalities described below are characteristic of diabetic ketoacidosis, the most severe disorder along the continuum of glucose intolerance in IDDM patients. Patients identified before diabetic ketoacidosis evolves may have many of the same findings, although less severe.

In insulin-deficient states, the breakdown and mobilization of fatty acids are enhanced. They are metabolized by the liver to ketone bodies (acetone, ß-hydroxybutyric acid, and acetoacetic acid), which are released into the circulation. When ketone bodies are excreted into the urine, their presence there is called ketonuria. Without adequate insulin, this process progresses to diabetic ketoacidosis, in which accumulation of the acids contributes to acidosis. The most common causes of diabetic ketoacidosis are[65]

➤ Infections (30%).
➤ Noncompliance (20%).

**TABLE 16.** Typical Sliding Scale for Adjustment of Preprandial Supplementation with Regular Insulin[a]

| Blood Glucose Concentration (mg/dL) | Regular Insulin |
|---|---|
| <60 | ↓ by 2 U |
| 60–80 | ↓ by 1 U |
| 81–120 | No change |
| 121–170 | ↑ by 1 U |
| 171–220 | ↑ by 2 U |
| 221–270 | ↑ by 3 U |
| 271–320 | ↑ by 4 U[b] |

[a]The patient may be instructed not to increase the supplemental regular insulin dose unless the preprandial glucose concentration exceeds the target concentration for a given number of days (often 2–4). The algorithm assumes that exercise and diet have remained relatively constant. This protocol is relatively conservative; higher insulin doses may be needed for a given range in some patients.
[b]Some clinicians will ask patients to check their urine for ketones. If positive for two consecutive readings, patients are asked to report these results.

➤ Newly diagnosed IDDM (25%).

➤ Unknown or no precipitating event (25%).

Clinically, patients typically present with dehydration, lethargy, acetone-smelling breath, abdominal pain, tachycardia, orthostatic hypotension, tachypnea, and, occasionally, mild hypothermia and lethargy or coma. Because of the diabetic's tendency toward low temperatures, fever strongly suggests infection as a precipitant of diabetic ketoacidosis.

Chemically, diabetic ketoacidosis is characterized by a high glucose concentration. This concentration typically is 350–650 mg/dL (20–36 mmol/L). However, concentrations may range from 200 mg/dL (11 mmol/L) to greater than 1000 mg/dL (>56 mmol/L).[66] Patients who have continued to administer insulin, are pregnant, have not eaten adequately, or have vomited excessively generally present with lower glucose concentrations.[67] As insulin is given, the glucose concentrations decline at a rate of about 75–100 mg/dL/hr.

Diabetic ketoacidosis is also characterized by low bicarbonate (<10 mEq/L) and pH (<7.25). In addition to volume depletion, patients often have a deficit of total body sodium, potassium (200–400 mEq), and other electrolytes (e.g., phosphate and magnesium). These deficiencies primarily are due to glucosuria-induced osmotic diuresis.

In addition, total body phosphate often is depleted by about 0.15–1.5 mmol/kg due to extracellular shifting. Although phosphate salts usually are given to patients with hypophosphatemia, they probably do not influence the clinical course.[68]

Decreased vascular volume raises the glucose concentration further and may confound proper interpretation of electrolyte, BUN, and hematological results. Serum sodium concentrations often are low, not necessarily as a true reflection of total body stores but because of test interferences from high glucose and infrequently from high triglycerides (Chapters 1 and 6). Sodium results can be corrected (so that they can be interpreted relative to the usual normal reference range) by adding 2 mEq/L for every 100 mg/dL glucose above 200 mg/dL. Electrolyte imbalances may not be apparent early in the disorder with serum sodium, potassium, and perhaps other minerals in the normal or slightly high range due to hemoconcentration, but concentrations quickly fall on rehydration. Likewise, rehydration, along with insulin infusion, contributes later in the course to lowering glucose (Minicase 4, next page).

Potassium concentrations also may be elevated initially due to metabolic acidosis (Chapter 6). Correction of acidosis elicits the opposite effect. Potassium shifts intracellularly and out of the serum with insulin therapy, leading to a decrease in serum potassium concentrations.

Serum osmolality typically is 300–320 mOsm/kg;

normally, it is 280–295 mOsm/kg. Serum osmolarity (milliosmoles per liter), which is practically equivalent to osmolality (milliosmoles per kilogram), can be estimated by

serum osmolarity (mOsm/L) =

$$(2 \times \text{sodium}) + \frac{\text{glucose}}{18} + \frac{\text{BUN}}{2.8}$$

where glucose and BUN units are milligrams per deciliter.

Ketones are present in the blood and urine of patients in diabetic ketoacidosis, as the name of this disorder implies. Formation of ketone bodies (acetoacetate, acetone, and ß-hydroxybutyrate) is the main cause of acidosis in diabetic ketoacidosis. The usual, nitroprusside-based (nitroferricyanide) assays (Acetest, Ketostix, Labstix, and Multistix) do not detect ß-hydroxybutyrate and are 15–20 times more sensitive to acetoacetate than to acetone. In a few situations [e.g., severe hypovolemia, hypotension, low partial pressure of oxygen ($pO_2$), and alcoholism] where ß-hydroxybutyrate predominates, assessment of ketones may be falsely low. As diabetic ketoacidosis resolves, ß-hydroxybutyric acid is converted to acetoacetate, the assay-reactive ketone body. Therefore, a stronger reaction may be encountered in laboratory results. However, this reaction does not necessarily mean a worsening of the ketoacidotic state.

Ketones in the blood are measured or assayed by mixing serum with an equal volume of water or saline sequentially to achieve dilutions of 1:1, 1:2, 1:4, 1:8, etc. The tests are semiquantitative, with readings from 1+ to 4+. A positive nitroprusside ketone test at a dilution of 1:8 or higher should be interpreted as a clinically important degree of ketonemia.

Clinicians must keep in mind that ketonuria may also result from starvation, high-fat diets, fever, and anesthesia, but these conditions are not associated with hyperglycemia. Levodopa, mesna,[69] acetylcysteine (irrigation),[70] methyldopa, phenazopyridine, pyrazinamide, valproic acid, captopril,[71,72] and high-dose aspirin may cause false-positive results with urine ketone tests.[18] The influence of these drugs on serum ketone tests has not been studied extensively. If the ketone concentration is increased, a typical series of dipstick results is

1. Negative.
2. Trace or 5 mg/dL.
3. Small or 15 mg/dL.
4. Moderate or 40 mg/dL.
5. Large or 80 mg/dL.
6. Very large or 160 mg/dL.

Outside of diabetic ketoacidosis, urine ketone testing is done by IDDM patients when their fasting blood glucose concentration exceeds 240 mg/dL (>13.5 mmol/L) or when physiological (or emotional) stress is

## Minicase 4

Eugene T., a 45-year-old male with a 30-year history of IDDM, was brought into the emergency department after his wife found him to be "out of it" when attempting to wake him. Five days ago, he developed fever, nasal congestion, polyuria, and increasing nausea and abdominal aches. He took no medications except for insulin, captopril 25 mg twice a day for hypertension, multivitamins, and, recently, phenylephrine nasal spray. Over the past 3 days, he did not eat much.

To "adjust" for his decreased caloric intake, Eugene T. stopped injecting his usual insulin dose despite seeing increasing blood sugars with his glucometer (according to his meter's memory, fasting glucoses of 145, 180, 200, and 250 mg/dL). Physical examination revealed a lethargic male with a BP of 115/65 (which dropped to 95/50 when sitting), HR 105, respiratory rate 30 (deep and regular), and oral temperature 101.4 °F (38.6 °C). His skin turgor was poor, and his mucous membranes were dry. Eugene T. had a fruity aromatic odor to his breath and was disoriented and confused. His lab results were as follows:

- Sodium, 143 mEq/L (136–145 mEq/L).
- Potassium, 3.5 mEq/L (3.5–5.0 mEq/L).
- Chloride, 99 mEq/L (96–106 mEq/L).
- BUN, 38 mg/dL (8–20 mg/dL).
- SCr, 2.8 mg/dL (0.7–1.5 mg/dL).
- Phosphorus, 2.7 mg/dL (2.6–4.5 mg/dL).
- Amylase, 350 IU/L (44–128 IU/L).
- pH, 7.15 (7.36–7.44).
- Bicarbonate, 9.0 mEq/L (24–30 mEq/L).
- Hct, 52% (42–52%).
- WBCs, $16 \times 10^3$ cells/mm³ ($4.8–10.8 \times 10^3$ cells/mm³).
- Calcium, 9 mg/dL (8.5–10.8 mg/dL).
- Glucose, 650 mg/dL (70–110 mg/dL).
- Ketones, 3+ @1:8 serum dilution (normal = 0).
- Osmolality, 335 mOsm/kg (280–295 mOsm/kg).
- Triglycerides, 174 mg/dL (10–160 mg/dL).
- Lipase, 1.4 U/mL (<1.5 U/mL).
- Magnesium, 2 mEq/L (1.5–2.2 mEq/L).

A urine screen with Multistix indicated a "large" (160 mg/dL) amount of ketones, the highest designation on the strip.

*Based on clinical and lab findings, what is the most likely diagnosis for Eugene T.? What precipitated this metabolic disorder? Can interpretation of any results be influenced by his acidosis or hyperglycemia? Are there potential drug interferences with any lab tests?*

**Discussion:** Eugene T., an IDDM patient, developed diabetic ketoacidosis from an infection and discontinuation of his insulin. Diabetic ketoacidosis rarely occurs in patients with NIDDM. Clinically, the patient's presentation is classic. His decreased skin turgor, dry mucous membranes, tachycardia (HR of 105), and orthostatic hypotension are consistent with dehydration, a common condition in patients with diabetic ketoacidosis. His breathing is rapid and deep. Although he is not coma-

tose, he is lethargic, confused, and disoriented.

Chemically, Eugene T. probably has a *total body* deficit of sodium and potassium despite *serum* concentration results within normal limits. Orthostatic hypotension is consistent with decreased intravascular volume, causing hemoconcentration of these minerals. Therefore, these values do not reflect total body stores, and the clinician can expect them to decline rapidly if unsupplemented fluids are infused. Although the patient's phosphorus concentration is in the normal range (lower end), it likely will decrease after rehydration and insulin. Serial testing should be done every 3–4 hr during the first 24 hr.

Serial glucose, ketones, and acid–base measurements, typical of diabetic ketoacidosis, should show gradual improvement with proper therapy. With use of the sodium correction factor (addition of 2 mEq/L to the sodium result for every 100 mg/dL of glucose above 200 mg/dL), Eugene T.'s sodium would have been 152 mEq/L had his glucose been normal, a value more consistent with the BUN and Hct concentrations. Another correction factor can be applied to adjust potassium. For reasons described in Chapter 6, Eugene T.'s potassium would have been 5.5–6.0 mEq/L had he not been acidemic. In other words, if his acidosis were corrected without rehydration, his potassium probably would rise above the normal range to 5.5–6.0 mEq/L. This situation does not occur in practice because rehydration is addressed concurrently.

Decreased intravascular volume has led to hemoconcentrated Hct and BUN. BUN is also elevated by decreased renal perfusion (prerenal azotemia), although intrinsic renal causes should be considered if SCr is also elevated. Fortunately, as is probably the case with Eugene T., high SCr may be an artifact caused by the influence of ketone bodies on the assay (Chapter 7). If so, SCr concentrations should decline with ketone concentrations.

Eugene T. also exhibits the typical leukocytosis that often accompanies diabetic ketoacidosis, even in the absence of infection. His osmolarity based on the osmolarity estimation formula would be $(2 \times 143) + (650/18) + (38/2.8) = 335.7$ mOsm/L, approximately equal to the laboratory result. This value is slightly higher than normal for diabetic ketoacidosis (300–320 mOsm/kg).

Finally, Eugene T. had a 3+ serum ketone reading at a dilution of 1:8, not unexpected given the overall severity of his diabetic ketoacidosis. A urine screen also indicated the presence of ketones. Even if the captopril he was taking had falsely "elevated" the urine ketone screen, the results still would have to be interpreted as real and significant, given the serum ketones and all of the other signs and symptoms. For academic purposes, the impact of the drug could be tested (Chapter 3) after the diabetic ketoacidosis resolves.

A serum amylase and lipase were measured to rule out pancreatitis, usually suspected with abdominal pain. However, elevated amylase probably originated from the salivary glands because Eugene T.'s lipase was normal. This finding is seen in 20% of diabetic ketoacidosis patients (Chapter 11).

unusually high (e.g., during an acute infection). If ketonuria is present, serum ketones should be measured to assess the severity of the ketosis.

### Hyperosmolar Nonketotic Hyperglycemia Syndrome

If a patient presents with extreme hyperglycemia (600–2000 mg/dL or 34–112 mmol/L) but with insignificant ketonemia and a normal or slightly low bicarbonate concentration, the patient is not experiencing diabetic ketoacidosis but hyperosmolar nonketotic hyperglycemia syndrome. As with diabetic ketoacidosis, patients experience dehydration, hypovolemia, disorientation, and, in severe cases, coma. The onset of the syndrome is often more insidious than with diabetic ketoacidosis, with polyuria worsening over many days or weeks.

This syndrome occurs most often in elderly patients with NIDDM who do not drink enough to keep up with the osmotic diuresis. In many cases, patients are taking drugs that cause glucose intolerance (e.g., diuretics, steroids, and phenytoin). Stroke and infection are nondrug predisposing factors. Initially, electrolytes are within normal ranges, but the BUN routinely is elevated. Serum osmolalities characteristically are higher than those in diabetic ketoacidosis—in the range of 320–400 mOsm/kg. Electrolytes (e.g., magnesium, phosphorus, and calcium) should be monitored until stable.

## Diagnosis of Hypoglycemia

Plasma glucose concentrations less than 50 mg/dL (<2.8 mmol/L) with concurrent signs and symptoms of sweating, hunger, anxiety, trembling, blurred vision, weakness, headache, and/or altered consciousness are diagnostic of hypoglycemia. Actually, any glucose concentration below the normal range could be called hypoglycemia, but the subnormal concentration is not important unless signs and symptoms manifest. Concentrations below 40 mg/dL (<2.25 mmol/L) generally cause symptoms, and concentrations below 20 mg/dL (<1.1 mmol/L) lead to seizures and coma. Most signs and symptoms are from adrenergic discharge or neuroglycopenia. Sweating is mediated through the cholinergic nervous system and is one sign not masked by beta-blockers.

Hypoglycemia as the cause of symptoms is confirmed if correction of the glucose concentration abolishes the symptoms. Normal individuals usually do not manifest hypoglycemia except during pregnancy, strenuous exercise, or prolonged fasting. Commonly, hypoglycemia is the result of an insulin overdose in a patient with unstable IDDM. Hypoglycemia may be categorized into two types: postprandial and fasting.

Table 17 lists medications and other agents that may induce hypoglycemia. The only important artifactual cause of hypoglycemia, as measured by usual laboratory procedures, is improper collection and storage.

**TABLE 17.** Agents with Potential to Induce Hypoglycemia[18,37,51,73–75]

| Agents that may directly cause hypoglycemia |
| --- |
| Acute alcohol ingestion |
| Beta-blocking agents[a] |
| Disopyramide |
| Insulin |
| Monoamine oxidase inhibitors |
| Pentamidine |
| Salicylates (overdose) |
| Sulfonylureas |
| **Medications that may potentiate hypoglycemic effect of sulfonylurea agents[b]** |
| Chloramphenicol |
| Cimetidine |
| Clofibrate |
| Phenylbutazone |
| Sulfonamides |

[a]Also may mask most signs and symptoms of hypoglycemia. Cardioselective beta-blockers (e.g., atenolol and metoprolol) have less potential.

[b]Metformin does not potentiate hypoglycemic effects of sulfonylureas, nor does it cause hypoglycemia by itself.

### Postprandial Hypoglycemia

Most episodes of the postprandial type have no demonstrable pathological cause and are not considered a health risk to the patient. Postprandial hypoglycemia may reflect an abnormal secretion pattern (a delay or increased duration) of insulin in response to a high-carbohydrate meal. Symptoms generally last no more than 30 min and resolve without treatment. Furthermore, postprandial hypoglycemia can occur after GI surgery.

### Fasting Hypoglycemia

In contrast, fasting hypoglycemia may be secondary to insulin-secreting tumors (insulinomas), adrenal insufficiency, hypopituitarism, alcoholism with starvation, severe liver damage, and, of course, hypoglycemic drugs. The underlying problem usually involves undermobilization of glucose or overproduction (or overdose) of insulin. Patients may experience mental confusion and delirium. If untreated, hypoglycemia may progress and cause seizures, brain damage, coma, and death.

Patients with persistent fasting hypoglycemia should be assumed to have insulinoma until another diagnosis can be proved. In normal patients, insulin secretion is almost entirely suppressed when glucose concentrations fall below 45 mg/dL (<2.5 mmol/L). The diagnosis of insulinoma requires determination of serum insulin concentrations. Fasting insulin concentrations normally are 8–15 µU/mL and correlate with glucose concentrations. A serum insulin:glucose ratio greater than 0.3 when glucose is above 50 mg/dL indicates inappropriate hyperinsulinism, which is usually caused by an insulin-secreting tumor.

The C-peptide concentrations (fasting normal range:

0.5–2.5 ng/mL or 0.14–0.70 pmol/mL) may also be useful. Within the pancreatic beta cells, proinsulin is cleaved to produce insulin and C-peptide (connecting peptide). Patients with inappropriately high serum insulin and C-peptide concentrations at the time of hypoglycemia most likely have an insulinoma. If the C-peptide concentration is not concomitantly high, then the patient or caregiver may intentionally or unintentionally be administering excessive insulin.

# ESTROGEN AND PROGESTERONE RECEPTORS

Estrogen and progesterone receptor assays are useful in the prognosis and treatment of gynecological malignancies, especially breast cancer. Before the discussion on chemical and clinical considerations of the hormone receptor assays, this section briefly reviews the normal endocrine actions and metabolism of these hormones. Because estrogen is more important but similar in its role to progesterone, estrogen physiology is emphasized.

## Physiology

Estrogen and progesterone are the ovarian hormones responsible for the regulation of the female reproductive system. The uterus, vagina, oviduct, and mammary glands are estrogen-dependent tissues. The hypothalamus and anterior pituitary also are sensitive to the effects of estrogen. Besides maintaining the integrity of the female reproductive system, estrogens exert metabolic effects in the skin, bone, and liver that can be likened to those of glucocorticoids.

Estrogen and progesterone receptors probably are created in the cytoplasm of gynecological endocrine cells, but they quickly enter the nucleus.[76] A full biological response to estrogen requires that a sufficient number of estrogen receptor complexes enter the cell nucleus and that the nuclear receptor sites remain occupied for a critical period. In fact, the relative potency of the estrogenic compounds is based on their dissociation rates from nuclear receptor sites. In general, estrogens enhance and progestins suppress the synthesis of both estrogen and progesterone receptors.[76]

Aside from the natural products, birth control pills and postmenopausal replacement products contain synthetic estrogenic compounds (e.g., ethinyl estradiol, mestranol, diethylstilbestrol, and dienestrol). Estrogens in low doses may promote the growth of estrogen-dependent neoplastic cells; however, higher doses inhibit their growth. Therefore, estrogen therapy or receptor blockade has been used with varying degrees of success in many gynecological carcinomas. Investigators have correlated the presence of certain hormone receptors within tumor tissue to treatment outcome and prognosis.

## Estrogen and Progesterone Receptor Assays
*Positive: >10 femtomoles (fmol)/mg; intermediate:*
*3–10 fmol/mg; negative: <3 fmol/mg*

The presence or absence of estrogen and progesterone receptors in a tumor is prognostic for the potential responsiveness to endocrine therapy of a primary or metastatic breast tumor and, possibly, an endometrial tumor. Some evidence also suggests the usefulness of these assays in ovarian cancer. Assays are performed on a tissue slice or cytoplasm extract from the tumor itself. Most assays, which are biochemical in nature, were thought to measure receptors in the cytosol but actually may measure the unoccupied fraction of the nuclear receptors.[77]

In general, tumors that are positive for estrogen receptors respond better to hormonal manipulation than tumors with negative estrogen receptor assay results. This response occurs because estrogen (and progesterone) controls tumor growth in hormone receptor-positive patients, while hormone receptor-negative tumors grow independently of these hormones.

### Breast Cancer

The use of estrogen receptor assays has improved the selection of breast cancer patients for estrogen therapy. For both stage I (negative-axillary lymph nodes) and stage II (positive-axillary lymph nodes), the recurrence rate is higher for estrogen receptor-negative patients. Sixty-six percent of estrogen receptor-positive patients experience tumor shrinkage and/or clinical improvement from high-dose estrogen therapy or endocrine-ablative surgery. If progesterone receptors are also present in tumor tissue, the probability of a desirable response to endocrine therapy increases to 80%. Conversely, patients with negative estrogen and progesterone assays or a negative estrogen receptor assay alone have poor response rates to estrogen therapy (<10%).[78] In such patients, other chemotherapy should be considered.

Both estrogens and antiestrogen drugs are useful for estrogen receptor assay-positive patients. High-dose estrogen therapy for breast cancer is primarily palliative and requires nonhormonal chemotherapy regimens. Antiestrogens such as tamoxifen decrease estrogen-induced tumor flare, hypercalcemia, and the possibility of precipitating cardiovascular accidents. As an antiestrogen, tamoxifen binds to estrogen receptors, but this drug–receptor complex elicits few estrogenic effects. Therefore, it impedes the growth of estrogen-sensitive breast carcinomas.

### Endometrial Cancer

Although less clear than for breast cancer, both the estrogen and progesterone receptor assays are clinically useful indicators of prognosis in patients with endometrial cancer.[77] The progesterone receptor assay appears to correlate to prognosis more strongly than the estrogen receptor assay or conventional parameters. For example, absence or low concentration of receptor is associated with an increased risk of recurrence. In endometrial cancer, a positive progesterone receptor assay appears to identify responders to progestin therapy more precisely. Concomitant estrogen receptor assay results do not improve predictive usefulness. Some investigators argue that a much higher than usual cutoff point for positivity (>30 fmol/mg versus the usual cutoff of >10 fmol/mg) should furnish more useful prognostic and therapeutic information.[79]

### Ovarian Cancer

Estrogen and progesterone receptors are present in tumors in about 50% of patients with ovarian cancer, and androgen receptors are detected in 90%. Earlier studies revealed that progesterone receptor assay-positive patients survive somewhat longer than progesterone receptor assay-negative patients.[80] A more recent study suggested that the distinction is more dramatic with a higher cutoff point for positivity (≥50 fmol/mg).[81] These authors recommended that quantitative (instead of qualitative) receptor data be evaluated in future studies.

Most studies of ovarian cancer have not considered receptor status in the selection of endocrine therapy. Therefore, information is scarce on receptors with respect to endocrine therapy response. Androgen receptors are present in most ovarian cancer tissue. Since proliferation of androgen receptor-positive tumors is inhibited by antiandrogenic drugs, investigators have been enticed to search for answers regarding patient selection for endocrine therapy based on androgen and other receptor assay results.

### Limitations of Receptor Assays

Several factors can confound interpretation of receptor assay results:

1. Patients should not be empirically started on tamoxifen if a receptor assay is planned. Antiestrogens taken within 2 months prior to the assay may cause a false-negative result. The enzyme immunoassay method, however, may not be affected by prior tamoxifen therapy.
2. Oral contraceptives and menopausal estrogens are associated with lower receptor concentrations.
3. Insufficient tumor tissue in the specimen or specimens that have been fixed or that contain significant amounts of blood may lead to false-negative results.
4. Receptor-binding proteins are thermolabile, so biopsy samples that are not rapidly frozen (<15 min) will have the number of measurable receptors vastly and falsely decreased.

## DIABETES INSIPIDUS

Diabetes insipidus is a syndrome in which the body's inability to conserve water manifests as excretion of very large volumes of dilute urine. This section explores related pathophysiology, types of diabetes insipidus, and interpretation of test results to evaluate this disorder.

### Physiology

Normally, serum osmolality is maintained around 285 mOsm/kg and is determined by the amounts of sodium, chloride, bicarbonate, glucose, and urea in the serum. The excretion of these solutes along with water is a primary factor in determining urine volume and concentration (discussion on specific gravity in Chapter 7). In turn, the amount of water excreted by the kidneys is determined by renal function and antidiuretic hormone (ADH), also known as vasopressin.

ADH is synthesized in the hypothalamus and stored in the posterior pituitary gland. This hormone is released into the circulation following physiological stimulation, such as a change in serum osmolality or blood volume, detected by the osmoregulatory centers in the hypothalamus.[82] Congestive heart failure lowers the osmotic threshold for ADH release, while nausea, but not vomiting, strongly stimulates ADH. In general, α-adrenergic agonists stimulate ADH release while ß-adrenergic agonists inhibit release. ADH acts on the distal renal tubule and the collecting duct to cause water reabsorption. Chlorpropamide potentiates the effect of ADH on renal concentrating ability. When ADH is lacking or the renal tubules do not respond to the hormone, polyuria ensues. If the polyuria is severe enough, a diagnosis of diabetes insipidus is considered.

### Clinical Diagnosis

Diabetes insipidus should be differentiated from other causes of polyuria such as osmotic diuresis (e.g., hyperglycemia, mannitol, and contrast media), renal tubular acidosis, diuretic therapy, and psychogenic polydipsia.[83,84] For a diagnosis of diabetes insipidus, urine excretion must be at least 2 L (30 mL/kg) in 24 hr and the specific gravity must be less than 1.010 or the urine osmolality must be less than 300 mOsm/kg.[85]

Diabetes insipidus usually is caused by a defect in the secretion (neurogenic, also called central) or renal activity (nephrogenic) of ADH. It also can be caused by a defect in thirst (dipsogenic) or psychological function (psychogenic), with resultant excessive intake of water. Although diabetes insipidus typically does not lead to significant morbidity, the underlying cause should be sought to ensure proper prognosis and therapy. The specific type of diabetes insipidus often can be identified by the clinical setting. If the diagnosis is equivocal, a therapeutic trial with an antidiuretic drug or measurement of plasma ADH is necessary.[83–86]

Clinically, the easiest way to make the diagnosis is to monitor closely the effects of a therapeutic trial of vasopressin or its analog, desamino-D-arginine-vasopressin (DDAVP). The trial uses intramuscular vasopressin tannate in oil, 5 U every 24–48 hr, or DDAVP, 1–2 μg subcutaneously every 12 hr. If, after several days, thirst, polydipsia, and polyuria cease (without excessive fluid retention), the diagnosis is neurogenic diabetes insipidus. If signs and symptoms do not improve, nephrogenic diabetes insipidus is most likely.[85]

### Central Diabetes Insipidus

Central diabetes insipidus (ADH deficiency) may be the result of any disruption in the pituitary–hypothalamic regulation of ADH. Patients often present with a sudden onset of polyuria (in the absence of hyperglycemia) and preference for iced drinks. Tumors or metastases in or around the pituitary or hypothalamus, head trauma, neurosurgery, genetic abnormalities, meningitis, tuberculosis, and aneurysms are some of the known causes. In addition, phenytoin and alcohol inhibit ADH release from the pituitary. In response to deficient secretion of ADH and subsequent hyperosmolality of the plasma, thirst is stimulated. Thirst induces water intake, which leads to polyuria in the absence of effective ADH.

### Nephrogenic Diabetes Insipidus

In nephrogenic diabetes insipidus (ADH resistance), the secretion of ADH is normal but the renal tubule does not respond to ADH. Causes of nephrogenic diabetes insipidus include chronic renal failure, pyelonephritis, hypokalemia, hypercalciuria, malnutrition, genetic defects, and sickle cell disease. Additionally, lithium, demeclocycline, and methoxyflurane occasionally cause this disorder.

Lithium leads to polyuria in about 20% of patients. Typically, polyuria begins after 2–3 months of therapy. This antimanic drug appears to exert its nephrotoxicity by entering collecting duct cells through sodium channels. Lithium impairs ADH's ability to produce cyclic adenosine monophosphate (AMP).

Amiloride, a potassium-sparing diuretic, is useful in lithium-induced diabetes insipidus because it closes the sodium channels in the collecting duct cells and decreases lithium accumulation. Chlorpropamide potentiates ADH's effect on the collecting tubules. Given in doses of 250 mg daily, it rarely causes hypoglycemia but is sometimes effective in treating partial diabetes insipidus (Chapters 6 and 7).

### Diabetes Insipidus of Pregnancy

A transient diabetes insipidus, originally thought to be a form of nephrogenic diabetes insipidus, may develop during late pregnancy from excessive vasopressinase (ADHase) activity. This kind of diabetes insipidus is associated with preeclampsia with liver involvement. Fortunately, vasopressinase does not metabolize DDAVP (or desmopressin acetate), which is, therefore, the treatment of choice.[87]

### Laboratory Diagnosis

Until recently, a specific diagnosis of diabetes insipidus was made by performing a water deprivation test followed by administration of vasopressin. With the advent of more sensitive and specific assays, many clinicians avoid iatrogenic dehydration and rely on measuring plasma vasopressin concentrations to distinguish neurogenic from nephrogenic forms. In otherwise healthy adults, the average basal plasma vasopressin concentration is 1.3–4.0 pg/mL or ng/L.

In the presence of dilute urine, a normal or high basal plasma vasopressin concentration almost always indicates nephrogenic diabetes insipidus. If the basal plasma vasopressin concentration is low (<1 pg/mL) or unmeasurable, the result is inconclusive and a dehydration test should be done. If the diagnosis is ambiguous based on clinical setting and basal plasma vasopressin concentrations, the plan in Figure 4 should elucidate the diagnosis, even in a patient with a less common form of diabetes insipidus.

The theory behind the water deprivation test is that, in normal individuals, dehydration stimulates ADH release and the urine becomes concentrated. An injection of vasopressin at this point does not further concentrate the urine. In contrast, the urine of patients with central diabetes insipidus will not be maximally concentrated after fluid deprivation but will be after vasopressin injection.

To perform the test, patients are deprived of fluid intake (up to 18 hr) until the urine osmolality of three consecutive samples varies by no more than 30 mOsm/kg. Urine osmolality and/or specific gravity are measured hourly. At this time, 5 U of aqueous vasopressin are administered subcutaneously, and urine osmolality is measured 1 hr later. Plasma osmolality is measured before the test, when urine osmolality has stabilized and after vasopressin has been administered.

In healthy individuals, fluid deprivation for 8–12 hr results in normal serum osmolality and a urine osmolality of about 800 mOsm/kg. Their urine osmolality plateaus after 16–18 hr. In central diabetes insipidus, urine osmolality plateaus after 4–8 hr, and urine osmolality remains low while serum osmolality increases. In nephrogenic diabetes insipidus, the vasopressin injection has little effect.

In addition to being inconvenient and expensive, dehydration procedures are reliable only if the diabetes insipidus is severe enough that—even with induced dehydration—the urine still cannot be concentrated. Table 18 (page 272) presents a summary of typical results of a

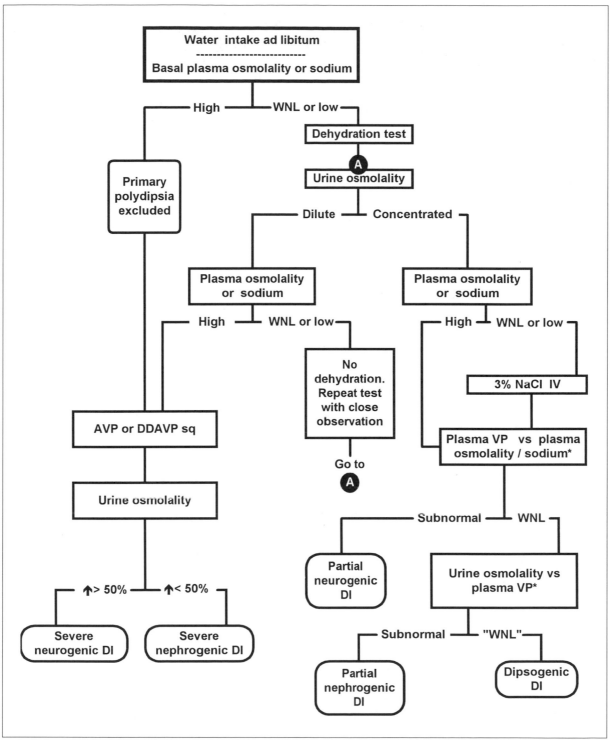

**FIGURE 4.** Evaluation of diabetes insipidus if diagnosis is ambiguous based on the clinical setting and basal plasma vasopressin concentrations. Plasma osmolality and sodium are considered high if they exceed the upper limit of normal for the laboratory (usually 295 mOsm/kg and 145 mEq/L, respectively). Urine is considered diluted if its osmolality is less than 300 mOsm/kg; it is concentrated if its osmolality is greater than 300 mOsm/kg. If indicated, hypertonic saline is infused at 0.1 mL/kg/min for 2 hr. The vasopressin (aqueous Pitressin, AVP) dose is 1 U, while the DDAVP dose is 1 µg subcutaneously. WNL = within normal limits; VP = vasopressin = ADH; DI = diabetes insipidus. *Interpretation of plasma VP versus plasma osmolality/sodium and urine osmolality versus plasma VP requires use of a nomogram. (Adapted, with permission, from Reference 85.)

**TABLE 18.** Differential Diagnosis of Diabetes Insipidus Based on Water Deprivation Test[83,84,88]

| Diagnosis | Urine Specific Gravity | Average Urine Osmolality (mOsm/kg) | Plateau Urine Osmolality (mOsm/kg) | Average Serum Osmolality (mOsm/kg) | Change in Urine Osmolality After Vasopressin |
|---|---|---|---|---|---|
| Normal individuals | >1.015 | 300–800 | <1600 | 280–295 | Little change |
| Central diabetes insipidus | <1.010 | <300 | <300 | Normal or increased | Increases |
| Nephrogenic diabetes insipidus | <1.010 | <300 | <300 | Normal or decreased | Little change |

water deprivation test.

Accurate interpretation requires consideration of potential confounding factors. If the laboratory cannot ensure accurate and precise plasma (not serum) osmolality measurements, plasma sodium should be used. Patients should be observed for nonosmotic stimuli, such as vasovagal reactions, that may affect ADH release. Lastly, if the patient has previously received ADH therapy, ADH antibodies may cause results falsely suggestive of nephrogenic diabetes insipidus.[85]

## SUMMARY

Endocrine disorders often result from a deficiency or excess of a hormone. Laboratory tests that measure the actual hormone, precursors, or metabolites can help to elucidate whether and why a hormonal or metabolic imbalance exists. Tests used to assess thyroid, glucose, sex hormone, and water homeostasis or receptors have been discussed.

Thyroid tests can be divided into those that (1) measure the concentration of products secreted by the thyroid gland ($T_3$ and $T_4$), (2) evaluate the integrity of the hypothalamic–pituitary–thyroid axis (TSH and TRH), (3) assess inherent thyroid gland function (radioactive iodine uptake test), and (4) detect antibodies to thyroid tissue (thyroid microsomal antibody). TSH concentrations usually are undetectable or less than 0.3 mU/L (newer assays), and $T_4$ concentrations usually are high in patients with overt hyperthyroidism. TSH concentrations are low or undetectable in patients with hypothyroidism from hypothalamic or pituitary insufficiency and in patients with nonthyroidal illness. In contrast, TSH concentrations are high and $T_4$ concentrations are low in patients with primary hypothyroidism.

The fasting plasma glucose and the 2-hr postprandial glucose concentrations are the most commonly performed tests for evaluation of glucose homeostasis. If elevated (>140 mg/dL) blood glucose persists, diabetes mellitus is likely; however, other causes of hyperglycemia (e.g., drugs) should be considered. Glycated hemoglobin ($Hgb_{A1c}$) assesses average glucose control over the previous 2–3 months, while fructosamine assesses average control over the previous 2–3 weeks.

Diabetic ketoacidosis and hyperosmolar nonketotic hyperglycemia are the most severe disorders along the continuum of glucose intolerance. Extreme hyperglycemia (600–2000 mg/dL) with insignificant ketonemia/acidosis is consistent with hyperosmolar nonketotic hyperglycemia, while less severe (350–650 mg/dL) hyperglycemia with ketonemia and acidosis is characteristic of diabetic ketoacidosis. Conversely, hypoglycemia (glucose <50 mg/dL) most often is seen in patients with IDDM who have injected excessive insulin relative to their caloric intake.

The presence or absence of estrogen and progesterone receptors in tumors is prognostic in determining the potential responsiveness to endocrine therapy of a primary or metastatic tumor from the breast and possibly from the ovary and endometrium. In general, tumors that are positive for estrogen receptors respond better to hormonal manipulation than tumors with negative results from the estrogen receptor assay.

Diabetes insipidus is a syndrome in which the body's inability to conserve water manifests as excretion of very large volumes of dilute urine. It most often is caused by a defect in the secretion (neurogenic, also called central) or renal activity (nephrogenic) of the antidiuretic hormone ADH. Urine and plasma osmolality are key tests. With the advent of high-performance assays, the use of plasma vasopressin concentrations to distinguish neurogenic from nephrogenic may obviate the need for iatrogenic dehydration procedures.

## REFERENCES

1. Greenspan FS, Rapoport B. Thyroid gland. In: Greenspan FS, Forsham PH, eds. Basic and clinical endocrinology, 2nd ed. Los Altos, CA: Lange Medical Publications; 1986:143–201.
2. Larsen PR. Thyroid-pituitary interaction: feedback regulation of thyrotropin secretion by thyroid hormones. *N Engl J Med*. 1982; 306:23–32.
3. Kaptein EM. Clinical application of free thyroxine determinations. *Clin Lab Med*. 1993; 13:653–72.
4. Thomas JA, Keenan EJ. Thyroid and antithyroidal drugs. In: Thomas JA, Keenan EJ, eds. Principles of endocrine pharmacology. New York: Plenum; 1986:69–91.
5. Nelson JC, Wilcox RB, Pandin MR. Dependence of free thyroxine estimates obtained with equilibrium tracer di-

alysis on the concentration of thyroxine-binding globulin. *Clin Chem.* 1992; 38:1294–1300.

6. Singer PA. Thyroid function tests and effects of drugs on thyroid function. In: Lavin N, ed. Manual of endocrinology and metabolism. Boston, MA: Little, Brown; 1986:341–54.

7. Klee GG, Hay ID. Assessment of sensitive thyrotropin assays for an expanded role in thyroid function testing: proposed criteria for analytic performance and clinical utility. *J Clin Endocrinol Metab.* 1987; 64:461–71.

8. Ingbar SH, Woeber KA. The thyroid gland. In: Williams RH, ed. Textbook of endocrinology, 6th ed. Philadelphia, PA: W. B. Saunders; 1981:117–248.

9. Mokshagundam S, Barzel US. Thyroid disease in the elderly. *J Am Geriatr Soc.* 1993; 41:1361–9.

10. Safrit H. Thyroid disorders. In: Fitzgerald PA, ed. Handbook of clinical endocrinology. Greenbrae, CA: Jones Medical Publications; 1986:122–69.

11. Hershman JM. Hypothyroidism and hyperthyroidism. In: Lavin N, ed. Manual of endocrinology and metabolism. Boston, MA: Little, Brown; 1986:365–78.

12. Tunbridge WMG, Evered DC, Hall R, et al. The spectrum of thyroid disease in a community: the Whickham survey. *Clin Endocrinol (Oxf).* 1977; 7:481–93.

13. Becker DV, Bigos ST, Gaitan E, et al. Optimal use of blood tests for assessment of thyroid function. *JAMA.* 1993; 269:2736–7.

14. Spencer CA. Thyroid profiling for the 1990s: free $T_4$ estimate or sensitive TSH measurement. *J Clin Immunoassay.* 1989; 12:82–5.

15. Surks MI, Hupart KH, Pan C, et al. Normal free thyroxine in critical nonthyroidal illnesses measured by ultrafiltration of undiluted serum and equilibrium dialysis. *J Clin Endocrinol Metab.* 1988; 67:1031–9.

16. Wong TK, Pekary AE, Hoo GS, et al. Comparison of methods for measuring free thyroxine in nonthyroidal illness. *Clin Chem.* 1992; 38:720–4.

17. Klee GG, Hay ID. Role of thyrotropin measurements in the diagnosis and management of thyroid disease. *Clin Lab Med.* 1993; 13:673–82.

18. Young DS. Effects of drugs on clinical laboratory tests, 3rd ed. Washington, DC: American Association for Clinical Chemistry Press; 1990.

19. Khanderia U, Jaffe CA, Theisen V. Amiodarone-induced thyroid dysfunction. *Clin Pharm.* 1993; 12:774–9.

20. Okamura K, Ikenoue H, Shiroozu A, et al. Reevaluation of the effects of methylmercaptomidazole and propylthiouracil in patients with Graves' hyperthyroidism. *J Clin Endocrinol Metab.* 1987; 65:719–23.

21. Franklyn JA. The management of hyperthyroidism. *N Engl J Med.* 1994; 330:1731–8.

22. Finucane P, Rudra T, Hsu R, et al. Thyrotropin response to thyrotropin-releasing hormone in elderly patients with and without acute illness. *Age Ageing.* 1991; 20:85–9.

23. Toft AD. Thyroxine therapy. *N Engl J Med.* 1994; 331:174–80.

24. Nicoloff JT, Spencer CA. The use and misuse of the sensitive thyrotropin assays. *J Clin Endocrinol Metab.* 1990; 71:553–8.

25. McClelland P, Stott A, Howel-Evans W. Hyperthyrotropinaemia during thyroxine replacement therapy. *Postgrad Med J.* 1989; 65:205–7.

26. Reinwein D, Benker G, Lazarus JH, et al. A prospective randomized trial of antithyroid drug dose in Graves' disease therapy. *J Clin Endocrinol Metab.* 1993; 76:1516–21.

27. Liewendahl K, Helenius T, Lamberg BA, et al. Free thyroxine, free triiodothyronine, and thyrotropin concentrations in hypothyroid and thyroid carcinoma patients receiving thyroxine therapy. *Acta Endocrinol.* 1987; 116:418–24.

28. Stall GM, Harris S, Sokoll LJ, et al. Accelerated bone loss in hypothyroid patients overtreated with L-thyroxine. *Ann Intern Med.* 1990; 113:265–9.

29. Vanelle JM, Poirier MF, Benkelfat C, et al. Diagnostic and therapeutic value of testing stimulation of thyroid-stimulating hormone by thyrotropin-releasing hormone in 100 depressed patients. *Acta Psychiatr Scand.* 1990; 81:156–61.

30. Ingbar SH. Diseases of the thyroid. In: Braunwald E, Isselbacher KJ, Petersdorf RG, et al., eds. Harrison's principles of internal medicine, 11th ed. New York: McGraw-Hill; 1987:1732–52.

31. Hershman JM, Chopra IJ, Van Herle AJ, et al. Thyroid disease. In: Hershman JM, ed. Endocrine pathophysiology: a patient-oriented approach, 2nd ed. Philadelphia, PA: Lea & Febiger; 1982:34–68.

32. Utiger RD. Thyrotropin-receptor mutations and thyroid dysfunction. *N Engl J Med.* 1995; 332:183–5.

33. Sacher RA, McPherson RA. Widman's clinical interpretation of laboratory tests, 10th ed. Philadelphia, PA: F. A. Davis; 1991.

34. Wallach J. Interpretation of diagnostic tests: a synopsis of laboratory medicine, 5th ed. Boston, MA: Little, Brown; 1992.

35. Refetoff S, Weiss RE, Usala SJ. The syndromes of resistance to thyroid hormone. *Endocr Rev.* 1993; 14:348–99.

36. Wood JM, Gordon DL, Rudinger AN, et al. Artifactual elevation of thyroid-stimulating hormone. *Am J Med.* 199; 90:261–2.

37. Porte D, Halter JB. The endocrine pancreas and diabetes mellitus. In: Williams RH, ed. Textbook of endocrinology, 6th ed. Philadelphia, PA: W. B. Saunders; 1981:715–842.

38. Bennett PH. Definition, diagnosis, and classification of diabetes mellitus and impaired glucose tolerance. In: Kahn CR, Weir GC, eds. Joslin's diabetes mellitus, 13th ed. Philadelphia, PA: Lea & Febiger; 1994:193–200.

39. Karam JH, Salber PR, Forsham PH. Pancreatic hormones and diabetes mellitus. In: Greenspan FS, Forsham PH, eds. Basic and clinical endocrinology, 2nd ed. Los Altos, CA: Lange Medical Publications; 1986:523–74.

40. Howanitz PJ, Howanitz JH. Carbohydrates. In: Henry JB, ed. Clinical diagnosis and management by laboratory methods, 17th ed. Philadelphia, PA: W. B. Saunders; 1984:165–203.

41. Lorenzi M. Diabetes mellitus. In: Fitzgerald PA, ed. Handbook of clinical endocrinology. Greenbrae, CA: Jones Medical Publications; 1986:337–409.

42. Dinneen S, Gerich J, Rizza R. Carbohydrate metabolism in non-insulin-dependent diabetes mellitus. *N Engl J Med.* 1992; 327:707–13.

43. Ensinck JW, Williams RH. Disorders causing hypoglycemia. In: Williams RH, ed. Textbook of endocrinology, 6th ed. Philadelphia, PA: W. B. Saunders; 1981:843–74.

44. Young CW, Karam JH. Hypoglycemic disorders. In: Greenspan FS, Forsham PH, eds. Basic and clinical endocrinology, 2nd ed. Los Altos, CA: Lange Medical Publications; 1986:575–86.

45. Atkinson MA, Maclaren NK. The pathogenesis of insulin-dependent diabetes mellitus. *N Engl J Med.* 1994; 331:1428–36.

46. Rowley MJ, Mackay IR, Chen Q-Y, et al. Antibodies to glutamic acid decarboxylase discriminate major types of

diabetes mellitus. *Diabetes.* 1992; 41:548–51.

47. Geffner ME, Lippe BM. The role of immunotherapy in type I diabetes mellitus. *West J Med.* 1987; 146:337–43.

48. Godsland IF, Crook D, Simpson R, et al. The effects of different formulations of oral contraceptive agents on lipid and carbohydrate metabolism. *N Engl J Med.* 1990; 323:1375–81.

49. Pollak PT, Sami M. Acute necrotizing pneumonitis and hyperglycemia after amiodarone therapy: case report and review of amiodarone-associated pulmonary disease. *Am J Med.* 1984; 76:935–9.

50. Kondziela JR, Kaufmann MW, Klein MJ. Diabetic ketoacidosis associated with lithium: case report. *J Clin Psychiatry.* 1985; 46:492–3.

51. Stahl-Bayliss CM, Kalman CM, Laskin OL. Pentamidine-induced hypoglycemia in patients with acquired immune deficiency syndrome. *Clin Pharmacol Ther.* 1986; 39:271–5.

52. Friedel HA, Buckley MMT. Torsemide: a review of its pharmacological properties and therapeutic potential. *Drugs.* 1991; 41:81–103.

53. Goldstein DE, Little RR, Wiedmeyer HM, et al. Glycated hemoglobin: methodologies and clinical applications. *Clin Chem.* 1986; 32(10 Suppl):B64–70.

54. Yarrison G, Allen L, King N, et al. Lipemic interference in Beckman Diatrac hemoglobin $A_{1c}$ procedure removed. *Clin Chem.* 1993; 39:2351–2.

55. Ardawi MS, Nasrat HA, Bahnassy AA. Fructosamine in obese normal subjects and type 2 diabetes. *Diabet Med.* 1994; 11:50–6.

56. Cefalu WT, Ettinger WH, Bell-Farrow AD, et al. Serum fructosamine as a screening test for diabetes in the elderly: a pilot study. *J Am Geriatr Soc.* 1993; 41:1090–4.

57. Smolowitz JL, Zaldivar A. Evaluation of diabetic patients' home urine glucose testing technique and ability to interpret results. *Diabetes Educ.* 1992; 18:207–10.

58. Rotblatt MD, Koda-Kimble MA. Review of drug interference with urine glucose tests. *Diabetes Care.* 1987; 10:103–10.

59. Sylvester ACJ, Price CP, Burrin JM. Investigation of the potential for interference with whole blood glucose strips. *Ann Clin Biochem.* 1994; 31:94–6.

60. Meters for glucose monitoring. *Med Lett.* 1992; 34:115–6.

61. National Diabetes Data Group. Classification and diagnosis of diabetes mellitus and other categories of glucose intolerance. *Diabetes.* 1979; 28:1039–57.

62. Genuth S. Classification and diagnosis of diabetes mellitus. *Med Clin North Am.* 1982; 66:1191–207.

63. The Diabetes Control and Complications Trial Research Group. The effect of intensive treatment of diabetes on the development and progression of long-term complications in insulin-dependent diabetes mellitus. *N Engl J Med.* 1993; 329:977–86.

64. Albisser AM, Sperlich M. Adjusting insulins. *Diabetes Educ.* 1992; 18:211–9.

65. Lebovitz HE. Diabetic ketoacidosis. *Lancet.* 1995; 345:767–72.

66. Jenkins D, Close CF, Krentz AJ, et al. Euglycemic diabetic ketoacidosis: does it exist? *Acta Diabetol.* 1993; 30:251–3.

67. Burge MD, Hardy KJ, Schade DS. Short term fasting is a mechanism for the development of euglycemic ketoacidosis during periods of insulin deficiency. *J Clin Endocrinol Metab.* 1993; 76:1192–8.

68. Fisher JN, Kitabchi AE. A randomized study of phosphate therapy in the treatment of diabetic ketoacidosis. *J Clin Endocrinol Metab.* 1983; 57:177–80.

69. Goren MP, Pratt CB. False-positive ketone tests: a bedside measure of urinary mesna. *Cancer Chemother Pharmacol.* 1990; 25:371–2.

70. Holcombe BJ, Hopkins AM, Heizer WD. False positive tests for urinary ketones. *N Engl J Med.* 1994; 330:578. Letter.

71. Graham P, Naidoo D. False-positive Ketostix in a diabetic on antihypertensive therapy. *Clin Chem.* 1987; 33:1490.

72. Warren SE. False-positive urine ketone test with captopril. *N Engl J Med.* 1980; 303:1003–4.

73. Cate EW, Rogers JF, Powell JR. Inhibition of tolbutamide elimination by cimetidine but not ranitidine. *J Clin Pharmacol.* 1986; 26:373–7.

74. Lager I, Blohme G, Smith U. Effect of cardioselective and non-selective beta-blockade on the hypoglycaemic response in insulin-dependent diabetics. *Lancet.* 1979; 1(8114):458–62.

75. Strathman I, Schubert EN, Cohen A, et al. Hypoglycemia in patients receiving disopyramide phosphate. *Drug Intell Clin Pharm.* 1983; 17:635–8.

76. Brenner RB, West NB, McClellan MC. Estrogen and progestin receptors in the reproductive tract of male and female primates. *Biol Reprod.* 1990; 42:11–9.

77. Kauppila A. Oestrogen and progestin receptor as prognostic indicators in endometrial cancer. *Acta Oncol.* 1989; 28:561–6.

78. Thomas JA, Keenan EJ. Estrogens and antiestrogenic drugs. In: Thomas JA, Keenan EJ, eds. Principles of endocrine pharmacology. New York: Plenum; 1986:135–65.

79. Palmer DC, Muir IM, Alexander AI, et al. The prognostic importance of steroid receptors in endometrial carcinoma. *Obstet Gynecol.* 1988; 72:388–93.

80. Rao BR, Slotman BJ. Action and counter-action of hormones in human ovarian cancer. *Anticancer Res.* 1989; 9:1005–8.

81. Slotman BJ, Kuhnel R, Rao BR, et al. Importance of steroid receptors and aromatase activity in the prognosis of ovarian cancer: high tumor progesterone receptor levels correlate with longest survival. *Gynecol Oncol.* 1989; 33:76–81.

82. Lightman S. Central nervous system control of fluid balance: physiology and pathology. *Acta Neurochir Suppl.* 1990; 47:90–4.

83. Fitzgerald PA. Pituitary disorders. In: Fitzgerald PA, ed. Handbook of clinical endocrinology, Greenbrae, CA: Jones Medical Publications; 1986:22–9.

84. Ramsay DJ. Posterior pituitary gland. In: Greenspan FS, Forsham PH, eds. Basic and clinical endocrinology, 2nd ed. Los Altos, CA: Lange Medical Publications; 1986:132–42.

85. Robertson GL. Differential diagnosis of polyuria. *Ann Rev Med.* 1988; 39:425–42.

86. Lightman SL. Molecular insights into diabetes insipidus. *N Engl J Med.* 1993; 328:1562–3.

87. Krege J, Katz VL, Bowes WA Jr. Transient diabetes insipidus of pregnancy. *Obstet Gynecol Surv.* 1989; 44:789–95.

88. Sowers JR, Zieve FJ. Clinical disorders of vasopressin. In: Lavin N, ed. Manual of endocrinology and metabolism. Boston, MA: Little, Brown; 1986:65–74.

*The contribution of material written by Diana Laubenstein, Pharm.D., in the first edition of this book is acknowledged.*

## QuickView—Total Serum T$_4$

| Parameter | Description | Comments |
|---|---|---|
| **Common reference ranges** | | |
| Adults and children | 4–12 µg/dL<br>(51–154 nmol/L) | Affected by TBG changes with nonthyroidal illness<br>SI conversion factor = 12.87 (nmol/L) |
| Newborn/3–5 days | 16–26/9–20 µg/dL | Affected by TBG changes with nonthyroidal illness<br>SI conversion factor = 12.87 (nmol/L) |
| **Critical value** | Not established | Extremely high or low values should be reported quickly, especially in newborns |
| **Natural substance?** | Yes | Only 0.02% of T$_4$ is unbound |
| **Inherent activity?** | Only free portion | *Total* assumed to correlate with *free* T$_4$ activity |
| **Location** | | |
| Production and storage | Thyroid gland | Bound mostly to thyroglobulin |
| Secretion/excretion | From thyroid to blood | About 33% converted to T$_3$ outside thyroid |
| **Major causes of . . .** | | |
| High results | Hyperthyroidism | Not truly a cause but a reflection of high result |
| | T$_4$ supplements<br>Other causes (Table 2) | |
| Associated signs and symptoms | Signs and symptoms of hyperthyroidism | Nervousness, weight loss, heat intolerance, HR increase, diaphoresis |
| Low results | Hypothyroidism | Not truly a cause but a reflection of low result |
| | Other causes (Table 1) | |
| Associated signs and symptoms | Signs and symptoms of hypothyroidism | Lethargy, constipation, dry skin, cold intolerance, slow speech, confusion |
| **After insult, time to . . .** | | |
| Initial elevation or depression | Weeks to months | Increases within hours in *acute* T$_4$ overdose |
| Peak values | Weeks to months | Increases within hours in *acute* T$_4$ overdose |
| Normalization | Usually same time as onset | Assumes insult removed or effectively treated |
| **Drugs often monitored with test** | Levothyroxine (T$_4$) | Other drugs (Tables 1 and 2) |
| **Causes of spurious results** | Increased or decreased TBG leads to falsely increased or decreased total serum T$_4$<br>Nonthyroidal illness leads to falsely increased or decreased total serum T$_4$ | Factors affecting TBG (Table 6) |

## QuickView—Total Serum T$_3$

| Parameter | Description | Comments |
|---|---|---|
| **Common reference ranges** <br> **Adults and children** | 78–195 ng/dL <br> (1.2–3.0 nmol/L) | Affected by TBG changes <br> SI conversion factor = 0.0154 (nmol/L) |
| **Critical value** | Not established | Extremely high or low values should be reported quickly |
| **Natural substance?** | Yes | Only 0.2% of T$_3$ is unbound |
| **Inherent activity?** | Only free portion | *Total* assumed to correlate with *free* T$_3$ activity |
| **Location** <br> **Production and storage** <br> **Secretion/excretion** | <br> Liver and kidneys; thyroid gland <br> From thyroid, liver, and kidneys to blood | <br> Bound mostly to thyroglobulin |
| **Major causes of . . .** <br> **High results** | Hyperthyroidism <br><br> T$_4$/T$_3$ supplements <br> Other causes (Table 2) | Not truly a cause but a reflection of high result |
|     Associated signs and symptoms | Signs and symptoms of hyperthyroidism | Nervousness, weight loss, heat intolerance, tachycardia, diaphoresis |
| **Low results** | Hypothyroidism <br><br> Other causes (Table 1) <br> Propranolol <br> Propylthiouracil <br> Glucocorticoids | Not truly a cause but a reflection of low result <br><br> Inhibit peripheral conversion of T$_4$ to T$_3$ |
|     Associated signs and symptoms | Signs and symptoms of hypothyroidism | Lethargy, constipation, dry skin, cold intolerance, slow speech, confusion |
| **After insult, time to . . .** <br> **Initial elevation or depression** | Weeks to months | Increases within hours in *acute* T$_4$ or T$_3$ overdose |
| **Peak values** | Weeks to months | Increases within hours in *acute* T$_4$ or T$_3$ overdose |
| **Normalization** | Usually same time as onset | Assumes insult removed or effectively treated |
| **Drugs often monitored with test** | Levothyroxine (T$_4$) and triiodothyronine (T$_3$) | Other drugs (Tables 1 and 2) |
| **Causes of spurious results** | Increased or decreased TBG leads to falsely increased or decreased total serum T$_3$ <br> Nonthyroidal illness leads to falsely increased or decreased total serum T$_3$ | Factors affecting TBG (Table 6) |

## QuickView—Free T$_4$

| Parameter | Description | Comments |
|---|---|---|
| **Common reference ranges** <br> **Adults and children** | 0.8–2.7 ng/dL <br> (10–35 pmol/L) | Higher in infants <1 month; direct equilibrium dialysis assay not affected by TBG changes or severe nonthyroidal illness <br> SI conversion factor = 12.87 (pmol/L) |
| **Critical value** | Not established | Extremely high or low values should be reported quickly |
| **Natural substance?** | Yes | Only 0.02% of T$_4$ is unbound |
| **Inherent activity?** | Probably | Some influence on basal metabolic rate; T$_3$ most active |
| **Location** <br> **Production and storage** <br> **Secretion/excretion** | <br> Thyroid gland <br> From thyroid to blood | <br> Bound mostly to thyroglobulin <br> 33% converted to T$_3$ outside thyroid |
| **Major causes of . . .** <br> **High results** | Hyperthyroidism <br><br> T$_4$ supplements <br> Other causes (Table 2) | Not truly a cause but a reflection of high result |
| **Associated signs and symptoms** | Signs and symptoms of hyperthyroidism | Nervousness, weight loss, heat intolerance, tachycardia, diaphoresis |
| **Low results** | Hypothyroidism <br><br> Other causes (Table 1) | Not truly a cause but a reflection of low result |
| **Associated signs and symptoms** | Signs and symptoms of hypothyroidism | Lethargy, constipation, dry skin, cold intolerance, slow speech, confusion |
| **After insult, time to . . .** <br> **Initial elevation or depression** | Weeks to months | Increases within hours in *acute* T$_4$ over dose |
| **Peak values** | Weeks to months | Increases within hours in *acute* T$_4$ overdose |
| **Normalization** | Usually same time as onset | Assumes insult removed or effectively treated |
| **Drugs often monitored with test** | Levothyroxine (T$_4$) | Other drugs (Tables 1 and 2) |
| **Causes of spurious results** | Rare with direct equilibrium dialysis assay (Table 5) | Decreased direct equilibrium dialysis assay for free T$_4$ with decreased or normal TSH may occur in patients taking T$_3$ |

## QuickView—TSH

| Parameter | Description | Description |
|---|---|---|
| **Common reference ranges** <br> **Adults and children** | 0.3–5.0 µU/mL | Sometimes reported in mU/L |
| **Critical value** | Not established | Extremely high or low values should be reported quickly |

*continued*

## QuickView—TSH *continued*

| Parameter | Description | Comments |
|---|---|---|
| Natural substance? | Yes | |
| Inherent activity? | Yes | Stimulates thyroid to secrete hormones |
| **Location** | | |
| Production and storage | Anterior pituitary | |
| Secretion/excretion | Unknown | |
| **Major causes of . . .** | | |
| High results | Primary hypothyroidism | Causes of primary hypothyroidism (Table 1) |
| | Antithyroid drugs | |
| Associated signs and symptoms | Signs and symptoms of hypothyroidism | Lethargy, constipation, dry skin, cold intolerance, slow speech, confusion |
| Low results | Primary hyperthyroidism | Must be ≤0.05 for definitive diagnosis of (primary hyperthyroidism); may be decreased or normal in secondary or tertiary hypothyroidism |
| | Other causes (Table 2) | |
| Associated signs and symptoms | Signs and symptoms of hyperthyroidism | Nervousness, weight loss, heat intolerance, HR increase, diaphoresis |
| **After insult, time to . . .** | | |
| Initial elevation or depression | Weeks to months | Decreases within hours in *acute* $T_4$ overdose |
| Peak values | Weeks to months | Decreases within hours in *acute* $T_4$ overdose |
| Normalization | Usually same time as onset | Assumes insult removed or effectively treated |
| Drugs often monitored with test | Levothyroxine ($T_4$) and triiodothyronine ($T_3$) | Also antithyroid drugs (methimazole and propylthiouracil) |
| Causes of spurious results | Increased TSH: dopamine antagonists<br>Decreased TSH: dopamine agonists<br><br>Above TSH measurements are accurate here | Metoclopramide and domperidone<br>Dopamine, bromocriptine, levodopa, glucocorticoids<br>But may confound diagnosis<br>These drugs affect TSH, but the change is not reflective of primary hypo- or hyperthyroidism; therefore, the results are not truly spurious |

## QuickView—Glucose, Plasma

| Parameter | Description | Comments |
|---|---|---|
| **Common reference ranges** | | |
| Adults and children | Fasting: 70–110 mg/dL<br>    (3.9–6.1 mmol/L)<br>2-hr postprandial: <150 mg/dL<br>    (8.4 mmol/L)<br>Full-term infant normal: 20–90 mg/dL | Multiply by 0.056 for SI units (mmol/L) |
| Critical values | No previous history: >200 mg/dL<br>Anytime: <50 mg/dL | In known diabetic, increased glucose is not immediate concern unless symptomatic; increased glucose is not critical if decreasing in series |
| Natural substance? | Yes | Always present in blood |

## QuickView—Glucose, Plasma *continued*

| Parameter | Description | Comments |
|---|---|---|
| Inherent activity? | Yes | Major source of energy for cellular metabolism |
| **Location** | | |
| Production/intake | Liver and muscle | Dietary intake |
| Storage | Liver and muscle | As glycogen |
| Secretion/excretion | Mostly metabolized for energy | Levels >180 mg/dL spill into urine |
| **Major causes of . . .** | | |
| High results | Diabetes mellitus<br>Drugs<br>Excess intake | IDDM and NIDDM<br>Steroids, thiazides, adrenalin |
| Associated signs and symptoms | Polyuria, polydipsia, polyphagia, weakness | Long-term: damage to kidneys, retina, neurons, and vessels |
| Low results | Insulin secretion/dose excessive relative to diet<br>Sulfonylureas<br>Insulinomas | Most common in diabetics |
| Associated signs and symptoms | Hunger, sweating, weakness, trembling, headache, confusion, seizures, coma | From neuroglycopenia and adrenergic discharge |
| **After insult, time to . . .** | | |
| Initial elevation or depression | IDDM: months to elevation<br>NIDDM: years to elevation<br>After insulin: minutes to decrease<br>After meal: 15–30 min to elevation<br>After epinephrine or glucagon: minutes<br>After steroids and growth hormone: hours | |
| Normalization | After insulin: minutes<br>After exercise: minutes to hours | Depends on insulin type<br>Depends on intensity and duration |
| Drugs often monitored with test | Insulin, sulfonylureas, biguanides (e.g., metformin) | Also diazoxide, L-asparaginase, total parenteral nutrition |
| Causes of spurious results | High dose vitamin C<br>Metronidazole | With some glucometers<br>With some automated assays |

## QuickView—Hgb A$_{1c}$

| Parameter | Description | Comments |
|---|---|---|
| **Common reference ranges**<br>Adults and teenagers | 3–6% | Fasting not required; represents average glucose levels past 8 weeks |
| Critical value | Not applicable | Reflects long-term glycemic control; >13% suggests poor control |
| Natural substance? | Yes | Subunit of Hgb |
| Inherent activity? | Yes | Oxygen carrier; also carries glucose |

*continued*

## QuickView—Hgb A~1c~ *continued*

| Parameter | Description | Comments |
|---|---|---|
| **Location** | | |
| **Production** | Bone marrow | In newborns in liver and spleen |
| **Storage** | Not stored | Circulates in blood |
| **Secretion/excretion** | Older cell removed by spleen | Transformed to bilirubin |
| **Major causes of . . .** | | |
| **High results** | Diabetes mellitus<br>Chronic hyperglycemia | Any cause of prolonged hyperglycemia |
| **Associated signs and symptoms** | Signs and symptoms of diabetes | |
| **Low results** | Not clinically useful | |
| **After insult, time to . . .** | | |
| **Initial elevation** | 2–4 months | Initial insult is chronic hyperglycemia |
| **Normalization** | 2–4 months | Assumes sudden and persistent euglycemia |
| **Drugs often monitored with test** | Insulin, sulfonylureas, biguanides | Also diet and exercise |
| **Causes of spurious results** | Alcoholism, uremia, increased triglycerides, hemolysis, polycythemia | Also seen in pregnant and splenectomized patients |

# Chapter 13

# Metabolic Disorders

*Scott L. Traub*

Hypercholesterolemia, a disorder of cholesterol metabolism, clearly is a major factor in the development of coronary artery disease. With the increasing focus on heart disease and overall preventive health, practitioners are being called on to assess such factors as cholesterol and triglycerides. Recent technological advances and increased promotion of low-cholesterol diets have prompted both patients and health care providers to learn about the effects of cholesterol and other lipids. The understanding of lipid disorders continues to grow significantly each year.

Porphyrias are metabolic disorders of heme synthesis in which there are an overproduction, accumulation, and excretion of porphyrins and their intermediary precursors. While these conditions are less common than hyperlipidemia, they can cause neurological complications. This chapter first describes the physiology involved in cholesterol, triglyceride, and heme synthesis and then discusses the laboratory tests used to diagnose and monitor related disorders.

## OBJECTIVES

Upon completion of this chapter, the reader should be able to

1. Cite genetic abnormalities and secondary causes associated with lipid disorders (i.e., hyperlipidemia).
2. Correlate blood cholesterol and various lipoprotein concentrations with the risk of developing atherosclerotic cardiovascular disease.
3. Given a case study, interpret laboratory results from a lipid profile and discuss how they should guide treatment choices.
4. Differentiate among hepatic and erythropoietic porphyrias based on symptomatology and blood and excretion patterns of heme precursors measured by various laboratory tests.

## LIPID DISORDERS

This section primarily covers the physiology of choles-

terol and triglyceride metabolism, their actions as part of lipoproteins of various densities, disorders of lipids and lipoproteins, and risks and diseases that occur secondary to elevated concentrations of these products. The effects of diet, exercise, and drugs on these lipids also are discussed. A detailed interpretation of test results with regard to cardiovascular prognosis and specific treatment options is beyond the scope of this chapter. However, References 1–3 offer additional information.

### Physiology

Triglycerides, the esterified form of glycerol and fatty acids, constitute the main form of lipid storage in humans. Triglycerides serve as a reservoir of fatty acids to be used as fuel for gluconeogenesis or for direct combustion as an energy source. Endogenous triglycerides are mainly synthesized in the liver from accumulated fatty acids. In contrast, dietary fat is incorporated into chylomicrons in the small intestine and is known as exogenous triglyceride.

Cholesterol serves as a structural component of cell wall membranes and is a precursor for the synthesis of steroid hormones and bile acids. It may be dietary in origin or synthesized in the liver and intestine. Cholesterol is continuously undergoing synthesis, degradation, and recycling. Most cholesterol synthesis occurs between midnight and 3 a.m.[4] Like cholesterol, phospholipids become constituents of cell wall membranes; most phospholipids originate in the liver and intestinal mucosa. Phospholipids act as donors of phosphate groups for intracellular metabolism and blood coagulation.

Triglyceride, cholesterol, and phospholipid molecules are complexed with specialized proteins (apoproteins) to form lipoproteins, the transport form in which lipids are measured in the blood. Lipoproteins are classified by their density and chemical composition. Table 1 (next page) summarizes their characteristics.

High serum concentrations of low-density lipoproteins (LDL) are associated with an increased risk of coronary heart disease, since most of the cholesterol in plasma is carried in LDL.[7] Conversely, elevated concentrations

**TABLE 1.** Characteristics of Lipoproteins[3,5,6]

| Lipoprotein | Triglycerides (%) | Cholesterol (%) | Origin | Comments |
|---|---|---|---|---|
| Chylomicrons | 80–95 | 3–7 | Intestines | Primarily triglycerides |
| Very low-density lipoproteins (VLDL) | 45–65 | 16–24 | Liver and intestines | Primarily triglycerides |
| Intermediate-density lipoproteins (IDL) or remnants | 15–32 | 30–50 | Chylomicrons and VLDL | Transitional forms |
| Low-density lipoproteins (LDL) | 4–10 | 46–58 | End-product VLDL | Major carrier of cholesterol |
| High-density lipoproteins (HDL) | 2–7 | 18–25 | Intestines and liver | Removes cholesterol from atherosclerotic plaques in arteries |

**TABLE 2.** Characteristics of Familial Hyperlipoproteinemias[5,8]

| Genetic Disorder | Elevated Lipoprotein | Plasma Cholesterol (mg/dL) | Plasma Triglyceride (mg/dL) | Clinical Manifestations and Genetics |
|---|---|---|---|---|
| Familial lipoprotein lipase deficiency (type 1) | Chylomicrons | Normal[a] | >1000[a] | Abdominal pain and/or pancreatitis; hepatosplenomegaly; eruptive xanthomas; lipemia retinalis Monogenic, recessive |
| Familial hypercholesterolemia (type 2a) | LDL | >300 | Normal | Premature atherosclerosis and tendinous xanthomas Monogenic, dominant |
| Familial dysbetalipoproteinemia (type 3) | IDL | >300 | >300 | Coronary and peripheral atherosclerosis; tuberous xanthomas; tendinous xanthomas; palmar and plantar xanthomatous streaks; glucose intolerance (25%); hypothyroid (25%) Monogenic, recessive |
| Familial hypertriglyceridemia (type 4) | VLDL | Normal or 300–800 | 200–500 | Commonly associated with obesity, hyperglycemia, and insulin resistance Adult onset; monogenic, dominant |
| Familial hyperlipoproteinemia (type 5) | Chylomicrons and VLDL | >300 | >500 | Pancreatitis and eruptive xanthomas; rare Monogenic, dominant |
| Familial combined hyperlipidemia (types 2a, 2b, 4, and 5) | LDL and VLDL | 250–600 | 200–600 | Premature atherosclerosis Monogenic, dominant |
| Polygenic hypercholesterolemia (type 2b) | LDL and VLDL (inconsistent) | >300 | Normal or >300 | Premature atherosclerosis Monogenic, dominant |

[a]Conversion factor for cholesterol in International System (SI) units (millimoles per liter) is 0.026. Conversion factor for triglyceride in SI units (millimoles per liter) is 0.011.

of high-density lipoproteins (HDL) have been associated with a low incidence of coronary heart disease,[8] while a low HDL (<35 mg/dL) is considered an independent risk factor for the development of coronary heart disease.[1] Moreover, some evidence suggests that high concentrations of serum triglycerides, which are carried mainly in very low-density lipoproteins (VLDL), may be involved in the pathogenesis of coronary atherosclerosis (Triglycerides section).[9]

## Primary Lipid Disorders

Hyperlipidemias (elevated concentrations of any lipoprotein type), when classified according to etiology, fall into a primary or secondary category. Primary disorders are caused by genetic defects in the synthesis or metabolism of the lipoproteins. Table 2 shows the characteristics of the major familial hyperlipoproteinemias. Familial (genetic) disease should be strongly suspected in a patient with an elevated total serum cholesterol concentration greater than 300 mg/dL (>7.8 mmol/L). In such cases, family members should be screened.

## Secondary Lipid Disorders

Secondary hyperlipidemias are disorders precipitated by other disease states, medications, or lifestyle (Table 3). For example, recent studies have shown that various oral contraceptives affect lipoproteins differently. Combination oral contraceptives do not routinely cause an increase in total serum cholesterol, but they do increase triglyceride concentrations. Effects on HDL are variable, depending on oral contraceptive components.[10]

Another study found a statistically significant but weak positive relationship between the cumulative dose of amiodarone and total serum cholesterol that was independent of thyroid function.[11] As shown in Table 3, hypothyroidism—which can be induced by amiodarone—is associated with hyperlipidemia, specifically hypercholesterolemia. Withdrawal or treatment of the precipitating factor usually leads to a reversal of secondary hyperlipidemia.

Lifestyle (diet and exercise) also may affect a patient's lipoprotein concentrations. Besides being an independent risk factor for coronary heart disease, obesity causes an increase in serum triglycerides (primarily VLDL). Likewise, a sedentary lifestyle may increase serum triglyceride concentrations by decreasing peripheral utilization of fat and glucose and by increasing VLDL production by the liver.[3] In contrast, exercise increases HDL, a beneficial type of cholesterol; independently, exercise increases longevity.[14]

A diet that is high in saturated fats and cholesterol increases total serum cholesterol concentrations (especially LDL). In fact, age-adjusted coronary heart disease mortality rates have declined by 50% over the past four decades, probably because of decreases in animal fats in the diet along with better control of hypertension and smoking cessation.[3] One vice, light to moderate alcohol intake (one to two glasses of beer or wine or 1–2 ounces of liquor per day), compared with abstention from alcohol increases HDL and is associated with lower mortality from coronary heart disease.[15,16]

**TABLE 3.** Secondary Causes of Hyperlipidemia and Associated Changes in Lipoprotein Component (If Known)[5,10–13,a]

| Disorder or Condition | Drug or Diet |
|---|---|
| Acromegaly | Alcohol[c] (↑ VLDL, ≈ LDL, ↑ HDL) |
| Acute hepatitis | Amiodarone |
| Cholestasis | Contraceptives (estrogen and progestin) |
| Cushing's syndrome | Corticosteroids (↑ VLDL, ↑ LDL, ≈ HDL) |
| Diabetes mellitus (↑ VLDL, ≈/↑ LDL, ↓ HDL) | Danazol (↑ LDL, ↓ HDL)[d] |
| Glycogen storage disease | Diet high in saturated fats and cholesterol |
| Hypothyroidism (≈/↑ VLDL, ↑ LDL, ↓ HDL) | Estrogens (↑ VLDL, ↓ LDL, ↑ HDL) |
| Myeloma or lymphoma | Etretinate (↑ VLDL, ↑ LDL, ↓ HDL) |
| Myocardial infarction[b] (↑ VLDL, ↓ LDL, ↓ HDL) | Isotretinoin (↑ VLDL, ↑ LDL, ↓ HDL) |
| Nephrotic syndrome (↑ VLDL, ↑ LDL, ↓ HDL) | Parenteral lipid emulsions (↑ VLDL, ≈ LDL, ≈ HDL) |
| Obesity (↑ VLDL, ↑ LDL, ↓ HDL) | Progestins (≈ VLDL, ↑ LDL, ↓ HDL) |
| Porphyria, acute intermittent | Tamoxifen |
| Sedentary lifestyle | Thiazide diuretics (↑ VLDL, ↑ LDL, ≈/↓ HDL) |
| Systemic lupus erythematosus | |
| Uremia (↑ VLDL) | |

[a] ↑ = increase; ↓ = decrease; ≈ = no change.
[b] Total cholesterol starts to fall 24 hr after an acute myocardial infarction and reaches its lowest point in 4–9 days; it then returns to baseline after 6–8 weeks.[13]
[c] Moderate intake.
[d] Total cholesterol not affected.

## Laboratory Tests for Lipids and Lipoproteins

Hypercholesterolemia and hypertriglyceridemia clearly are major contributors to coronary artery disease and peripheral vascular disease. Fortunately, several laboratory tests can be used to assess the concentrations of various lipids in the blood, making early detection and monitoring possible. For instance, total serum cholesterol is used initially to screen for atherosclerotic risk. After a patient fasts, triglycerides and LDL can be measured to confirm a diagnosis and monitor drug therapy, if necessary. HDL, the beneficial type of cholesterol, also can be measured. In combination, the results of these tests are used to determine a diagnosis. Some of them can even be performed by patients with new home testing devices.

### Total Serum Cholesterol

*For nonfasting adults >20 years without coronary heart disease: desirable, <200 mg/dL or <5.17 mmol/L; borderline high, 200–239 mg/dL or 5.17–6.18 mmol/L; or high, >239 mg/dL or >6.18 mmol/L (ranges from American Heart Association[1])*

Although there is some controversy concerning the elderly (>70 years),[17,18] lowering elevated serum cholesterol concentrations generally decreases death from coronary artery disease and may cause regression of atherosclerotic lesions.[19] In young healthy adults, total serum cholesterol is a strong predictor of clinically evident cardiovascular disease occurring 25 or more years later.[20]

Therefore, the total serum cholesterol concentration is used as an initial screening test for assessing atherosclerotic risk. Despite popular belief, a fasting sample is not necessary because total serum cholesterol is not affected by a single meal. Factors that may interfere with its accurate assessment include pregnancy, recent weight loss, vigorous exercise, and acute myocardial infarction. Total serum cholesterol may also be lowered by corticosteroids. Although low total serum cholesterol usually is considered a sign of good health, it can be a sign of hyperthyroidism, malnutrition, chronic anemia, cancer, or severe liver disease.

The National Institutes of Health and the American Heart Association recommend that all adults (≥20 years) have a baseline total serum cholesterol measured and then repeated every 5 years. If the value is greater than 200 mg/dL (>5.17 mmol/L), the measurement should be repeated in 1–8 weeks and the results of the two measurements averaged. If the two values vary by more than 30 mg/dL (>0.8 mmol/L), a third measurement should be taken and all three values averaged to obtain the patient's baseline.[1]

In addition to total serum cholesterol, clinicians should evaluate triglycerides, LDL, and HDL in patients with one or more of the following criteria:

1. A *high* total serum cholesterol.
2. A *borderline high* total serum cholesterol and evidence of definite coronary heart disease (prior

**TABLE 4.** Risk Factors for Atherosclerotic Vascular Disease from High Cholesterol (Primarily LDL)[1,a]

| |
|---|
| Age: ≥45 years for men or ≥55 years for women |
| Family history of premature (<55 years) coronary heart disease |
| Myocardial infarction or myocardial ischemia (angina pectoris) |
| Cigarette smoking (more than 10 cigarettes a day) |
| Uncontrolled hypertension |
| HDL cholesterol <35 mg/dL on at least two occasions |
| Obesity (>30% over lean body weight) |
| History of cerebrovascular or occlusive peripheral vascular disease |
| Diabetes mellitus |

[a]*When risk is assessed, an HDL ≥60 mg/dL is considered a negative factor that, if present, "neutralizes" one (of the above) existing positive risk factors.*

myocardial infarction or definite myocardial ischemia).

3. A *borderline high* total serum cholesterol and the presence of two coronary heart disease risk factors (listed in Table 4).

Methods used to assay total serum cholesterol vary greatly in laboratories. Therefore, clinicians should become familiar with the method used by their laboratory as well as with potential causes of misleading or erroneous results. Serum or heparinized plasma is the typical specimen collected. Prolonged tourniquet application should be avoided because venous stasis may cause total serum cholesterol concentrations to increase 5–10%.

### Triglycerides

*For adults >20 years:[1] desirable, <200 mg/dL or <2.26 mmol/L; borderline high, 200–400 mg/dL or 2.26–4.52 mmol/L; high, 400–1000 mg/dL or 4.52–11.3 mmol/L; or very high, >1000 mg/dL or >11.3 mmol/L*

Disorders leading to hypertriglyceridemia involve chylomicrons and/or VLDL. VLDL, LDL, and HDL are present in the fasting state, but chylomicrons and intermediate-density lipoproteins are present only in postprandial or pathological states. Triglycerides in the form of chylomicrons appear in the plasma as soon as 2 hr after a meal, reach a maximum at 4–6 hr, and persist for up to 14 hr.[6] To avoid inflation of concentrations, measurement of triglycerides and lipoproteins is recommended after an overnight fast. Triglyceride concentrations occasionally become transiently or persistently elevated in patients receiving intermittent or constantly infused intravenous lipids, respectively. However, lipid emulsion regimens usually are not changed unless there is risk of pancreatitis. Heparin, a common additive to parenteral nutrition solutions, may facilitate faster metabolism of chylomicrons and reduce triglyceride concentrations by a stimulatory effect on lipoprotein lipase.

As a secondary disorder, hypertriglyceridemia is associated with obesity, uncontrolled diabetes mellitus, liver disease, alcohol ingestion, and uremia. Combination oral contraceptives, corticosteroids, antihypertensive agents, and isotretinoin also may elevate triglyceride concentrations (Table 3).

Consideration of hypertriglyceridemia, without other lipid abnormalities, as an independent risk factor for coronary heart disease is controversial.[21] However, high triglyceride concentrations along with low HDL may add to the risk of coronary heart disease.[22] It is *not* controversial that hypertriglyceridemia (concentrations >1000 mg/dL or >11.3 mmol/L) may precipitate pancreatitis (Chapter 11). In fact, many patients with hypertriglyceridemia have intermittent episodes of epigastric pain due to recurrent pancreatic inflammation. A reduction of the triglyceride concentration through diet or drugs (usually initiated when triglycerides remain >600 mg/dL or >6.8 mmol/L) may prevent the progression to pancreatitis. Gemfibrozil and nicotinic acid (if LDL also is elevated) are drugs of choice.

Extremely high concentrations of VLDL, the primary carrier lipoprotein of triglycerides, also may lead to eruptive cutaneous xanthomas on the elbows, knees, and buttocks. The xanthomas may disappear once triglyceride concentrations fall below 2000 mg/dL (<22.6 mmol/L). Hypertriglyceridemia may also manifest as lipemia retinalis (a whitish cast in the vascular bed of the retina). This sign is due to triglyceride particles scattering light in the blood and is seen in the retinal vessels during an eye exam. In patients with lipemia retinalis, triglyceride concentrations may be 3000 mg/dL (34 mmol/L) or greater.[2,23] A concentration this high requires immediate action because it causes hyperviscosity of the blood with the risk of thrombus formation.

Most patients with a high triglyceride concentration are inactive and obese. Many are also hypertensive and insulin resistant and have low HDL. In patients with a triglyceride concentration of 250–750 mg/dL (2.8–8.5 mmol/L), a 10–20-lb weight loss usually leads to a marked reduction in triglyceride concentrations and an increase in HDL (if low). Finally, hyperuricemia is strongly associated with high triglycerides, obesity, and myocardial infarction.[24,25]

There are several assay interferences regarding triglycerides. The triglyceride assay itself is susceptible to interference by glycerol, which may be a component of medications or used as a lubricant in laboratory equipment.[26] An excess of triglycerides in the blood can lead to errors in other laboratory measurements. Lipemic samples can cause falsely low serum amylase results, underestimation of electrolytes, and erratic interferences with many other tests.[27] The potential interference with amylase is especially clinically relevant since high triglyceride concentrations can cause pancreatitis, and accurate amylase concentrations are crucial to diagnosis.

Fortunately, most technologists can identify lipemic samples (milky serum). The appearance of a patient's serum sample before and after 12–16 hr of refrigeration can indicate triglyceride-rich serum. If the sample shows a uniform turbidity (opalescence), VLDL has increased without a concurrent increase in chylomicrons. A "cream" supernatant layer atop a clear solution indicates chylomicronemia, without an excess of both chylomicrons and VLDL.[5]

### Low-Density Lipoprotein Cholesterol

*For fasting adults >20 years without coronary heart disease or other atherosclerotic disease:[1] desirable, <130 mg/dL or <3.36 mmol/L; borderline high, 130–159 mg/dL or 3.36–4.11 mmol/L; or high, >159 mg/dL or >4.11 mmol/L*
*For fasting adults >20 years with coronary heart disease or other atherosclerotic disease:[1] desirable, ≤100 mg/dL or ≤2.6 mmol/L*

Reference ranges for normal LDL concentrations are higher in the United States than in the rest of the world. This difference probably is due to the high calorie, fat, and cholesterol content of the American diet. Therefore, normal LDL concentrations do not imply a lack of atherosclerotic risk.

The LDL must be measured while the patient is in a fasting state. This measurement should be performed twice, at least 1–8 weeks apart, and the values averaged. Patients should not change their dietary habits between tests. Patients whose LDL cholesterol is less than 130 mg/dL (<3.36 mmol/L) should have their total serum cholesterol measured every 5 years. By use of the following formula (all in milligrams per deciliter), LDL may be estimated in patients with a triglyceride concentration less than 400 mg/dL (<4.52 mmol/L) and without type 3 hyperlipoproteinemia (Table 2):

LDL = total serum cholesterol − HDL − (0.16 × triglycerides)

Table 5 (next page) lists the treatment recommendations from the 1993 report of the expert panel of the National Cholesterol Education Program.[1] Some clinicians start hypolipidemic drug therapy in patients with symptomatic coronary artery disease before cholesterol reaches the concentrations defined by the American Heart Association. One study found that drugs such as pravastatin slow progression of atherosclerosis and reduce the incidence of adverse cardiovascular events as early as 6 months after starting therapy, even when cholesterol concentrations are well within current low-risk limits. Male patients with a serum cholesterol concentration of 155–310 mg/dL (4–8 mmol/L) were included.[28]

For monitoring during long-term drug or dietary therapy, most patients can be assessed based on their total serum cholesterol concentration. This method obviates the need for a fasting sample and the expense of further lipoprotein analysis. A total serum cholesterol concentration of 240 mg/dL (6.22 mmol/L) is comparable to an

**TABLE 5.** LDL-Based Treatment Recommendations of the Expert Panel of the National Cholesterol Education Program[1]

| AVD Present[a] | Risk Factors[b] | LDL Concentration (mg/dL) to Consider Starting Treatment[c] | | LDL Goal |
|---|---|---|---|---|
| | | Special Diet | Drugs[d] | |
| No | None or one | ≥160 (≥4.14) | ≥190 (≥4.92) | <160 (<4.14) |
| No | Two or more | ≥130 (≥3.36) | ≥160 (≥4.14) | <130 (<3.36) |
| Yes | None or any | >100 (>2.60) | ≥130 (≥3.36) | ≤100 (≤2.60) |

[a]Atherosclerotic vessel disease (AVD) includes angina, myocardial infarction, and stroke. An increased (≥60 mg/dL) HDL concentration is a negative risk factor (discussed previously) and negates one of the positive factors.
[b]Risk factors in Table 4.
[c]Amount in parentheses is in SI units of millimoles per liter.
[d]Concentration achieved after adequate trial of dietary therapy.

LDL cholesterol concentration of 160 mg/dL (4.14 mmol/L), and a total serum cholesterol concentration of 200 mg/dL (5.17 mmol/L) is comparable to an LDL concentration of 130 mg/dL (3.36 mmol/L). Therefore, in borderline to high-risk patients, an actual LDL measurement is recommended only once yearly.[1,23]

### High-Density Lipoprotein Cholesterol
*For fasting adults >20 years:[1] desirable, >35 mg/dL or*
*>0.91 mmol/L on at least two separate occasions*

Based on epidemiological evidence, HDL seems to act as an antiatherogenic factor. An HDL concentration lower than 35 mg/dL (<0.91 mmol/L) on at least two separate occasions has been shown to be a risk factor for the development of atherosclerotic disease. The blood need not be drawn after a 12-hr fast; however, a fast is required because HDL is usually ordered in combination with LDL.

Examples of this atherogenic potential are best illustrated with the coronary arteries. Concentrations less than 35 mg/dL (<0.91 mmol/L) are associated with an increased risk of myocardial infarction. Similarly, low HDL is also associated with an increased risk of coronary angioplasty restenosis.[29] HDL is negatively correlated with triglycerides, smoking, and obesity. In contrast, HDL is positively correlated with physical activity. Generally, the ideal LDL:HDL ratio is less than 3. An LDL:HDL ratio greater than 4 is considered atherogenic[1,2] (Minicases 1 and 2, pages 287 and 288).

### Home Testing of Cholesterol

Patients now can use a home testing device to measure their serum cholesterol.[30] The test takes about 12–15 min to perform and requires that the patient lance a finger for a drop of blood. Whether this test is simple enough for persons to perform and read accurately is unknown. The test should not be performed within 4 hr of taking acetaminophen or 500 mg or more of vitamin C because either drug can cause falsely low results.

## Effects of Hypolipemic Medications

Although this book does not have a therapeutic focus, clinicians must be aware of how antihyperlipidemic drugs can influence laboratory test results. Obviously, if therapy is successful, these drugs should lower total serum cholesterol and/or triglycerides. A recent study found that 3-hydroxy-3-methylglutaryl coenzyme A reductase inhibitors (HMG Co-A RIs), fibric acid derivatives, and nicotinic acid raise HDL concentrations in patients whose baseline concentrations are less than 39 mg/dL (<1.0 mmol/L) but not in patients with baseline HDL greater than 39 mg/dL. Furthermore, among patients with a baseline HDL less than 39 mg/dL, HMG Co-A RIs did not significantly lower triglyceride concentrations and fibric acid analogs did not significantly reduce LDL cholesterol.[31] Depending on the patient's baseline HDL (and other lipid profile), treatment goals may be refined based on the study's findings. The effects on specific lipoproteins are discussed below.

### Bile Acid Binders

Agents that bind bile acids (e.g., cholestyramine and colestipol) lower LDL concentrations by 15–30% but may raise triglycerides by 5–15%, especially if hypertriglyceridemia exists.[4,32] Because these products stay within the enterohepatic circulation, they do not directly cause other systemic effects that may be reflected in laboratory data. They do, however, interfere with the absorption of fat-soluble vitamins and drugs (e.g., digoxin, thyroid supplements, and warfarin) and may affect serum concentrations of these drugs or prothrombin times.

### Niacin

Although niacin is associated with more bothersome side effects (e.g., flushing, pruritis, and gastrointestinal distress) than other agents, it has a desirable antilipidemic profile. In therapeutic doses, this B vitamin lowers total serum cholesterol (by 15–30%), LDL, and triglycerides (by 15–40%) and tends to raise HDL (by 7–20%).[4,32] Niacin may increase serum glucose, uric acid, and liver function tests (LFTs)[4,33] and decrease serum thyroxine (T$_4$) and thyroxine-binding globulin without clinical hypothyroidism.[34] Flushing can be relieved by taking one baby or adult aspirin before each dose.

### 3-Hydroxy-3-methylglutaryl Coenzyme A Reductase Inhibitors

By inhibiting the enzyme that catalyzes the rate-limiting step in cholesterol synthesis, lovastatin, pravastatin, simvastatin, and fluvastatin lower total cholesterol (17–34%) and LDL (24–40% depending on the dose) and usually have no effect on or raise HDL.[4,7] In some cases, lovastatin also decreases high triglyceride concentrations (5–15%). At recommended doses, fluvastatin is less effective than older HMG Co-A RIs, has variable effects on triglycerides, and can slightly decrease HDL.[35] With all HMG Co-A RIs, maximum effects usually are seen after 4–6 weeks.

Patients on these agents may develop increases in transaminases and creatine phosphokinase (CPK) (Chapter 10) with myopathy. Lovastatin causes elevations in CPK concentrations of at least twice the upper limit of normal in about 11% of patients. Some manufacturers recommend that LFTs be performed before the initiation of therapy, at 6 and 12 weeks after initiation, and then semiannually. If transaminases (aspartate aminotransferase and alanine aminotransferase) rise to three times the up-

per limit of normal or higher, manufacturers recommend withdrawal of the drug. Many clinicians will not order CPK levels unless the patient complains of myalgias.

Little data exist on the newer agents regarding this effect. These agents not only improve biochemical indices of atherogenic risk but, not surprisingly, have slowed progression and reduced development of new lesions in the coronary arteries.[36,37] HMG Co-A RIs as a class probably have this potential. One study showed that 5–6 years of simvastatin use led to a desirable change in lipid profile and a decreased coronary death rate (5 versus 8.5% for placebo).[38]

### Fibric Acid Derivatives

The fibric acid derivatives gemfibrozil and clofibrate reduce VLDL and triglycerides. Gemfibrozil appears to be more effective in lowering triglycerides (>30%). Moreover, total serum cholesterol often is decreased (5–15%). In some patients, these derivatives increase HDL. LDL occasionally may increase when triglycerides decline.[39] Gemfibrozil is preferred to clofibrate, which some clinicians feel is less effective and is associated with more trans-

---

**Minicase 1**

George L., a 56-year-old, 5-ft 9-in, 250-lb male stockbroker, visited his doctor because of first-time angina on exertion. He had just finished eating in a fast food restaurant and was carrying a heavy box of brochures from his car to his colleague's car when the chest pressure started. He rushed right over to his physician's office, arriving within 1 hr. His chest discomfort was associated with sweating, nausea, and dyspnea.

George L. was a long-term smoker and did very little exercise. His father died of a heart attack at age 58. He had no family history of diabetes or lipid disorders. His electrocardiogram at the office was normal, except for mild tachycardia (heart rate 90), which he attributed to being nervous. His blood pressure was 150/86, and his glucose was 180 mg/dL. He was on no medications except for occasional antacids taken for epigastric burning.

George L. stated that this episode was not like indigestion. He also stated that if his cholesterol was high, he should not be bothered about special diets because he would not comply. As part of the workup, his physician measured serum lipids. After the tachycardia and chest discomfort resolved, the doctor sent George L. home and told him not to exert himself. He also gave him a prescription for sublingual nitroglycerin. The next day, results from the office visit were as follows: total serum cholesterol, 225 mg/dL; triglycerides, 600 mg/dL; LDL, 140 mg/dL; and HDL, 40 mg/dL. Prior to this reading, George L. had never had his lipid concentrations measured.

*Was it appropriate to order a lipid profile? How should the lipid profile be interpreted?*

**Discussion:** Patients with coronary artery disease (myocardial infarction or angina) should have a lipid profile performed. However, in the case of George L., the triglyceride, lipoprotein, and glucose results are unin-

terpretable because he had eaten about 1–2 hr beforehand. This recent meal may explain why his triglyceride, LDL, and glucose concentrations may be elevated. Total cholesterol concentrations are not significantly affected by a recent meal.

Even before this episode, George L. was at high risk for atherosclerotic heart disease. He is an overweight, male smoker, older than 45 years, who lives a sedentary lifestyle. His father died rather prematurely of atherosclerotic vessel disease, although his age at death (58) does not meet the official criteria for a risk factor (<55 years old).

George L.'s total cholesterol was 225 mg/dL, which is in the borderline high category. His LDL of 140 mg/dL also is in the borderline high category but is not a fasting level. However, according to the recent expert panel consensus guidelines, George L. falls into the "artherosclerotic vessel disease present" category, and he has several risk factors. A special diet should be started even if his LDL is only higher than 100 mg/dL. His entire lipid profile should be run again after a 12-hr fast.

Unfortunately, George L. will not agree to diet management; although he may be willing to lose weight, it could take months. Therefore, if repeat fasting values are in the same range, he appears to be a candidate for drug therapy (LDL ≥130 mg/dL). The lipid profile should be repeated again in about 3–4 weeks to confirm the patient's previous value before committing to drug therapy. George L.'s HDL is 40 mg/dL, which is close to the "high-risk" category (<35 mg/dL). But, again, this value also should be measured after a 12-hr fast. If repeat fasting values are similar, the goal should be to lower LDL to less than 100 mg/dL and raise the HDL. If achieved, the risk of future coronary episodes may be reduced by inhibiting progression or inducing regression of atherosclerosis.[19,41–43]

Henrietta F., a 42-year-old, 5-ft 8-in, 125-lb premeno-
pausal female, had her lipid profile results forwarded to
the clinic after her attendance at a local health fair. Her
fasting concentrations were a total serum cholesterol of
205 mg/dL and triglycerides of 400 mg/dL. She followed
a reasonable, low-fat diet, hiked often, and had no major
medical problems except for chronic asthma. For this condition, she took 5–10 mg of prednisone per day. She was
also taking vitamins, calcium, and an oral contraceptive.

Henrietta F. did not smoke, rarely drank alcohol, and
did not have a family history of diabetes, hyperlipidemias,
pancreatitis, or coronary heart disease. At her office visit,
she had a perfectly normal physical exam. Her fasting
glucose was 100 mg/dL; electrolyte, hematology, liver,
renal, and thyroid tests were all normal.

*How should the lipid results be interpreted? What
should be done next?*

**Discussion:** Henrietta F. is young, asymptomatic, and pre-
menopausal; watches her cholesterol intake; is active; is
not hypertensive; and has no familial risk factors. She
should have normal total serum cholesterol and triglyceride concentrations, but her triglyceride concentration is
in the *high* category and her total serum cholesterol is

barely in the *borderline high* category. These tests should
be repeated, and secondary causes of the elevations
should be eliminated. Regarding secondary causes, she
has no occult thyroid, renal, or liver disease. Henrietta F.
is, however, using drugs that can cause an elevation in
these tests. Oral contraceptives usually have more of an
effect on triglycerides, but they can also increase total
serum cholesterol concentrations.

Although Henrietta F. is on a relatively low, barely
supraphysiological, dose of prednisone, it may be having
some impact on her total serum cholesterol and triglyceride concentrations. If her repeat tests are elevated, her
oral contraceptive should be stopped and concentrations
repeated in 4–6 weeks. If her concentrations do not decline, withdrawal of or alternatives to prednisone should
be considered. For example, inhaled steroids may keep
her asthma in check. Concentrations should be repeated
again 4–6 weeks after prednisone is stopped. A measurement of cholesterol subtypes (HDL, LDL, and VLDL) also
may help to assess cardiovascular risk, since elevated concentrations of HDL (the "protective" cholesterol) may be
contributing to the high total serum cholesterol. If so, perhaps no action should be taken at this time.

aminase and CPK elevations (with myositis and flu-like
symptoms) and cholelithiasis. Periodic (every 6–12
months) LFTs and CPK measurements should be done
in patients receiving these drugs.

### *Probucol*

Probucol typically lowers total serum cholesterol, LDL
(≤10%), and HDL (15%). Its antiatherogenic effects may
occur despite its inability to lower cholesterol concentrations in some patients.[4,32,40] Therefore, LDL (and total
serum cholesterol) determinations may be less useful in
adjusting therapy. Transient eosinophilia and increases in
CPK, uric acid, glucose, and LFTs rarely occur.

## PORPHYRIAS

*Erythrocytes—normal range for coproporphyrin: 0.5–2 µg/dL or
0.75–3 nmol/L; and normal range for protoporphyrin: 4–52
µg/dL or 7.2–93.6 nmol/L
Urine—normal range for δ-amino levulinic acid: 1.5–7.5 mg/
24 hr or 11–57 µmol/24 hr; normal range for porphobilinogen:
<2 mg/24 hr or <8.8 µmol/24 hr; normal range for
coproporphyrin: 50–160 µg/24 hr or 0.075–0.24 µmol/24 hr;
and normal range for uroporphyrin: 10–30 µg/24 hr or 0.012–
0.037 µmol/24 hr
Feces—normal range for coproporphyrin: <500 µg/24 hr or
<0.75 µmol/24 hr; and normal range for protoporphyrin: <600
µg/24 hr or <1.1 µmol/24 hr*

Porphyrias are metabolic disorders of heme synthesis in
which there are an overproduction, accumulation, and
excretion of porphyrins and their intermediary precursors. Porphyrias may be either genetic (usually autosomal

dominant) or acquired (e.g., lead poisoning) disturbances
in the synthesis of heme. They manifest as neurological
and psychiatric dysfunction and/or dermatological lesions.
This section opens with a discussion of heme synthesis.
Then the relationship between test results and clinical
findings seen in the various porphyrias is discussed.[44]

### Heme Synthesis

Heme is a necessary component of all aerobic cells, and it
is essential to life. The synthesis of heme (Figure 1) is
initiated by glycine (Gly) and succinyl coenzyme-A
(SCoA); they serve as raw materials for the formation of
δ-aminolevulinic acid (ALA). A series of biochemical steps
form protoporphyrin, which chelates ferrous iron to become heme.

When functioning normally, heme's biosynthetic
pathway generates enough heme for myoglobin and hemoglobin (Hgb). It also generates enough heme for cyto-
chromes (including $P_{450}$), catalase, peroxidase, and other
oxidative enzymes involved in drug metabolism. Any sur-
plus forms a cellular pool of free heme that controls the
production of the enzyme ALA–synthetase via negative
feedback. The first reaction, Gly/SCoA to ALA, is the
rate-limiting step for the entire pathway.[45] Synthesis of
heme occurs in the liver as well as the bone marrow, where
it affords oxygen-carrying capacity to erythrocytes as Hgb.

Certain drugs and other substances influence heme
synthesis dramatically. Some drugs (e.g., barbiturates,
phenytoin, sulfonylureas, and rifampin) induce the production of cytochrome $P_{450}$, a substance rich in hemo-
proteins, and deplete cellular heme stores. Theoretically,

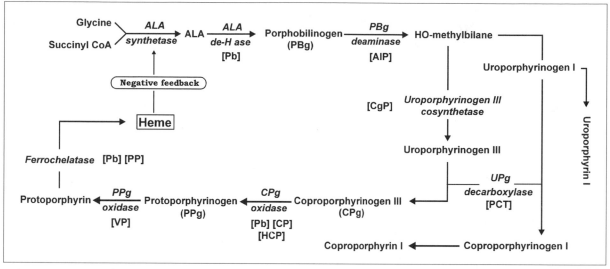

**FIGURE 1.** Heme synthesis and sites of enzyme deficiency for specific porphyrias. ALA = δ-aminolevulinic acid; [ ] = site of enzyme defect or inhibition for specific porphyria; Pb = lead poisoning; AIP = acute intermittent porphyria; CgP = congenital (erythropoietic) porphyria; PP = protoporphyria; VP = variegate porphyria; CP = coproporphyria (erythropoietic); HCP = hereditary coproporphyria; PCT = porphyria cutanea tarda. (Compiled from References 45–48.)

through negative feedback mechanisms, ALA–synthetase activity is stimulated, more porphyrins (or precursors) are produced, and disease manifests in susceptible people. Griseofulvin may directly increase ALA–synthetase activity, and iron products and steroids have induced the enzyme synergistically.[44,47] Conversely, hematin and carbohydrates seem to inhibit heme synthesis, and both are used in treating acute attacks even though some studies failed to show clinical benefit from hematin in acute hepatic porphyria (although there was biochemical improvement).[43]

## Laboratory Diagnosis

The two major classes of genetic porphyrias are *erythropoietic*, in which the primary biochemical abnormality occurs in the red blood cell, and *hepatic*, in which the important findings are in the urine or stool. Protoporphyria has characteristics of both classes.

In general, porphyrias that cause excessive synthesis of ALA and porphobilinogen (PBg) are associated with neurological problems.[47] These substances are water soluble and fat insoluble; therefore, excess amounts are found in the urine as opposed to the feces. Porphyrias that lead to excessive production of intermediate products further down the metabolic pathway (coproporphyrin and protoporphyrin) are associated with dermatological manifestations. These products are fat soluble; therefore, they are preferentially excreted in the bile and sought in the feces.

Coproporphyrin is also water soluble; of the porphyrins, it is found in normal urine in the highest concentration. Deficiency of heme in nerve cells and a direct toxic effect of ALA and PBg have been postulated as the cause of neuropathy.[48] The porphyrins are pigmented compounds. Urine that appears bright burgundy or turns red on standing may indicate a porphyria disorder. (Other causes of urine color changes can be found in Chapter 7.)

Table 6 (next page) summarizes typical diagnostic test results in the porphyrias. Although the types of porphyria have been grouped into three classes in this table, other classification systems may be used. Moreover, porphyria can be acquired, as in lead poisoning and anemias.

Although there are many approaches to the diagnosis of porphyria, Figure 2 (next page) shows one practical way to evaluate patients with consistent history and physical examinations. It is based on urinary ALA and PBg, tests that are available in many hospital laboratories.

### Hepatic Porphyrias

Hepatic porphyrias are characterized by acute intermittent abdominal pain, neuropathies, and psychiatric disturbances. These symptoms are caused by visceral (gut), peripheral, or central (brain) nerve-cell dysfunction or destruction. Specific signs and symptoms include nausea, vomiting, constipation, pain or numbness in the extremities, tachycardia, dark urine, and mental changes.

The laboratory diagnosis is made on the basis of increased concentrations of PBg and ALA in the urine. Hyponatremia and hypomagnesemia are associated laboratory findings. Barbiturates and other drugs (Table 7, page 291) may trigger or worsen hepatic porphyrias. Except for porphyria cutanea tarda, urine concentrations of porphyrins and precursors may be absent unless the patient is having an acute attack.[49]

*Acute intermittent porphyria.* Acute intermittent porphyria causes the most severe attacks and is more common in women than men. Its onset occurs as early as puberty. In

**TABLE 6.** Age at Onset and Accumulation and Excretion Patterns of Porphyrias[a]

| Class or Type of Porphyria | Age at Onset (years) | Urine ALA | Urine PBg | Urine UP | Urine CP | Feces CP | Feces PP | Erythrocytes UP | Erythrocytes CP | Erythrocytes PP |
|---|---|---|---|---|---|---|---|---|---|---|
| **Erythropoietic porphyria** | | | | | | | | | | |
| Congenital porphyria | Congenital | N | N | II | I | I/II | N or I | II | I | N or I |
| **Hepatic porphyrias** | | | | | | | | | | |
| Acute intermittent porphyria | 13–30 | (I/II) | (II) | (I) | N or (I) | N | N | N | N | N |
| Hereditary coproporphyria | <10 | (II) | (I) | N or (I) | II | II | N or I | N | N | N |
| Variegate porphyria | <30 | (II) | (II) | N or I | (I/II) | I[b] | II | N | N | N |
| Porphyria cutanea tarda | >40 | N | N | II[c] | I | N or I | N or I | N | N | N |
| **Erythrohepatic porphyria** | | | | | | | | | | |
| Protoporphyria | <6 | N | N | N | N or I | (I) | II | N | N | II |

[a] UP = uroporphyrin; CP = coproporphyrin; PP = protoporphyrin; N = normal concentrations; I = increased concentrations, II = markedly increased concentrations; ( ) = increased concentrations during acute attacks (may be normal during remission). During acute attacks, urine ALA is 20–100 mg/day (150–760 μmol/day) and urine PBg is 50–200 mg/day (220–880 μmol/day). (Compiled from References 44–51.)
[b] Fecal PP > CP in variegate, but fecal PP < CP in cutanea tarda.
[c] Urine UP:CP ratio is <1 in variegate but >7.5 in cutanea tarda.

addition to neurological and psychiatric problems, sinus tachycardia and hypertension are common symptoms. Buildup of PBg and ALA probably leads to signs and symptoms.

*Hereditary coproporphyria.* Hereditary coproporphyria manifests neuroviscerally and cutaneously. As the name

implies, coproporphyrin accumulation is the principal problem; however, elevated PBg and ALA contribute to manifestations.

*Variegate porphyria.* Variegate porphyria presents like hereditary coproporphyria, except that dermatological problems are so severe that scarring is not uncommon. Large

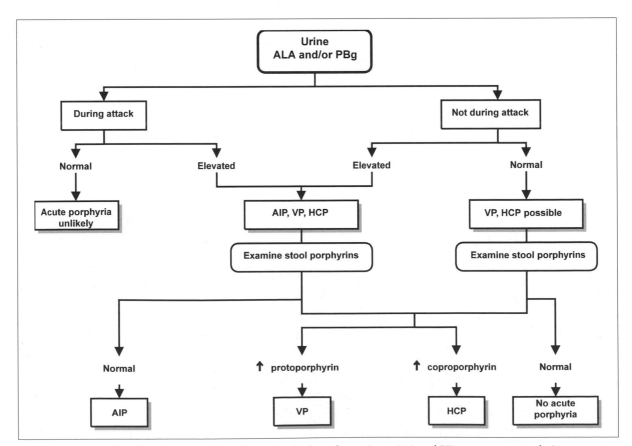

**FIGURE 2.** Approach to the diagnosis of hepatic porphyrias based on urinary ALA and PBg measurements during an acute attack and between attacks. VP = variegate porphyria; HCP = hereditary coproporphyria; AIP = acute intermittent porphyria. (Adapted, with permission, from Reference 44.)

**TABLE 7.** Unsafe and Safe Drugs in Patients with Hepatic Porphyrias[a]

---

**Unsafe drugs**
  Alcohol
  Barbiturates
  Carbamazepine
  Danazol
  Ergots
  Estrogens and progesterones
  Griseofulvin
  Meprobamate
  Sulfonamide antibiotics
  Valproic acid
**Safe drugs**
  Acetaminophen
  Aminoglycoside antibiotics
  Aspirin
  Atropine
  Beta-lactam antibiotics
  Glucocorticoids
  Insulin
  Opiates
  Phenothiazines

---

[a]*Hepatic porphyrias include acute intermittent porphyria, hereditary coproporphyria, and variegate porphyria.*

amounts of fecal protoporphyrin, the prototypical finding, are accompanied by elevated ALA and PBg in the urine.

*Porphyria cutanea tarda and pseudoporphyria.* Hallmarks of porphyria cutanea tarda, as the name implies, are cutaneous lesions that occur late in life. The advent of oral contraceptives, however, has increased the incidence of porphyria cutanea tarda in younger women. Excessive iron and alcohol intake also can precipitate an attack. In porphyria cutanea tarda, decreased uroporphyrinogen decarboxylase causes uroporphyrin accumulation, leading to the development of characteristic skin lesions in sun-exposed areas. Phlebotomy and chloroquine are used to treat this form.

A disorder resembling porphyria cutanea tarda, pseudoporphyria, occasionally occurs in patients being hemodialyzed for chronic renal failure. Rarely, drugs such as amiodarone, cyclosporine, dapsone, diflunisal, furosemide, ketoprofen, nalidixic acid, naproxen, pyridoxine, and tetracycline also can induce it.[52] Diagnosis depends on the concentrations of plasma porphyrins, because little urine is produced. Patients with normal concentrations have pseudoporphyria; the name of the diagnosis with elevated concentrations has not been universally accepted.[50]

### Erythropoietic Porphyrias

In contrast to hepatic types, erythropoietic porphyrias are manifested by photosensitivity, burning, and pruritus. Congenital porphyria is the primary disorder in this class. Elevated concentrations of uroporphyrin and coproporphyrin in the urine and erythroid cells are diagnostic for erythropoietic disorders. Fecal porphyrins also may be elevated. Any drug that is oxidized by the cytochrome $P_{450}$ system may precipitate an acute attack. Oral ß-carotene reduces photosensitivity.

### Acquired Porphyrias

Porphyrin imbalance occurs in other diseases in which heme synthesis is disturbed, such as poisoning from polychlorinated benzenes or lead, hepatic tumors, liver disease, alcoholism, chronic renal failure during hemodialysis, and anemias. Patients with lead poisoning have increased (300–3000 mg/dL) free erythrocyte protoporphyrin and urinary ALA and coproporphyrin, and they develop many of the noncutaneous signs and symptoms of the porphyrias.[48] Despite these findings, only an elevated blood (or urine) lead concentration makes the diagnosis definitive.

In iron deficiency anemia, protoporphyrin in red cells is markedly increased. In fact, increases in protoporphyrin occur before changes appear in peripheral blood. Although erythrocyte protoporphyrin is rarely used in diagnosis, it may help when interpretation of serum iron and iron-binding capacity (Chapter 14) is confounded by premature iron therapy.[48]

### Reference Ranges, Specimen Collection, Storage, and Spurious Results

Factors such as wide and variable reference ranges and specimen-handling problems can cause erroneous interpretation of test results. The normal ranges listed at the beginning of this section vary widely among laboratories. Furthermore, to obtain valid results, proper collection and storage are critical.

Urine collections for porphyrins should be alkalinized, but urine for PBg and ALA should be acidified. Urine should be collected in dark containers, because some substances (e.g., ALA) deteriorate quickly on exposure to light. Patients taking ofloxacin and, possibly, other fluoroquinolones may have falsely elevated coproporphyrin concentrations in their urine when measured by some high performance liquid chromatography methods.[53]

## SUMMARY

If total serum cholesterol is lowered and HDL is raised, death from coronary artery disease decreases. Hypertriglyceridemia increases the risk of pancreatitis. Hyperlipidemia may be primary (genetic or familial) or secondary to other diseases or drugs. Measurement of the specific lipoproteins (LDL, HDL, and VLDL) that carry cholesterol and triglycerides assists with diagnostic, prognostic, and therapeutic decisions. When diet and exercise fail to correct hyperlipidemia, antilipemic agents are used.

Porphyrias are metabolic disorders of heme synthesis in which there are an overproduction, accumulation, and excretion of porphyrins and their intermediary precursors. In general, porphyrias that cause excessive synthesis of ALA and PBg are associated with neurological problems; those that lead to excessive production of porphyrins are associated with dermatological manifestations.

# REFERENCES

1. National Cholesterol Education Program. Summary of the second report of the National Cholesterol Education Program expert panel on detection, evaluation and treatment of high blood cholesterol in adults. *JAMA.* 1993; 269: 3015–23.
2. Brewer HB Jr. Clinical significance of plasma lipid levels. *Am J Cardiol.* 1989; 64:3–9G.
3. Schaefer EJ, Lichtenstein AH, Lamon-Fava S, et al. Lipoproteins, nutrition, aging, and atherosclerosis. *Am J Clin Nutr.* 1995; 61(Suppl):726–40S.
4. Choice of cholesterol-lowering drugs. *Med Lett.* 1993; 35: 19–22.
5. Brown MS, Goldstein JL. The hyperlipoproteinemias and other disorders of lipid metabolism. In: Braunwald E, Isselbacher KJ, Petersdorf RG, et al., eds. Harrison's principles of internal medicine, 11th ed. New York: McGraw-Hill; 1987:1650–61.
6. Koay ESC. Plasma lipid profiles: the expanding repertoire of tests, their clinical significance and pitfalls. *Ann Acad Med (Singapore).* 1989; 18:436–43.
7. Dart AM. Managing elevated blood lipid concentrations: who, when and how? *Drugs.* 1990; 39:374–87.
8. Gordon DJ, Probstfield JL, Garrison RJ, et al. High-density lipoprotein cholesterol and cardiovascular disease. Four prospective American studies. *Circulation.* 1989; 79:8–15.
9. Blankenhorn DH, Alaupovic P, Wickham E, et al. Prediction of angiographic change in native human coronary arteries and aortocoronary bypass grafts: lipid and nonlipid factors. *Circulation.* 1990; 81:470–6.
10. Godsland IF, Crook D, Simpson R, et al. The effects of different formulations of oral contraceptive agents on lipid and carbohydrate metabolism. *N Engl J Med.* 1990; 323: 1375–81.
11. Wiersinga WM, Trip MD, van Beeren MH, et al. An increase in plasma cholesterol independent of thyroid function during long-term amiodarone therapy. *Ann Intern Med.* 1991; 114:128–32.
12. Chait A, Brunzell JD. Acquired hyperlipidemia (secondary dyslipoproteinemias). *Endocrinol Metab Clin North Am.* 1990; 19:259–78.
13. Jackson R, Scragg R, Marshall R, et al. Changes in serum lipid concentrations during the first 24 hours after myocardial infarction. *Br Med J.* 1987; 294:1588–9.
14. Lee IM, Hsieh CC, Paffenbarger RS Jr. Exercise intensity and longevity in men: the Harvard alumni health study. *JAMA.* 1995; 273:1179–84.
15. Suh I, Shaten BJ, Cutler JA, et al. Alcohol use and mortality from coronary heart disease: the role of high-density lipoprotein cholesterol. *Ann Intern Med.* 1992; 116:881–7.
16. Gaziano JM, Buring JE, Breslow JL, et al. Moderate alcohol intake, increased levels of high-density lipoprotein and its subfractions, and decreased risk of myocardial infarction. *N Engl J Med.* 1993; 329:1829–34.
17. Krumholtz HM, Seeman TE, Merrill SS, et al. Lack of association between cholesterol and coronary heart disease mortality and morbidity and all-cause mortality in persons older than 70 years. *JAMA.* 1994; 272:1335–40.
18. Young DS. Effects of drugs on clinical laboratory tests, 3rd ed. Washington, DC: American Association for Clinical Chemistry Press; 1990.
19. Kane JP, Malloy MJ, Ports TA, et al. Regression of coronary atherosclerosis during treatment of familial hypercholesterolemia with combined drug regimens. *JAMA.* 1990; 264:3007–12.
20. Klag MJ, Ford DE, Mead LA, et al. Serum cholesterol in young men and subsequent cardiovascular disease. *N Engl J Med.* 1993; 328:313–8.
21. NIH Consensus Development Panel. Triglyceride, high-density lipoprotein, and coronary heart disease. *JAMA.* 1993; 269:505–10.
22. Criqui MH, Heiss G, Cohn R, et al. Plasma triglyceride level and mortality from coronary heart disease. *N Engl J Med.* 1993; 328:1220–5.
23. Consensus Conference. Treatment of hypertriglyceridemia. *JAMA.* 1984; 251:1196–1200.
24. Frohlich ED. Uric acid: a risk factor for coronary heart disease. *JAMA.* 1993; 270:378–9. Editorial.
25. Agamah ES, Srinivasad SR, Webber LS, et al. Serum uric acid and its relation to cardiovascular disease risk factors in children and young adults from a biracial community: the Bogalusa heart study. *J Lab Clin Med.* 1991; 118:241–9.
26. Klotzsch SG, McNamara JR. Triglyceride measurements: a review of methods and interferences. *Clin Chem.* 1990; 36:1605–13.
27. Hulley SB, Newman TB. Cholesterol in the elderly: is it important? *JAMA.* 1994; 272:1372–3. Editorial.
28. Jukema JW, Bruschke AV, van Boven AJ, et al. Effects of lipid lowering by pravastatin on progression and regression of coronary artery disease in symptomatic men with normal to moderately elevated serum cholesterol levels. The Regression Growth Evaluation Statin Study (REGRESS). *Circulation.* 1995; 91:2528–40.
29. Shah PK, Amin J. Low high density lipoprotein level is associated with increased restenosis rate after coronary angioplasty. *Circulation.* 1992; 85:1279–85.
30. Home testing of cholesterol. *Med Lett.* 1994; 36:85–6.
31. Kolovou GD, Fostinis YP, Bilianou HI, et al. Response of high-density lipoproteins to hypolipidemic drugs according to their initial level. *Am J Cardiol.* 1995; 75:293–5.
32. O'Connor P, Feely J, Shepherd J. Lipid lowering drugs. *Br Med J.* 1990; 300:667–72.
33. Henkin Y, Johnson KC, Segrest JP. Rechallenge with crystalline niacin after drug-induced hepatitis from sustained-release niacin. *JAMA.* 1990; 264:241–3.
34. Cashin-Hemphill, Spencer CA, Nicoloff JT, et al. Alterations in serum thyroid hormonal indices with colestipol-niacin therapy. *Ann Intern Med.* 1987; 107:324–9.
35. Sprecher DL, Abrams J, Allen JW. Low-dose combined therapy with fluvastatin and cholestyramine in hyperlipidemic patients. *Ann Intern Med.* 1994; 120:537–43.
36. Waters D, Higginson L, Gladstone P, et al. Effects of monotherapy with HMG-CoA reductase inhibitor on the progression of coronary atherosclerosis as assessed by serial quantitative arteriography: the Canadian coronary atherosclerosis intervention trial. *Circulation.* 1994; 89:959–68.
37. Blankenhorn DH, Azen SP, Kramsch M, et al. Coronary angiographic changes with lovastatin therapy: the monitored atherosclerosis regression study MARS. *Ann Intern Med.* 1993; 119:969–76.
38. Scandinavian simvastatin survival study group. Randomised trial of cholesterol lowering in 4444 patients with

coronary heart disease: the Scandinavian simvastatin survival study 4S. *Lancet.* 1994; 344:1383–9.

39. Vega DL, Grundy SM. Gemfibrozil therapy in primary hypertriglyceridemia associated with coronary heart disease: effects on metabolism of low-density lipoproteins. *JAMA.* 1985; 253:2398–403.

40. Steinberg D, Witztum JL. Lipoproteins and atherogenesis: current concepts. *JAMA.* 1990; 264:3047–52.

41. Brown G, Albers JJ, Fisher LD, et al. Regression of coronary artery disease as a result of intensive lipid-lowering therapy in men with high levels of apolipoprotein B. *N Engl J Med.* 1990; 323:1289–98.

42. Ornish D, Brown SE, Scherwitz LW, et al. Can lifestyle changes reverse coronary heart disease? *Lancet.* 1990; 336:129–33.

43. Watts GF, Lewis B, Brunt JNH, et al. Effects on coronary artery disease of lipid-lowering diet, or diet plus cholestyramine, in the St. Thomas' atherosclerosis regression study. *Lancet.* 1992; 339:563–9.

44. Tefferi A, Solberg LA, Ellefson RD. Porphyrias: clinical evaluation and interpretation of laboratory tests. *Mayo Clin Proc.* 1994; 69:289–90.

45. Rimington C. Hemebiosynthesis and porphyrias: 50 years in retrospect. *J Clin Chem Clin Biochem.* 1989; 27:473–86.

46. Meyer UA. Porphyrias. In: Braunwald E, Isselbacher KJ, Petersdorf RG, et al., eds. Harrison's principles of internal medicine, 11th ed. New York: McGraw-Hill; 1987:1638–43.

47. Werman HA. The porphyrias. *Emerg Med Clin North Am.* 1989; 7:927–42.

48. Moore MR, McColl KEL, Fitzsimons EJ, et al. The porphyrias. *Blood Rev.* 1990; 4:88–96.

49. Kushner JP. Laboratory diagnosis of the porphyrias. *N Engl J Med.* 1991; 324:1432–4.

50. Straka JG, Rank JM, Bloomer JR. Porphyria and porphyrin metabolism. *Annu Rev Med.* 1990; 41:457–69.

51. Wallach J. Interpretation of diagnostic tests: a synopsis of laboratory medicine, 5th ed. Boston, MA: Little, Brown; 1992.

52. Suarez SM, Cohen PR, DeLeo VA. Bullous photosensitivity to naproxen: "pseudoporphyria." *Arthritis Rheum.* 1990; 33:903–8.

53. Schoenfeld N, Mamet R. Interference of ofloxacin with determination of urinary porphyrins. *Clin Chem.* 1994; 40:417–9.

*The contribution of material written by Diana Laubenstein, Pharm.D., in the first edition of this book is acknowledged.*

## QuickView—Serum Triglycerides

| Parameter | Description | Comments |
|---|---|---|
| **Common reference ranges** | | |
| Adults | Desirable: <200 mg/dL<br>Borderline high: 200–400 mg/dL<br>High: 400–1000 mg/dL<br>Very high: >1000 mg/dL | SI conversion factor: 0.0113 (mmol/L) |
| Pediatrics | 1–9 years: 25–125 mg/dL<br>    0.28–1.41 mmol/L<br>10–19 years: 25–140 mg/dL<br>    0.28–1.58 mmol/L | |
| **Critical value** | >1000 | High risk of pancreatitis |
| **Natural substance?** | Yes | Required |
| **Inherent activity?** | No, but intermediary for other active substances | Needed for formation of other lipids and fatty acids |
| **Location** | | |
| Production | Liver and intestines | From ingested food |
| Storage | Fat | |
| Secretion/excretion | Excreted in bile | Also recycled to liver |
| **Major causes of . . .** | | |
| High results | Excess fat intake<br>Genetic defects<br>Drugs<br>Alcohol | Associated with obesity, diabetes, steroids, estrogens, and renal disease |
| Associated signs and symptoms | Pancreatitis, xanthomas, lipemia retinalis | Atherosclerotic vascular disease? |
| Low results | Not clinically important | Usually considered sign of good health |
| Associated signs and symptoms | None | |
| **After insult, time to . . .** | | |
| Initial elevation | Days to weeks | Single meal has major effect on triglyceride concentration within 2 hr |
| Peak values | Days to weeks | Increases with aging |
| Normalization | Days to weeks | After diet changes or drugs |
| **Drugs often monitored with test** | Hypolipidemics | Statins, niacin, fibric acids |
| **Causes of spurious results** | Glycerol, recent meal, alcohol, lipid emulsion | |

## QuickView—Total Serum Cholesterol

| Parameter | Description | Comments |
|---|---|---|
| **Common reference ranges** | | |
| Adults | Desirable: <200 mg/dL<br>Borderline high: 200–239 mg/dL<br>High: >239 mg/dL | SI conversion factor: 0.0259 (mmol/L) |
| Pediatrics | 0–1 month: 45–100 mg/dL<br>    1.17–2.59 mmol/L<br>1–9 years: 45–240 mg/dL<br>    1.17–6.22 mmol/L<br>10–19 years: 115–215 mg/dL<br>    2.98–5.57 mmol/L | |
| **Critical value** | Not acutely critical | Depends on risk factors, LDL, and HDL |

## QuickView—Total Serum Cholesterol *continued*

| Parameter | Description | Comments |
|---|---|---|
| **Natural substance?** | Yes | Required |
| **Inherent activity?** | No, but intermediary for other active substances | Needed for cell wall, steroid, and bile acid production |
| **Location** | | |
| **Production** | Liver and intestines | Ingested in diet |
| **Storage** | Fat | |
| **Secretion/excretion** | Excreted in bile | Also recycled to liver |
| **Major causes of . . .** | | |
| **High results** | Excess fat intake (especially saturated fats) Genetic defects Drugs | Tables 2 and 3 |
| **Associated signs and symptoms** | Atherosclerotic vascular disease | Angina, myocardial infarction, stroke |
| **Low results** | Hyperthyroidism Malnutrition Anemia Liver disease | Usually considered sign of good health |
| **Associated signs and symptoms** | None | |
| **After insult, time to . . .** | | |
| **Initial elevation** | Days to weeks | Single meal has little effect on total cholesterol concentration |
| **Peak values** | Days to weeks | Can increase with aging; does not change acutely |
| **Normalization** | Weeks to months | After diet changes or drugs |
| **Drugs often monitored with test** | Hypolipidemics | Statins, niacin, fibric acids, binding resins |
| **Causes of spurious results** | Prolonged tourniquet application | Causes venous stasis (increase 5–10%) |

# Chapter 14

# Hematology: Red and White Blood Cell Tests

*Nancy S. Jordan*

This chapter reviews the functions of erythrocytes [red blood cells (RBCs)] and their disorders, primarily anemias. It also discusses the functions and common disorders of leukocytes [white blood cells (WBCs)]. Blood disorders can be functional (qualitative), quantitative, or neoplastic (uncontrolled proliferation of bone marrow cells). Practitioners must understand the purpose of blood cells before interpreting laboratory test results used to detect and monitor these disorders. Therefore, the physiology of blood cell development is introduced before specific tests are discussed in detail. For teaching purposes, each test is defined and described. Its interpretation and application in diagnosing and monitoring various blood disorders are then discussed. (Platelets are discussed in Chapter 15.)

## OBJECTIVES

Upon completion of this chapter, the reader should be able to

1. Describe the physiology of blood cell development and bone marrow function.

2. Discuss the interpretation and alterations of hemoglobin (Hgb), hematocrit (Hct), and various RBC indices in the evaluation of macrocytic; microcytic; and normochromic, normocytic anemias.

3. Describe circumstances when a Schilling test is needed to assess vitamin $B_{12}$ deficiency and how it is conducted.

4. Interpret results of the erythrocyte sedimentation rate (ESR) test.

5. Name the different types of leukocytes and their primary functions.

6. Interpret alterations in the WBC count and differential and the $CD_4$ lymphocyte count in acute bacterial infections, parasitic infections, and

human immunodeficiency virus (HIV) infection.

## PHYSIOLOGY OF BLOOD CELLS AND BONE MARROW

The cellular components of blood are derived from pluripotential stem cells located in the bone marrow (Figure 1, next page). Bone marrow is one of the largest organs in the human body. Bone marrow is a hematopoietic and reticuloendothelial organ. It normally produces 2.5 billion RBCs, 1 billion granulocytes, and 2.5 billion platelets/kg of body weight daily.[1] Production can vary greatly, from nearly zero to 5–10 times normal. Usually, however, levels of circulating cells remain in a relatively narrow range. As a reticuloendothelial organ, bone marrow is involved in processing antigens, cellular immune reactions, antibody synthesis, and the recognition and removal of aging and abnormal cells and particulate matter from the blood.[1]

In the bone marrow, stem cells are believed to undergo differentiation—a process called hematopoiesis—until they are committed to develop further into leukocytes, erythrocytes, or platelets. Many regulatory proteins are involved in the maintenance of hematopoiesis. Their functions and interrelationships are not fully understood. The proteins that stimulate hematopoiesis, called hematopoietins or colony-stimulating factors (csf), include granulocyte-macrophage csf, megakaryocyte csf, interleukin 2, erythropoietin, and thrombopoietin. Inhibitors of hematopoiesis are not as well defined but appear to include certain interferons and lymphotoxins.

Unipotential stem cells undergo further differentiation in the bone marrow until they develop into mature cells. Many developmental stages along the way can be identified by differing morphological characteristics. Generally, only mature cellular forms are found in the circu-

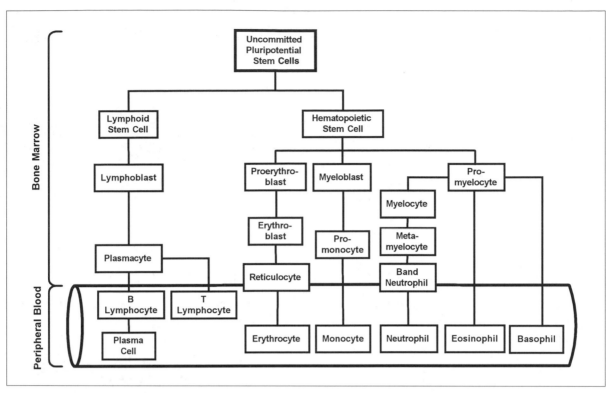

**FIGURE 1.** One possible scheme of hematopoiesis.

lating blood. From this blood, clinical specimens are usually taken.

The reticulocyte is the final cell form that precedes development of the mature RBC or erythrocyte. During the entire maturation process, Hgb is produced and incorporated into the cell.[2] The reticulocyte does not contain a nucleus but possesses nucleic acids that can be considered remnants of the nucleus or endoplasmic reticulum, while the mature erythrocyte contains neither an organized nucleus nor nucleic acids. Normally, few reticulocytes are present in circulating blood. They persist in the circulation for 1–2 days before maturing into erythrocytes.[2] Mature erythrocytes have a 120-day lifespan and are lost from the circulation by senescence.[1]

## COMPLETE BLOOD COUNT

The CBC is perhaps the most commonly ordered laboratory test. It supplies useful information regarding the concentration of the different cellular and noncellular elements of blood and applies to multiple disorders. CBC is a misnomer since concentrations, not counts, are measured and provided. Functionally, the CBC can be thought of as a complete blood analysis because a series of tests are performed. Moreover, information besides concentrations are reported.

Most clinical laboratories utilize an automated method to determine the CBC. Results are usually accurate, reproducible, and rapidly obtained. Numerous measured and calculated values are included in a CBC (Table

1). These results traditionally include

- ➢ RBC count.
- ➢ WBC count.
- ➢ Hgb.
- ➢ Hct.
- ➢ RBC indices [mean cell volume (MCV), mean cell Hgb (MCH), and mean cell Hgb concentration (MCHC)].
- ➢ Reticulocyte count.
- ➢ RBC distribution width (RDW).
- ➢ Platelet count and mean platelet volume (MPV).

When a "CBC with differential" is ordered, various types of WBCs are also analyzed (White Blood Cell Count and Differential section). The reliability of the results can be doubtful if (1) the integrity of the specimen is questionable (inappropriate handling or storage) or (2) the specimen contains substances that interfere with the automated analysis. Grossly erroneous results are usually flagged for verification by another method. Manual microscopic review of the blood smear can also intercept incorrect automated results.[3]

### Red Blood Cell Count
*Normal range: 4.6–6.2 × 10⁶ cells/mm³ or 4.6–6.2 × 10¹²* 
*cells/L for males or 4.2–5.4 × 10⁶ cells/mm³ or 4.2–5.4 × 10¹²* 
*cells/L for females[5]*

The RBC count is an actual count of red corpuscles in a given amount of blood (a cubic millimeter or liter). The

**TABLE 1.** Reference Ranges and Interpretive Comments on Common Hematological Tests (Typical CBC)

| Test Name | Reference Range[a] | SI Units[b] | Comments[c] |
|---|---|---|---|
| RBC count | $4.6–6.2 \times 10^6$ cells/mm$^3$ for males<br>$4.2–5.4 \times 10^6$ cells/mm$^3$ for females | $4.6–6.2 \times 10^{12}$ cells/L<br>$4.2–5.4 \times 10^{12}$ cells/L | |
| WBC count | $4.8–10.8 \times 10^3$ cells/mm$^3$ | $4.8–10.8 \times 10^9$ cells/L | Elevated by large numbers of giant platelets and platelet clumps. Decreased with cold agglutinins |
| Hgb | 14–18 g/dL for males<br>12–16 g/dL for females | 8.7–11.2 mmol/L<br>7.4–9.9 mmol/L | Amount of Hgb in given volume of whole blood. Indication of oxygen-transport capacity of blood. Elevated in hyperlipidemia |
| Hct | 42–52% for males<br>37–47% for females | 0.42–0.52<br>0.37–0.47 | Percentage volume of blood comprised of erythrocytes—usually approximately three times Hgb |
| RBC indices<br>  Mean cell volume (MCV) | 80–96 fL for males<br>82–98 fL for females | | Hct/RBC: increased in vitamin B$_{12}$ and folate deficiency, cold agglutinins, reticulocytosis, hyperglycemia, and leukemic cells. Decreased in iron deficiency |
|   Mean cell Hgb (MCH) | 27–33 pg/cell | | Hgb/RBC: increased in vitamin B$_{12}$ and folate deficiency, cold agglutinins, and hyperlipidemia. Decreased in iron deficiency |
|   Mean cell Hgb concentration (MCHC) | 31–35 g/dL | 310–350 g/L | Hgb/Hct: amount of Hgb in terms of percentage volume of cell. Increased in hyperlipidemia and cold agglutinins. Decreased in iron deficiency |
| Reticulocyte count | 0.5–2.5% of RBCs | 0.005–0.025 | Increased in acute blood loss and hemolysis. Decreased in untreated iron, vitamin B$_{12}$, and folate deficiency |
| RBC distribution width (RDW) | 11–16% | 0.11–0.16 | Measure of variation in red cell volumes: the larger the percent, the greater the variation in size of red cells. Increased in early iron deficiency anemia and mixed anemias |
| Platelet count | 140,000–440,000/μL | | Elevated in presence of red cell fragments and microcytic erythrocytes. Decreased in presence of large numbers of giant platelets and platelet clumps |
| Mean platelet volume (MPV) | 7–11 fL | | Chapter 15 |

[a]*Reference ranges—Holyoke Hospital, Inc.*
[b]*International System units here and in other tables adapted from* N Engl J Med. *1992; 327:718–24.*
[c]*Adapted from References 3 and 4. Text offers further explanation and detail.*

count is now done by automated methods so that results are accurate, reproducible, and quickly derived. After puberty, females have slightly lower counts (and Hgb), partly because of their menstrual blood loss and because of higher androgen (an erythropoietic stimulant) concentrations in men. In all anemias, the RBC count by definition is below the normal range. This decrease causes a proportionate decrease in Hct and Hgb.

## White Blood Cell Count
*Normal range: $4.8–10.8 \times 10^3$ cells/mm$^3$ or $4.8–10.8 \times 10^9$ cells/L*

The WBC count is an actual count of the number of leukocytes in a given amount of blood. Unlike RBCs, leukocytes develop into several mature forms. The various percentages of immature and mature WBCs, also called the WBC differential, are discussed later in this chapter.

## Hemoglobin
*Normal range: 14–18 g/dL or 8.7–11.2 mmol/L for males
or 12–16 g/dL or 7.4–9.9 mmol/L for females*

The laboratory value designated by Hgb is the amount contained in a given volume (100 mL or 1 L) of whole blood (plasma plus within the RBCs). The Hgb concentration provides a direct indication of the oxygen-transport capacity of the blood.[5] As a substance contained in RBCs, Hgb is proportionately low in patients with anemia.

## Hematocrit
*Normal range: 42–52% or 0.42–0.52 for males or 37–47%
or 0.37–0.47 for females*

Hct is the percentage volume of blood that is composed of erythrocytes. It is also known as the packed cell volume. To perform the Hct test, a blood-filled capillary tube is centrifuged to settle the erythrocytes. Then, the percentage volume of the tube that is composed of erythrocytes is calculated.[5] The Hct is usually about three times the value of the Hgb, but disproportion can occur when cells are substantially abnormal in size or shape. Like Hgb, Hct is low in patients with anemia.

## Red Blood Cell Indices

Because the following laboratory tests specifically assess RBCs, they are called RBC indices. These indices are useful in the evaluation of anemias, polycythemia, and nutritional disorders. Essentially, they assess the size and Hgb content of the RBC. They are not measured but are calculated from Hgb, RBC count, and Hct using predetermined formulas.

### Mean Cell Volume
*Normal range: 80–96 fL for males or 82–98 fL for females*

The MCV is an estimate of the average volume of RBCs. It is derived by dividing the Hct by the RBC count. Abnormally large cells have an increased MCV and are called macrocytic. Vitamin $B_{12}$ and folate deficiency cause the formation of macrocytic erythrocytes and correspond to a true increase in MCV. On the other hand, reticulocytosis—an increase in the number of reticulocytes in the peripheral blood—causes a false increase in MCV. Reticulocytes are larger than mature erythrocytes, so an increase in circulating reticulocytes can lead to an increased MCV.[5]

Likewise, cold agglutinins that cause clumping (agglutination) of erythrocytes also cause false elevations when automated methods interpret these clumps to be individual cells. The MCV also may be falsely increased in hyperglycemia. When erythrocytes are mixed with diluting fluids to perform the test, the cells swell because the fluids are relatively hypotonic compared to the patient's blood.

Abnormally small cells (with a decreased MCV) are called microcytic. The most common cause of microcytosis is iron deficiency. A decrease in the MCV implies some abnormality in Hgb synthesis.[5]

### Mean Cell Hemoglobin
*Normal range: 27–33 pg/cell*

MCH is the percent volume of Hgb per RBC. It is calculated by dividing the Hgb by the RBC count. MCH can be falsely increased in patients with hyperlipidemia, but it can be truly increased in the presence of folate deficiency. As expected, MCH is decreased in iron deficiency, when the iron is insufficient to manufacture the usual amount of Hgb in RBCs. A low MCH corresponds with hypochromic (pale) RBCs, as seen in iron deficiency anemia.

### Mean Cell Hemoglobin Concentration
*Normal range: 31–35 g/dL or 310–350 g/L*

The MCHC is the Hgb divided by the Hct. As alluded to previously, this calculation is usually around 33 g/dL (330 g/L) because the Hct is usually three times the Hgb. Iron deficiency is the only anemia in which the MCHC is *routinely* low, although it can also be decreased in other disorders of Hgb synthesis.[5] Like MCH, it can be falsely elevated in hyperlipidemia due to specimen turbidity.

## Reticulocyte Count
*Normal range: 0.5–2.5% of RBCs or 0.005–0.025*

The reticulocyte count is an indirect measurement of recent RBC production. In the basal state, approximately 1% of circulating RBCs is replaced daily. This replacement results in a reticulocyte count of 1%. In anemia, the reticulocyte count reflects not only the level of bone marrow production but also a decline in the total number of mature erythrocytes that normally dilute the reticulocytes.[5] Therefore, in a person whose bone marrow production is unchanged but whose Hct has fallen from 46 to 23%, the reticulocyte count doubles.

A corrected reticulocyte count is one that has been adjusted to a normal Hct to eliminate the increase in count seen on the basis of changes in the dilution effect alone.[5] In persons with anemia secondary to *acute* blood loss or hemolysis, even the corrected reticulocyte count is increased. This increase reflects an attempt by the bone marrow to compensate for the lack of circulating erythrocytes. Because RBC production is increased to far above basal activity, more reticulocytes "escape" into the circulation earlier than normal. In contrast, persons with *untreated* anemia secondary to iron, folate, or vitamin $B_{12}$ deficiency are unable to increase their reticulocyte count appropriate to the degree of their anemia.

The reticulocyte count can be useful in identifying drug-induced bone marrow suppression where the percentage of circulating reticulocytes should be close to zero. It can also be used to monitor an anemic patient's response to vitamin or iron therapy. In such patients, supplementation of the lacking factor causes rapid (5–7 days) elevation of the reticulocyte count.

## Red Blood Cell Distribution Width
*Normal range: 11–16% or 0.11–0.16*

The RDW is an indication of the variation in red cell volume.[6] As this value increases, so does the variability in the size (width) of RBCs. This value is used primarily with other tests to diagnose iron deficiency anemia. The RDW increases in early iron deficiency, often before other tests show signs of this kind of anemia. However, it is not specific for iron deficiency anemia.

In a patient with signs and symptoms of anemia, a high RDW suggests a mixed anemia (both macrocytic and microcytic) despite a normal MCV. Although RBCs are both small and large, the average or mean size (volume) is normal.

## Platelet Count and Mean Platelet Volume
*Normal ranges: 140,000–440,000/μL and 7–11 fL, respectively*

These tests, often included in the CBC with differential, are discussed in detail in Chapter 15.

## LABORATORY ASSESSMENT OF ANEMIA

The functions of the erythrocyte are to transport and protect Hgb, the molecule used for oxygen transport.[2] Anemia can be defined as a decrease in either the RBC count or the Hgb concentration. Therefore, the practitioner is usually dealing with anemia when assessing RBCs.

Anemia can be caused by decreased production and/or increased destruction of erythrocytes as well as acute blood loss. Normal amounts of vitamin $B_{12}$, folic acid, and iron are essential for the normal development of erythrocytes. Both vitamin $B_{12}$ and folic acid play essential roles in nucleic acid synthesis. Iron and vitamin deficiencies delay and distort the development of the erythrocyte in the bone marrow.

Anemia is not a disease in itself but one manifestation of an underlying disease process. Appropriate treatment of the anemic patient depends on the exact cause of the condition.

Signs and symptoms of anemia depend on its severity and the rapidity with which it has developed. Severe, acute blood loss results in more dramatic symptoms than an anemia that took months to develop, because there may not have been time for adequate compensatory adjustments. Patients with mild anemia are often asymptomatic (i.e., absence of pallor, weakness, and fatigue), but severely symptomatic patients manifest shortness of breath, tachycardia, and palpitations even at rest. This contrast should be kept in mind when interpreting test results.

Use of erythrocyte morphology is one common method to "narrow down" the possible etiology of anemia. This method is useful because different causes of anemia lead to different erythrocyte morphology. Figure 2 outlines this approach. Only a few common causes of anemia are included, but others can be fit into this outline. Other laboratory tests that are useful in differentiating the anemias are listed in their appropriate locations.

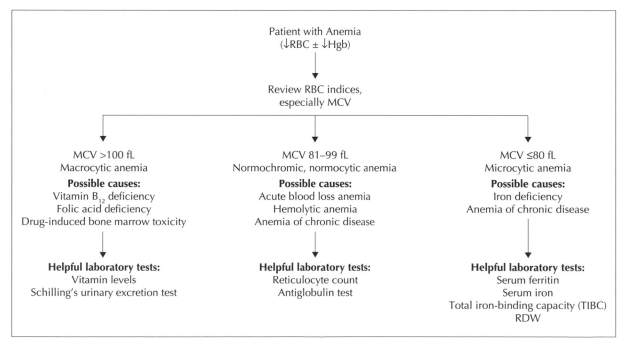

**FIGURE 2.** Use of erythrocyte morphology in differential diagnosis of anemia.

Usual laboratory findings are also tabulated in each section.

## Macrocytic Anemia

Macrocytic anemia is associated with abnormally enlarged erythrocytes. The two most common causes are vitamin $B_{12}$ and folic acid deficiencies. Drugs that cause macrocytic anemia mainly interfere with proper utilization, absorption, and metabolism of these vitamins (Table 2).

### Vitamin $B_{12}$ Deficiency

Vitamin $B_{12}$ is also known as cyanocobalamin. It is stored primarily in the liver, which contains approximately 1 µg of vitamin/g of liver tissue.[7] To be absorbed from the intestinal tract, vitamin $B_{12}$ must be bound to intrinsic factor, which is produced by the parietal cells of the stomach. Vitamin $B_{12}$ present in food is first bound to intrinsic factor in the proximal small bowel. The intrinsic factor–vitamin $B_{12}$ complex is then absorbed in the ileum. The absorbed vitamin binds to serum proteins and is transported to the liver, bone marrow, and other sites.[7]

The normal daily requirement of vitamin $B_{12}$ is 2–5 µg.[7] The body has $B_{12}$ stores of approximately 2–5 mg. Therefore, if vitamin $B_{12}$ absorption suddenly ceased in a patient with normal liver stores, several years would pass before any abnormalities occurred due to vitamin deficiency.

*Causes.* Vitamin $B_{12}$ deficiency can be caused by

- ➤ Inadequate dietary intake.
- ➤ Defective production of intrinsic factor.

**TABLE 2.** Pathophysiology of Drug-Induced Macrocytic Anemia[a]

---

**Marrow toxicity and interference with folate metabolism**
Alcohol

**Marrow toxicity**
Antineoplastic agents (6-mercaptopurine, 5-fluorouracil, cyclophosphamide, methotrexate, hydroxyurea)
Zidovudine (AZT)

**Altered folate metabolism**
Anticonvulsants (phenytoin, primidone, phenobarbital)
Methotrexate
Oral contraceptives
Pentamidine
Sulfasalazine
Sulfamethoxazole
Triamterene
Trimethoprim

**$B_{12}$ malabsorption**
Colchicine
Neomycin
Para-aminosalicylic acid

**Impaired $B_{12}$ utilization**
Nitrous oxide

---

[a]*Adapted from Reference 4.*

- ➤ Defective or deficient absorption of the intrinsic factor–vitamin $B_{12}$ complex.

Inadequate dietary intake is a rare cause of vitamin $B_{12}$ deficiency, occurring only in individuals who abstain totally from all animal food, including milk and eggs. On the other hand, defective production of intrinsic factor is a common cause of the deficiency.[7] The gastric mucosa can fail to secrete intrinsic factor because of atrophy (especially in the elderly).

Pernicious anemia is a disease characterized by atrophic gastritis in which antibodies against intrinsic factor and gastric parietal cells have been isolated. It is not clear whether the gastritis results from or is caused by antibody formation. Gastrectomy, removal of all or part of the stomach, can lead to vitamin $B_{12}$ deficiency because the procedure removes the production site of intrinsic factor. Defective or deficient absorption of the intrinsic factor–vitamin $B_{12}$ complex can be caused by inflammatory disease of the small bowel, ileal resection, and bacterial overgrowth in the small bowel.[7,8] Administration of colchicine, neomycin, and para-aminosalicylic acid can lead to impaired absorption of vitamin $B_{12}$ (Table 2).

*Clinical and laboratory diagnosis.* Since vitamin $B_{12}$ is necessary for deoxyribonucleic acid (DNA) synthesis in all cells, deficiency leads to symptoms involving many organ systems. The most notable symptoms involve the[7,9]

- ➤ Gastrointestinal (GI) tract (e.g., loss of appetite, smooth and/or sore tongue, and diarrhea or constipation).
- ➤ Central nervous system (CNS) (e.g., paresthesias in fingers and toes, loss of coordination of legs and feet, tremors, irritability, somnolence, and abnormalities of taste and smell).
- ➤ Hematopoietic system (anemia).

A maturation arrest occurs in the immature cells in the bone marrow. The morphological result is that larger cells are produced, and they have characteristics specific to this maturation arrest. The anemia that results is called a macrocytic, megaloblastic (morphological characteristics of maturation arrest) anemia.[7] Visual inspection of smears of both peripheral blood and bone marrow reveals characteristic megaloblastic changes in the appearance of erythrocytes and WBCs. The development of neutrophils is also affected, resulting in macrocytic cells with hypersegmented nuclei. A mild pancytopenia, decreased numbers of all blood elements, also occurs. The usual laboratory test results found with vitamin $B_{12}$ deficiency are listed in Table 3.

*Schilling test.* The Schilling urinary excretion test is important in determining the cause of low vitamin $B_{12}$ concentrations. This test is often performed in two parts. For

**TABLE 3.** Laboratory Findings for Vitamin B$_{12}$ Deficiency Anemia

| Test | Result[a] |
|------|---------|
| RBC | ↓ |
| Hgb | ↓ |
| Hct | ↓ |
| MCV | ↑ |
| MCH | ↑ |
| MCHC | → |
| Reticulocytes | →↓ |
| Serum vitamin B$_{12}$[b] | ↓ |

[a] ↑ = increased; ↓ = decreased; → = no change.
[b] Normal range: 205–876 pg/mL or 151–646 pmol/L. Vitamin B$_{12}$ must fall below 140 pg/mL or 103 pmol/L to be considered a true deficiency.

a regular Schilling test, the patient ingests cobalt-labeled vitamin B$_{12}$. After 1 hr, 1000 μg of unlabeled vitamin B$_{12}$ is injected intramuscularly (IM) and a 24-hr urine collection is begun.[7] The IM dose saturates the tissue binding sites of vitamin B$_{12}$.[10] Because these sites are then unable to take up any more vitamin B$_{12}$, the orally administered vitamin is excreted in the urine. The amount of vitamin B$_{12}$ absorbed after the oral dose can then be calculated.

Under normal conditions, the 24-hr urinary excretion of vitamin B$_{12}$ is 8–40% of the oral dose.[10] The urine collection must be verified as complete, because incomplete collection can lead to a falsely low-percentage excretion of the orally administered vitamin.

If the test shows deficient oral absorption, a Schilling test with intrinsic factor can be performed to determine whether the vitamin B$_{12}$ deficiency is due to a lack of intrinsic factor or a defect in ileal absorption.[7] This test is performed like the first Schilling test, except that the oral vitamin B$_{12}$ dose is given concomitantly with an oral dose of intrinsic factor (usually derived from pork).[7] If the absorption difficulty is corrected with the addition of exogenous intrinsic factor, the problem is usually attributable to intrinsic factor deficiency. If the problem is not corrected, other causes must be investigated (e.g., bacterial overgrowth in the small intestine, inflammatory bowel disease, and small bowel resection).[7]

The Schilling test is becoming unpopular with clinical laboratories because of difficulty in performing the procedure and regulatory problems involving radioactive substances. Detection of antibodies to parietal cells and/or intrinsic factors is often performed instead. Fifty percent of adults with pernicious anemia have intrinsic factor antibody.[11]

Parietal cell antibodies are present in 80% of adults with pernicious anemia and chronic gastritis. Unfortunately, parietal cell antibody is nonspecific by itself. It is found in 20–30% of patients with various autoimmune disorders and in 16% of asymptomatic people older than 60 years.[12]

### Folic Acid Deficiency

Folic acid is also called pteroylglutamic acid. Folates refer to a family of compounds related to folic acid that have multiple glutamic acid residues as opposed to the single residue of folic acid.[2] The folates present in food are mainly in a polyglutamic acid form and must be broken down in the intestine to the glutamate form to be absorbed efficiently.

The principal form of folate in serum, erythrocytes, and the liver is 5-methyltetrahydrofolate.[2] The liver is the chief storage site. Adult daily requirements are approximately 50 μg of folic acid, equivalent to about 400 μg of food folates.[7] Folic acid, like vitamin B$_{12}$, is necessary for DNA synthesis.

*Causes.* Folic acid deficiency can be caused by

> ➤ Inadequate dietary intake.
> ➤ Defective absorption.
> ➤ Defective conversion to the active form of the vitamin.

Inadequate dietary intake is the major cause. Folates are found in green, leafy vegetables such as spinach, lettuce, and broccoli. Development of a deficiency state takes 3–6 months once folic acid absorption ceases.[7]

Inadequate intake can have numerous causes. Alcoholics classically have poor nutritional intake of folic acid (Minicase 1, next page). Certain physiological states, such as pregnancy, require an increase in folic acid. Malabsorption syndromes (mentioned in the section on vitamin B$_{12}$) can also lead to defective absorption of folic acid. Celiac sprue can lead to folate malabsorption as well.[8]

Certain medications (e.g., methotrexate, trimethoprim–sulfamethoxazole, and triamterene) can act as folic acid antagonists by interfering with the conversion of folic acid into its metabolically active form, tetrahydrofolic acid. Phenytoin and phenobarbital administration can interfere with the intestinal absorption or utilization of folic acid[9,13] (Table 2).

*Clinical and laboratory diagnosis.* Since folic acid is necessary for DNA synthesis, lack of it causes a maturation arrest in the bone marrow similar to that caused by vitamin B$_{12}$ deficiency. Folic acid deficiency is also characterized by a macrocytic, megaloblastic anemia.[7] However, with folic acid deficiency, pancytopenia does not develop as consistently as it does with vitamin B$_{12}$ deficiency. Table 4 (next page) shows the usual laboratory results for patients with folate deficiency.

Signs and symptoms of folate deficiency are similar to those seen in vitamin B$_{12}$ deficiency. In folate deficiency,

---

### ✎ Minicase 1

A 41-year-old male alcoholic, Frederick M., was admitted to the hospital because of pneumonia. His physical exam revealed an emaciated patient with ascites, dyspnea, fever, cough, and weakness. No cyanosis, jaundice, or peripheral edema was evident. His peripheral neurological exam was within normal limits. Electrolytes, blood urea nitrogen (BUN), serum creatinine (SCr), and glucose were also normal. The following CBC was obtained:

| Test Name | Result | Reference Range |
|---|---|---|
| RBC | $3.06 \times 10^6$ cells/mm³ | $4.6$–$6.2 \times 10^6$ cells/mm³ for males |
| WBC | $4.6 \times 10^3$ cells/mm³ | $4.8$–$10.8 \times 10^3$ cells/mm³ |
| Hgb | 12.3 g/dL | 14–18 g/dL for males |
| Hct | 33.9% | 42–52% for males |
| MCV | 110.8 fL | 80–96 fL for males |
| MCH | 40.2 pg/cell | 27–33 pg/cell |
| MCHC | 36.3 g/dL | 31–35 g/dL |
| RDW | 15.4% | 11–16% |
| Platelet count | 174,000/µL | 140,000–440,000/µL |
| Segs | 68% | 45–73% |
| Bands | 6% | 3–5% |
| Lymphocytes | 11% | 20–40% |
| Monocytes | 11% | 2–8% |
| Eosinophils | 2% | 0–4% |
| Basophils | 2% | 0–1% |

*What abnormalities are present? What is the likely cause?*

**Discussion:** The most remarkable finding is the macrocytic anemia, evidenced by the low RBC, Hgb, and Hct and the markedly increased MCV and MCH. These findings are typical of folic acid deficiency, a common condition in alcoholics.

---

diarrhea is more common than constipation. Typically, slowly progressing weakness, dyspnea, headache, palpitations, and syncope occur. Irritability, forgetfulness, and insomnia can occur in patients with deficiency of vitamin $B_{12}$ or folate. If these signs and symptoms are caused by the latter, the CNS symptoms disappear within 24 hr of starting folate therapy. Peripheral neurological deficits rarely manifest in patients with pure folic acid deficiency, as they do in vitamin $B_{12}$ deficiency.

**TABLE 4.** Laboratory Findings for Folic Acid Deficiency Anemia

| Test | Result[a] |
|---|---|
| RBC | ↓ |
| Hgb | ↓ |
| Hct | ↓ |
| MCV | ↑ |
| MCH | ↑ |
| MCHC | → |
| Reticulocytes | →↓ |
| Serum folic acid[b] | ↓ |

[a] ↑ = increased; ↓ = decreased; → = no change.
[b] Normal range: ≥3.3 ng/mL or >7.5 nmol/L.

## Microcytic Anemia

Microcytic anemia is associated with abnormally small erythrocytes. Iron deficiency is the primary cause of microcytic anemia (Figure 2). Iron is necessary for Hgb synthesis. Daily requirements are approximately 1 mg of elemental iron for each 1 mL of RBCs produced, so daily requirements are approximately 20–25 mg for erythropoiesis.[2] Most required iron is obtained by recycling. Only about 5% of the daily requirement (1 mg) is newly absorbed to compensate for losses to fecal and urinary excretion, sweat, and desquamated skin.[2]

Menstruating women require more iron because of increased losses. Iron requirements vary among women, but 2 mg/day is probably an average. Orally ingested iron is absorbed in the GI tract, which should permit just enough to prevent excess or deficiency. Typically, 5–10% of oral intake is absorbed (normal daily dietary intake: 10–20 mg).[2]

RBCs have a lifespan of approximately 120 days. When old erythrocytes are taken up by phagocytic cells (macrophages) in the liver, spleen, and bone marrow, the Hgb molecule is broken down and iron is extracted and stored with proteins. This iron–protein complex within the macrophage is known as ferritin[2] (Figure 3). In the normal adult, approximately 500–1500 mg is stored as ferritin and 2500 mg of iron is contained in Hgb. While ferritin is primarily stored in macrophages, small amounts can be found in plasma. Therefore, serum ferritin con-

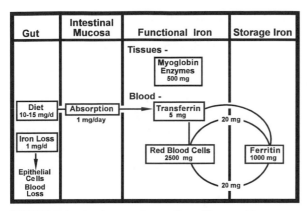

**FIGURE 3.** Intake, loss, and recycling of iron and iron storage forms.

centrations reflect total body iron stores and can be used for evaluating patients with hypochromic, microcytic anemia.

When the total quantity of extracted iron exceeds the amount that can be stored as ferritin, the excess iron is stored in an insoluble form called hemosiderin. Hemosiderin can be seen through a regular light microscope. Other proteins and some enzymes contain small amounts of iron as well.[2] For example, transferrin is a protein that transports iron from macrophage storage sites to the bone marrow, where it is incorporated into RBC precursors.[2]

*Causes.* Iron deficiency is usually due to inadequate dietary intake and/or increased iron requirements. Poor dietary intake, especially in situations that require increased iron (e.g., pregnancy), is a common cause. Other causes of iron deficiency include

> Blood loss due to excessive menstrual discharge.
> Peptic ulcer disease.
> Hiatal hernia.
> Gastrectomy.
> Gastritis due to the ingestion of alcohol, aspirin, and nonsteroidal anti-inflammatory drugs (NSAIDs).
> Bacterial overgrowth of the small bowel.
> Inflammatory bowel disease.
> Occult bleeding from GI carcinoma.

*Clinical and laboratory diagnosis.* The first change observed in the development of iron deficiency anemia is a loss of storage iron. If the deficiency continues, a loss of plasma iron occurs.[2] The decrease in plasma iron stimulates an increase in transferrin synthesis. When enough iron has been depleted that supplies for erythropoiesis are inadequate, anemia develops.[2] The RBCs are smaller than usual (microcytic—low MCV) and not as heavily pigmented as normal RBCs (hypochromic—low MCH) because they contain less Hgb than normal erythrocytes. Clinically, patients present with progressively worsening weakness, fatigue, pallor, shortness of breath, tachycardia, and pal-

pitations. Numbness, tingling, and glossitis may exist.

Laboratory results for iron deficiency anemia are listed in Table 5. After iron therapy, the maximal daily rate of Hgb regeneration is 0.3 g/dL.

*Serum ferritin (normal range: >10–20 ng/mL or >10–20 µg/L).* Loss of storage iron was traditionally evaluated by a liver or bone marrow biopsy. Serum ferritin has been largely replaced by these invasive tests as an indirect measure of iron stores. Serum ferritin concentrations are markedly reduced in iron deficiency anemia (3–6 µg/L).

*Serum iron (normal range: 50–150 µg/dL or 9–26.9 µmol/L) and total iron-binding capacity (TIBC) (normal range: 250–410 µg/dL or 45–73 µmol/L).* The serum iron concentration measures iron bound to transferrin. This value represents about one-third of the TIBC of transferrin.[2]

The TIBC measures the iron-binding capacity of transferrin protein. In iron deficiency anemia, TIBC is increased due to a compensatory increase in transferrin synthesis.[2] This increase leads to a corresponding decrease in the percent saturation, which can be calculated. For example, a person with a serum iron concentration of 100 µg/dL and a TIBC of 300 µg/dL has a transferrin saturation of 33%. Iron deficient erythropoiesis exists whenever the percent saturation is 15% or less.[5]

Other disease states besides iron deficiency that can alter serum iron and TIBC are infections, malignant tumors, and uremia.[2,5] Serum iron and TIBC both decrease in these disorders, unlike in iron deficiency anemia where serum iron decreases but TIBC increases. Anemia from

**TABLE 5.** Laboratory Findings for Iron Deficiency Anemia

| Test | Result[a] |
|---|---|
| RBC | ↓ |
| Hgb | ↓ |
| Hct | ↓ |
| MCV | ↓ |
| MCH | ↓ |
| MCHC | ↓ |
| Reticulocytes | → ↓ |
| Serum iron | ↓ |
| Total iron-binding capacity | ↑ |
| Transferrin saturation | ↓ |
| Ferritin | ↓ |
| RDW | ↑ |

[a] ↑ = increased; ↓ = decreased; → = no change.

these diseases is sometimes called anemia of chronic disease.

*RDW (normal range: 11–16%).* Since iron deficiency anemia leads to production of smaller cells (decreased MCV), the RDW increases in early iron deficiency. As iron deficiency develops, a mixture of red cell volumes appears as smaller, iron deficient cells are produced. However, older, larger cells are still in circulation. The RDW increases in iron deficiency before any other blood cell parameter becomes abnormal. Therefore, an isolated, increased RDW in the presence of other normal red cell indices can be an early sign of deficiency. Unfortunately, an increase in RDW is not specific for iron deficiency anemia. An increased RDW also may be present in a mixed anemia (simultaneous microcytic and macrocytic anemia).

## Normochromic, Normocytic Anemia

This classification encompasses numerous etiologies. Three causes are discussed: acute blood loss anemia, hemolytic anemia, and anemia of chronic disease.

### Acute Blood Loss Anemia

Patients who suffer from acute hemorrhage can have a dramatic drop in their RBC count. In this situation, the Hct is not a reliable indicator of the extent of anemia. It is a measure of the concentration of Hgb, not the total body amount of Hgb. The RBC count can be markedly reduced, while the Hct may be normal or even slightly increased. Usually, however, it is decreased. Hemorrhage evokes vasoconstriction, and it initially prevents extravascular fluid from replacing intravascular fluid loss.

In patients with normal bone marrow, the production of RBCs increases in response to hemorrhage, resulting in reticulocytosis. Each unit of packed RBCs administered should increase the Hgb by 1 g/dL if the bleeding has stopped. Table 6 shows the usual laboratory findings in acute blood loss anemia, while Minicase 2 (page 308)

demonstrates the use of them in diagnosis.

### Hemolytic Anemia

Hemolysis is the lysis of erythrocytes. If hemolysis is rapid and extensive, severe anemias can develop. RBC indices remain unchanged. Patients with normal bone marrow respond with an increase in erythrocyte production to replace the lysed cells. Reticulocytosis is present. Specialized tests, called antiglobulin tests, can be useful in determining immune causes of hemolytic anemia.[14] Plasma (free) Hgb measures the concentration of Hgb circulating in the plasma unattached to RBCs. It is almost always elevated in the presence of intravascular hemolysis.

Haptoglobin, an acute-phase reactant, binds free Hgb and carries it to the reticuloendothelial system. In the presence of intravascular hemolysis, haptoglobin is decreased. Concomitant corticosteroid therapy may confound interpretation, since many diseases associated with in vivo hemolysis are treated with steroids. Serum haptoglobin may be normal or elevated in hemolysis if the patient is receiving steroids. If the increase in serum haptoglobin is from steroids, other acute-phase reactants such as prealbumin (Chapter 11) will often be elevated. Serum haptoglobin is also elevated in patients with biliary obstruction and nephrotic syndrome. It is variably decreased in folate deficiency, sickle cell anemia, thalassemia, hypersplenism, liver disease, and estrogen therapy or pregnancy.

Immune hemolytic anemias are caused by the binding of antibodies and/or complement components to the erythrocyte cell membrane. Antiglobulin tests are also sometimes referred to as Coombs' tests. Other laboratory

**TABLE 6.** Laboratory Findings for Acute Blood Loss Anemia

| Test | Result[a] |
|---|---|
| RBC | ↓ |
| Hgb | ↓ |
| Hct | → ↓ |
| MCV | → |
| MCH | → |
| MCHC | → |
| Reticulocytes | ↑ |

[a]↑ = increased; ↓ = decreased; → = no change.

**TABLE 7.** Laboratory Findings for Hemolytic Anemia

| Test | Result[a] |
|---|---|
| RBC | ↓ |
| Hgb | ↓ |
| Hct | ↓ |
| MCV | → |
| MCH | → |
| MCHC | → |
| Reticulocytes | ↑ |
| Antiglobulin test (in immune types) | positive |
| Serum haptoglobin[b] | ↓ |
| Plasma (free) Hgb[c] | ↑ |

[a]↑ = increased; ↓ = decreased; → = no change.
[b]Normal range: 27–140 mg/dL or 0.3–1.4 g/L.
[c]Normal range: <3 mg/dL or <0.47 µmol/L.

test results for hemolytic anemia are listed in Table 7. The method used to detect antibodies bound to erythrocytes is a direct antiglobulin test (DAT). The method used to detect antibodies present in serum is an indirect antiglobulin test (IAT). Chapter 2 describes the agglutination technology used for DAT and IAT. In both tests, results are reported as either positive or negative.

The DAT is performed by combining a patient's RBCs with antiglobulin serum, which contains antibodies against human immunoglobulins and complement.[14] Antiglobulin serum is produced by immunizing rabbits or goats with human serum or serum components. The resulting serum is combined with the patient's RBCs. If they are coated with antibody or complement, the antibodies in the antiglobulin serum combine with the immunoglobulins coating the RBCs, leading to the agglutination of the RBCs. The DAT is the only test that provides definitive evidence of immune hemolysis.[15] The DAT can also be used to investigate possible blood transfusion reactions.[14]

The IAT detects antibodies in the patient's serum. Serum is combined with normal erythrocytes, which are subjected to the DAT to detect if any serum antibodies have coated the erythrocytes. The IAT is important in blood typing.[14]

The antiglobulin tests are very sensitive, but a negative result does not eliminate the possibility of antibodies bound to erythrocytes. An estimated 100–150 molecules of antibody must be bound to each erythrocyte for detection by the antiglobulin test.[14] Smaller numbers of antibodies give a false-negative reaction.

Numerous conditions and medications can be associated with immune hemolytic anemia (Table 8). Medications induce antibody formation, by three mechanisms, that results in a hemolytic anemia.

**TABLE 8.** Causes of Immune Hemolytic Anemia[a]

**Neoplasm**
Chronic lymphocytic leukemia
Lymphoma
Multiple myeloma

**Collagen vascular disease**
Systemic lupus erythematosis
Rheumatoid arthritis

**Medication**
Autoimmune type—levodopa, mefenamic acid, methyldopa, procainamide
Innocent bystander type—cefotaxime, ceftazidime, ceftriaxone, chlorpromazine, doxepin, fluorouracil, isoniazid, quinidine, quinine, rifampin, sulfonamides, thiazides
Hapten type 1—cephalosporins and penicillins

**Infections**
*Mycoplasma*
Viruses

[a]Adapted from References 15 and 16.

*Autoimmune type.* Methyldopa, an infrequently used antihypertensive drug, can induce the formation of antibodies directed specifically against normal RBC proteins. This autoimmune state can persist for up to 1 month after drug administration has been discontinued. This mechanism is known as a true autoimmune type of antibody formation.[2]

*Innocent bystander type.* Antibodies to the drugs quinine and quinidine are examples of the immune complex (innocent bystander) mechanism.[2] Each drug forms a drug–protein complex with plasma proteins, to which antibodies are formed. This drug–plasma protein–antibody complex attaches to erythrocytes and fixes complement, which leads to lysis of the RBCs.[7] In this situation, the RBC is an innocent bystander. Other drugs implicated in causing this type of hemolytic anemia (in addition to those listed in Table 8) include chlorpromazine, isoniazid, mefenamic acid, para-aminosalicylic acid, rifampin, sulfonamides, sulfonylureas, and temafloxacin (no longer marketed in the United States).[7,17,18]

*Hapten type 1.* The hapten (penicillin) type 1 mechanism is involved when a patient has produced antibodies to penicillin. If the patient receives high-dose penicillin at a future date, some penicillin can bind to the RBC membrane. The antipenicillin antibodies, in turn, bind to the penicillin bound to the RBC, and hemolysis can result.

## Anemia of Chronic Disease

Mild to moderate anemia often accompanies numerous infections, inflammatory traumatic illnesses, or neoplastic diseases that last over 1–2 months.[19] Chronic infections include pulmonary abscesses, tuberculosis (TB), endocarditis, pelvic inflammatory disease, and osteomyelitis. Chronic inflammatory illnesses (e.g., rheumatoid arthritis and systemic lupus erythematosus) and hematological malignancies (e.g., Hodgkin's disease, leukemia, and multiple myeloma) are also associated with anemia. Because these disorders as a group are common, anemia due to chronic disease is also quite common. While anemia of chronic disease is more commonly associated with normocytic, normochromic anemia, it can also cause microcytic anemia. Table 9 (next page) shows the usual laboratory results found in anemia of chronic disease.

The pathogenesis of this anemia is not totally understood. Various investigations have found that the erythrocyte lifespan is shortened and that the bone marrow does not increase erythrocyte production to compensate for the decreased longevity.[19] Iron utilization is also impaired.

Erythrocytes are frequently normal size; however, microcytosis can develop. One distinguishing feature between early iron deficiency anemia and a microcytic anemia of chronic disease is the normal serum ferritin that is present in the latter.[19]

### Minicase 2

Brian O., a 39-year-old male with a long history of alcohol abuse, cirrhosis, and esophageal varices, was brought to the emergency department by concerned family members. The family said that he suddenly began coughing up bright red blood. As Brian O. was moved to a bed in the emergency department, he began coughing and vomiting large amounts of bright red blood. A stat CBC revealed the following:

| Test Name | Result | Reference Range |
|---|---|---|
| RBC | $2.91 \times 10^6$ cells/mm³ | $4.6–6.2 \times 10^6$ cells/mm³ for males |
| WBC | $6.6 \times 10^3$ cells/mm³ | $4.8–10.8 \times 10^3$ cells/mm³ |
| Hgb | 8.9 g/dL | 14–18 g/dL for males |
| Hct | 29.6% | 42–52% for males |
| MCV | 92.4 fL | 80–96 fL for males |
| MCH | 30.6 pg/cell | 27–33 pg/cell |
| MCHC | 33.1 g/dL | 31–35 g/dL |
| RDW | 14.1% | 11–16% |
| Platelet count | 80,000/µL | 140,000–440,000/µL |

*What does the CBC indicate?*

**Discussion:** The CBC is consistent with acute blood loss. The RBC, Hgb, and Hct are all markedly decreased (as usual) in acute blood loss, and the red cell indices are within normal limits. The platelet count is also decreased, which may have led to increased blood loss. In fact, Brian O. was experiencing acute, dramatic blood loss due to bleeding from his esophageal varices.

## ERYTHROCYTE SEDIMENTATION RATE

*Normal range:[20] 1–15 mm/hr in males or 1–20 mm/hr in females (increases with age)*

ESR is discussed separately because numerous physiological and disease states are associated with its alteration (Table 10). Anemia, pregnancy, and various inflammatory diseases (including infections) can elevate the ESR. Sickle cell disease, high doses of corticosteroids, microcytosis, and congestive heart failure can decrease the ESR. However, aspirin and NSAIDs have no effect on it.[21]

Although the ESR may be used to confirm a diagnosis supported by other tests, it is rarely used alone for a specific diagnosis. Rather, the ESR is useful for monitoring the activity of inflammatory conditions (e.g., temporal arteritis, polymyalgia rheumatica, rheumatoid arthritis, and osteomyelitis).[21] (The reader is referred to Chapter 17 for more information on ESR related to these conditions.) The ESR is often higher when the disease is active and falls when the intensity of the disease decreases.

Erythrocytes normally settle slowly in plasma but settle rapidly when they aggregate. Aggregation is caused by electrostatic forces. Each cell normally has a net negative charge and repels other erythrocytes because like charges repel each other. Many plasma proteins are positively charged and can neutralize the surface charge on the RBC, thereby promoting erythrocyte aggregation. The proteins known as acute-phase reactants (e.g., fibrinogen) enhance erythrocyte aggregation.[21] Other proteins can also cause aggregation of RBCs.

A common way to determine the ESR is the Westergren method. Anticoagulated blood is diluted and

**TABLE 9.** Laboratory Findings for Anemia of Chronic Disease

| Test | Result[a] |
|---|---|
| RBC | ↓ |
| Hgb | ↓ |
| Hct | ↓ |
| MCV | →↓ |
| MCH | →↓ |
| MCHC | →↓ |
| Reticulocytes | →↓ |
| Serum iron | ↓ |
| TIBC | ↓ |
| Ferritin | → |

[a] ↑ = increased; ↓ = decreased; → = no change.

**TABLE 10.** Conditions that May Alter ESR

| Increased ESR | Decreased ESR |
|---|---|
| Advanced age | Congestive heart failure |
| Female gender | Corticosteroids |
| Infection (osteomyelitis) | Microcytic anemia |
| Macrocytic anemia | Sickle cell anemia |
| Normocytic anemia | |
| Pregnancy | |
| Rheumatoid arthritis | |

placed in a glass tube of standard size. After 1 hr, the distance from the meniscus to the top of the erythrocytes is recorded as the ESR in millimeters per hour.[21]

A corrected sedimentation rate, called the zeta-sedimentation rate or ratio, has been developed to eliminate the effect of anemia on the ESR.[20] The patient's blood is spun in a special centrifuge. The level of erythrocytes in the centrifuged tube is recorded as if it were the Hct. This value is called the zeta crit, and its normal range is 40–52%. It is linearly related to increases in the fibrinogen concentration.[22] Elevations above the normal range are interpreted in the same manner as an elevated ESR by traditional methods.

# WHITE BLOOD CELL COUNT AND DIFFERENTIAL

WBCs can be divided into two major categories on the basis of their differing functions:[14]

> Phagocytes (leukocytes that engulf and digest other cells).
> Lymphocytes and plasma cells (leukocytes involved in the recognition and destruction of foreign proteins).

The functions are interrelated, as are the cells that perform them. The different types of leukocytes function as members of an elaborate team to eliminate invading bacteria and foreign proteins from the body.

When a WBC count and differential is ordered for a patient, the resulting laboratory report is a tally of the total WBCs in a given volume of blood plus the relative percentages each cell type contributes to the total. Therefore, the percentages of the WBC subtypes must add up to 100%. If one cell type increases, percentages of all other types must decrease proportionately. This decrease is not necessarily associated with any pathology. Table 11 is a general breakdown of the different types of WBCs and

**TABLE 11.** Normal WBC Count and Differential

| Cell Type | Normal Range |
|---|---|
| Total WBC count | 4800–10,800/mm³ |
| Polymorphonuclear neutrophils (segs, PMNs, polys) | 45–73% |
| Bands (stabs) | 3–5% |
| Lymphocytes | 20–40% |
| Monocytes | 2–8% |
| Eosinophils | 0–4% |
| Basophils | 0–1% |

their usual percentages in peripheral blood.

Absolute counts are sometimes calculated and compared with reference ranges. For example, the absolute segmented neutrophil count is the percentage of "segs" multiplied by the WBC count. The reference range for absolute counts can be estimated by multiplying the normal range of percentages for the particular type of WBC by the upper and lower limits of the total WBC count.

The WBC count and differential is one of the most widely performed clinical laboratory tests. In the past, differentials were determined by a manual count of a standard number of cells. This method is imprecise and inaccurate when compared to reference methods. The main reason for this inaccuracy is sampling error. When a manual differential is performed, typically 100–200 cells are viewed. This procedure can lead to an unacceptable false-negative rate for the detection of small populations of abnormal cells. To achieve an acceptable level of precision, 1000 cells should be counted. However, this procedure is too time consuming, labor intensive, and expensive.[23]

Currently, clinical laboratories commonly use an automated method for determining the WBC differential. These instruments count thousands of cells and can report not only the relative percentages of the various WBC types but also the absolute numbers. When reviewing a WBC differential, one must be aware of not only the relative percentages of cell types but also the absolute numbers. The percentages viewed in isolation can lead to incorrect conclusions. Minicase 3 demonstrates this principle.

Automated methods are useful in leukopenic patients because few cells are present and a manual examination of them is especially difficult. However, automated differentials have some disadvantages. A band count cannot be performed because bands are indistinguishable from mature neutrophils. Therefore, a total neutrophil count is generated that includes the bands. This limitation should not be of any clinical significance in most situations.

False-negative results can occur. Lymphoma cells, atypical lymphocytes, and various types of immature granulocytes may not be detected in small numbers. Likewise, false-positive results can occur. However, positive results generally provoke a warning, requiring subsequent manual review of the blood smear.[23]

## Phagocytes

Phagocytes include granulocytes (neutrophils, eosinophils, and basophils) and monocyte macrophages.[23] Neutrophils are further divided into polymorphonuclear (PMN) leukocytes and band leukocytes.

### Granulocytes

Granulocytes derive their name from the presence of gran-

### Minicase 3

A 46-year-old male, David D., presented to the emergency department with a temperature of 104 °F (40 °C), diarrhea, and abdominal pain. He had a history of alcohol abuse. Urine and blood cultures were obtained, and David D. was given broad-spectrum antibiotics. The following CBC was obtained:

| Test Name | Result | Reference Range |
|---|---|---|
| RBC | $3.18 \times 10^6$ cells/mm³ | $4.6$–$6.2 \times 10^6$ cells/mm³ for males |
| WBC | $118.9 \times 10^3$ cells/mm³ | $4.8$–$10.8 \times 10^3$ cells/mm³ |
| Hgb | 9.9 g/dL | 14–18 g/dL for males |
| Hct | 29.5% | 42–52% for males |
| MCV | 92.8 fL | 80–96 fL for males |
| MCH | 31.1 pg/cell | 27–33 pg/cell |
| MCHC | 33.6 g/dL | 31–35 g/dL |
| Platelet count | 69,000/µL | 140,000–440,000/µL |
| Segs | 21% | 45–73% |
| Bands | 12% | 3–5% |
| Metamyelocytes | 5% | 0% |
| Myelocytes | 5% | 0% |
| Promyelocytes | 8% | 0% |
| Lymphocytes | 6% | 20–40% |
| Atypical lymphocytes | 0% | 0–6% |
| Monocytes | 2% | 2–8% |
| Eosinophils | 1% | 0–4% |
| Basophils | 10% | 0–1% |
| Blasts | 30% | 0% |

*What does his CBC reveal?*

**Discussion:** This CBC is grossly abnormal, showing marked leukocytosis with elevations in the absolute neutrophil and lymphocyte counts. However, the percentages of these cells are markedly decreased. When the absolute numbers are calculated (i.e., $118.9 \times 21\% = 25,000$ segmented neutrophils/mm³), neutrophilia is found. Although bands are also neutrophilic leukocytes, it is common to use only segs in determining the absolute neutrophil count. The normal range varies but is usually around 2160–7880 segs/mm³.

At first, one might expect that David D.'s condition could be consistent with an overwhelming infection. However, he has a marked number of immature WBC forms in the peripheral blood—metamyelocytes, myelocytes, promyelocytes, and blasts. These forms are not present in a normal WBC differential. David D. also has normochromic, normocytic anemia (RBCs, Hgb, and Hct are low; MCV and MCH are normal) and thrombocytopenia (low platelet count).

Further analysis of this patient's CBC and bone marrow biopsy reveals that he has chronic myelogenous leukemia with a blast (myeloblast) crisis. The anemia is likely myelophthisic, which can occur partly from the "crowding out" of red cell precursors by hoards of WBCs or other cells in the bone marrow.

ules within the cytoplasm. When a peripheral smear of blood is prepared, three types of granulocytes can be microscopically identified by the staining characteristics of their cytoplasmic granules:[5]

> ➤ Neutrophils retain neutral stains and appear light tan.
> ➤ Eosinophils retain acidic dyes and appear red orange.
> ➤ Basophils retain basic dyes and appear dark blue to purple.

The granulocytes function as a line of defense against bacteria and other invading organisms. To do so, granulocytes must accumulate in sufficient numbers at the right place, become attached to the foreign substances, and then engulf, dissolve, and dispose of them.[24]

Granulocytes are formed in large numbers in the bone marrow. They probably arise from stem cells, undergo numerous maturation steps in the marrow, and finally form mature granulocytes that are released into the peripheral blood. Production time from immature granulocyte precursors to release of mature granulocytes into the circulation is estimated to be 2 weeks.[1]

Once these mature cells are released into the peripheral blood, approximately half of them are freely circulating. The other half are marginated along blood vessel walls. Granulocytes remain in the circulation for less than 1 day, and then they migrate into various body tissues. After migrating out of the circulation, granulocytes have a lifespan of 2–3 days. They are destroyed either during their defense activities or by the body because they have aged.[24]

*Neutrophils [PMN leukocytes (normal range: 45–73%)] and bands (normal range: 3–5%).* PMN leukocytes are also called polys, PMNs, and segs. Bands, a slightly immature form of neutrophil, frequently appear in small amounts in peripheral blood. Bands, also called stabs, derive their name from the morphology of their nucleus, which has not yet segmented into multiple lobes as in the seg form. The nucleus appears as a curved band across the cytoplasm. Less mature forms of the neutrophil, such as the metamyelocyte and myelocyte, are normally not in the peripheral blood. The neutrophil is a phagocytic cell that exists to ingest and digest foreign proteins (e.g., bacteria and fungi). Certain body constituents, such as dead cells, are also phagocytized by neutrophils.[24]

The concept of "left shift" originally connoted an increase in the number of immature WBCs in the peripheral blood. Over many years, the term has been used in different ways. Some clinicians use "shift to the left" to mean that the percentage of segs and/or bands (neutrophils) has increased. The inference is that, given the proper clinical setting, the shift may have been caused by infection or another type of inflammation. The term "left" reflects the order in which various types of WBCs are listed across the page from left to right, with segs and bands on the left side. The headings on a typical differential report look like

Segs \ Bands \ Lymphocytes \ Monocytes \ Eosinophils \ Basophils

The very immature forms (e.g., metamyelocytes and blasts) are usually not listed unless they are seen in the blood. Occasionally, a few appear in the results, especially if the marrow is hyperproductive. When they make up more than a few percent of the WBCs, hematological malignancy is suspected.

During an acute infection, theoretically the first change in the differential should be an increase in the percentage of segs. This increase occurs because these already mature neutrophils, which have been waiting (noncirculating) along the inner walls of blood vessels, detach (or demarginate) soon after the insult. To replenish and increase the supply of segs, bands are produced in and released from the bone marrow more rapidly. More neutrophils than usual enter the bloodstream as bands (sometimes called bandemia). Typically, there may be 10–20% bands.

Therefore, the second change in the differential should be an increase in bands. As these bands mature into segs, the number of segs will increase. If the infection has been treated properly, the outpouring of bands should cease and the left shift will be comprised mainly of an increased percentage of segs (typically 70–85%). If the infection is not treated properly, both segs and bands are likely to remain elevated. Rarely, if the infection is overwhelming and the signs and symptoms suggest it is worsening, bands may paradoxically decrease due to "exhausted" marrow. The prognosis is poor in this case.

Whenever the segs and/or bands are elevated, the percentage of lymphocytes decreases proportionately. Only 10–15% lymphocytes may appear in these patients, but the "lymphopenia" is not real because of a concomitant increase in total WBCs. This increase brings the absolute lymphocyte (WBC × % lymphocytes) count into the normal range.

Although the previous situation might describe events in the theoretical infection, it is uncommon to see this utopian pattern in clinical practice. Too many physiological, pharmacological, and logistical events affect WBC production. In fact, some clinicians feel that a high *total* WBC count and fever are better indicators of infection than a "left shifted" differential.[25]

*Eosinophils (normal range: 0–4%) and basophils (normal range: 0–1%).* The functions of eosinophils and basophils are not completely known. Eosinophils are present in large numbers in the intestinal mucosa and lungs, two locations where foreign proteins enter the body.[3] Eosinophils can phagocytize, kill, and digest bacteria and yeast. They provide defense against parasites and are involved in hypersensitivity reactions. In both situations, they become elevated.[1] Other causes of eosinophilia are listed in Table 12.

Basophils are present in small numbers in the peripheral blood. They contain heparin, histamine, and leukotriene B$_4$.[26,27] Many signs and symptoms of allergic responses can be attributed to specific mast cell and basophil products.[26] Basophils are probably involved in immediate hypersensitivity reactions [e.g., extrinsic (allergic) asthma] in addition to delayed hypersensitivity reactions.[1,27] Basophils may be increased in chronic inflammation and leukemia.

*Granulocyte disorders.* Granulocytes can suffer from three major types of disorders:

> ➤ Qualitative.
> ➤ Quantitative.
> ➤ Myeloproliferative.

Qualitative disorders involve defects in the phagocytic activity or digestive capability of neutrophils.[23] Since routine laboratory values do not detect these abnormalities, qualitative defects will not be discussed further.

Quantitative disorders involve too few or too many granulocytes.[23] Possible causes are listed in Table 12 (next page). Neutropenia is said to exist when the neutrophil count is less than 1500 cells/mm$^3$.[30] When the neutrophil count is less than 500 cells/mm$^3$, normal defense mechanisms are greatly impaired and the patient is at increased risk of bacterial infections. When infections occur in such patients, they can be very difficult to treat—even with effective antibiotics—because the phagocytic activity of the neutrophils is impaired.

Neutrophilia (increased neutrophils), another kind of quantitative disorder, can be caused by a shift of granulocytes from the marginated pool (cells stuck to vessel

**TABLE 12.** Quantitative Disorders of WBCs[a]

| Abnormality | Typical Cutoff[b] (cells/mm$^3$) | Possible Causes |
|---|---|---|
| Neutrophilia | >12,000 | Acute bacterial infection<br>Trauma<br>Myocardial infarction<br>Chronic bacterial infection<br>Epinephrine, corticosteroids, lithium<br>Leukemia |
| Neutropenia | <1500 | Radiation exposure<br>Medications:<br>    Antineoplastic drugs (in association with anemia and thrombocytopenia)<br>    Captopril<br>    Cephalosporins<br>    Chloramphenicol (in association with anemia and thrombocytopenia)<br>    Ganciclovir<br>    Methimazole<br>    Penicillins<br>    Phenothiazines<br>    Phenylbutazone<br>    Procainamide<br>    Ticlopidine<br>    Tricyclic antidepressants<br>    Vancomycin<br>    Zidovudine<br>Overwhelming acute bacterial infection<br>Vitamin B$_{12}$ or folate deficiency<br>Salmonellosis<br>Pertussis |
| Eosinophilia | >350 | Allergic disorders (asthma)<br>Parasitic infections<br>Leukemia<br>Medications:<br>    Angiotensin-converting enzyme inhibitors<br>    Antibiotics (or any allergic reaction to a drug) |
| Eosinopenia | <50 | Acute infection |
| Basophilia | >300 | Chronic inflammation<br>Leukemia |
| Monocytosis | >800 | Recovery stage of acute bacterial infection<br>TB, disseminated<br>Endocarditis<br>Protozoal or rickettsial infection<br>Leukemia |
| Lymphocytosis | >4000 | Infectious mononucleosis<br>Viral infections (e.g., rubella, varicella, cytomegalovirus, mumps)<br>Pertussis<br>TB<br>Lymphoma<br>Syphillis |
| Lymphopenia | <1000 | HIV Type 1<br>Radiation exposure<br>Corticosteroids<br>Lymphoma (Hodgkin's disease)<br>Aplastic anemia |

[a]*Adapted from References 10, 24, and 26–29.*
[b]*Actual cutoffs can be calculated by multiplying the upper and lower limits of the total WBCs by the limits of normal (percent) of the specific type of WBCs.*

walls) and bone marrow into the circulation. This shift can be caused by acute infections, trauma, or administration of epinephrine or corticosteroids. Chronic neutrophilia is due to sustained overproduction, usually caused by chronic bacterial infections or neoplasms.[23,27]

Agranulocytosis is a term for severe granulocytopenia. Granulocytopenia can result from decreased production caused by disorders of the bone marrow, exposure to radiation, use of certain medications, or increased peripheral destruction of granulocytes (Table 12). Increased utilization due to overwhelming infection or immune disorders is a common cause of peripheral destruction[23] (Minicase 4).

Myeloproliferative disorders involve an uncontrolled proliferation of bone marrow cells.[23] Leukemia is a common type of myeloproliferative disorder. In leukemia, the cells that proliferate abnormally can be granulocytes or lymphocytes and either mature or immature forms. There are many different types of leukemia; however, only one type of leukocyte (mature or immature) usually undergoes uncontrolled proliferation. Large numbers of these abnormal cells gain access to the bloodstream and can be visualized on a smear of peripheral blood.

Because of the massive proliferation of leukocytes, the bone marrow frequently cannot produce adequate numbers of other cellular components of blood. This situation results in anemia, due to the low level of erythrocytes, as well as thrombocytopenia and bleeding, due to the low level of platelets. In addition, even though the bone marrow is producing numerous leukocytes, these

---

### ✎ Minicase 4

A 26-year-old female, Holly H., was hospitalized with sinusitis. The clinician subsequently reviewed her medical record. She had acquired immunodeficiency syndrome (AIDS), been febrile, and recently received granulocyte csf. The following CBC was obtained:

| Test Name | Result | Reference Range |
|---|---|---|
| RBC | $3.47 \times 10^6$ cells/mm³ | $4.2–5.4 \times 10^6$ cells/mm³ for females |
| WBC | $1.5 \times 10^3$ cells/mm³ | $4.8–10.8 \times 10^3$ cells/mm³ |
| Hgb | 10.1 g/dL | 12–16 g/dL for females |
| Hct | 31.3% | 37–47% for females |
| MCV | 90.2 fL | 82–98 fL for females |
| MCH | 29.1 pg/cell | 27–33 pg/cell |
| MCHC | 32.2 g/dL | 31–35 g/dL |
| RDW | 15.2% | 11–16% |
| Platelet count | 353,000/μL | 140,000–440,000/μL |
| Segs | 15% | 45–73% |
| Bands | 9% | 3–5% |
| Metamyelocytes | 2% | 0% |
| Lymphocytes | 35% | 20–40% |
| Atypical lymphocytes | 5% | 0–6% |
| Monocytes | 0% | 2–8% |
| Eosinophils | 34% | 0–4% |

*What hematological abnormalities are apparent from these results? How might they affect treatment of Holly H.'s acute infection?*

**Discussion:** Holly H. has leukopenia, a reduction in the numbers of all WBCs. She also has normocytic, normochromic anemia. The only blood cell line not suppressed is her platelets. The total WBC count is low: $1.5 \times 10^3$ cells/mm³. The percent and absolute number of segmented neutrophils are only 15% (normal range: 45–73%) and 225 or 15% of 1500 (normal range: 2160–7880 cells/mm³), respectively. The percent of bands is higher than normal at 9% (normal range: 3–5%), and the absolute number is slightly below normal at 135 or 9% of 1500 (normal range: 144–540 cells/mm³). Although the percent of lymphocytes is normal (35%), lymphocytopenia is present. The absolute number is low: $35\% \times 1.5 \times 10^3$ = 525 (normal range: 960–4320 cells/mm³). The absolute eosinophil count is only slightly elevated at 510 (normal range: <432 cells/mm³), even though the percent is dramatically elevated.

Metamyelocytes, immature WBCs, are normally not present in peripheral blood. The granulocyte csf may be stimulating this cell line production so that a few escape into the circulation. For the same reason, a higher than normal percent of bands is found in the blood. Patients with infections typically have an elevated WBC count and a shift to the left in the differential. AIDS patients often do not have this normal response.

Holly H. is highly susceptible to infections. Due to her neutropenia, they will be difficult to treat adequately. Aggressive antimicrobial therapy is necessary. Knowledge of Holly H.'s AIDS, current therapy with granulocyte csf, and neutropenia reemphasizes the likelihood of an infection that is difficult to treat. Unusual pathogens (e.g., *Rhizopus* sp. and *Aspergillus* sp.) may be the cause of her sinusitis. Additionally, one cannot expect a correction of her neutropenia or immunological defects due to AIDS. Long-term suppressive antimicrobial therapy may be required.

cells are frequently abnormal and do not fight infection effectively. Therefore, leukemic patients are at risk for numerous bacterial, fungal, and parasitic infections.[31–33]

### Monocyte Macrophages

Monocytes are actually immature cells released from the bone marrow into the circulation. Monocytes leave the circulation in 16–36 hr and enter the tissues, where they mature into macrophages. Macrophages are present in lymph nodes, alveoli of the lungs, spleen, liver, and bone marrow.[24] These tissue macrophages participate in the removal of foreign substances from the body. They are involved in the destruction of old erythrocytes, denatured plasma proteins, and plasma lipids. Tissue macrophages also salvage iron from the Hgb of old erythrocytes and return the iron to transferrin for delivery to the bone marrow.[24] Using mechanisms not fully understood, tissue macrophages are involved in the immune system.[1]

## Lymphocytes and Plasma Cells
*Normal range for lymphocytes: 20–40%*

Lymphocytes and plasma cells make up the second major group of leukocytes. These cells give specificity and memory to the body's defense against foreign invaders.[28] The two types of lymphocytes are

> ➤ T lymphocytes (T cells).
> ➤ B lymphocytes (B cells).

With the help of T cells, B cells recognize foreign substances and are transformed into plasma cells, capable of producing antibodies (discussed later). Table 12 lists the types of disorders in which lymphocytes are increased or decreased.

### T Lymphocytes

T lymphocytes are responsible for cell-mediated immunity. This immunity involves delayed hypersensitivity (seen with skin tests for TB, mumps, and *Candida*), rejection of transplanted organs, and defense against fungal and viral infections.[34] T cells may also have a defensive role against neoplastic growth. They regulate humoral (B-cell-mediated) immunity and are the most common lymphocytes found in blood and lymph.[28] Table 13 shows normal ranges for various types and ratios of T cells.

HIV Type 1 (HIV-1), the causative agent of AIDS, infects a specific type of T cell ($CD_4$ cells). This infection leads to destruction of this subset of T cells, an imbalance of the remaining T cells, and susceptibility to numerous opportunistic infections and even cancer.[29] (Chapter 16 presents more information about AIDS.)

### B Lymphocytes and Plasma Cells

As explained previously, B cells recognize foreign substances and bacteria, most likely with the help of T cells,

**TABLE 13.** Typical Normal Ranges for CD Lymphocytes[a]

| Cell | Normal Range |
|------|--------------|
| $CD_4$ lymphocyte (absolute count | 440–1600 cells/mm³ |
| $CD_4$ lymphocyte (percentage of total lymphocytes) | 29–61% |
| $CD_8$ lymphocyte (absolute count) | 170–940 cells/mm³ |
| $CD_8$ lymphocyte (percentage of total lymphocytes) | 11–39% |
| $CD_4$:$CD_8$ ratio | 0.9–5.0 |

[a]*Actual values vary among laboratories.*

and are transformed into plasma cells. Plasma cells then produce antibodies, also known as immunoglobulins. These immunoglobulins can be divided into five classes based on their structure. Listed in order of greatest to least frequency in the blood, these groups are

> ➤ Immunoglobulin G (IgG).
> ➤ Immunoglobulin M (IgM).
> ➤ Immunoglobulin A (IgA).
> ➤ Immunoglobulin E (IgE).
> ➤ Immunoglobulin D (IgD).

The two antibodies most commonly associated with the development of immunity to foreign proteins, viruses, and bacteria are IgM and IgG (Chapters 16 and 17). IgE is associated with the development of allergic phenomena. IgA is secreted into the lumen of the GI tract, and IgD is bound to the lymphocyte cell membrane.[34]

The functions and interactions of T cells, B cells, and antibodies are complex and not completely understood. For the smooth functioning of the entire system, T cells, antibodies, and phagocytes must interact. If one small part of this intricate puzzle is missing, the system does not work as it should.

### Lymphocyte Disorders

Quantitative lymphocyte disorders involve problems of too few or too many lymphocytes (Table 12). Lymphopenia and hypogammaglobulinemia (a decrease in the total quantity of immunoglobulin) can result from radiation exposure. Corticosteroid use causes a shift of lymphocytes from the intravascular to the extravascular space, which leads to lymphopenia.[28] HIV-1 virus infection also leads to lymphopenia. Other viral infections (e.g., infectious mononucleosis, hepatitis, mumps, varicella, rubella, herpes simplex, herpes zoster, and influenza) increase the number of circulating lymphocytes (lymphocytosis).[32,34]

*HIV-1 virus.* The HIV-1 virus interacts with the $CD_4$ molecule. This molecule is primarily found on the surface of certain T lymphocytes (known as T-helper or $CD_4$ lymphocytes). Other leukocytes, such as monocyte macrophages, also have populations of cells with $CD_4$ molecules on the cell surface.

HIV-1 infection decreases the percent and number of $CD_4$ lymphocytes as the virus infects and destroys the cells. This decrease, in turn, alters the ratio of T-helper lymphocytes to $CD_8$ (suppressor T cell) lymphocytes. As HIV infection progresses, the $CD_4$ lymphocyte count falls and the $CD_4$:$CD_8$ ratio drops.

The $CD_4$ lymphocyte count seems to correlate with overall prognosis; therefore, it has been used as a surrogate marker in numerous drug trials in HIV-infected patients. Additionally, as the $CD_4$ count falls below certain levels, the HIV-infected patient is at increased risk for developing opportunistic infections due to *Pneumocystis carinii* and *Mycobacterium avium intracellularae*. By monitoring the $CD_4$ counts, the clinician can institute appropriate prophylactic therapy when the count reaches a particular level. The $CD_4$ count can also be useful in determining when to institute antiretroviral therapy (HIV is a retrovirus). Table 14 describes the therapeutic applications of the $CD_4$ count.

Although Table 14 recommends that asymptomatic patients with $CD_4$ counts greater than 500 cells/mm³ not be treated, some clinicians still begin zidovudine therapy in HIV-infected patients (Minicase 5, next page). Furthermore, some clinicians initiate therapy with concomitant zidovudine and didanosine or zidovudine and zalcitabine in patients with $CD_4$ counts less than 200 cells/

mm³, regardless of symptoms. The reason is that some data show greater $CD_4$ count elevations and other benefits with combination therapy.[35]

*Lymphomas.* Immunoproliferative disorders are neoplasms of lymphocytes or plasma cells. Examples include leukemias and lymphomas. Unlike leukemias, lymphomas often release only a few malignant cells into the bloodstream.[28]

Neoplasms derived from B or T cells or their precursors form various lymphomas, often grouped together and referred to as non-Hodgkin's lymphomas.[18] Hodgkin's disease is another type of neoplasm that also arises in the lymph nodes. The exact cell type that proliferates to cause this disease is not definitely known. Many symptoms of lymphomas result from the expansion of lymph nodes and compression of nearby organs. Late in the disease, some lymphomas change to a form in which many immature leukocytes are produced and the bone marrow is infiltrated.[28] In this end stage, patients have the same complications as leukemia sufferers.

### Plasma Cell Disorders

Multiple myeloma is the prototypical dyscrasia of the plasma cells. In this disorder, uncontrolled proliferation of differentiated plasma cells produces nonfunctional immunoglobulins. Only one type of immunoglobulin accumulates excessively. Myeloma proteins are called monoclonal because they are the progeny of a single, autonomously multiplying cell. The excessive immunoglobulins that can be measured by electrophoresis are usu-

**TABLE 14.** Therapeutic Utility of $CD_4$ Count in HIV-Infected Adults[a]

| Antiretroviral History[b] | Disease Status | $CD_4$ Cell Count (cells/mm³) | Therapeutic Suggestion |
|---|---|---|---|
| NPAT | No symptoms | >500 | Do not treat |
| NPAT | No symptoms | 200–500 | Zidovudine or no treatment |
| NPAT | Symptoms | 200–500 | Zidovudine |
| NPAT | No symptoms | <200 | Zidovudine |
| NPAT | Symptoms | <200 | Zidovudine |
| PAT | Stable | ≥300 | Continue zidovudine |
| PAT | Progressing | <300 | Continue zidovudine or change to didanosine |
| PAT | Progressing | 50–500 | Change to didanosine or zalcitabine |
| PAT | Progressing | <50 | Change to didanosine or zalcitabine |
| ZI | Stable | >500 | Change to didanosine or zalcitabine |

[a]*Recommendations from the 1993 National Institute of Allergy and Infectious Diseases' State-of-the-Art Conference.*
[b]*NPAT = no previous antiretroviral therapy; PAT = previous antiretroviral therapy; ZI = zidovudine intolerant.*

---

**✎ Minicase 5**

CBC results were obtained for a 55-year-old female, Julie L., with chronic renal failure due to AIDS and diabetes mellitus. She undergoes hemodialysis three times a week and has been treated with zidovudine for 2 years. The CBC results were as follows:

| Test Name | Result | Reference Range |
|---|---|---|
| RBC | $3.01 \times 10^6$ cells/mm³ | $4.2–5.4 \times 10^6$ cells/mm³ for females |
| WBC | $4 \times 10^3$ cells/mm³ | $4.8–10.8 \times 10^3$ cells/mm³ |
| Hgb | 9.2 g/dL | 12–16 g/dL for females |
| Hct | 27.6% | 37–47% for females |
| MCV | 91.7 fL | 82–98 fL for females |
| MCH | 30.6 pg/cell | 27–33 pg/cell |
| MCHC | 33.3 g/dL | 31–35 g/dL |
| RDW | 15.4% | 11–16% |
| Platelet count | 199,000/μL | 140,000–440,000/μL |
| Segs | 53% | 45–73% |
| Bands | 9% | 3–5% |
| Lymphocytes | 15% | 20–40% |
| Atypical lymphocytes | 2% | 0–6% |
| Monocytes | 8% | 2–8% |
| Eosinophils | 13% | 0–4% |
| CD₄ lymphocytes | 550 cells/mm³ | 440–1600 cells/mm³ |
| SCr | 3.2 mg/dL | 0.7–1.5 mg/dL |
| BUN | 7.5 mg/dL | 8–20 mg/dL |

*What hematological abnormalities are evident? How are they interpreted in light of this patient's condition?*

**Discussion:** The WBC count is slightly low, and the absolute neutrophil count (53% × 4000 cells/mm³ = 2120 cells/mm³; normal range: 2160–7880 cells/mm³) is also slightly low. Moreover, lymphocytopenia is present (absolute lymphocyte count: 15% × 4000 = 600 cells/mm³; normal range: 960–4320 cells/mm³), which is typical in patients with advanced HIV. Julie L. has anemia (low RBCs, Hgb, and Hct) typical of patients with chronic renal failure (ane-

mia of chronic disease). She also has a mild eosinophilia (absolute count: 520; normal range: <432 cells/mm³), although it is not apparent from other signs and symptoms. It is probably not clinically significant unless Julie L. has other evidence of a parasitic infection or allergic reaction.

Julie L.'s CD₄ count is 550 cells/mm³. Treatment should not be changed if her antiretroviral disease (AIDS) is not progressing. If it is progressing, either didanosine or zalcitabine or one of the newer antiretrovirals should replace zidovudine therapy or be added to it.

---

ally IgG or IgA. Other laboratory findings associated with multiple myeloma include Bence Jones proteins in urine, hypercalcemia, increased ESR, and findings consistent with normochromic, normocytic anemia and coagulopathies.

## SUMMARY

In this chapter, the functions and some common disorders of erythrocytes and leukocytes were reviewed. Erythrocytes transport Hgb. Anemias are common disorders involving erythrocytes. Determination of the etiology of the anemia is essential for proper patient therapy. In this regard, use of erythrocyte morphology is helpful.

Anemias can be classified as macrocytic, microcytic, or normochromic, normocytic based on RBC indices. Macrocytic anemias are frequently caused by vitamin B₁₂ or folic acid deficiencies. Serum vitamin B₁₂ and folate concentrations, which are low in these cases, can be useful in the diagnosis of these anemias. The Schilling urinary excretion test can determine the cause of vitamin

B₁₂ deficiency so that appropriate treatment can be instituted.

The most common cause of microcytic anemia is iron deficiency. Serum iron and ferritin concentrations are low, and the TIBC and RDW are usually elevated. In chronic disease anemia, which is normocytic, both serum iron and TIBC are low.

Lastly, normochromic, normocytic anemias can be caused by acute blood loss, hemolysis, or chronic disease. The antiglobulin tests are positive in most immune-mediated hemolytic anemias. The reticulocyte count renders an external view of the activity of RBC production in the bone marrow.

The ESR is a commonly performed but nondiagnostic test. It can be useful in monitoring inflammatory and rheumatic disease activity and the patient's response to therapy. It is of little use in diagnosing or monitoring anemias.

Granulocyte disorders can be qualitative, quantitative, or myeloproliferative. Quantitative disorders can be detected by the WBC count with differential. Quantitative changes can be caused by numerous medications, inflammatory diseases, infections, and neoplastic illnesses. Quantitative disorders of lymphocytes can be caused by radiation exposure, neoplasms, medications, and various infections (e.g., HIV-1 infection and lymphoma).

## REFERENCES

1. Gulati GL, Ashton JK, Hyun BH. Structure and function of the bone marrow and hematopoiesis. *Hematol Oncol Clin North Am.* 1988; 2:495–511.

2. Erslev AJ, Gabuzda TG. The pathophysiology of blood. Philadelphia, PA: W. B. Saunders; 1979:23–112.

3. Gulati GL, Hyun BH. The automated CBC. A current perspective. *Hematol Oncol Clin North Am.* 1994; 8:593–603.

4. Colon-Otero G, Menke D, Hook CC. A practical approach to the differential diagnosis and evaluation of the adult patient with macrocytic anemia. *Med Clin North Am.* 1992; 76:581–97.

5. Hillman RS, Finch CL. Red cell manual. Philadelphia, PA: F. A. Davis; 1974:52–74.

6. Massey AC. Microcytic anemia: differential diagnosis and management of iron deficiency anemia. *Med Clin North Am.* 1992; 76:549–66.

7. Nelson DA, Davey FR. Erythrocytic disorders. In: Henry JB, ed. Clinical diagnosis and management by laboratory methods. Philadelphia, PA: W. B. Saunders; 1984:652–703.

8. Phillips DL, Keeffe EB. Hematologic manifestations of gastrointestinal disease. *Hematol Oncol Clin North Am.* 1987; 1:207–28.

9. Babior BM, Bunn HF. Megaloblastic anemias. In: Braunwald E, Isselbacher KJ, Petersdorf RG, et al., eds. Harrison's principles of internal medicine. New York: McGraw-Hill; 1986:1498–1504.

10. Ravel R. Clinical laboratory medicine: Diagnosis of malabsorption. In: Ravel R, ed. Clinical laboratory medicine: clinical application of laboratory data. Chicago, IL: Year Book Publishers; 1978:294–302.

11. Bunting RW, Bitzer AM, Kennedy RM, et al. Prevalence of intrinsic factor antibodies and vitamin $B_{12}$ malabsorption in older patients admitted to a rehabilitation hospital. *J Am Geriatr Soc.* 1990; 38:743–7.

12. Davidson RJ, Atrah O, Sewell HF. Longitudinal study of circulating gastric antibodies in pernicious anemia. *J Clin Pathol.* 1989; 42:1092–5.

13. Troutman WG. Drug-induced diseases. In: Knoben JE, Anderson PO, eds. Handbook of clinical drug data. Hamilton, IL: Drug Intelligence Publications; 1988:64–77.

14. Lee CL, Henry JB. Immunohematology. In: Henry JB, ed. Clinical diagnosis and management by laboratory methods. Philadelphia, PA: W. B. Saunders; 1984:970–1015.

15. Tabbara IA. Hemolytic anemias. Diagnosis and treatment. *Med Clin North Am.* 1992; 76:649–68.

16. Foerster J. Autoimmune hemolytic anemias. In: Lee GR, Bithell TC, Foerster J, et al., eds. Wintrobe's clinical hematology. Philadelphia, PA: Lea & Febiger; 1993:1171.

17. Cooper RA, Bunn HF. Hemolytic anemias. In: Braunwald E, Isselbacher KJ, Petersdorf RG, et al., eds. Harrison's principles of internal medicine. New York: McGraw-Hill; 1986:1506–18.

18. Blum MD, Graham DJ, McCloskey CA. Temafloxacin syndrome: review of 95 cases. *Clin Infect Dis.* 1994; 18:946–50.

19. Lee GR. The anemia of chronic disorders. In: Lee GR, Bithell TC, Foerster J, et al., eds. Wintrobe's clinical hematology. Philadelphia, PA: Lea & Febiger; 1993:840–51.

20. Nelson DA, Morris MW. Basic methodology. In: Henry JB, ed. Clinical diagnosis and management by laboratory methods. Philadelphia, PA: W. B. Saunders; 1984:578–625.

21. Sox HC, Liang MH. The erythrocyte sedimentation rate: guidelines for rational use. *Ann Intern Med.* 1986; 104:515–23.

22. Wintrobe MW. The diagnostic and therapeutic approach to hematologic problems. In: Lee GR, Bithell TC, Foerster J, et al. Wintrobe's clinical hematology. Philadelphia, PA: Lea & Febiger; 1993:30–1.

23. Krause JR. The automated white blood cell differential. A current perspective. *Hematol Oncol Clin North Am.* 1994; 8:605–16.

24. Erslev AJ, Gabuzda TG. The pathophysiology of blood. Philadelphia, PA: W. B. Saunders; 1979:113–31.

25. Bentley SA. Alternatives to neutrophil band count. *Arch Pathol Lab Med.* 112:883–4.

26. Serafin WE, Austen KF. Mediators of immediate hypersensitivity reactions. *N Engl J Med.* 1987; 317:30–4.

27. Nelson DA, Davey FR. Hematopoiesis. In: Henry JB, ed. Clinical diagnosis and management by laboratory methods. Philadelphia, PA: W. B. Saunders; 1984:626–51.

28. Erslev AJ, Gabuzda TG. The pathophysiology of blood. Philadelphia, PA: W. B. Saunders; 1979:132–56.

29. Ho DD, Pomerantz RJ, Kaplan JC. Pathogenesis of infection with human immunodeficiency virus. *N Engl J Med.* 1987; 317:278–86.

30. Liu PI. Blue book of diagnostic tests. Philadelphia, PA: W. B. Saunders; 1986:61–4.

31. Strausbaugh LJ. Hematologic manifestations of bacterial and fungal infections. *Hematol Oncol Clin North Am.* 1987; 1:185–206.

32. Baranski B, Young N. Hematologic consequences of viral infections. *Hematol Oncol Clin North Am.* 1987; 1:167–83.

33. Weinstein HJ. The acute leukemias. In: Wyngaarden JB, Smith LH Jr, eds. Cecil textbook of medicine. Philadelphia, PA: W. B. Saunders; 1985:986–92.

34. Roitt IM. Essential immunology. Oxford, England: Blackwell Scientific Publications; 1977:21–100.

35. Fischl M. Combination antiretroviral therapy for HIV infection. *Hosp Pract.* 1994; 29:43–8.

## QuickView—RBC Count (Concentration)[a]

| Parameter | Description | Comments |
|---|---|---|
| **Common reference ranges** | | |
| Adults | Males: $4.6–6.2 \times 10^6$ cells/mm$^3$ $4.6–6.2 \times 10^{12}$ cells/L Females: $4.2–5.4 \times 10^6$ cells/mm$^3$ $4.2–5.4 \times 10^{12}$ cells/L | |
| Pediatrics | Birth: $5.0–6.3 \times 10^6$ cells/mm$^3$ 1 year: $3.5–5.0 \times 10^6$ cells/mm$^3$ 8 years: $4.0–5.1 \times 10^6$ cells/mm$^3$ | Ranges for males and females do not significantly differ until after menarche |
| **Critical value** | Sudden decrease >1 and/or symptomatic | Signs and symptoms: weakness, dypsnea, increased heart rate |
| **Natural substance?** | Yes | |
| **Inherent activity?** | Yes | Carrier of oxygen, Hgb, and pH buffer |
| **Location** | | |
| Production | Bone marrow | Mainly vertebrae, ribs, sternum, and pelvis |
| Storage | None | |
| Natural removal (old/damaged cells) | Spleen/reticuloendothelium system | Lifespan of 120 days; heme metabolized to bilirubin |
| **Major causes of . . .** | | |
| High results | Polycythemia vera Secondary polycythemia (SP) | SP caused by chronic obstructive pulmonary disease, cardiac shunting, vigorous exercise, and high altitude |
| Associated signs and symptoms | Related to blood hyperviscosity Signs and symptoms of secondary disease | Headache, tinnitus, venous thrombosis, itching Splenomegaly and ruddy cyanosis |
| Low results | Acute/chronic blood loss Nutritional deficiencies | GI ulcer, surgery, penetrating wounds Iron, folate, or vitamin $B_{12}$ deficiency; malnutrition |
| Associated signs and symptoms | Signs and symptoms of anemia; hemorrhage | Pallor, weakness, dyspnea, increased heart rate, decreased blood pressure |
| **After insult, time to . . .** | | |
| Initial elevation/depression | Weeks to months | Minutes to hours for acute blood loss |
| Peak/nadir values | Months to years/weeks to months | Hours to days for acute blood loss |
| Normalization after treatment | Immediate after phlebotomy/blood 4–8 months after oral nutrient supplementation | After oral iron, folate, vitamin $B_{12}$, and reticulocytes start to rise in 5–7 days, peak in 10–14 days, and then fall to normal; RBCs continue to climb |
| **Drugs often monitored with test** | Anticoagulants, NSAIDs, cytotoxic cancer drugs, iron, folate, vitamin $B_{12}$ | As part of CBC, Hgb and Hct monitored more often |
| **Causes of spurious results** | Hemolytic anemia | Agglutination of red cells decreased |

[a]Except for normal ranges, the above entries also reflect Hgb and Hct.

## QuickView—WBC Count (Concentration)

| Parameter | Description | Comments |
|---|---|---|
| **Common reference ranges** | | |
|    **Adults** | $4.8–10.8 \times 10^3$ cells/mm$^3$ <br> $4.8–10.8 \times 10^9$ cells/L | |
|    **Pediatrics** | Birth: $9.0–30 \times 10^3$ cells/mm$^3$ <br> 14 days: $5.0–20 \times 10^3$ cells/mm$^3$ <br> 1 year: $6.0–18 \times 10^3$ cells/mm$^3$ <br> 4 years: $5.0–15 \times 10^3$ cells/mm$^3$ <br> 8–21 years: $4.5–13 \times 10^3$ cells/mm$^3$ | |
| **Critical value** | $<2.5$ or $>20 \times 10^3$ cells/mm$^3$ | Depends on acuity of change |
| **Natural substance?** | Yes | |
| **Inherent activity?** | Yes | Immune defense: humoral and cellular |
| **Location** | | |
|    **Production** | Bone marrow, lymph nodes, spleen | |
|    **Storage** | Bone marrow, lymph nodes, spleen | |
|    **Natural removal (old/damaged cells)** | Recycled by phagocytes | Lifespan: granulocytes, 12 hr; lymphocytes, 100–300 days |
| **Major causes of . . .** | | |
|    **High results** | Inflammation <br> Infection <br> Leukemia <br> Lymphoma <br> Postmyocardial infarction | Strenuous exercise, corticosteroids, lithium, uremia, posthemorrhage |
|      **Associated signs and symptoms** | Signs and symptoms of cause | |
|    **Low results** | Gram-negative sepsis <br> Aplastic anemia | Vitamin B$_{12}$ or folate deficiency, radiation, cytotoxic drugs, hypersplenism |
|      **Associated signs and symptoms** | Signs and symptoms of cause | Increased risk of infection |
| **After insult, time to . . .** | | |
|    **Initial elevation/depression** | Elevation: hours to days <br> Depression: days to weeks (varies greatly) | |
|    **Peak/nadir values** | Varies greatly; reflects above | |
|    **Normalization after treatment** | Often same as time to onset | Varies greatly |
| **Drugs often monitored with test** | Antibiotics, cytotoxics, chloramphenicol, clozapine | Any drug that is a relatively common cause of neutropenia or agranulocytosis |
| **Causes of spurious results** | No important causes | |

# Chapter 15

# Hematology: Blood Coagulation Tests

*James B. Groce III and Barry L. Carter*

Normal hemostasis results from a complex interaction among the vascular subendothelium, platelets, coagulation factors, and proteins that promote clot degradation as well as inhibitors of these substances. Bleeding can result from acquired deficiencies or physiological disorders of platelets or clotting components. Excessive clotting can result from abnormalities of the vascular endothelium, alterations in blood flow, or deficiencies in clotting inhibitors.[1,2]

Practitioners routinely monitor coagulation tests for patients receiving anticoagulants, thrombolytics, or antiplatelet agents. However, bleeding abnormalities are associated with primary coagulopathies and numerous drugs. Therefore, coagulation tests should be monitored periodically for patients in these situations.

This chapter reviews normal coagulation physiology, common tests used to assess coagulation, and factors (including drugs) that alter coagulation tests.

## OBJECTIVES

Upon completion of this chapter, the reader should be able to

1. Discuss normal platelet physiology and the role of platelets in hemostasis.
2. Describe the coagulation cascade system, including the intrinsic, extrinsic, and common pathways.
3. Discuss normal physiology of coagulation inhibition.
4. Discuss the fibrinolytic system and how it promotes clot degradation.
5. List the laboratory tests used to assess platelets and discuss factors, such as drugs, that may influence their results.
6. List the laboratory tests used to assess coagulation and explain their use in evaluating anticoagulant therapy.
7. Define International Normalized Ratio (INR) and recognize both the advantages and disadvantages of INR determinations.
8. List the laboratory tests used to assess clot degradation and disseminated intravascular coagulation (DIC) and discuss their limitations.
9. Given results of laboratory tests used for evaluating coagulation and anticoagulant therapy in a case description, properly interpret the results and suggest followup action.
10. Briefly discuss the availability and use of bedside testing devices for anticoagulant therapy.

## PHYSIOLOGICAL PROCESS OF HEMOSTASIS

Hemostasis is the process that halts bleeding following vascular injury. Normal hemostasis involves the complex relationship among substances that promote clot formation (platelets and the coagulation cascade), inhibit coagulation, and dissolve the formed clot. Each substance is briefly reviewed.

### Clot Formation

#### Platelets

Platelets are 2–4-$\mu$, disk-shaped structures that are nonnucleated and do not reproduce themselves. Platelets contain mitochondria and glycogen granules that provide energy. Lysosomal granules, nonribosomal endoplasmic reticulum, and contractile actinomycin are found within platelets.

Most platelets are formed in the extravascular spaces of bone marrow from megakaryocytes. The lungs and other tissues can retain megakaryocytes and produce platelets.[3] The megakaryocytes produce 35,000 platelets/$\mu$L of blood per day and up to eight times this amount during stress. Megakaryocyte production and maturation are promoted by the hormone thrombopoietin, which recently was purified and cloned.[4] Two-thirds of the platelets are found in the circulation and one-third in the spleen (in splenectomized patients, however, nearly 100% are in the circulation).

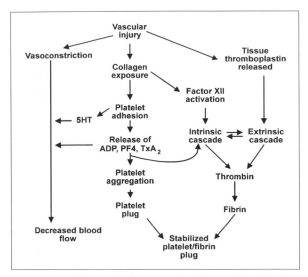

**FIGURE 1.** Relationship between platelets and the clotting cascade in the generation of a stabilized fibrin clot. 5HT = serotonin; ADP = adenosine diphosphate; PF4 = platelet factor 4; TxA₂ = thromboxane A₂.

The average platelet lifespan is 8–12 days, and about 10% turn over each day.[3] Transfused platelets have a shorter lifespan (4–5 days). The size of platelets does not change as they age. Upon aging, platelets are destroyed by the spleen, liver, and bone marrow. Additionally, platelet function is affected by numerous factors:[5]

> ➤ Drugs.
> ➤ Common foods.
> ➤ Vitamins.
> ➤ Spices.
> ➤ Systemic conditions such as chronic renal disease and hematological disorders (e.g., myeloproliferative and lymphoproliferative diseases, dysproteinemias, and the presence of antiplatelet antibodies).

The surface of normal blood vessels does not stimulate platelet adhesion. However, vascular injury is often caused by rheological damage, trauma, or the rupture of plaque from the vessel wall, resulting in endothelial damage. Subendothelial structures, such as collagen, basement membrane, and fibronectin, then become exposed (Figure 1). Collagen is a potent stimulator of platelet adhesion.[6–10] Circulating

von Willebrand factor acts as a binding ligand between the subendothelium and glycoprotein Ib receptors on the platelet surface and contributes to platelet adhesion.

Once adhesion occurs, platelets change shape and activation occurs.[6,8] Collagen, adenosine diphosphate (ADP), thrombin, thromboxane A₂, and prostaglandin H₂ stimulate the change in platelet shape from ovoid disks to spheres with pseudopods.[8] These stimulators cause the platelets to aggregate, change shape, and release their contents, which include ADP, serotonin (5HT), platelet factor 3 (PF3), and platelet factor 4 (PF4). Following platelet adhesion to the subendothelium, platelet aggregation completes the formation of the homeostatic plug. Platelets bind to one another at glycoprotein IIa/IIIb receptor sites, with fibrinogen acting as the primary binding ligand.

ADP and thromboxane A₂ recruit additional platelets, which aggregate to the platelets that are already bound to the subendothelial tissues. In addition to promoting aggregation, thromboxane A₂, 5HT, and other substances are potent vasoconstrictors that limit blood flow to the damaged site. When vascular damage is minimal, the vasoconstriction and platelet aggregation (formation of a platelet plug) may be sufficient to limit bleeding.

However, the platelet plug is not stable and can be dislodged. To form a more permanent fibrin plug, the clotting system must be stimulated. By releasing PF3, platelets initiate the clotting cascade and concentrate clotting factors at the site of the vascular (endothelial) injury.

Prostaglandins play an important role in platelet function. Figure 2 displays a simplified version of the complex arachidonic acid pathways that occur in platelets and

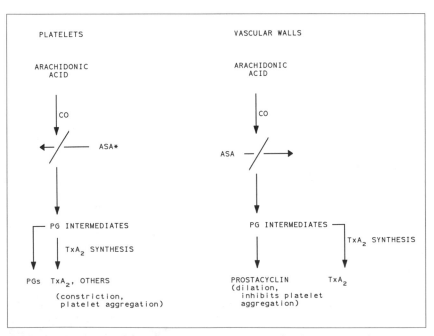

**FIGURE 2.** Formation of thromboxane A₂ (TxA₂), prostaglandins (PGs), and prostacyclin in platelets and vascular endothelial cells. CO = cyclo-oxygenase; ASA* = low-dose, irreversible, inactivation of platelet cyclo-oxygenase; ASA/ = high-dose inactivation of platelet cyclo-oxygenase.

on the vascular endothelium. Thromboxane $A_2$, a potent stimulator of platelet aggregation and vasoconstriction, is formed in platelets. In contrast, prostacyclin ($PGI_2$) (located on the vessel surface) is a potent inhibitor of platelet aggregation and a potent vasodilator that limits excessive platelet aggregation.

Cyclo-oxygenase and $PGI_2$ are clinically important. An aspirin dose of 80 mg/day acetylates and inhibits cyclo-oxygenase in the platelet irreversibly because the platelet cannot regenerate this enzyme.[9,10] Platelets are rendered incapable of forming arachidonic acid and prostaglandins. Therefore, this effect of aspirin lasts for the lifespan of the exposed platelets (up to 12 days).

Vascular endothelial cells also contain cyclo-oxygenase, which converts arachidonic acid to $PGI_2$. Aspirin in high doses inhibits the production of $PGI_2$. However, because the vascular endothelium can regenerate $PGI_2$, aspirin's effect there is much shorter than its effect on platelets. Thus, aspirin's effect at high doses may both inhibit platelet aggregation (platelet effect) and block the aggregation inhibitor $PGI_2$. This phenomenon is the rationale for using aspirin 80–325 mg/day to help prevent myocardial infarction.

In summary, a complex interaction between the platelet and blood vessel wall maintains hemostasis. Once platelet adhesion occurs, the clotting cascade may become activated. After thrombin and fibrin are generated, the platelet plug becomes stabilized with insoluble fibrin at the site of vascular injury.

### Coagulation Cascade

The coagulation cascade (Figure 3) generates fibrin, which forms an insoluble mesh surrounding the platelet plug. Platelets concentrate clotting factors at the site of vascular injury. The platelet surface has receptors that bind and activate factors XII, XI, IX, and X; prekallikrein; and prothrombin.[11]

The coagulation system is called a cascade because each activated factor serves as a catalyst to the next reaction. Therefore, small amounts of activated clotting factors early in the cascade result in very large concentrations of thrombin and fibrin. The nomenclature for the coagulation proteins is shown in Table 1 (next page). The coagulation cascade is typically divided into the intrinsic, extrinsic, and common pathways.

*Intrinsic pathway.* All components for initiation of the intrinsic pathway are present in the blood in their inactive forms. In this pathway, factor XII becomes activated when exposed to collagen in damaged vascular subendothelium. In the presence of prekallikrein and a kininogen, activated factor XII activates factor XI; in the presence of calcium, factor XI activates factor IX. Activated factor IX, in turn, activates factor X in the presence of platelet membrane lipoprotein, factor VIII, and calcium.

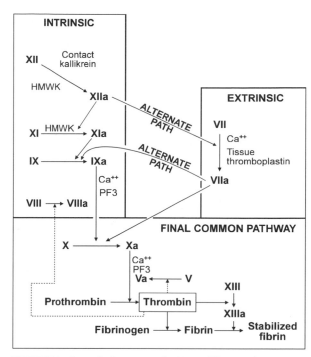

**FIGURE 3.** Coagulation cascade. Dotted lines indicate thrombin's feedback action, which modifies factors V and VIII. HMWK = high molecular weight kininogen. (Reproduced, with permission, from Reference 11.)

*Extrinsic pathway.* The extrinsic pathway is initiated when tissue thromboplastin is released from damaged cells and then activates factor VII in the presence of calcium. Tissue thromboplastin is a complex mixture of substances located in the vascular intima.[11] It activates factor VII and, in the presence of calcium, factor X.

*Common pathway.* Both the intrinsic and extrinsic pathways activate factor X in the final common pathway. Prothrombinase, with a phospholipid (e.g., PF3), is a complex that forms when factors Xa and V, platelet phospholipid, and calcium combine to become an enzyme-like substance.[11] This complex converts prothrombin to thrombin. In addition to the direct effects and feedback mechanisms of thrombin shown in Figure 3, thrombin also stimulates platelet aggregation and activates protein C and the fibrinolytic system. Thrombin cleaves other prothrombin molecules to form additional thrombin. It also cleaves fibrinogen in several steps that eventually result in a stable, insoluble fibrin plug.

## Inhibition of Coagulation

Numerous mechanisms limit coagulation.[12–15] Factors V and VIII are destroyed by protein C, which is activated by negative feedback from high concentrations of thrombin. Thrombin activates protein C by cleaving a heavy chain from the molecule.[15] Normal blood flow also dilutes activated clotting factors and results in their degradation in various tissues (e.g., liver) and by proteases.

**TABLE 1.** International Nomenclature and Corresponding Half-Lives for Hemostatic Proteins[a]

| Coagulation Factor | Names | Half-Life (hr) |
|---|---|---|
| I | Fibrinogen | 90 |
| II | Prothrombin and prethrombin | 60 |
| III | Tissue factor and tissue thromboplastin | |
| IV | Calcium | |
| V | Proaccelerin and accelerator globulin | 12–36 |
| VI | Not assigned | |
| VII | Proconvertin and serum prothrombin conversion accelerator | 4–6 |
| VIII | Antihemophilic factor and platelet co-factor I | 12 |
| IX | Plasma thromboplastin component, Christmas factor, antihemophilic factor B, platelet cofactor II | 24 |
| X | Stuart-Prower factor, Stuart factor, autoprothrombin III | 45–72 |
| XI | Plasmin thromboplastin antecedent and antihemophilic factor C | 48–84 |
| XII | Hageman factor, glass factor, contact factor | 48–52 |
| XIII | Fibrin stabilizing factor and fibrinase | 72–124 |
| | Prekallikrein and Fletcher factor | 35 |
| | High molecular weight kininogen and Fitzgerald factor | 156 |

[a]*Adapted, with permission, from Reference 11.*

bin are also limited to the injury site by protease inhibitors, enhancement of the thrombin–ATIII complex, and binding of thrombin to thrombomodulin. This, in turn, activates protein C to destroy factors V and VIII and also induces the release of tissue plasminogen activator (tPA) from the endothelium. Therefore, thrombin initiates negative feedback mechanisms controlling its own generation.

ATIII, a naturally occurring glycoprotein, inactivates thrombin. Heparin (either natural or exogenous) serves as a cofactor for the reaction between ATIII and serine proteases in the clotting cascade that includes thrombin and activated factors IX–XII (discussed previously).[1,12] Heparin and ATIII combine one to one, and the complex almost instantaneously neutralizes the activated clotting factors and halts the coagulation cascade.

Protein C, a vitamin K-dependent protein, inactivates factors Va and VIIIa in the presence of phospholipid and calcium ions.[11,12,15] Before this reaction can occur, protein C must be activated. Circulating protein S increases the rate at which activated protein C inactivates factor Va. Thrombin binds to thrombomodulin and forms a complex that markedly accelerates the activation of protein C.

However, in areas of low flow or venous stasis, clotting factors may not be readily cleared. Other mechanisms that limit coagulation include natural inhibitors and the fibrinolytic system.

Antithrombin III (ATIII) and proteins C and S are naturally occurring inhibitors of coagulation. These substances are, in part, responsible for preventing uncontrolled coagulation of blood. Most patients who are deficient in these proteins have recurrent thromboembolic events, often at a young age.[1,2,12–17]

The complex mechanisms that limit thrombus formation are shown in Figure 4. Coagulation—thrombus extension—is limited due to resistance of intact endothelium to thrombus formation. Platelet aggregation is prevented by active clearance of vasoactive amines, complexation of thrombin with ATIII, and the explosive thrombin-mediated synthesis and release of the platelet aggregation inhibitor PGI$_2$. The effects of throm-

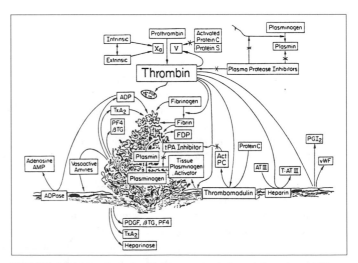

**FIGURE 4.** Mechanisms for limiting coagulation. Adenosine AMP = cyclic adenosine monophosphate; vWF = plasma cofactor VIII/von Willebrand factor; PDGF = platelet-derived growth factor; βTG = β-thromboglobulin; PF4 = platelet factor 4; TxA$_2$ = thromboxane A$_2$. (Reproduced, with permission, from Reference 9.)

Since thrombomodulin is located on the endothelial cell surface, it is not present at the site of vascular injury.[12] However, thrombomodulin at adjacent, noninjured tissue activates protein C and prevents the propagation of the clot onto normal tissues. Activated protein C also increases fibrinolysis. It neutralizes an inhibitor of the naturally occurring fibrinolytic protein, tPA, which results in enhanced conversion of plasminogen to plasmin (Clot Degradation section).[15]

Studies have found that the uncommon complication of skin necrosis may occur when warfarin is started in patients with depressed concentrations of protein C.[2,15] Protein C has a very short half-life (6 hr). Clotting factors IX and X are associated with the antithrombotic effects of warfarin, but their half-lives are 20–30 hr.[1,2] Therefore, initiation of warfarin depresses protein C more rapidly than factors IX and X. This inequity results in a relative hypercoagulable state that may manifest as skin necrosis.

Other thrombin inhibitors include $\alpha_1$-proteinase inhibitor and heparin cofactor II as well as $\alpha_2$-macroglobulin, which inhibits both thrombin and plasmin.[12]

## Clot Degradation

*Fibrinolysis* is the mechanism by which formed thrombi are lysed to prevent excessive clot formation and vascular occlusion. As discussed previously, fibrin is formed in the final common pathway of the clotting cascade. During fibrinolysis, fibrin in a formed clot is broken down. A natural or extrinsic activator of the fibrinolytic system, tPA, is produced by the vascular endothelial cells. Drugs or exogenous activators (e.g., streptokinase, anistreplase, urokinase, and recombinant tPA) also activate fibrinolysis. Various other activators of plasminogen are referred to as intrinsic (e.g., kallikrein). They include activated factor XII, activated protein C, and a plasma protein termed "activator" (Figure 5).

Plasmin is the enzyme that eventually breaks down

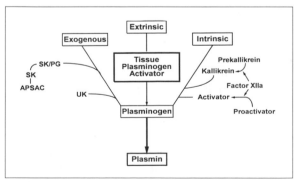

**FIGURE 5.** Exogenous, extrinsic, and intrinsic pathways for activation of plasminogen. APSAC = anistreplase; SK = streptokinase; SK/PG = streptokinase–plasminogen complex; UK = urokinase. (Reproduced, with permission, from Reference 18.)

fibrin into fibrin degradation products (FDPs). However, plasmin must first be formed from plasminogen (Figure 5).[10,18] The fibrin located in the clot binds circulating plasminogen. The release of tPA from the adjacent vascular endothelium is stimulated by thrombin, causing the conversion of plasminogen to plasmin (Figure 4). Plasmin that is released from the clot enters the circulation and is rapidly inactivated by $\alpha_2$-antiplasmin and $\alpha_2$-macroglobulin.[11] Pharmacological inhibitors of fibrinolysis include tranexamic acid, aminocaproic acid, and aprotinin.

## TESTS TO EVALUATE HEMOSTASIS

For the purpose of discussion, bleeding disorders are divided into tests to assess

- ➤ Platelets.
- ➤ Coagulation.
- ➤ Clot degradation.

Tests to assess platelets include platelet count, volume [mean platelet volume (MPV)], function [e.g., bleeding time (BT) and platelet aggregation], and others. Thrombin time (TT), Reptilase, prothrombin time (PT)/INR, activated partial thromboplastin time (aPTT), activated clotting time (ACT), fibrinogen assay, and others are laboratory tests that assess coagulation. Clot degradation is assessed with tests for FDPs and the D-dimer.

In addition, general hematological values such as hemoglobin (Hgb), hematocrit (Hct), red blood cell count, and white blood cell count should be obtained when evaluating blood and coagulation disorders (Chapter 14). Even the results of urinalysis and stool guaic tests may be important. Table 2 is a summary of common tests used to evaluate bleeding disorders and monitor anticoagulant therapy.

### Platelet Tests

#### Platelet Count
*Normal range: 140,000–440,000/μL*

The only test to determine the number (actually, the concentration) of platelets in a blood sample is the platelet count, although various methods are used. Platelet counts can be performed by manual or automated methods. When the platelet count is 50,000–500,000/μL, the automated methods are more accurate. Values outside this range exceed the accuracy of the instrumentation. In such cases, manual counts using phase-contrast microscopy are the most reliable.[19] Hct values below 20 or above 50 also cause a loss of reliability and necessitate manual platelet counts. The coefficient of variation (CV) is 16% for phase-contrast microscopy and may be up to 25% for ordinary light microscopy.

Automated platelet counts can be performed on whole blood or platelet-rich plasma. Most instrumenta-

**TABLE 2.** Summary of Coagulation Tests Done in Hemorrhagic Disorders and Anticoagulant Drug Monitoring[a]

| Disorder or Drug | Platelet Count | BT | PT | aPTT | Comments |
|---|---|---|---|---|---|
| Thrombocytopenic purpura | *Low* | *Prolonged* | WNL | WNL | |
| Glanzmann's thrombasthenia | *WNL* | WNL or prolonged | WNL | *WNL* | *Platelets appear normal* |
| von Willebrand's disease | WNL | *Prolonged* or WNL | WNL | *WNL or prolonged* | |
| Fibrinogen deficiency | WNL | WNL | *Prolonged* | Prolonged | BT prolonged if severe, *fibrinogen levels decreased*, TT prolonged |
| Warfarin therapy | WNL | WNL | *Prolonged* | WNL or prolonged | BT prolonged if overdosed |
| Heparin therapy | WNL | WNL or prolonged | WNL or prolonged | *Prolonged* | Platelet count may decrease[b] |
| Vascular purpura | WNL | WNL | WNL | WNL | |

[a]*Italic type indicates most useful diagnostic or therapeutic tests; WNL = within normal limits.*
[b]*Significant thrombocytopenia may occur as a heparin side effect in 1–5% of patients.*

tion that performs hematological profiles provides platelet counts. Platelets are passed through a tube, generating an electric pulse each time one passes, and each pulse is counted. When the platelet count is 50,000–500,000/µL, the CV may be as low as 4%.[19]

*Thrombocythemia.* An abnormal platelet count can have many causes. Stress or infection is associated with thrombocytosis, an elevation in the platelet count. Additionally, thrombocytosis may be caused by

> Splenectomy.
> Trauma.
> Asphyxiation.
> Rheumatoid arthritis.
> Iron-deficiency anemia.
> Posthemorrhagic anemia.
> Cirrhosis.
> Chronic pancreatitis.
> Tuberculosis.
> Recovery from bone marrow suppression.

Values of 500,000–800,000/µL are not uncommon.

Thrombocythemia refers to an excess of platelets, often greater than 800,000/µL of whole blood. Thrombocythemia may be seen with essential thrombocythemia, polycythemia vera, chronic myelogenous leukemia, or myelosclerosis. In addition to arterial and venous thrombosis, patients with thrombocythemia may have abnormalities in platelet function studies as well as spontaneous bleeding.

*Thrombocytopenia.* The definition of thrombocytopenia

is a platelet count below 150,000/µL. Several diseases, such as thrombotic thrombocytopenic purpura (TTP), idiopathic thrombocytopenic purpura (ITP), disseminated intravascular coagulation (DIC), and hemolytic-uremic syndrome, result in rapid destruction of platelets.[3,10,20] TTP and hemolytic-uremic syndrome have been associated with several drugs, including antineoplastic agents.[21] Diseases such as aplastic anemia, leukemia, and metastatic carcinoma may decrease the production of platelets.

Numerous drugs have been associated with thrombocytopenia (Table 3); however, heparin and antineoplastics are common causes. Thrombocytopenia is also common with radiation therapy. Autoimmune diseases such as ITP result from antibodies to platelets that lead to their destruction. Many drugs associated with thrombocytopenia alter platelets by the formation of antibodies to platelets (e.g., heparin, penicillin, and gold).

Immunoassay techniques can now measure drug-directed platelet antibodies, but these methods are not commonly used to assess drug-induced thrombocytopenia. Other causes of thrombocytopenia include viral infections; pernicious, aplastic, and folate/$B_{12}$-deficiency anemias; complications of pregnancy; massive blood transfusions; exposure to dichlorodiphenyltrichloroethane (DDT); and human immunodeficiency virus (HIV) infections.

When the platelet count falls below 20,000/µL, the patient is at risk of spontaneous bleeding. Therefore, therapy with platelet concentrations is often initiated. Bleeding may occur at higher platelet counts (e.g., 50,000/µL) if trauma occurs.

Heparin has been associated with thrombocytopenia

**TABLE 3.** Partial List of Agents Associated with Thrombocytopenia[a]

| | |
|---|---|
| Aldesleukin | Nalidixic acid |
| Allopurinol | Penicillamine |
| Amphotericin B | Penicillins |
| Amrinone | Pentamidine |
| Antineoplastics | Phenylbutazone |
| Antiviral agents | Phenytoin |
| Azathioprine | Propylthiouracil |
| Carbamazepine | Quinacrine |
| Cephalosporins | Quinidine |
| Chloramphenicol | Quinine |
| Chlorpropamide | Radiation |
| Etretinate | Sulfonamides |
| Gold compounds | Tamoxifen |
| Griseofulvin | Thiazide diuretics |
| $H_2$ antagonists | Tolbutamide |
| Heparin | Trimethoprim |
| Interferons | Trimetrexate |
| Methimazole | Valproic acid |

[a]*Most drugs listed cause an idiosyncratic, drug-induced thrombocytopenia. Exceptions include amrinone, antineoplastics, and possibly amphotericin B, which cause a direct toxic effect that may be dose related.*

in up to 30% of patients who receive the drug.[1,2] Reliable estimates of the incidence are 1–5%. Two types of thrombocytopenia exist:

1. A mild thrombocytopenia occurs within the first 4 days of therapy as the result of a direct effect on platelet sequestration and clumping. Patients remain asymptomatic, and the low count is often transient.

2. A severe thrombocytopenia does not occur until 6–12 days after the start of heparin and rapidly recurs with rechallenge. For about 5 days after the drug is stopped, platelet counts remain low. This form of thrombocytopenia is an immune-mediated phenomenon resulting from platelet aggregation caused by heparin binding to immunoglobulin G (IgG) antibodies. This delayed thrombocytopenia may result in thrombosis, which can cause gangrene, stroke, myocardial infarction, and DIC.

Although much less common, cases of thrombocytopenia associated with low-dose heparin prophylaxis (5000 U every 8–12 hr subcutaneously) have been reported. There may be no difference in the risk of drug-induced thrombocytopenia with heparin derived from either bovine lung or porcine intestine.[22] Recent evidence also suggests that the incidence of heparin-induced thrombocytopenia is lower with a low molecular weight heparin (LMWH) since it binds less to platelets.[23]

In all patients receiving heparin, platelet counts should be monitored at least every 2–3 days. Some experts recommend daily platelet counts for the first 3 weeks. Shorter treatment courses of heparin and warfarin dosed concomitantly on day 1 may eliminate this requirement. If the platelet count falls below 100,000/μL, heparin should be discontinued.

### *Mean Platelet Volume*
*Normal range: 7–11 fL but varies with laboratory*

MPV, the relationship between platelet size and count, is most likely to be used by clinicians in assessing disturbances of platelet production. MPV is useful in distinguishing between hypoproductive and hyperdestructive causes of thrombocytopenia (Figure 6). Despite the widespread availability of platelet indices, many clinicians do not use them in clinical decisionmaking. In the past, this disuse was attributed to difficulties with the laboratory measurement of indices. Laboratory measurement has now overcome methodological problems that once stymied the role of MPV determinations in the diagnosis of pathological thrombopoiesis.[24]

Many laboratories routinely report the MPV as part of the complete blood count (CBC) (Chapter 14), especially if a differential is requested. In general, lower platelet counts are common with higher platelet volumes (i.e.,

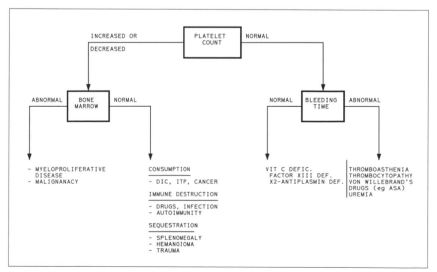

**FIGURE 6.** Assessment of abnormalities of homeostasis based on platelet count, bone marrow exam, and BT.

an inverse relationship exists between the platelet count and the MPV). Although MPV is most valuable in distinguishing hypoproductive from hyperdestructive causes of thrombocytopenia, a definitive diagnosis cannot be made based on MPV alone. In thrombocytopenia, an elevated MPV suggests no problem with platelet production (in fact, production is reflexively increased). Conversely, a normal or low MPV suggests impaired thrombopoiesis.

Determination of MPV requires a blood collection tube containing an anticoagulant. Usually, such tubes contain the anticoagulant ethylenediamine tetraacetic acid (EDTA).[25] Heparin should not be used because it may interfere with the method of measuring platelet volume by causing platelets to clump. Citrated anticoagulants also should not be used because platelets tend to maintain their normal discoid shape within citrated anticoagulant tubes.[26]

Currently, MPV is not widely used but may evolve into a valuable screening test for the disorders listed in Table 4. Interesting data relating MPV to these disorders are now surfacing. For example, the MPV is often elevated at the time of myocardial infarction, although it is not specific enough to be of diagnostic value. Two recent studies[27,28] suggested that a high MPV at 6 months postinfarction is a predictor of reinfarction. Moreover, the magnitude of the changes was similar to established coronary risk factors such as fibrinogen.

MPV is also altered in the presence of other disease states. For example, a fall in MPV is common in patients with enlarged spleens (hypersplenism) due to preferential sequestering of larger platelets within the spleen. Hypersplenism is associated with slightly low MPVs, whereas elevated MPVs are seen with immune thrombocytopenic purpura.[29] In myoproliferative disorders, MPVs usually stay within the reference range.[29] Concomitant increases in large and small platelets account for an overall net zero increase in size. During the third trimester of pregnancy, an increase in platelet size in preeclamptic patients results from increased platelet consumption.[30] Finally, MPV is elevated in hyperthyroid patients and declines to normal as they become euthyroid. Hypothyroid patients often have a high platelet count and a low MPV.[31,32]

The inverse relationship of a high MPV and a low platelet count is demonstrated in other conditions including respiratory disease,[33] renal failure,[34] and sepsis.[35] Unlike most other conditions that demonstrate the inverse relationship of MPV and platelet count, both are low in HIV infection. These decreases suggest an impairment of synthesis and maturation of megakaryocytes as well as enhanced platelet destruction in the bloodstream.[36] Administration of erythropoietin stimulates megakaryocyte cell line production that leads to an increase in MPV. Thrombopoietin probably causes the same effect.[37–40] The relatively recent discovery of thrombopoietin may lead to advances in the treatment of thrombocytopenia caused by deficient production of platelets (e.g., in patients undergoing bone marrow transplantation or cancer chemotherapy).[4]

### Platelet Function

Abnormalities of platelet function may be either *inherited* or *acquired*. Bleeding as a result of an inherited versus acquired abnormality may be difficult to prove. Common bleeding sites in patients with inherited disorders of platelet function include ecchymosis of the skin, epistaxis, gingival bleeding, and menorrhagia.[5] Less common bleeding disorders are gastrointestinal hemorrhage and hematuria. Hematomas and hemarthroses (the predominant sites of bleeding in patients with inherited familial clotting disorders) are rare, except after trauma.[41]

Although the *sites* of bleeding are predictable, the *severity* is not predictable in patients with inherited disorders of platelet function.[41] Unfortunately, the risk of bleeding and bleeding patterns in patients with acquired platelet dysfunction are less predictable and more difficult to distinguish. Because both inherited and acquired etiologies increase the risk of bleeding, patients that have overt bleeding without a clear cause or without an invasive procedure should be suspect for one of these platelet function disorders.[41]

*Bleeding time (normal range: 2–9 min).* Tissue and vascular injury causes platelets to aggregate at the site of injury. Various aspects of platelet function can be determined with BT and more specific aggregation studies. Although BT is an indirect test of primarily platelet aggregation, low platelet counts and other factors can prolong test results. The ability of platelets to perform this function can be assessed with the BT test.

BT is the single best screening test for disorders of platelet function.[42] However, technical difficulty in performing this test may significantly affect results. BT may

**TABLE 4.** Conditions that Alter MPV[a]

| Increase in MPV | Decrease in MPV |
| --- | --- |
| Diabetes | Host chemotherapy |
| Hereditary | Hyperplasia |
| Hyperthyroidism | Hypersplenism |
| Immune thrombocytopenic purpura | Hypothyroidism |
| Myocardial infarction | Marrow aplasia |
| Pregnancy-induced hypertension | Reactive thrombocytosis |
| Renal failure | |
| Respiratory disease | |
| Sepsis | |

[a]*Reference ranges for MPV vary among laboratories and are inversely proportional to the platelet count; however, a common reference range is 7–11 fL in patients with a normal platelet count.*[21]

be prolonged if platelet counts are less than 80,000/μL. In these cases, if platelet function is normal, BT reference ranges should be adjusted[43] (Table 5).

Some platelet disorders can prolong BT. Common hereditary disorders include Glanzmann's thrombasthenia and Bernard-Soulier syndrome. An increased BT or a BT increased out of proportion to platelet count suggests von Willebrand's disease or dysfunctioning platelets. BT also may be useful in determining the success of therapy in patients with prolonged BT due to uremia, von Willebrand's disease, congenital platelet disorders, or severe anemia.[44] Patients may also have congenital platelet function defects related to platelet adhesion, aggregation, or release.[45]

Some patients with acquired disorders of platelet function may have deficient platelet aggregation but a normal BT.[4] Conversely, certain systemic disorders, such as chronic renal failure and DIC,[46,47] have been shown to prolong BT. Lastly, patients with coronary artery disease (CAD) undergoing cardiopulmonary bypass have longer than expected BTs relative to their degree of thrombocytopenia.[48]

Most acquired disorders affecting BT are related to drugs that decrease platelet numbers or reduce platelet function. The most notable drug that affects platelet function is aspirin. After the administration of aspirin, some patients appear to have excessive increases in BT.[49] After the ingestion of 650 mg of aspirin, the average BT in normal patients increases and stays increased for as long as 4–7 days. However, this rise occurs in only 50% of persons taking this dose.[50,51]

Aspirin irreversibly acetylates cyclo-oxygenase (Figure 2). Platelets cannot synthesize new cyclo-oxygenase, and the effect of aspirin persists for the lifespan of the exposed platelets. The prolongation of BT caused by aspirin is somewhat shorter than the platelet lifespan (8–12 days), because platelets formed after aspirin exposure are not affected. In other words, platelets formed after aspirin is no longer present can confer some aggregability before all aspirin-exposed platelets are eliminated. Aspirin's ability to prolong BT is enhanced immediately after alcohol consumption.[52] Heparin may also prolong BT but not by affecting platelet aggregation.[53] Although BT is influenced by some drugs, it is not used to monitor drug therapy.

The increase in BT caused by aspirin may have beneficial effects. Numerous studies examined the use of as-

pirin to prevent either myocardial infarction (e.g., high-risk patients with unstable angina) or reinfarction in patients who have suffered a myocardial infarction.[54] In one arm of the Physicians' Health Study, otherwise healthy male physicians were given either placebo or 325 mg of aspirin every other day.[55] The risk of myocardial infarctions in the aspirin-treated group was so significantly reduced that investigators terminated this arm of the study early. The role of aspirin in the prevention of *recurrent* myocardial infarction is now universally accepted.

The combined use of warfarin and aspirin may be synergistic and superior to either agent alone in prevention of myocardial infarction. Elevations in activated clotting factor VII are associated with risk of ischemic heart disease.[56] This clotting factor's activity is most rapidly and extensively reduced by warfarin. Because of this consideration, investigators have speculated whether warfarin would be of benefit in myocardial infarction prevention.

On theoretical grounds, one could predict that a reduction of thrombin generation by warfarin could cause secondary decreases in thrombin-mediated platelet aggregation. The Coumadin–Aspirin Reinfarction Study is currently examining this possibility in a randomized, double-blind, active-controlled evaluation of 6000 patients to determine both the efficacy and safety of such regimens. Controversy exists about whether 80 mg/day of aspirin is optimal for inhibition of platelet aggregation because higher doses have proven beneficial in patients with cardiovascular disease. In the study, patients are randomized to one of three treatment regimens:

> Warfarin 3 mg plus aspirin 80 mg.
> Aspirin 160 mg.
> Warfarin 1 mg plus aspirin 80 mg.

Upon completion of the study, this vexing medical question may be answered.

Other drugs that may prolong BT are listed in Table 6 (next page). While nonacetylated salicylates do not impair platelet aggregation or affect BT, all other nonsteroidal anti-inflammatory drugs (NSAIDs) reversibly inhibit platelet cyclo-oxygenase and inhibit aggregation as long as the drug remains in the plasma. Therefore, the clinician can estimate the time it takes for BT to normalize after withdrawing these drugs (by knowing their respective half-lives).

*Platelet aggregation.* The ability of platelets to aggregate is measured by preparing a specimen of platelet-rich plasma and warming it to 98.6 °F (37 °C) with constant stirring. This test is performed with an aggregometer that measures light transmission through a sample of platelets in suspension.[19] After a baseline reading is obtained, a platelet-aggregating agonist (e.g., epinephrine, collagen, ADP, or arachidonic acid) is added. As platelets aggregate, more light passes through the sample. The change in optical density can be measured photometrically and recorded as

**TABLE 5.** Prolongation of BT in Thrombocytopenia[a]

| Platelet Count (per μL) | BT (min) |
| --- | --- |
| 80,000 | ~10 |
| 40,000 | ~20 |
| <10,000 | >30 |

[a]*Adapted, with permission, from Reference 43.*

**TABLE 6.** Medications and Drug Classes that May Cause Abnormalities of Platelet Function[a]

| Medication | Abnormality | |
| --- | --- | --- |
| | Abnormal BT | Abnormal Platelet Aggregation |
| Aspirin | ✓ | ✓ |
| Anticoagulants | ✓ | ✓ |
| Beta-blocking agents | | ✓ |
| Calcium channel blockers | ✓ | ✓ |
| Cephalosporins | ✓ | ✓ |
| Chemotherapeutic agents | ✓ | ✓ |
| Clofibrate | | ✓ |
| Dextran | ✓ | ✓ |
| Dipyridamole[b] | | |
| Ethanol | ✓ | ✓ |
| Nitrofurantoin | ✓ | ✓ |
| Nitroglycerin | ✓ | ✓ |
| Nonsteroidal anti-inflammatory agents | ✓ | ✓ |
| Phenothiazines | | ✓ |
| Quinidine | ✓ | |
| Thrombolytic agents | ✓ | |
| Ticlopidine | ✓ | ✓ |

[a]Adapted from Reference 5.
[b]This medication has not been demonstrated to cause abnormal platelet function, but it has been used extensively as an antithrombotic agent.

an aggregation curve, which is then printed on a plotter.

Interpretation of platelet aggregation tests involves a comparison of the patient's curves with the corresponding curves of a normal control. Minor differences in the slope (rate) and extent (plateau) of aggregation of as much as 25% are not significant.[57] To eliminate the optical problems of turbidity with lipemia plasma, the patient and the normal control should be fasting. Patients should not take aspirin or NSAIDs because they may interfere with test results.

Lumiaggregometry measures platelet aggregation, but it also measures the platelet secretion reaction. This measurement simplifies the diagnosis of platelet dysfunction.[19] The lumiaggregometer measures light transmission through platelets and the emission luminescence generated by adenosine triphosphate during the platelet release reaction.

The shape of the aggregation curve depends on the agonist(s) used and the type of platelet abnormality. By examining the pattern of aggregation, the shape of the

curve, and the platelet release reaction, the laboratory can detect several functional platelet disorders—either inherited or acquired. A decrease in platelet aggregation may be seen in thrombasthenia, Wiskott-Aldrich syndrome, ITP, and uremia[58] (Figure 6).

The platelet retention (adhesion) test was once thought to measure the adhesion reaction. However, the current method of passing blood through a column of glass beads actually measures both the adhesion and aggregation reactions.[19] This test adds little information to the aggregation tests described previously. As blood passes through the column, normal platelets adhere to the glass surface. The platelet count is measured before and after passage, and the percent retention is calculated. Normal platelet retention is 31–83%. Von Willebrand's disease and Glanzmann's thrombasthenia may cause diminished platelet retention along with prolongation of some coagulation tests (Table 2).

### Other Platelet Tests

The measurement of platelet-specific substances, such as PF4 and ß-thromboglobulin, can now be performed by radioimmunoassay or enzyme immunoassay.[19] High concentrations of these substances may be observed with CAD, acute myocardial infarction (AMI), and thrombosis, where platelet lifespan is reduced. Since numerous drugs can potentially cause thrombocytopenia, detection of antibodies directed by specific drugs against platelets may help to determine the culprit.

Platelet survival can be measured by injecting radioisotopes that label the platelets. Serial samples can then determine platelet survival, which is normally 8–12 days.

## Coagulation Tests

Careful blood collection and laboratory quality control are critical for reliable coagulation test results. Blood is collected in syringes or vacuum tubes that contain heparin, EDTA, or sodium citrate. Because heparin and EDTA interfere with several clotting factors, with few exceptions, only sodium citrate is used for coagulation and platelet tests. Factors that promote clotting and interfere with coagulation studies include[59]

➢ Tissue trauma (searching for a vein).
➢ Prolonged use of tourniquet.
➢ Small-bore needles.
➢ Vacuum tubes.

Ideally, blood should be collected through a butterfly needle with a syringe and then transferred to the appropriate blue-top glass tube containing an anticoagulant substance. This method eliminates the activation of platelets due to excessive turbulence caused by vacuum tubes.

The maximum time before a sample must be centrifuged and the temperature it must be stored at are critical and depend on the type of test being performed. Errors in coagulation can be large unless quality assurance is strict with collection, reagents, controls, and equipment.

Coagulation tests can assess bleeding or clotting disorders. This discussion focuses on commonly used tests but does not cover outdated ones such as whole blood clotting time. In Minicase 1 (page 333), the common screening tests are discussed. Other sophisticated tests that might be used to assess a bleeding disorder include assays for specific clotting factors. (Coagulation tests related to liver disease are discussed in Chapter 11.)

Coagulation studies may be used to assess certain bleeding disorders; the hemophilias are the most common. Hemophilia A (factor VIII deficiency) or hemophilia B (factor IX deficiency) occurs in one out of every 5000 males.[60] These deficiencies, inherited sex-linked recessive traits, primarily affect males and cause over 90% of hemophilia cases. Other rare bleeding disorders include von Willebrand's disease and deficiencies in fibrinogen or factors II, V, VII, X, XI, XIII, and/or a combination of these factors.

Patients with thrombotic disorders may have their hypercoagulability evaluated with specific assays for[1,2,12]

> ➤ ATIII.[13]
> ➤ Protein C.[15,17]
> ➤ Protein S.[14,16]

Normal reference ranges for these three tests are often reported as a percent of normal activity. For ATIII, the normal activity level is 70–145%. For proteins C and S, normal activity levels are 58–201 and 83–167%, respectively. Protein C activity level is performed utilizing a chromogenic assay. Protein S activity level is performed via a clot-based assay. As alluded to previously, deficiencies result in frequent, recurrent thromboembolic events in most patients with these disorders. Because these deficiencies are rare, their respective assays are not discussed here.

### Thrombin Time
*Normal range: 25–35 sec but varies*

Also known as thrombin clotting time, this test uses human or bovine thrombin mixed with the patient's plasma. TT measures the time required for a plasma sample to clot after the addition of thrombin and is compared to that of a normal plasma control. Deficiencies in both the intrinsic and extrinsic systems do not affect TT. TT assesses only the final phase of the common pathway or essentially the ability to convert fibrinogen to a fibrin clot.

Prolongation of TT (e.g., ≥3 sec beyond the control value) may be caused by afibrinogenemia, dysfibrinogenemia, heparin, or the presence of FDPs that are produced with thrombolytic therapy (e.g., streptokinase). In thrombolytic therapy, laboratory monitoring may not prevent bleeding or ensure thrombolysis. However, some clinicians recommend measuring TT, fibrinogen, plasminogen activation, or FDPs to document that a "lytic state" has been achieved. Typically, TT is greater than 120 sec 4–6 hr after "adequate" thrombolytic therapy.

### Reptilase Test
*Normal range: 18–22 sec*

Additional tests can be performed to rule out the presence of circulating coagulation inhibitors such as heparin.[61] The Reptilase test is a variation of the TT test in which venom from the pit viper is used instead of thrombin. Both thrombin and the venom convert fibrinogen to fibrin. FDPs inhibit conversion by Reptilase, but heparin does not. Therefore, Reptilase time is used to evaluate fibrinogen status in heparinized patients. If heparin is the only cause of a prolonged TT, Reptilase time will be normal.

### Prothrombin Time/International Normalized Ratio
*Normal range for PT: 10–13 sec but varies*
*Normal range for INR: varies*

The PT, also called protime, test has an interesting history that has led to a great deal of confusion.[62,63] Much of this confusion resulted from the use of different reagents with different sensitivities. This longstanding confusion contributed to the revision of the therapeutic range for anticoagulant therapy in the United States in the mid-1980s.[1,2,63,64]

*Assay performance and standardization.* PT measures deficiencies in prothrombin (factor II) and factors VII, IX, and X. This test is conducted by adding a tissue thromboplastin reagent and calcium chloride to the patient's plasma. This method is Quick's test, first described in 1935.[65] The time it takes for the blood to clot is the PT, which is measured by automated instrumentation. When rabbit brain thromboplastin is used, the normal value is 10–12 sec; the reference range depends on the specific reagent and instrumentation used.

The most commonly used thromboplastin in North America is derived from rabbit brain, which is less sensitive than human brain thromboplastin. Furthermore, the lack of standardization among rabbit thromboplastins from different manufacturers and different lots may markedly affect sensitivity and precision.[66-68]

The accuracy of PT determinations is also affected when different instrumentation is used. Therefore, a PT of 18 sec from one laboratory may not represent the same degree of anticoagulation as a PT of 18 sec from another laboratory (Table 7). In a study conducted by the New York State Department of Health, blood samples were mailed to 340 laboratories. The CVs ranged from 5 to 6% with mechanical methods and from 7 to 11% with manual methods.[68]

In recent years, attempts have been made to standardize the PT. Two international committees proposed the use of the INR. The INR is the PT ratio that would result if the World Health Organization (WHO) international reference thromboplastin were used to test the sample.[2,64] To convert a PT ratio to an INR, the sensitivity of the thromboplastin must be known. The sensitivity should be expressed as an International Sensitivity Index (ISI). The ISI is a value assigned to each lot of commercially prepared thromboplastin reagent. When used as an exponent to the observed PT ratio (a patient's PT in seconds divided by the mean normal PT obtained with a specific reagent/instrument combination; Table 7), the ISI reliably produces the same result that would have been obtained if the primary International Reference Preparation of WHO had been used as the reagent.[69]

The accuracy of manufacturers' ISI calibrations over the last few years has been questioned.[70] The calibration of the ISI value may impact the accuracy of normalizing PTs. In addition, consideration must be given to the variability in PTs caused by differing lab instrumentation when paired to specific reagents. Because of this problem, thromboplastin manufacturers should describe in their product literature the variability introduced by use of their reagent with different instruments for PT determinations.[71] ISI values for North American rabbit brain thromboplastin have been variously reported as 2.2–2.6[67] and 1.8–2.8.[72] For bovine brain, 1.0–1.1 has been reported.[72]

Additional inaccuracy in normalizing PTs occurs with thromboplastins that have especially high ISI values (>2.0). An Australian study urged caution when interpreting INRs obtained with ISI values greater than 2.0, citing these high values to be the likely cause of bleeding be-cause the patient may not be detected as overanticoagu-lated.[73] Finally, if heparin-sensitive thromboplastin reagents are used, falsely elevated PT/INR values may result. These inaccurate values might suggest sufficient anticoagulation and result in the premature discontinuation of heparin. This additional variability in the response of some thromboplastins introduced by concomitant heparin therapy was just elucidated.[74] In the United States, several manufacturers currently sell thromboplastins with ISI values greater than 2.5.[72,75,76] Standard curves have been devised to convert common reagents (e.g., Dade, Simplastin, and Ortho values) into INRs.[75]

*Monitoring warfarin therapy.* The PT/INR is used to monitor warfarin therapy. Laboratory monitoring of warfarin therapy is performed by measuring the PT. Because commercially available PT reagents vary markedly in their responsiveness, a standardized reporting system became necessary. Standardization is achieved by converting the PT ratio with any local thromboplastin into the INR (Table 7). When warfarin therapy is monitored, INR is used more often to correct for PT ratios obtained with thromboplastin reagents with varying degrees of responsiveness.

Current American College of Chest Physicians' and National Heart, Lung and Blood Institute guidelines recommend an INR of 2.0–3.0 for all indications (including recurrent systemic embolism), except mechanical prosthetic heart valves (an INR of 2.5–3.5 is recommended).[2,64] The Fourth American College of Chest Physicians' Conference consensus report, the most comprehensive guide for the clinical management of patients requiring antithrombotic therapy, recommended that all laboratories convert to the INR system of reporting. This document cited the reporting of a PT ratio and its corresponding INR as potentially dangerous.[77,78]

Despite this recommendation, a majority of laboratories still report PT ratios or, worse still, PT percentages or PT in seconds.[72] Therefore, clinicians continue to use

**TABLE 7.** Variability in International Sensitivity Index (ISI) Thromboplastin Reagents Using Blood from Single Patient

| Thromboplastin | Patient's PT (sec) | Mean Normal (sec) | PT Ratio[a] | ISI | INR[b] |
|---|---|---|---|---|---|
| A | 16 | 12 | 1.3 | 3.2 | 2.6 |
| B | 18 | 12 | 1.5 | 2.4 | 2.6 |
| C | 21 | 13 | 1.6 | 2.0 | 2.6 |
| D | 24 | 11 | 2.2 | 1.2 | 2.6 |
| E | 38 | 14.5 | 2.6 | 1.0 | 2.6 |

[a]$PT\ ratio = \left[ \dfrac{patient's\ PT\ (sec)}{mean\ normal\ PT\ (sec)} \right]$

[b]$INR = (PT\ ratio)^{ISI}$

Example: $\left[ \dfrac{24\ sec}{11\ sec} \right]^{1.2} = 2.58 \approx 2.6$

## Minicase 1

Harry C., a 36-year-old male, was hospitalized with a longstanding history of alcohol abuse. Physical examination revealed a cachectic-appearing male with spider-hemangiomas, petechial hemorrhages, and asterixis. The patient was taking cimetidine and phenytoin. He denied taking over-the-counter medications.

The following laboratory parameters were determined for Harry C:

| Laboratory Study | Normal Results | Patient Results |
|---|---|---|
| PT | 10–13 sec | 14.8 sec |
| INR | – | 1.49 |
| aPTT | 21–45 sec | 54 sec |
| CBC | | |
| Hgb | 14–18 g/dL | 11 g/dL |
| Hct | 42–52% | 33% |
| Platelet count | 140,000–440,000/μL | 87,000/μL |
| MPV | 7–11 fL | 19 fL |
| Aspartate aminotransferase (AST) | 8–42 IU/L | 85 IU/L |
| Alanine aminotransferase (ALT) | 3–30 IU/L | 25 IU/L |
| Albumin | 3.5–5 g/dL | 1.4 g/dL |

*What specific test(s) may be performed to assess the pertinent patient findings from the physical examination? How might these tests relate to normal hemostasis?*

**Discussion:** Specific studies for bleeding disorders include the PT/INR and aPTT; they should be used as a preliminary screening for Harry C. His elevations above baseline are consistent with coagulopathies common in patients who abuse ethanol. This increase occurs because clotting factors that affect these tests are manufactured in the liver.

Platelet count determination and general hematologic values (Hgb and Hct) are consistent with physical examination findings (petechial hemorrhages), revealing the patient to be thrombocytopenic and anemic. As expected, the lowered platelet count and higher platelet volume demonstrate the inverse relationship that typically exists when thrombocytopenia occurs (MPV section). Liver func-

tion tests (LFTs) would further substantiate the suspected etiology of the patient's petechial hemorrhages. The typical AST/ALT "split" (i.e., a doubling of the AST relative to ALT) is consistent with the patient's history of alcohol abuse.

These findings suggest liver impairment and, when paired with Harry C.'s albumin, indicate the possibility of clotting abnormalities (demonstrated objectively by his prolonged PT and aPTT). Table 2 summarizes common tests to evaluate bleeding disorders and monitor anticoagulant therapy.

With this patient, history is important. Cimetidine and phenytoin have been associated with thrombocytopenia, which could also account for petechial hemorrhages. Harry C. denies using aspirin, but many patients unknowingly ingest it in over-the-counter products such as brand-name aspirin and cold preparations.

PT ratio values. This situation is unfortunate since variability among reagents and labs still exists.[68]

Heparin may also prolong PT, especially in higher doses.[79–81] Patients who have significant prolongation of their aPTT values (>150 sec) are likely to have their PTs prolonged an average of 2.5 sec. When heparin dosage is therapeutic, minimal prolongation of the PT should be expected (1.2–1.8 sec).[80] These "crossover" effects may have to be considered frequently because oral and parenteral anticoagulants are usually given concomitantly for several days. However, this influence of heparin on PT is infrequently of clinical significance when the heparin is dosed to maintain an aPTT between 1.5 and 2.5 times the patient's control value. Numerous drugs, disease states, and other factors prolong PTs—in patients receiving warfarin—by various mechanisms of action (Table 8, next page).

Minicase 1 (above) presents each test of blood coagulation that is already described and other tests that follow.

### Activated Partial Thromboplastin Time
*Normal range: 21–45 sec but varies*

The aPTT measures the intrinsic clotting system (factors VIII, IX, XI, and XII) as well as factors in the final common pathway (factors II, V, and X). It is determined by adding partial thromboplastin (rabbit brain phospholipid that mimics platelet phospholipid), calcium chloride, and a particulate activator to the patient's plasma.[61] This activator substance simulates a surface on which contact activation can occur. The activator can be kaolin, diatomaceous earth, silica, or elegiac acid. The typical control range is 35–45 sec, but it may be 26–38 sec in some laboratories.

The sensitivity as well as the precision of the aPTT test depends on the reagents and instrumentation.[68,82–84] Various multicenter surveys of laboratories have found CVs from 5 to 17%.[68,84] The use of the ratio of the patient's aPTT to the control value may reduce the CV.[68] The issue of the aPTT control value is the same as for the PT

**TABLE 8.** Factors Altering Pharmacokinetics and Pharmacodynamics of Warfarin[a]

| Gut | Plasma | Liver | Hemostatic Plug |
|---|---|---|---|
| **Anticoagulant effect potentiated**<br>Low vitamin K intake<br>Reduced vitamin K absorption in fat malabsorption<br><br>**Anticoagulant effect counteracted**<br>Increased vitamin K intake<br>Reduced absorption of warfarin by cholestyramine | **Anticoagulant effect unchanged**<br>Displacement of warfarin from albumin binding does not influence anticoagulant effect of warfarin | **Anticoagulant effect potentiated**<br>Drugs<br>  Amiodarone<br>  Anabolic steroids<br>  Cimetidine<br>  Clofibrate<br>  Disulfiram<br>  Erythromycin<br>  Fluconazole<br>  Isoniazid<br>  Ketoconazole<br>  Metronidazole<br>  Omeprazole<br>  Oral fluoroquinolones<br>  Phenylbutazone<br>  Phenytoin<br>  Piroxicam<br>  Quinidine<br>  Sulfinpyrazone<br>  Tamoxifen<br>  Thyroxine<br>  Trimethoprim–sulfamethoxazole<br>  Vitamin E (mega dose)<br>Liver disease<br>Hypermetabolic states<br>  Pyrexia<br>  Thyrotoxicosis<br><br>**Anticoagulant effect counteracted**<br>Drugs<br>  Barbiturates<br>  Carbamazepine<br>  Griseofulvin<br>  Penicillin<br>  Rifampin<br>Alcohol | **Impaired hemostatic plug formation**<br><br>**Impaired coagulation**<br>Reduced vitamin K dependent<br><br>**Coagulation factors**<br><br>**Reduction in concentration of other coagulation factors**<br><br>**Other anticoagulants:**<br>Heparin and ancrod<br><br>**Impaired platelet function**<br>Thrombocytopenia<br>Aspirin<br>Other NSAIDs<br><br>**Ticlopidine**<br><br>**Moxalactam**<br><br>**Carbenicillin and high doses of other penicillins** |

*[a]Adapted from Reference 78.*

control. Some clinicians have argued that a ratio of the patient's aPTT to the patient's own baseline may be more appropriate, but this issue is unresolved.[1] As with PT reagents, aPTT reagents lack standardization among manufacturers and between lots produced by the same manufacturer. This inter- and intrapatient variability in aPTT results makes interinstitutional comparisons very difficult.

In addition to detecting clotting factor deficiencies, aPTT monitors heparin therapy. The current recommendation for the therapeutic range of heparin is an aPTT ratio of 1.5–2.5 times control. Given the inter- and intrapatient variability that can result from aPTT reagents, alternative means of monitoring heparin therapy are being scrutinized. This 1.5–2.5 aPTT ratio corresponds to[85–87]

> A whole blood heparin concentration of 0.2–0.4 U/mL by assay using the protamine titration method.

> A plasma heparin concentration of 0.35–0.7 U/mL by assay using the inhibition of factor Xa.

Heparin should be given by continuous intravenous (IV) infusion using an individualized, weight-based dosing approach. Various methods may be used.[85–92] Most methods rely on a weight-based approach, typically 15–25 U/kg of body weight per hour. To achieve an immediate anticoagulant effect, an initial heparin bolus (70–100 U/kg) is administered. Coagulation tests (e.g., aPTT) should be drawn 6 hr after continuous IV heparin is begun and after each subsequent dosage adjustment, since this interval approximates four half-lives of heparin (the time to achieve steady-state pharmacokinetics).[90]

Some authors advocate serial aPTT determinations during the initial 24 hr of heparinization.[91] The latest study using serial aPTT determinations is called GUSTO-III. GUSTO-III is comparing the safety and efficacy of

| GUSTO III Heparin Infusion Adjustment Nomogram | | | | |
|---|---|---|---|---|
| aPTT (sec) | Heparin Bolus (units) | Stop Drip (min) | Rate Change (cc / hour) | Repeat aPTT |
| < 40 | 3,000 | 0 | +2 (↑100 U/hr) | 6 hours |
| 40 - 49 | 0 | 0 | +1 (↑ 50 U/hr) | 6 hours |
| 50 - 75 | 0 | 0 | 0 (no change) | Next a.m. |
| 76 - 85 | 0 | 0 | -1 (↓ 50 U/hr) | Next a.m. |
| 86 - 100 | 0 | 30 | -2 (↓ 100 U/hr) | 6 hours |
| 101 - 150 | 0 | 60 | -3 (↓ 150 U/hr) | 6 hours |
| > 150 | 0 | 60 | -6 (↓ 300 U/hr) | 6 hours |

**FIGURE 7.** GUSTO-III trial heparin adjustment nomogram for heparin dilution of 50 U/mL and standard laboratory reagents with a mean control aPTT of 26–36 sec. The infusion rate may be adjusted *only* upward in response to the 6-hr post-thrombolytic aPTT unless overt bleeding is seen or the aPTT is greater than 150.

reteplase (a new plasminogen activator thrombolytic) with alteplase in patients with AMI. An aPTT is drawn before heparin; at 6, 12, and 24 hr after heparin is started; and then daily. Heparin is given in both study groups and is adjusted with a nomogram (Figure 7). A similar nomogram was used in earlier trials (GUSTO-I, GUSTO-IIa, and TIMI-9A), but the target aPTT range has been lowered from approximately 60–85 sec to 50–75 sec based on data of the earlier studies.[93-95]

Because use of a nomogram allows quick fine tuning of anticoagulation by nurses without continuous physician input, many hospitals have adopted one of the GUSTO nomograms as their standard protocol for dosing heparin in patients with AMI. Some hospitals use the nomogram in patients with noncoronary thrombosis (e.g., deep veinous thrombosis and pulmonary embolism), although its efficacy and safety have not been well studied in these disorders. The initial heparin infusion rate has traditionally been 20 mL/hr (1000 U/hr) using a heparin concentration of 50 U/mL; however, the GUSTO-III trial uses a starting dose of 800 U/hr (1000 U/hr in patients ≥80 kg).

Subcutaneous doses of heparin, usually 5000 U every 8 hr or 7500 U every 12 hr, have been used for prophylaxis against thromboembolic disease after total hip replacement surgery and in acute spinal cord injury patients.[92] The dosage of subcutaneous heparin in this regimen is sometimes adjusted to keep the aPTT in the upper normal range (31–36 sec) at the midpoint of the dosing interval. However, some clinicians do not adjust subcutaneous heparin requirements with an aPTT value.

aPTT determinations obtained earlier than 6 hr, while not at steady state, may be combined with heparin concentrations for dosage individualization using non-steady-state concentrations. This approach has been demonstrated to reduce the incidence of subtherapeutic aPTT ratios significantly during the first 24 hr of therapy.[85,96]

This finding is important because the recurrence rate of thromboembolic disease increased when aPTT values were not maintained above 1.5 times the patient's baseline aPTT during the first 24 hr of treatment.[97,98]

*Warfarin effect on aPTT.* Although warfarin also elevates the aPTT, aPTT is not used to monitor warfarin therapy. Hauser and Rozek[99] found a strong correlation between the increase in PT and a corresponding increase in aPTT with warfarin therapy. With an average PT ratio of 1.8, aPTT was 1.9 times the aPTT baseline (55 versus 31 sec). Therefore, if warfarin is started in a patient receiving heparin, the clinician should expect some elevation in aPTT.

Heparin concentration measurements may provide a target plasma therapeutic range, especially in unusual coagulation situations such as pregnancy (where the reliability of clotting studies is questionable).[100] Patients may have therapeutic heparin concentrations measured by whole blood protamine sulfate titration or by the plasma anti-Xa heparin assay. However, they may have aPTTs not significantly prolonged above baseline. This difference has been referred to as a dissociation between the aPTT and the heparin concentration.[101] Many of these patients have very short pretreatment aPTT determinations.

Current recommendations suggest that such patients be managed by monitoring their heparin concentrations using a heparin assay to avoid unnecessary dosage escalation without compromising efficacy.[101,102] These patients, referred to as "pseudo-heparin resistant," may be identified as having a poor aPTT response (but an adequate heparin concentration >0.3 U/mL via plasma anti-Xa assay) despite high doses of heparin (>50,000 U/24 hr; usual dose is 20,000–30,000 U/24 hr) (Minicase 2, next page).[102] When higher doses of heparin (>1500 U/hr) are required to maintain therapeutic aPTT values, high concentrations of heparin-binding protein, thrombocytosis, or ATIII deficiency may exist.[101]

Heparin alone has minimal anticoagulant effects; when it is combined with ATIII (normal range: 70–145%), the inhibitory action of ATIII on coagulation enzymes results in the inhibition of thrombus propagation. Patients who are ATIII deficient (<50%) may be difficult to anticoagulate, as seen with DIC (Minicase 3, next page). The DIC syndrome is associated not only with obvious hemorrhage but also with occult diffuse thrombosis.

Another use for heparin concentrations is to demonstrate both efficacy and safety with LMWH. For prophylaxis against deep vein thrombosis following hip or

## ✎ Minicase 2

Brian M., a 36-year-old male with a history of deep vein thrombosis, presented to the emergency department with signs and symptoms of the same condition. A routine heparin regimen was started. The patient had the following laboratory determinations performed 6 hr after initiation of heparin:

| Laboratory Study | Normal Results | Pretreatment Patient Results | Postheparin Patient Results |
|---|---|---|---|
| PT | 10–13 sec | 11.1 sec | 12.3 sec |
| INR | varies | 0.98 | 1.18 |
| aPTT | 21–45 sec | 19 sec | 23 sec |
| ATIII | 70–145% | 57% | 50% |

*What might account for this patient's postheparin elevation in PT? Why was the aPTT not prolonged? What is the role of AIIII here?*

**Discussion:** Brian M. was started on a continuous IV heparin infusion with plans to convert to long-term warfarin, per the institution's protocol. Subsequent postheparin laboratory determinations revealed a hypercoagulable state consistent with thromboembolic disease. Circulating procoagulants account for the patient's low pretreatment aPTT. ATIII—the cofactor with which heparin binds to exert its anticoagulant effect—is depressed, making the patient hypercoagulable. Subsequent to the initiation of heparin, the ATIII concentration declined further. This drop reflected the binding of ATIII to heparin.

Despite a normal dosing protocol for heparin, Brian M.'s initial aPTT value (obtained 6 hr after the loading dose and continuous maintenance infusion of heparin) remained low. One might be suspicious of pseudo-heparin resistance or dissociation of the aPTT responsiveness after adequate treatment with heparin. To assess the likelihood of this situation, a heparin concentration measurement could be obtained (discussed later) to demonstrate adequate heparinization despite a subtherapeutic aPTT determination.

Prior to initiation of concomitant warfarin therapy, Brian M.'s PT increased slightly to 12.3 sec. Minimal prolongation of the PT may be expected from heparin's influence. This degree of elevation is consistent with this observation. The patient's PT/INR should be followed, with the desired endpoint of warfarin therapy being an INR of 2–3.

## ✎ Minicase 3

Teresa G., a 36-year-old female in her third trimester of pregnancy, was hospitalized with clinical suspicion of DIC because of acute onset of respiratory failure, circulatory collapse, and shock. The following laboratory values for Teresa G. were obtained:

| Laboratory Study | Normal Results | Patient Results |
|---|---|---|
| PT | 10–13 sec | 16 sec |
| aPTT | 21–45 sec | 59 sec |
| TT | 25–35 sec | 36 sec |
| CBC | | |
| Hgb | 12–16 g/dL | 9.8 g/dL |
| Hct | 37–47% | 27.7% |
| Platelet count | 140,000–440,000/µL | 64,000/µL |
| MPV | 7–11 fL | 17 fL |
| FDP (latex) | 2–7 µg/mL | 120 µg/mL |
| ATIII | 70–145% | 57% |
| D-dimer | <200 ng/mL | 2040 ng/mL |

*What laboratory tests are used to determine if a patient is experiencing DIC? What are the expected laboratory results for these tests?*

**Discussion:** Teresa G.'s PT and aPTT are prolonged. Laboratory findings of DIC may be highly variable, complex, and difficult to interpret. Both PT and aPTT should be prolonged but this may not occur.[107] Because of this consideration, the usefulness of both PT and aPTT determinations may be unreliable. TT is prolonged as expected. The platelet count is typically and dramatically decreased. The patient's MPV is inversely related to her decreased platelet count as expected, suggesting a hyperdestructive phenomenon versus a hypoproliferative state. FDPs are elevated, but this rise is not solely pathognomonic for DIC. ATIII determination reveals a considerable decrease consistent with DIC. Decreased ATIII is useful and reliable for diagnosis of DIC in the absence of D-dimer testing ability. The role of ATIII concentrate (human ATIII, Thrombate III) replacement therapy in congenital ATIII deficiency is well established. The role of the concentrate in acquired ATIII deficiencies by DIC is currently being investigated.

knee replacement surgery, enoxaparin (a LMWH) may be used. No monitoring is necessary since neither PT nor aPTT times are significantly prolonged at recommended doses of enoxaparin.[103] However, both efficacy and safety can be demonstrated by performing a heparin level (if necessary). A therapeutically effective serum concentration range is approximately 0.2–0.4 plasma anti-Xa U/mL at prophylactic doses.[104]

Recently, a modified version of the aPTT, the Heptest, was studied. This test measures several clotting factors, but it is specific for anti-Xa activity.[105] The role of this test has not yet been determined for monitoring heparin therapy.

*Bleeding risk and test results.* The major determinants of oral anticoagulant-induced bleeding are the

> ➤ Intensity of the anticoagulant effect.
> ➤ Underlying patient characteristics.
> ➤ Use of drugs that interfere with hemostasis (Tables 3 and 6).
> ➤ Length of therapy.

In terms of treatment decisionmaking for anticoagulant therapy, bleeding risk cannot be considered alone. The potential decrease in thrombosis must be balanced against the potential increased bleeding risk.[106]

The risk of bleeding associated with continuous IV heparin in patients with acute thromboembolic disease is approximately 5%. Some evidence suggests that this bleeding increases with an increase in heparin. However, evidence also suggests that serious bleeding can occur in patients prone to bleeding even when the anticoagulant response is in the therapeutic range.[106]

The risk of bleeding is usually higher earlier in therapy, when both heparin and warfarin are given together, which may be related to excessive anticoagulation. Patients who have a coexisting disease that elevates the PT, the aPTT, or both (e.g., liver disease) are often at much higher risk of bleeding. In these patients, the use and intensity of anticoagulation that should be employed are controversial.

*Diagnostic followup.* If TT, PT, or aPTT is prolonged and if circulating inhibitors or bleeding disorders are suspected, further tests are usually performed. For example, hemophilia or autoimmune diseases may be associated with inhibitors such as antifactor VIII and the lupus anticoagulant. When dysfibrinogenemia or afibrinogenemia causes prolonged TT, PT, and aPTT values (Table 2), it may be necessary to measure fibrinogen.[61] Fibrinogen levels are recommended by some clinicians to measure the lytic state with nonspecific thrombolytic agents (e.g., streptokinase). However, due to nonavailability of the fibrinogen test in many hospitals and delays in turnaround time, this measurement is not routinely done.

### Activated Clotting Time
*Normal range: 80–130 sec but varies*

ACT[61] (also known as activated coagulation time) is frequently used to monitor heparin therapy[1,88] during procedures that require high-dose heparin (e.g., cardiopulmonary bypass surgery and angioplasty). Because the ACT device is considered a near-patient testing apparatus, it may be run directly in the operating room as well as in the angioplasty suite by nonlaboratory-trained personnel. This advantage has placed ACT devices in other locations where rapid bedside testing is desirable (e.g., hemodialysis unit, operating room, and cardiac catheterization laboratories).

ACT responsiveness remains linear in proportion to an increasing dose of heparin. Corresponding ACT values up to 400 sec demonstrate this dose–response relationship, but ACT lacks reproducibility for values in excess of 600 sec. The variability in ACT test results is significantly increased by variations in

> ➤ Blood volume to be tested.
> ➤ Speed and direction of sample tube agitation.
> ➤ Technique.

While normal adult values are 80–130 sec, a measure of adequate heparinization would be prolonged ACT values of 150–190 sec.[91]

### Fibrinogen Assay
*Normal range: 200–400 mg/dL*

Thrombin time (TT) is the most sensitive test for fibrinogen deficiency, and it is prolonged when fibrinogen concentrations are below 100 mg/dL.[61] However, the actual fibrinogen concentration occasionally must be determined. A common method is the Dade fibrinogen assay. Erroneous results can be caused by (1) improper specimen collection with the wrong blood:anticoagulant ratio or (2) lack of correction of citrate volume for a low or high Hct. Additionally, heparin concentrations greater than 1 U/mL of the patient's blood volume may result in falsely low fibrinogen concentration measurements.

### Other Coagulation Studies

Assays for specific clotting factors can be performed to determine whether a deficiency exists.[61] Factor assays using the aPTT test include factors VIII, IX, XI, and XII as well as prekallikrein. Factors II, V, VII, and X can be determined with assays that use the PT.

## Clot Degradation Tests

### Fibrin Degradation Products
*Normal range: 2–7 μg/mL but varies*

Excessive activation of thrombin leads to overactivation of the fibrinolytic system and increased production of

FDPs. Excessive degradation of fibrin and fibrinogen also increases FDPs. This increase can be observed with DIC or thrombolytic drugs—FDP values may be in excess of 40 µg/mL. FDPs can be monitored during thrombolytic therapy, but they may not be predictive of clot lysis.[107,108]

FDPs can be measured by immunological techniques in which immunoglobulins to FDPs are produced in sheep, harvested, and coated onto latex particles.[56] In the semiquantitative Thrombo-Wellcotest, the concentration of FDPs is determined by the agglutination of the latex particles. Under normal conditions, FDPs should be below 2 µg/mL of plasma when using this test. However, this test is labor intensive and subject to observer variability.[109] A quantitative, automated assay for FDPs was recently described[108] in which the 95% confidence interval for normal subjects consisted of values between 2 and 7 µg/mL. False-positive reactions may occur in healthy women immediately before and during menstruation and in patients with advanced cirrhosis or metastatic cancer.

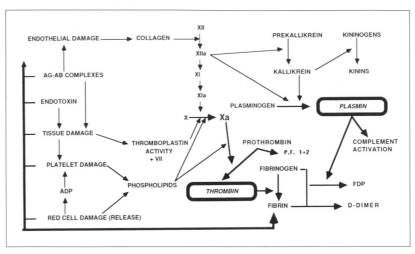

**FIGURE 8.** Triggering mechanisms for disseminated intravascular coagulation. (Reproduced, with permission, from Reference 107.)

### D-Dimer

*Normal range: <0.5 µg/mL or <200 ng/mL but varies with specific assay*

A newer test for DIC is the D-dimer assay. D-dimer is a neoantigen formed when thrombin initiates the transition of fibrinogen to fibrin and activates factor XIII to cross link the fibrin formed. This neoantigen is formed as a result of plasmin digestion of cross-linked fibrin. The D-dimer test is specific for FDPs, whereas the formation of FDPs (discussed previously) may be either fibrinogen or fibrin derived following plasmin digestion (Figure 8). Of the common tests used in assessing DIC patients, the D-dimer assay appears to be the most sensitive.[110] Because of this high predictive ability, the D-dimer is commonly used to confirm or rule out DIC. Table 9 provides a list of the laboratory parameters, including the D-dimer, used to diagnose DIC (Minicases 3 and 4).

## BEDSIDE PATIENT TESTING DEVICES

Several bedside/near-patient testing devices have been introduced over the past several years.[111] Various coagulation tests can be performed at the patient's bedside including aPTT, PT, ACT, fibrinogen assay, TT, and Heparin-Neutralizing Thrombin Time. To maximize the clinical relevance brought about by bedside/near-patient testing devices, new applications of the existing technologies must be investigated. Currently, investigations are underway to evaluate new test methods for these devices, which include the Heparin Management Test (an alternative to

**TABLE 9.** Laboratory Differential Diagnosis of DIC[a]

| DIC Monitoring Parameter | DIC | Primary Fibrinolysis | TTP | Chronic Liver Disease |
|---|---|---|---|---|
| FDP | ↑ | ↑ | WNL to ↑ | WNL to ↑ |
| D-dimer | ↑ | ↑ | WNL | WNL |
| PT | ↑ | ↑ | WNL | ↑ |
| aPTT | ↑ | ↑ | WNL | WNL to ↑ |
| Fibrinogen | ↓ | ↓ | WNL | Variable |
| Platelet count | ↓ | WNL | WNL to ↓ | ↓ |
| LFTs | WNL | WNL | WNL | ↑ |
| Blood urea nitrogen | ↑ | WNL | ↑ | WNL |

[a] ↓ = decrease; ↑ = increase; WNL = within normal limits.

### Minicase 4

Alfred F., a 44-year-old male, had clinical signs and symptoms and electrocardiogram findings consistent with acute anterior-wall myocardial infarction requiring emergent angioplasty. He received intracoronary streptokinase without successful opening of the coronary artery. Subsequently, Alfred F. was heparinized. The following pre- and post-therapy coagulation lab studies were obtained:

| Laboratory Study | Normal Results | Pretherapy | Post-Therapy |
| --- | --- | --- | --- |
| PT | 10–13 sec | 12.2 sec | 17 sec |
| aPTT | 21–45 sec | 39 sec | 69 sec |
| Fibrinogen | 200–400 mg/dL | 300 ng/mL | 22 ng/mL |
| FDP (latex) | 2–7 µg/mL | <10 µg/mL | >160 µg/mL |
| D-dimer | <200 ng/mL | <200 ng/mL | 300 ng/mL |
| Plasminogen | 68–150% | 70% | 22% |

*What might explain the elevated FDP? What accounts for the fall in the plasminogen level on completion of the lytic therapy? Finally, why is the D-dimer concentration not elevated in proportion to the greatly elevated FDP concentration?*

**Discussion:** The elevated post-therapy PT and aPTT are consistent with heparinization after intracoronary thrombolytic therapy. The FDP concentration is elevated because the streptokinase resulted in fibrinolysis. Many FDPs are generated in this setting. By the nature of thrombolytic therapy, plasminogen is converted to plasmin, accounting for the decline in the plasminogen percentage. Because thrombolytic therapy was unsuccessful in full clot lysis (resulting only in fibrinogen lysis), the D-dimer concentration is not greatly elevated. For this assay to have been more elevated, degradation products arising from cross-linked fibrin would have had to be present.

Fibrinogen concentrations should be followed periodically in patients receiving thrombolytic agents. Low levels may predict clot lysis with streptokinase and urokinase but not tPA (alteplase) or APSAC (anistreplase).[1,108]

ACT testing), detection of neutralizing antibodies to streptokinase, Lysis Onset Time,[112] and Heparin-Neutralizing Prothrombin Time.

In the clinical laboratory setting, considerable disease-state and drug-induced alterations can occur to the results obtained from such bedside/near-patient testing devices. For example, significant alterations of PT results may be seen in patients receiving heparin. This problem may be especially evident during the transition from heparin therapy to oral anticoagulation with warfarin during the period of overlap of these medications. In such patients, the accurate monitoring of therapy transition can be difficult because increased PT clotting times may be due to heparin in the blood rather than the therapeutic induction of anticoagulation.

The Heparin Neutralized Whole Blood PT (HNPT) test, developed for the Hemochron Blood Coagulation System, contains enough polybrene to neutralize up to 2 USP U/mL of heparin in whole blood. In the absence of heparin, the HNPT test yields equivalent results to the current whole blood PT test. The HNPT test reflects the level of the extrinsic clotting factor activity and the efficacy of oral anticoagulant therapy.[113] This method is one way that manufacturers have sought to strengthen the clinical utility of their devices and lab tests.

Finally, to assure clinically meaningful results, strict quality assurance indicators must be employed for bedside/near-patient testing devices. The user must be fully compliant with regulations of the Clinical Laboratory Improvement Amendment of 1988.

## SUMMARY

Many factors contribute to normal hemostasis, including interactions among vascular subendothelium, platelets, coagulation factors, natural anticoagulant proteins C and S, and substances that promote clot degradation such as tPA. In the clinical setting, the impact of these and other considerations must be evaluated. Disorders of platelets or clotting factors can result in bleeding, which may necessitate the monitoring of specific clotting tests. The MPV test is useful in distinguishing between hypoproductive versus hyperdestructive causes of thrombocytopenia.

Coagulation tests such as aPTT, ACT, and PT/INR are used to monitor heparin and warfarin therapies. In general, coagulation tests are used for patients receiving anticoagulants, thrombolytics, and antiplatelet agents. When fibrinolysis occurs, monitoring of FDPs is necessary. Other indications for routine use of these tests include primary coagulopathies and monitoring of drugs that may cause bleeding abnormalities. Finally, other available tests (e.g., D-dimer and ATIII level determinations) might improve diagnostic accuracy and resultant therapies.

## REFERENCES

1.  Carter BL, Jones ME, Waickman LA. Pathophysiology and treatment of deep-vein thrombosis and pulmonary embolism. *Clin Pharm.* 1985; 4:279–96.

2.  Carter BL. Therapy of acute thromboembolism with heparin and warfarin. *Clin Pharm.* 1991; 10:503–18.

3.  Fritsma GA. Platelet production and structure. In: Corriveau DM, Fritsma GA, eds. Hemostasis and thrombosis in the clinical laboratory. Philadelphia, PA: J. B. Lippincott; 1988:206–28.

4.  Schick BP. Clinical implications of basic research: hope for treatment of thrombocytopenia. *N Engl J Med.* 1994; 331:875–6.

5.  George JN, Shattil SJ. The clinical importance of acquired abnormalities of platelet function. *N Engl J Med.* 1991; 324:27–39.

6.  Vermylen J, Verstraete M, Fuster V. Role of platelet activation and fibrin formation in thrombogenesis. *J Am Coll Cardiol.* 1986; 8:2–9B.

7.  Heptinstall S, Hanley SP. Blood platelets and vessel walls. In: Bowie EJW, Sharp AA, eds. Hemostasis and thrombosis. London, England: Butterworth & Co.; 1985:36–74.

8.  Brace LD. Platelet physiology. In: Corriveau DM, Fritsma GA, eds. Hemostasis and thrombosis in the clinical laboratory. Philadelphia, PA: J. B. Lippincott; 1988:229–78.

9.  Harker LA, Fuster V. Pharmacology of platelet inhibitors. *J Am Coll Cardiol.* 1986; 8:21–32B.

10. Moake JL, Levine JD. Thrombotic disorders. In: Trench AH, ed. Clinical symposia, vol. 3. Summit, NJ: Ciba-Geigy Corp.; 1985:3–32.

11. Corriveau DM. Plasma proteins: factors of the hemostatic mechanism. In: Corriveau DM, Fritsma GA, eds. Hemostasis and thrombosis in the clinical laboratory. Philadelphia, PA: J. B. Lippincott; 1988:34–66.

12. High KA. Antithrombin III, protein C, and protein S: naturally occurring anticoagulant proteins. *Arch Pathol Lab Med.* 1988; 112:28–36.

13. Maung R, Kelly JK, Schneider MP, et al. Mesenteric venous thrombosis due to antithrombin III deficiency. *Arch Pathol Lab Med.* 1988; 112:3–9.

14. Comp PC, Esmon CT. Recurrent venous thromboembolism in patients with a partial deficiency of protein S. *N Engl J Med.* 1984; 311:1525–8.

15. Clouse LH, Comp PC. The regulation of hemostasis: the protein C system. *N Engl J Med.* 1986; 314:1298–1304.

16. Engesser L, Broekmans AW, Briet E, et al. Hereditary protein S deficiency: clinical manifestations. *Ann Intern Med.* 1987; 106:6–82.

17. Hubbard AR. Standardization of protein C in plasma: establishment of an international standard. *Thromb Haemost.* 1988; 59:464–7.

18. Crabbe SJ, Cloninger CC. Tissue plasminogen activator: a new thrombolytic agent. *Clin Pharm.* 1987; 6:33–86.

19. Fritsma GA. Tests of platelet number and function. In: Corriveau DM, Fritsma GA, eds. Hemostasis and thrombosis in the clinical laboratory. Philadelphia, PA: J. B. Lippincott; 1988:278–303.

20. Levin M, Walters MD, Barratt TM. Hemolytic uremic syndrome. *Adv Pediatr Infect Dis.* 1989; 4:51–81.

21. Fields SM, Lindley CM. Thrombotic microangiopathy associated with chemotherapy: case report and review of the literature. *Drug Intell Clin Pharm.* 1989; 23:582–8.

22. Bailey RT, Ursick JA, Helm KL, et al. Heparin-associated thrombocytopenia: a prospective comparison of bovine lung heparin manufactured by a new process and porcine intestinal heparin. *Drug Intell Clin Pharm.* 1986; 20:374–8.

23. Green D, Hirsh J, Heit J, et al. Low molecular weight heparin: a critical analysis of clinical trials. *Pharmacol Rev.* 1994; 46:89–109.

24. Jackson SR, Carter JM. Platelet volume: laboratory measurement and clinical application. *Blood Rev.* 1993; 7(2): 104–13.

25. Trowbridge EA, Reardon DM, Hutchinson D, et al. The routine measurement of platelet volume: a comparison of light-scattering and aperture impedence technologies. *Clin Phys Physiol Meas.* 1985; 6:221–38.

26. Thompson CB, Diaz D, Quinn PG, et al. The role of anticoagulation in the measurement of platelet volumes. *Am J Clin Pathol.* 1983; 80:327–32.

27. Martin JF, Bath DM, Burr ML. Influence of platelet size on outcome after myocardial infarction. *Lancet.* 1991; 338:1409–11.

28. Burr ML, Holliday RM, Fehily AM, et al. Hematological prognostic indices after myocardial infarction: evidence from the diet and reinfarction trial (PART). *Eur Heart J.* 1992; 13:166–70.

29. Baynes RD, Lamparelli RD, Bezwoda WR, et al. Platelet parameters, part II. Platelet volume-number relationships in various normal and disease states. *South Afr Med J.* 1988; 73:39–43.

30. Singer CRJ, Walker JJ, Cameron A, et al. Platelet studies in normal pregnancy and pregnancy induced hypertension. *Clin Lab Haematol.* 1986; 8:27–32.

31. Haubenstock A, Panzer S, Vierhapper H. Reversal of hyperthyroidism to euthyroidism leads to increased numbers of small size platelets. *Thromb Haemost.* 1988; 60:346–7.

32. Panzer S, Haubenstock A, Minar E. Platelets in hyperthyroidism: studies on platelet counts, mean platelet volume, 111-indium labeled platelet kinetics and platelet associated immunoglobulins G and M. *J Clin Endocrinol Metab.* 1990; 70:491–6.

33. Wedzicha JA, Cotter FE, Empey DW. Platelet size in patients with chronic airflow obstruction with and without hypoxemia. *Thorax.* 1988; 43:61–4.

34. Michalak E, Walkowiak B, Paradowski M, et al. The decreased circulating platelet mass and its relation to bleeding time in chronic renal failure. *Thromb Haemost.* 1991; 65:11–4.

35. Bessman JD, Gardner FH. Platelet size in thrombocytopenia due to sepsis. *Surg Gynecol Obstet.* 1983; 156:177–80.

36. Koenig C, Sidhu G, Schoentag RA. The platelet volume-number relationship in patients infected with the human immunodeficiency virus. *Am J Clin Pathol.* 1991; 96:500–3.

37. de Sauvage FJ, Hass PE, Spencer SD, et al. Stimulation of megakaryocytopoiesis and thrombopoiesis by the c-Mpl ligand. *Nature.* 1994; 369:533–8.

38. Lok S, Kaushansky K, Holly RD, et al. Cloning and expression of murine thrombopoietin cDNA and stimulation of platelet production in vivo. *Nature.* 1994; 369:565–8.

39. Kaushansky K, Lok S, Holly RD, et al. Promotion of megakaryocyte progenitor expansion and differentiation by the c-Mpl ligand thrombopoietin. *Nature.* 1994; 369:568–71.

40. Wendling F, Maraskovsky E, Debili N, et al. c-Mpl ligand is a humoral regulator of megakaryocytopoiesis. *Nature.* 1994; 369:571–4.

41. George JN, Caen JP, Nurden AT. Glanzmann's thrombasthenia: the spectrum of clinical disease. *Blood.* 1990; 75:1383–95.

42. Rodgers RPC, Levin J. A critical reappraisal of the bleeding time. *Semin Thromb Hemost.* 1990; 16:1–20.

43. Burns ER, Lawrence C. Bleeding time: a guide to its diagnostic and clinical utility. *Arch Pathol Lab Med.* 1989; 113:1219–24.

44. Hassouna HL. Specificity and sensitivity in coagulation testing. *Hematol Oncol Clin North Am.* 1993; 7:1194–1216.

45. Davis GL, Fritsma GA. Platelet disorders. In: Corriveau DM, Fritsma GA, eds. Hemostasis and thrombosis in the clinical laboratory. Philadelphia, PA: J.B. Lippincott; 1988:304–42.

46. Steiner RW, Coggins C, Carvalho ACA. Bleeding time in uremia: a useful test to assess clinical bleeding. *Am J Hematol.* 1979; 7:107–17.

47. Pareti FI, Capitanio A, Mannucci L, et al. Acquired dysfunction due to circulation of "exhausted" platelets. *Am J Med.* 1980; 69:235–40.

48. Holloway DS, Summaria L, Sandesara J, et al. Decreased platelet number and function and increased fibrinolysis contribute to postoperative bleeding in cardiopulmonary bypass patients. *Thromb Haemost.* 1988; 59:62–7.

49. Fiore LD, Brophy MT, Lopez A, et al. The bleeding time responses to aspirin: identifying the hyperresponders. *Am J Clin Pathol.* 1990; 94:292–6.

50. Mielke CH Jr, Kaneshiro MM, Maher IA, et al. The standardized normal ivey bleeding time and its prolongation by aspirin. *Blood.* 1969; 34:204–15.

51. Mielke CH Jr. Influence of aspirin on platelets and bleeding time. *Am J Med.* 1983; 74:Suppl(6A)72–8.

52. Deykin D, Janson P, McMahon L. Ethanol potentiation of aspirin-induced prolongation of the bleeding time. *N Engl J Med.* 1982; 306:852–4.

53. Heiden D, Mielke CH Jr, Rodvien R. Impairment by heparin of primary haemostasis and platelet [14C] 5-hydroxytryptamine release. *Br J Haematol.* 1977; 36:427–36.

54. Fuster V, Cohen M, Halperin J. Aspirin in the prevention of coronary disease. *N Engl J Med.* 1989; 321:183–5.

55. Steering committee of the Physician's Health Study research group. Final report on the aspirin component of the ongoing Physician's Health Study. *N Engl J Med.* 1989; 321:129–35.

56. Meade TW, Mellows S, Brozovic M, et al. Haemostatic function and ischaemic heart disease: principal results of the northwick park heart study. *Lancet.* 1986; 2:533–7.

57. Manner CE. Laboratory evaluation of platelets. In: Lotspeich-Steininger CA, Stein-Martin EA, Koepke JA, eds. Clinical hematology. Philadelphia, PA: J. B. Lippincott; 1992:671–9.

58. Hassouna HL. Laboratory evaluation of hemostatic disorders. *Hematol Oncol Clin North Am.* 1993; 7:1161–93.

59. Palkuti HS. Specimen collection and quality control. In: Corriveau DM, Fritsma GA, eds. Homeostasis and thrombosis in the clinical laboratory. Philadelphia, PA: J. B. Lippincott; 1988:6–91.

60. Weiss AE. The hemophilias. In: Corriveau DM, Fritsma GA, eds. Hemostasis and thrombosis in the clinical laboratory. Philadelphia, PA: J. B. Lippincott; 1988:128–68.

61. Fritsma GA. Clot-based assays of coagulation. In: Corriveau DM, Fritsma GA, eds. Hemostasis and thrombosis in the clinical laboratory. Philadelphia, PA: J. B. Lippincott; 1988: 92–197.

62. Loeliger EA. The optimal therapeutic range in oral anticoagulation: history and proposal. *Thromb Haemost.* 1979; 42:1141–52.

63. Poller L. Oral anticoagulants reassessed. *Br Med J.* 1982; 284:1425–6.

64. Hirsh J, Dalen JE, Deykin D, et al. Oral anticoagulants: mechanism of action, clinical effectiveness, and optimal therapeutic range. *Chest.* 1995; 108(Suppl 4):231–46s.

65. Quick AJ. The prothrombin in hemophilia and obstructive jaundice. *J Biol Chem.* 1935; 109:3–4.

66. Denson KWE. Thromboplastin—sensitivity, precision and other characteristics. *Clin Lab Haematol.* 1988; 10:315–28.

67. Poller L, Thomson JM, Taberner DA. Effect of automation on prothrombin time test in NEQAS surveys. *J Clin Pathol.* 1989; 42:97–100.

68. Naghibi F, Han Y, Dodds WJ, et al. Effects of reagent and instrument on prothrombin times, activated partial thromboplastin times and patient/control ratios. *Thromb Haemost.* 1988; 59:455–63.

69. Loeliger EA. ICSH/ICTH recommendations for reporting prothrombin time in oral anticoagulant controls. *J Clin Pathol.* 1985; 38:133–4.

70. McKernan A. The reliability of international normalized ratios during short-term oral anticoagulant treatment. *Clin Lab Haematol.* 1988; 10:63–71.

71. Poggio M. The effect of some instruments for prothrombin time testing on the international sensitivity index (ISI) of two rabbit tissue thromboplastin reagents. *Thromb Haemost.* 1989; 62:866–74.

72. Bussey HI. Reliance on prothrombin time ratios causes significant errors in anticoagulation therapy. *Arch Intern Med.* 1992; 152:278–82.

73. Moriarty HT, Lamp-Po-Tang PRL, Anastas N, et al. Comparison of thromboplastins using the ISI and INR system. *Pathology.* 1990; 22:71–6.

74. Schuff-Werner P, Schutz E, Gonska BD. Variation in the prothrombin-time ratio during oral anticoagulation. *N Engl J Med.* 1994; 330:570.

75. Package insert, Dade determination of INR. Deerfield, IL: Baxter Diagnostics; 1991.

76. Ansell J. Imprecision of prothrombin time ratios causes significant errors in anticoagulation. *Am J Clin Pathol.* 1992; 98:237–9.

77. Hirsh J. Substandard monitoring of warfarin in North America: time for a change. *Arch Intern Med.* 1992; 152: 257–8. Editorial.

78. Hirsh J, Dalen JE, Deykin D, et al. Oral anticoagulants: mechanism of action, clinical effectiveness and optimal therapeutic range. *Chest.* 1992; 102(Suppl 4):312–26s.

79. Sawyer WT, Raasch RH. Effect of heparin on prothrombin time. *Clin Pharm.* 1984; 3:192–4.

80. Lutomski DM, Djuric PE, Draeger RW. Warfarin therapy: the effect of heparin on prothrombin times. *Arch Intern Med.* 1987; 147:432–3.

81. Schultz NJ, Slaker RA, Rosborough TK. The influence of heparin on the prothrombin time. *Pharmacotherapy.* 1991; 11(4):312–6.

82. Poller L, Thomson JM, Palmer MK. Measuring partial thromboplastin-time: an international collaborative study. *Lancet.* 1976; 2:842–6.

83. Brandt JT, Triplett DA. Laboratory monitoring of heparin: effects of reagents and instruments on the activated partial thromboplastin time. *Am J Clin Pathol.* 1981; 76:530–7.

84. Gawoski JM, Arkin CF, Bovill T, et al. The effects of heparin on the activated partial thromboplastin time of the College of American Pathologists Survey specimens. *Arch Pathol Lab Med.* 1987; 111:785–90.

85. Groce JB, Gal P, Douglas JB, et al. Heparin dosage adjustment in patients with deep-vein thrombosis using heparin concentrations rather than activated partial thromboplastin time. *Clin Pharm.* 1987; 6:216–22.

86. Hyers TM, Hull RB, Weg JG. Antithrombotic therapy for venous thromboembolic disease. *Chest.* 1992; 102(Suppl 4):408–25s.

87. Brill-Edwards P, Ginsberg JS, Johnston M, et al. Estab-

lishing a therapeutic range for heparin therapy. *Ann Intern Med.* 1993; 119:104–9.

88. Hattersley PG, Mitsuoka JC, Ignoffo RJ, et al. Adjusting heparin infusion rates from the initial response to activated coagulation time. *Drug Intell Clin Pharm.* 1983; 17:632–4.

89. Hull RD, Raskob GE, Rosenbloom D, et al. Optimal therapeutic level of heparin therapy in patients with venous thromboembolism. *Arch Intern Med.* 1992; 152:1589–95.

90. Raschke RA, Reilly BM, Guidry JR, et al. The weight-based heparin dosing nomogram compared with a "standard care" nomogram: a randomized controlled trial. *Arch Intern Med.* 1993; 119:874–81.

91. Cipolle RJ, Rodvold KA. Heparin. In: Evans WE, Schentag JJ, Jusko WJ, eds. Applied pharmacokinetics. Vancouver, British Columbia: Applied Therapeutics; 1992:1–39.

92. Claggett GP, Anderson FA, Heit J. Prevention of venous thromboembolism. *Chest.* 1995; 108(Suppl 4):312–34s.

93. The GUSTO investigators. An international randomized trial comparing four thrombolytic strategies for acute myocardial infarction. *N Engl J Med.* 1993; 329:673–82.

94. The global use of strategies to open occluded coronary arteries (GUSTO) IIa investigators. Randomized trial of intravenous heparin versus recombinant hirudin for acute coronary syndromes. *Circulation.* 1994; 90:1631–7.

95. Antman EM, for the TIMI 9A investigators. Hirudin in acute myocardial infarction: safety report from the thrombolysis and thrombin inhibition in myocardial infarction (TIMI) 9A trial. *Circulation.* 1994; 90:1624–30.

96. Kandrotas RJ, Gal P, Douglas JB, et al. Rapid determination of maintenance heparin infusion rates with the use of non-steady-state heparin concentrations. *Ann Pharmacother.* 1993; 27:1429–33.

97. Basu D, Gallus A, Hirsh J, et al. A prospective study of the value of monitoring heparin treatment with the activated partial thromboplastin time. *N Engl J Med.* 1972; 287:324–7.

98. Hull RD, Raskob GE, Hirsh J, et al. Continuous intravenous heparin compared with intermittent subcutaneous heparin in the initial treatment of proximal-vein thrombosis. *N Engl J Med.* 1986; 315:1109–14.

99. Hauser VM, Rozek SL. Effect of warfarin on the activated partial thromboplastin time. *Drug Intell Clin Pharm.* 1986; 20:964–7.

100. Gal P, Kandrotas RJ. Heparin. In: Murphy JE, ed. Clinical pharmacokinetics. Bethesda, MD: American Society of Hospital Pharmacists; 1993:91–113.

101. Levine MN, Hirsh J, Gent M, et al. A randomized trial comparing activated partial thromboplastin time with heparin assay in patients with acute venous thromboembolism requiring large doses of heparin. *Arch Intern Med.* 1994; 154:49–56.

102. Hirsh J, Hull RD. Treatment of venous thromboembolism. *Chest.* 1986; 89(Suppl 5):426–33s.

103. Colwell CW, Spiro TE, Trowbridge AA, et al. Use of enoxaparin, a low-molecular-weight heparin, and unfractionated heparin for the prevention of deep venous thrombosis after elective hip replacement. *J Bone Joint Surg.* 1994; 76-A:3–14.

104. Frydman AM, Bara L, LeRoux Y, et al. The antithrombotic activity and pharmacokinetics of enoxaparin, a low molecular weight heparin, in humans given single subcutaneous doses of 20 to 80 mg. *J Clin Pharmacol.* 1988; 28:609–18.

105. Bara L, Combe-Tamzali S, Conard J, et al. Laboratory monitoring of a low molecular weight heparin (enoxaparin) with a new clotting test (Heptest). *Haemostasis.* 1987; 1:12–33.

106. Levine MN, Hirsh J, Landefeld S, et al. Hemorrhagic complications of anticoagulant treatment. *Chest.* 1992; 102 (Suppl 4):352–63s.

107. Bick RL. Disseminated intravascular coagulation: objective criteria for clinical and laboratory diagnosis and assessment of therapeutic response. *Clin Appl Thrombosis/Hemostasis.* 1995; 1(1):3–25.

108. Conrad J, Samama MM. Theoretic and practical considerations on laboratory monitoring of thrombolytic therapy. *Semin Thromb Hemost.* 1987; 13:212–22.

109. Sigal SH, Cembrowski GS, Shattil SJ, et al. Prototype quantitative assay for fibrinogen/fibrin degradation products: clinical evaluation. *Arch Intern Med.* 1987; 147:1790–3.

110. Bick RL. Disseminated intravascular coagulation: objective criteria for diagnosis and management. *Med Clin North Am.* 1994; 78:511–43.

111. Weibert RT, Adler DS. Evaluation of a capillary whole-blood prothrombin time measurement system. *Clin Pharm.* 1989; 8:864–7.

112. Product information. Raleigh, NC: Cardiovascular Diagnostics Technical Services; 1994.

113. Product information. Edison, NJ: ICT Commercial Group; 1994.

## QuickView—Platelet Count

| Parameter | Description | Comments |
|---|---|---|
| **Common reference ranges**<br>**Adults and pediatrics** | 140,000–440,000/μL | Automated methodology<br>Range to be determined in patients with suspected bleeding disorders, petechiae, DIC, or leukemia |
| **Critical value** | 20,000–50,000/μL | Risk of spontaneous bleeding increases greatly<br>Presents as petechiae, epistaxis, or gingival bleeding |
| | 500,000–800,000/μL | Reactive thrombocytosis (e.g., infection, acute blood loss, stress) or thrombocythemia (e.g., myeloproliferative disorders) |
| **Natural substance?** | Yes | |
| **Inherent activity?** | Yes | Hemostasis |
| **Location**<br>**Production** | Bone marrow | |
| **Storage** | Circulation and spleen | In splenectomized patients, 100% is in circulation |
| **Secretion/excretion** | Via spleen, liver, and bone marrow | Upon aging |
| **Major causes of . . .**<br>**Associated signs and symptoms** | Bleeding | As seen with thrombocytopenia |
| **After insult, time to . . .**<br>**Initial decline** | 2–4 days after initiation of therapy with heparin | Disappears in 1–5 days, even with heparin therapy |
| **Later decline** | 1–9 days (mean: 5.5) | Due to heparin-dependent IgG antibodies |
| **Initial elevation or positive result** | Variable | Phase reactant or myeloproliferative disorder |

## QuickView—PT

| Parameter | Description | Comments |
|---|---|---|
| **Common reference ranges**<br>**Adults and pediatrics** | 10–13 sec | Normal values vary from lab to lab, depending on technique used; each lab must determine its own expected values |
| **Critical value** | >1.5 upper limit of normal (off warfarin)<br>>2 times mean lab control (on warfarin) | Any corresponding INR >3 increases likelihood for bleed |
| **Major causes of . . .**<br>**High results** | Excessive warfarin–drug interactions | May be seen with liver dysfunction |
| **Associated signs and symptoms** | Bleeding and ecchymosis | With INR >6 |
| **Low results** | Noncompliance | May be seen rarely with warfarin resistance |
| **Associated signs and symptoms** | Clot formation and signs and symptoms related to ischemic organ(s) | In patients requiring warfarin anticoagulation; low results usually clinically insignificant in otherwise healthy patients |

*continued*

## QuickView—PT *continued*

| Parameter | Description | Comments |
|---|---|---|
| **After warfarin dose, time to . . .** | | |
| Initial elevation or positive result | 6 hr | Patient *not* fully anticoagulated; reflects decrease in factor VII |
| Peak value | 96 hr | Patient fully anticoagulated |
| Subtherapeutic value | ≤24 hr | With administration of vitamin K or fresh frozen plasma; may take longer with simple discontinuance of drug (estimated 1–3 days) |
| **Drugs often monitored with test** | Warfarin | |
| **Causes of spurious results** | Therapeutic or high levels of heparin may increase PT | Technique dependent<br>Seen with liver disease (increase) |

## QuickView—INR

| Parameter | Description | Comments |
|---|---|---|
| **Common reference ranges**<br>Adults and pediatrics | 2–3<br>2.5–3.5<br>1.0 (approximately) in healthy persons not receiving anticoagulants | Value (2–3) to be maintained for all thrombotic disorders except mechanical prosthetic valves (requires 2.5–3.5)<br>Intended for assessing patients on long-term oral anticoagulation<br>Must know ISI value of reagent to standardize PT with INR |
| **Critical value** | >2, without warfarin<br>>3–5, with warfarin | May indicate liver dysfunction<br>May indicate drug–drug interaction, excess dose, etc. |
| **Drugs often monitored with test** | Warfarin | Exclusively |
| **Causes of spurious results** | Therapeutic or high levels of heparin may increase INR | Technique dependent<br>Seen with liver disease (increase) |

## QuickView—aPTT

| Parameter | Description | Comments |
|---|---|---|
| **Common reference ranges**<br>Adults and pediatrics | 21–45 sec | Normal values vary from lab to lab depending on methodology, reagents, and instrument systems and their combinations; each lab must determine its own expected values |
| **Critical value** | Above upper limit of normal (not on heparin)<br>>150 sec (on heparin) | Increase may be seen with liver dysfunction |
| **Major causes of . . .** | | |
| High results | Excessive anticoagulation | Autoanticoagulation (i.e., liver dysfunction) |
| Associated signs and symptoms | Bleeding | Seen with normal results if patient at risk |
| Low results | Under anticoagulation or presence of procoagulants | Requires increased heparin dosage adjustment |
| Associated signs and symptoms | Thromboembolic disease | |

## QuickView—aPTT *continued*

| Parameter | Description | Comments |
|---|---|---|
| **After heparin dose, time to . . .** | | |
| Initial elevation or positive result | Immediately | Assumes bolus |
| | 6 hr | Without bolus |
| Steady-state values | 6 hr | |
| Subtherapeutic values | 1 hr | Upon discontinuing heparin |
| **Drugs often monitored with test** | Heparin | Exclusively |
| **Causes of spurious results** | Use of heparinized collection tubes (increase) | Increase may be seen with liver disease, lupus, and polycythemia |
| | Specimen collected from heparinized site | Increase may indicate factor deficiency |
| | | Technique dependent |

## QuickView—Heparin Concentration

| Parameter | Description | Comments |
|---|---|---|
| **Common reference ranges** | | |
| Adults and pediatrics | 0.2–0.4 U/mL | Whole blood value; labor intensive |
| | 0.35–0.7 U/mL | Plasma assay; automated, depends on adequate ATIII concentrations |
| | | Assays for anti-factor Xa activity |
| **Critical value** | >0.9 U/mL | Bleeding may increase |
| **Natural substance?** | Yes | Heparin is a natural substance, but assay measures exogenous heparin |
| **Inherent activity?** | Yes | Endogenous heparin has very local activity |
| **Location** | | |
| Production | Lungs and intestines | Nonpharmacological levels |
| Storage | Mast cells | Nonpharmacological levels |
| Secretion/excretion | Liver and kidneys | Nonpharmacological levels |
| **Major causes of . . .** | | |
| High results | Excess dosing | |
| Associated signs and symptoms | Bleeding | |
| Low results | Under anticoagulation | May be seen with suppression of vitamin K-dependent clotting factor X |
| | Increased clearance of heparin | |
| Associated signs and symptoms | Thromboembolic disease, shortness of breath, cough | Essentially signs and symptoms of thromboembolic disease in heart, lungs, brain, legs, etc. |
| **After dose, time to . . .** | | |
| Initial elevation or positive result | Immediately | Assumes bolus |
| Steady-state values | 6 hr | Without bolus |
| Subtherapeutic values | 1–2 hr | Upon discontinuing drug |
| **Drugs often monitored with test** | Heparin | Exclusively |
| **Causes of spurious results** | Sample from heparinized area | |
| | No heparin infusing | |
| | Vitamin K-dependent clotting factor X suppressed | |

## QuickView—D-Dimer

| Parameter | Description | Comments |
|---|---|---|
| **Common reference ranges** | | |
| **Adults and pediatrics** | <0.5 µg/mL | Specific for fibrin degradation secondary to coagulation activation |
| | <200 ng/mL | |
| **Critical value** | >0.5 µg/mL | Increased D-dimer suggestive of deep-venous thrombosis, pulmonary embolism, and DIC |
| | >200 ng/mL | |
| **Natural substance?** | Yes | |
| **Inherent activity?** | Yes | |
| **Major causes of . . .** | | |
| **High results** | Seen with DIC, PE, and thromboembolic disease | Positive rheumatoid factor and positive lupus procoagulant may interfere |
| **Associated signs and symptoms** | Thrombosis | |
| **Low results** | | D-dimer levels lower in serum than plasma |
| **Associated signs and symptoms** | None | |
| **After insult, time to . . .** | | |
| **Initial elevation or positive result** | 2–3 days | Postoperative in response to surgery |
| **Normalization** | Decreases progressively | |
| **Causes of spurious results** | Positive rheumatoid factor and lupus factor | Results in false positive |

# Chapter 16

# Infectious Diseases

*Nancy S. Jordan*

To practitioners already overwhelmed by the burgeoning number of antibiotics and by the confusing and changing names of bacteria, the topic of laboratory tests for infectious diseases may seem intimidating. Infectious disease is a rapidly changing area, especially with new challenges such as acquired immunodeficiency syndrome (AIDS) and the resurgence of tuberculosis (TB). Diagnostic techniques also change as technological advances are adapted for laboratory use.

This chapter describes some fundamental tests used in the diagnosis of infectious diseases and their clinical applications. Infectious diseases involving the gastrointestinal (GI) tract are discussed in Chapter 11.

## OBJECTIVES

Upon completion of this chapter, the reader should be able to

1. Discuss the types of clinical specimens often submitted for Gram's stain and the clinical utility of the information obtained from that stain.
2. Compare the techniques, limitations, and clinical implications of antimicrobial susceptibility testing (performed by the disk diffusion method) with those of the broth dilution method.
3. Given bacterial susceptibility results in the context of a clinical case study, select the one or more antibiotics most appropriate for the patient.
4. Discuss tests routinely performed on cerebrospinal fluid (CSF) when meningitis is suspected.
5. Discuss what a positive human immunodeficiency virus (HIV) antibody test means in terms of the risk of spreading the disease to others.

## BACTERIAL IDENTIFICATION

### Gram's Stain

Gram's stain is most commonly used to examine material from normally sterile body fluids (e.g., CSF, pleural fluid,

and urine), abscesses, wounds, sputum, and tissue.[1] A Danish physician, H. C. Gram, first described the stain in the late 1800s. This stain does not allow exact identification of the organism (e.g., *Escherichia coli* versus *Pseudomonas aeruginosa*), but it permits determination of shape and staining characteristics.

Gram's stain is the most common method of staining specimens in preparation for microscopic examination of bacteria. A slide with a dried sample suspected of containing organisms is fixed and stained with crystal violet and then iodine. Subsequently, the slide is decolorized with acetone/alcohol and counterstained with safranin (a pink dye).[1] Gram-positive bacteria stain purple, and Gram-negative bacteria stain pink. The entire process requires only a few minutes and can be performed in a laboratory, near the patient's bedside, or in the physician's office.

By viewing the Gram-stained specimen, the clinician can determine not only whether bacteria are present but also whether the bacteria are Gram positive, Gram negative, bacilli (rod shaped), or cocci (round). The test also reveals the quantity of organisms and any mixture of several different types of organisms. The presence of white blood cells (WBCs) suggests that the bacteria are likely to be pathogens (infecting organisms) as opposed to normal flora or nonpathogenic colonizers. Certain organisms, such as *Mycoplasma* and *Legionella* sp., cannot be visualized by Gram's stain.

The clinician can use the information obtained to design an empiric antibiotic regimen for the patient before the final culture and susceptibility results are known. The final report usually takes 1–2 days, but a clinician cannot wait 2 days before beginning therapy in a seriously ill patient. Therefore, Gram's stain can provide valuable guidance in choosing an appropriate antibiotic initially. This choice can then be revised (if necessary) when the final test results are known.

### Culture and Identification

Bacteria are identified by their Gram's stain, growth characteristics (e.g., type of media and aerobic versus anaerobic), colonial morphology, color, and biochemical profile.[1] Once a clinical specimen is received by the laboratory, it must be placed on or in media that provide the proper growth conditions for microorganisms potentially present in it. Many media can be used, but the number and types chosen for the culture of specimens must be individualized for each laboratory based on the typical patient population served and the usual microorganisms isolated.

Some common agars are blood and enteric. Blood agar is a medium that, when incubated in an anaerobic or carbon dioxide-supplemented atmosphere, can support the growth of most significant bacteria. Blood agar does not, however, support the growth of some organisms (e.g., *Haemophilus* sp., *Neisseria gonorrhoeae*, and *Legionella* sp.).[2] Chocolate agar, which is blood agar heated until chocolate in color, can support the growth of all bacteria that grow on blood agar plus *Haemophilus* sp. and *N. gonorrhoeae*.

Enteric agars (e.g., MacConkey) support the growth of Gram-negative bacilli and inhibit the growth of Gram-positive cocci. Furthermore, many types of enteric agars can preferentially support the growth of aerobic (e.g., *Salmonella* sp., *Shigella* sp., and Gram-positive bacteria) and anaerobic organisms (e.g., *Bacteroides fragilis*).

Some bacteria grow only in an aerobic (oxygen-containing) environment. These organisms are known as strict aerobes. Strict anaerobes grow only under anaerobic (lack of oxygen) conditions. On the other hand, many facultative anaerobes can grow in both aerobic and anaerobic conditions.[2] Therefore, the incubation conditions of the agar are important. Some agars should be incubated in air, others in air supplemented with carbon dioxide, and still others in anaerobic conditions.

After organisms are grown, a Gram's stain is prepared, the colonial morphology (what the bacterial colonies look like) is noted, and small samples of the bacteria are subjected to differentiating biochemical tests. These tests can determine if the organism ferments glucose, produces hydrogen sulfide, hydrolyzes urea, produces ornithine decarboxylase, etc.

Many identification systems simplify the culturing process by supplying prepackaged biochemicals in self-contained wells on a plastic card. Organisms are inoculated into each well and, after an appropriate time (usually <24 hr), the color changes that represent biochemical reactions are recorded. By combining the results of the biochemical reactions with the information already obtained, a clinician can identify the organism.

Table 1 lists, in an abbreviated form, common pathogenic bacteria and their Gram-stain characteristics and morphology. The table also identifies which organisms are primarily aerobic and which are anaerobic. All human microbial pathogens are not included, but the table provides a format for remembering a few bacteria and for

adding others. Clinicians must become familiar with these characteristics to make empiric antibiotic selection(s) (1) before culture results are available or (2) when a negative culture is inconsistent with the clinical setting.

## Empiric Antimicrobial Therapy

By knowing the characteristics of common bacteria and identifying them, one can more easily remember the activity spectrum of antimicrobial agents. It also helps to know where bacteria normally reside. This information makes it possible to (1) decide which pathogens probably caused a given infection and (2) design an empiric antimicrobial regimen for an infected patient.

When a patient is suffering from an infection, the clinician must consider several factors before instituting appropriate empiric antimicrobial therapy:

➤ The known or most probable site(s) of infection.

➤ The organisms that are most likely causing infection at the site(s).

**TABLE 1.** Common Human Bacterial Pathogens

| |
|---|
| **Gram-positive cocci** |
| *Staphylococcus* sp. |
| S. aureus |
| S. epidermidis |
| *Streptococcus* sp. |
| S. pneumoniae |
| S. pyogenes |
| *Enterococcus* sp. |
| E. faecalis |
| **Gram-negative cocci** |
| *Moraxella catarrhalis* |
| *Neisseria gonorrhoeae* |
| *Neisseria meningitidis* |
| **Gram-positive bacilli** |
| *Bacillus anthracis* |
| *Listeria monocytogenes* |
| *Corynebacterium diphtheriae* |
| *Clostridium* sp.[a] (*C. perfringens, C. difficile, C. tetani*) |
| **Gram-negative bacilli** |
| Enteric |
| *Bacteroides fragilis*[a,b] |
| *Campylobacter jejuni* |
| *Enterobacter aerogenes*[b] |
| *E. coli*[b] |
| *Klebsiella pneumoniae*[b] |
| *Proteus mirabilis*[b] |
| *Salmonella* sp. |
| *Shigella* sp. |
| *Serratia marcescens* |
| Nonenteric |
| *Acinetobacter* sp. |
| *Haemophilus influenzae* |
| *Legionella pneumophila* |
| *P. aeruginosa* |
| *Xanthomonas maltophilia* |

[a]*Strict anaerobes. All other organisms are strict aerobes or facultative anaerobes.*
[b]*Present in the GI tract as normal flora.*

**TABLE 2.** Bacteria and Infections They Commonly Cause

| Bacteria | Type or Site of Infection |
|---|---|
| **Gram-positive cocci** | |
| S. aureus | Skin, soft tissue, intravenous (IV) catheter, prosthetic device |
| S. epidermidis | Skin, soft tissue, IV catheter, prosthetic device |
| S. pneumoniae | Pneumonia |
| **Gram-negative cocci** | |
| N. gonorrhoeae | Urogenital infections |
| N. meningitidis | Bacteremia and meningitis |
| **Gram-positive bacilli** | |
| L. monocytogenes | Meningitis and bacteremia |
| C. perfringens | Intra-abdominal infections; usually part of abscess |
| C. difficile | Diarrhea and colitis |
| **Gram-negative bacilli[a]** | |
| B. fragilis | Intra-abdominal infections; usually part of abscess |
| E. aerogenes | Intra-abdominal infections and bacteremia |
| E. coli | Urinary tract infections, bacteremia, intra-abdominal infections |
| K. pneumoniae | Urinary tract infections, respiratory tract, intra-abdominal infections |
| P. mirabilis | Urinary tract infections, bacteremia, intra-abdominal infections |
| Salmonella sp. | Diarrhea |

[a]*All bacteria listed are enteric.*

➤ The usual antimicrobial susceptibility patterns of the suspected infecting bacteria.

Table 2 lists bacteria and the common infections they cause or site where they are found. Hospitals regularly compile cumulative susceptibility data of isolated microorganisms, commonly referred to as an antibiogram (Figure 1). Antibiograms are consulted to determine the usual antimicrobial susceptibility patterns of bacteria. However, antibiograms generated at one institution should not be applied to another setting, even in the same geographical area. Differing patterns of antimicrobial use and different patient populations may lead to different antibiograms. Many patient-specific variables can alter the likely infecting organisms and/or their antimicrobial susceptibilities.

Unfortunately, the culture result may show no growth despite overwhelming evidence of an infection (Table 3). Under such circumstances, the clinician must rely more on clinical experience and less on the inconsistent data (Chapter 1). A discussion of factors to consider in this clinical setting is beyond the scope of the text.

## ANTIMICROBIAL SUSCEPTIBILITY TESTING

In addition to identifying potential bacterial pathogens, a laboratory tests bacterial isolates for susceptibility to various antimicrobial agents. Before review of the methodology and interpretation of these data, two terms must be defined:

➤ Minimal inhibitory concentration (MIC).

➤ Minimal bactericidal concentration (MBC).

To determine the MIC and MBC for a particular organism, a standard inoculum of the microorganism (e.g., $5 \times 10^5$ cfu/mL) is added to serial (doubling) dilutions of antimicrobial agent. After incubation at 95 °F (35 °C) for 16–20 hr, the tubes of the bacteria–antimicrobial agent mixture are examined for cloudiness, which indicates

**TABLE 3.** Common Clinical and Laboratory Findings Associated with Infection

**Clinical**
    Localized
        Inflammation at site of infection: swelling, warmth, redness, pain
        Sputum production and cough
        Diarrhea
        Vaginal and urethral discharges
        Skin lesions
    Systemic
        Fever
        Chills and rigors
        Increased heart rate
        Increased respiratory rate
        Malaise
        Mental status changes
        Hypotension

**Laboratory**
    Increased WBCs with rise in immature forms (bands) or "shift to the left"
    Positive cultures and/or Gram stain
    Increased erythrocyte sedimentation rate
    Positive antigen or antibody titers

| Antibiotic Formulary Status Bold = FORMULARY Upper/Lower = RESERVED | Acinetobacter calcoaceticus (11) | Enterobacter aerogenes (12) | Enterobacter cloacae (30) | Escherichia coli (271) | Haemophilus influenzae (63) | Klebsiella pneumoniae (67) | Proteus mirabilis (37) | Pseudomonas aeruginosa (101) | Staphylococcus aureus (153) | Enterococci (gp D strep) (97) | Enterococcus faecium (12) | Usual dose | Cost/day includes administration costs |
|---|---|---|---|---|---|---|---|---|---|---|---|---|---|
| **AMPICILLIN** | | | | 73 | 73 | | 100 | | | 97 | | 1-2 gm IV Q6hr | $4 - 5 |
| **AMOXICILLIN - CLAVULANATE** | | | | | 95 | | | | | | | 250-500 mg PO TID | $4 - 6 |
| **CEFAZOLIN** | | | | 97 | | 97 | 100 | | 87 | | | 500 mg IV Q8 hr | $6 |
| **CEFOTETAN** | | | 63 | 100 | | 100 | 100 | | | | | 1-2 gm IV Q12 hr | $18 - 35 |
| Ceftazidime | 100 | 92 | | | | | | 98 | | | | 1-2 gm IV Q8 hr | $31 - 61 |
| Ceftriaxone | | 92 | 86 | 100 | 100 | 100 | 100 | | | | | 1-2 gm IV Q24 hr | $25- 50 |
| Cefuroxime | | 92 | 72 | 99 | 97 | 98 | 100 | | | | | 750 mg IV Q8 hr | $14 |
| Ciprofloxacin | 100 | 100 | 100 | 100 | | 100 | 100 | 95 | 90 | 78 | | 250-750 mg PO BID | $4 - 9 (only oral form available) |
| **CLINDAMYCIN** | | | | | | | | | 91 | | | 600 mg Q8 hr | IV - $9   PO - $8 |
| **ERYTHROMYCIN** | | | | | | | | | 72 | | | 500 mg Q6 hr | IV - $7   PO - $0.20 |
| **GENTAMICIN** | 91 | 100 | 100 | 100 | | 100 | 100 | 92 | | | | 80 mg IV Q8 hr | $5 |
| Imipenem | 100 | 100 | 100 | | | | | | 91 | | | 500 mg IV Q8-6 hr | $60 - 79 |
| **METRONIDAZOLE** | | | | | | | | | | | | 500 mg Q6 hr | IV - $7   PO - $.50 |
| **OXACILLIN** | | | | | | | | | 87 | | | 2 gm IV Q6 hr | $10 |
| **NITROFURANTOIN** | | 100 | | 99 | | | | | | 99 | 95 | 50 - 100 mg PO Q6hr for urine isolates only | $2 - 3 |
| **PENICILLIN G** | | | | | | | | | | | | 1 million units IV Q4 hr | $9 |
| **TETRACYCLINE** | | | 85 | 85 | | 92 | | | 92 | | | 250-500 mg PO Q6 hr | $0.20 |
| **TICARCILLIN** | 100 | 83 | 63 | 74 | | | 100 | 89 | | | | 3 gm IV Q4 | $48 |
| Ticarcillin-clavulanate | Activity superior to ticarcillin vs. staph, most gram neg. rods and anaerobes (including B. fragilis). Activity same as ticarcillin vs. Pseudomonas, Acinetobacter, Enterobacter. | | | | | | | | | | | 3.1 gm IV Q6 hr | $43 |
| Tobramycin | 100 | 100 | | | | | | 100 | | | | 80 mg IV Q8 hr | $18 |
| **TRIMETHOPRIM - SULFAMETHOXAZOLE** | 91 | 100 | 97 | 92 | 92 | 90 | 97 | | 94 | | | 20 ml IV Q12 hr / 1 DS Tab PO BID | IV - $3 / PO - $0.15 |
| Vancomycin | | | | | | | | | 99 | 100 | 92 | 1 gm IV Q12 hr | $15 |

**ANTIBIOTIC SUSCEPTIBILITIES Jan. - Dec. 1993** — Numbers are percent susceptible (# isolates). Pharmacy (x2549) / Microbiology (x5529)

**FIGURE 1.** Example of an antibiogram.

growth of the microorganism. The MIC is the lowest antibiotic concentration (or highest dilution) that inhibits visible growth of the bacteria. When the tubes are examined, the one containing the lowest concentration of antibiotic that is still clear (no growth) is the tube containing the MIC of antibiotic.[3]

The reported MIC value is not the "true" MIC. The true MIC is actually between the lowest test concentration that inhibits bacterial growth and the next lowest test concentration. For example, if antimicrobial concentrations of 1, 2, 4, and 8 µg/mL are tested and the tube containing 4 µg/mL has no visible bacterial growth but the 2-µg/mL solution has visible growth, the reported MIC will be 4 µg/mL. However, the true value is somewhere between 2 and 4 µg/mL. A dilution test may not yield the same result every time; acceptable variation is within one twofold dilution.

To determine the MBC, all tubes without visible growth are cultured to agar plates. The number of bacterial colonies that grow on the plates is compared with the number in the original inoculum. The MBC is the lowest antibiotic concentration that kills 99.9% of the bacteria.[3] The MIC is always equal to or lower than the MBC. For instance, the MIC of a bacteria to an antimicrobial agent might be 8 µg/mL, while the MBC is typically 16 µg/mL

(or higher). Therefore, a higher concentration of antimicrobial agent is required to kill an organism rather than merely inhibit its growth.

Bacterial susceptibility or resistance to a particular antimicrobial agent depends on the readily achievable serum concentrations obtained using normal doses of the agent in question. If the concentration of the agent represented by the MIC can be easily achieved in the patient's serum by usual doses of antibiotic and normal routes of delivery, the bacteria are considered susceptible to that agent. On the other hand, if the MIC exceeds usual serum concentrations of the antimicrobial agent, the organism is considered resistant.

Two terms regarding the MIC—$MIC_{50}$ and $MIC_{90}$—are not used on a patient's susceptibility report, but they are commonly used in literature reports and manufacturer advertising regarding susceptibility of bacteria to antimicrobial agents. The $MIC_{50}$ refers to the concentration of antimicrobial agent when 50% of the isolates of a particular microorganism are inhibited. The $MIC_{90}$ refers to the concentration when 90% of the isolates are inhibited.

The $MIC_{90}$ value is usually higher than the $MIC_{50}$, but they can be the same. For example, with a given organism, the $MIC_{50}$ for cefazolin might be 1 µg/mL and the $MIC_{90}$ might be 2 µg/mL. When susceptibility data are evaluated to determine the usefulness of an antimicrobial agent in treating infections from a particular organism, the $MIC_{90}$ and its relationship to readily achievable serum concentrations is more important than the $MIC_{50}$.

Two methods are commonly used for susceptibility testing of organisms that grow in the presence of oxygen:

➤ Broth dilution (automated microdilution) method.
➤ Disk diffusion method.

Aerobic susceptibility testing methods have been standardized. Performance of these tests and interpretation of the results should conform to nationally recognized standards, such as those established by the National Committee for Clinical Laboratory Standards.[4,5]

## Automated Microdilution Method

For most laboratories, the broth dilution (macrodilution) method described previously is impractical. The time and labor necessary for preparing multiple dilutions of multiple antibiotics for each microorganism are prohibitive. Automated microdilution methods (e.g., Vitek and Microscan) have been developed that use a smaller quantity of broth (50 µL as opposed to 1–2 mL) and are easier to perform than macrodilution. However, some organisms (e.g., *Haemophilus influenzae*, *N. gonorrhoeae*, and *Streptococcus pneumoniae*) cannot be tested by an automated microdilution method. Their growth characteristics prohibit its use. Both the broth dilution and disk diffusion methods can be used for susceptibility testing, but the materials and interpretive criteria for the results differ from those used for rapidly growing aerobic pathogens (e.g., staphylococci, *E. coli*, and *P. aeruginosa*).

For automated microdilution, commercially available microtiter plates or cassettes (with as many as 96 wells containing serial dilutions of multiple antimicrobial agents) are inoculated with a standardized amount of aerobic, rapidly growing bacteria (Figure 2). After incubation, the MIC of the bacteria to various antimicrobial agents can be read directly from the plate by instruments that measure the turbidity of the wells. Some of these methods can supply susceptibility information within 4–6 hr. Automated microdilution is preferable to macrodilution methods in the clinical laboratory because of its

➤ Ease of use.
➤ Accuracy.
➤ Reproducibility.
➤ Cost.

Using broth dilution methods, the laboratory can report bacteria as susceptible (S), intermediate (I), or resistant (R) based on the MIC of the organism and the usual serum concentration of antibiotic.

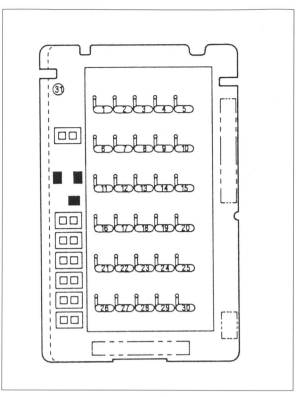

**FIGURE 2.** Example of a microtiter cassette used in automated systems that test for bacterial susceptibilities to various antimicrobials. (Reproduced, with permission, from Vitek Systems. Insert No. 012416-3. Hazelwood, MO: Vitek Systems, McDonnell Douglas; 1988.)

## Disk Diffusion Method

Before microdilution technology was developed, other methods were used to test an organism for susceptibility to numerous antimicrobial agents. The disk diffusion method described by Bauer and Kirby in 1966 is the basis for the disk diffusion technique commonly used today.[3]

Filter-paper disks impregnated with standard concentrations of antimicrobial agents are placed on an agar plate that has been inoculated with a standard concentration of bacteria (Figure 3, next page). The plate is incubated overnight. The bacteria multiply on the plate, and antibiotic diffuses out of the paper disk into the agar. Where the concentration of drug is high enough to inhibit bacterial growth, a clear zone of inhibition appears around the disk. The larger the zone, the more active the drug is at inhibiting bacterial growth.

For each antimicrobial agent, zone diameters have been ascertained that correspond to the MICs falling into S, I, and R ranges (based on usual achievable serum concentrations). For practical purposes, MICs cannot be determined with the disk diffusion method, but approximations can be made based on the size of the zone of inhibition.

The disk diffusion test is simple and easy to perform.

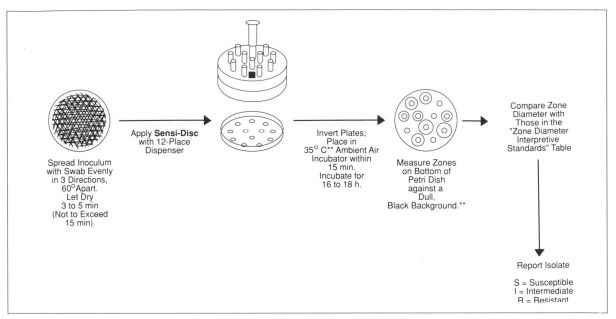

**FIGURE 3.** Typical susceptibility testing using the disk diffusion method. The diameter of the zones of growth inhibition around each disk is measured and compared with standards to determine the degree of susceptibility. **Additional steps may be performed for methicillin-resistant *S. aureus* isolates. (Adapted, with permission, from Power DA, McCuen PJ, eds. Manual of BBL products and laboratory procedures. Cockeysville, MD: Becton Dickinson Microbiology Systems; 1988:69.)

Compared to an automated microdilution method, disk diffusion also offers greater flexibility in the antibiotics selected for testing. Moreover, hospitals can individualize testing to correspond to the antibiotic formulary.

## Anaerobic Bacteria Tests

Anaerobic bacteria are often significant pathogens. Emerging resistance to antimicrobial agents is becoming a problem, especially *B. fragilis* sp. Antianaerobic activity of antimicrobial agents can vary widely within the same class of drugs. Therefore, the need for antimicrobial susceptibility testing of anaerobic organisms is increasing.[6]

Unfortunately, testing anaerobic organisms is technically more difficult and time consuming than testing rapidly growing aerobic organisms. Because of these limitations, clinical laboratories do not routinely test susceptibility of anaerobic isolates from patients. Antibiotic choices are frequently guided by the usual activity of an antibiotic against the isolated bacteria. This information is readily available in the medical literature. In certain clinical situations, susceptibility testing results are valuable in guiding therapy. These situations include[7]

> ➤ Known resistance of a particular organism.
> ➤ Failure of usual therapeutic regimens and persistence of the infection.
> ➤ A critical role of the antimicrobial agent in determining outcome.
> ➤ Severity of the infection.
> ➤ Long-term therapy required to treat the infection.

Examples of specific infections from which isolates should be tested include brain abscess, endocarditis, osteomyelitis, prosthetic device or vascular graft infections, and refractory or recurrent bacteremia.[7] More extensive discussion of anaerobic susceptibility testing may be found elsewhere.[7-9]

## E Test

The E test (AB Biodisk) is based on a combination of dilution and diffusion tests. Like MIC methods, the E test directly quantifies antimicrobial susceptibility in terms of discrete MIC values. The E test consists of a thin, plastic strip marked with an MIC reading scale on one side and with antibiotic impregnated on the other.[10] When the E strip is applied onto an inoculated agar plate, the antibiotic immediately diffuses into the agar and a continuous and exponential gradient of antibiotic concentrations forms underneath the carrier. After incubation, a symmetrical inhibition ellipse centered along the plastic strip is visible. The zone edge intersects the strip at the MIC value (in micrograms per milliliter) (Figures 4 and 5).

Although processed like a disk diffusion test, the E test differs by the use of a preformed and stable antibiotic concentration gradient. E test results correlate well with susceptibility results by other standard methods. The E test has the advantage of flexibility, similar to disk diffusion, because panels can be easily tailored to the needs of an institution.

Unfortunately, the E test is considerably more costly

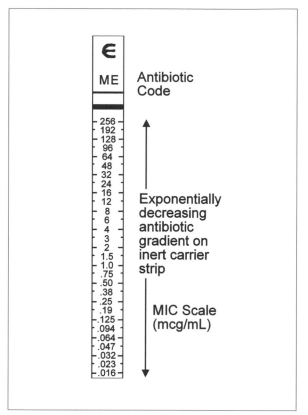

**FIGURE 4.** Diagram of E test strip and gradient.

MIC tests often require overnight incubation, a beta-lactamase test can be performed in minutes. Beta-lactamase tests can incorporate penicillin as a substrate along with an indicator system, which detects destruction of the beta-lactam ring by bacterial enzymes.[11] Nitrocefin, a chromogenic cephalosporin, changes color when its beta-lactam ring is hydrolyzed. Nitrocefin is commonly used to perform beta-lactamase tests.

A positive beta-lactamase test predicts resistance to penicillin, ampicillin, and amoxicillin among *Haemophilus* sp., *N. gonorrhoeae*, and *Moraxella catarrhalis*. For staphylococci and enterococci, a positive beta-lactamase test predicts resistance to penicillin, ampicillin, and extended-spectrum penicillins (e.g., ticarcillin, mezlocillin, and piperacillin).

Bacterial resistance to antimicrobial agents can be due to other mechanisms besides beta-lactamase. The beta-lactamase test should not be used to test enteric Gram-negative bacilli or *Pseudomonas* sp., because test results may not be predictive of susceptibility to the beta-lactam antibiotics often used for therapy.[4]

## Antimicrobial Drug Panels

Microbiology laboratories often limit the number of antimicrobial agents used for susceptibility testing to those expected to kill a particular organism. For example, when

than disk diffusion. It currently may be most suitable for use in susceptibility testing of fastidious organisms, such as *H. influenzae* and *S. pneumoniae*.[10,11] The E test may also be useful for susceptibility testing of anaerobic bacteria.[12]

The increased incidence of penicillin-resistant *S. pneumoniae* has led to a need for more intensive susceptibility testing of this organism when it is isolated from sterile body sites (e.g., blood and CSF). The E test can reliably detect penicillin or cephalosporin resistance. Additionally, the level of resistance is determined since an MIC is generated. This information serves as a valuable guide to proper antimicrobial therapy.[13]

## Beta-Lactamase Test

Many bacteria produce beta-lactamase enzymes that can inactivate numerous beta-lactam-containing antibiotics. While

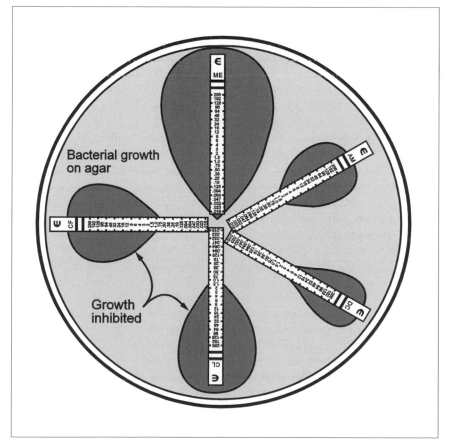

**FIGURE 5.** E test strips on agar showing inhibition of bacterial growth.

the antimicrobial susceptibility of Gram-negative bacilli (e.g., *E. coli*) is tested, it is impractical to test agents that have no appreciable activity against them (e.g., penicillin G, nafcillin, and vancomycin). Likewise, when the susceptibility of a Gram-positive coccus (e.g., *Staphylococcus aureus*) is tested, it is usually not practical to test drugs with limited antistaphylococcal activity (e.g., extended-spectrum penicillins and later-generation cephalosporins). Nevertheless, laboratories should comply with nationally recognized standards for the testing and reporting of antimicrobial susceptibility.

Table 4 illustrates some antimicrobial panels that are recommended for the susceptibility testing of various classes of bacteria.[4] These panels are based on the antimicrobial activity of the drugs, their clinical efficacy, prevalence of resistant organisms, cost, and current consensus recommendations for first- and second-choice agents.

In certain instances, susceptibility testing may be properly performed, yet its results do not reliably correlate with clinical efficacy. For example, cephalosporins, clindamycin, and trimethoprim–sulfamethoxazole should not be tested or reported against enterococci. Testing may indicate that the enterococcus is "susceptible," but these agents are clinically ineffective. Similarly, methicillin-resistant staphylococci may appear susceptible to drugs such as cephalosporins and beta-lactamase inhibitor combinations (e.g., ampicillin–sulbactam) based on in vitro susceptibility testing. However, methicillin-resistant staphylococci should be reported as resistant to these agents, regardless of the in vitro result, because clinical infections with methicillin-resistant staphylococci do not respond well to these drugs.

The previous examples demonstrate clinical selective reporting of susceptibility results. Another type of selective reporting takes drug pharmacokinetics into account. For instance, sulfisoxazole, nitrofurantoin, as well as norfloxacin (which are concentrated in the urine) susceptibilities should only be reported for urinary isolates, because these drugs rarely reach inhibitory concentrations at other sites.

Sometimes, reporting the susceptibility results of expensive, broad-spectrum antimicrobials may occur only when the organism is resistant to less expensive and/or narrower-spectrum agents. For example, if a Gram-negative bacillus such as *E. coli* is susceptible to cefazolin (a first-generation cephalosporin), susceptibility results for cefuroxime (a second-generation cephalosporin) and ceftriaxone (a third-generation cephalosporin) are not included on the susceptibility report. With this type of system, cefuroxime results are reported only if the organism is resistant to cefazolin. Ceftriaxone results are reported only if the organism is resistant to cefuroxime.

With *Pseudomonas* sp., if the organism is susceptible to gentamicin, tobramycin, and amikacin, results for tobramycin and amikacin are frequently not reported. The susceptibility results of the more expensive agents are reported only if the bacteria are resistant to gentamicin. If necessary, susceptibilities of nonreported antimicrobial agents can be obtained by contacting the microbiology department.

Laboratories, working in conjunction with hospital pharmacy departments and infectious disease specialists, have adopted these reporting procedures to prevent the prescribing of expensive antimicrobial agents when less expensive drugs should be effective. Pharmacy departments should take an active part in this decisionmaking process. Recommendations for selective reporting have been incorporated into Table 4.

## Serum Bactericidal Test (SBT)

The SBT measures the inhibitory and bactericidal activity of a patient's serum, during antimicrobial therapy, against the exact microorganism isolated from the patient.[14] The SBT is occasionally called a "Schlicter test," named after Schlicter and MacLean who used it in 1947 as an aid to determine effective therapy for endocarditis.

The SBT incorporates the interaction of the infecting microorganism, the antimicrobial agent(s), and the patient.[15] The SBT is a variation of the broth dilution test previously described. To perform the test, the infecting organism is inoculated into serial dilutions (Figure 6, page 356) of a sample of the patient's serum, collected while he or she is receiving antimicrobial therapy. Usually, a serum sample is obtained at the time of the expected peak antibiotic concentration. Occasionally, trough samples may be obtained just before the next dose of antibiotic.

Serum inhibitory and serum bactericidal titers are determined in the same manner as MICs and MBCs. In the case of the SBT, the result is expressed as a titer (e.g., 1:8 or 1:64). The patient's serum plus antibiotic can be diluted eight or 64 times (in these examples) and still kill the infecting organism. This test determines the susceptibility of the pathogen to an antibiotic and its metabolites as well as any synergistic or antagonistic effects of other drugs in the patient's serum. Theoretically, the combined effects of patient-specific absorption, distribution, metabolism, and elimination are also measured.

The SBT has been used to monitor antimicrobial therapy in patients with serious systemic infections such as endocarditis, osteomyelitis, and bacteremia (Minicase 1, page 356). Although useful in theory, this test raises controversy regarding its technical factors and clinical utility.[16] The most useful aspect is that it integrates serum concentration data (i.e., pharmacokinetics) with the MBC (i.e., pharmacodynamics) for a given organism. In addition, these tests have been used to detect additive or synergistic effects between antibiotic combinations.

The usefulness of the SBT as a predictor of successful therapy for serious infections remains controversial. Some studies have demonstrated that peak titers greater than 1:8 correlate with therapeutic efficacy. However, one

**TABLE 4.** Typical Antimicrobial Susceptibility Panels[a]

| Organism and Site | Antimicrobial Agents Used in Susceptibility Testing[b] |
|---|---|
| Gram-negative bacilli (not including *Pseudomonas* sp.) | |
| From blood and tissue | AMPICILLIN<br>CEFAZOLIN or CEPHALOTHIN<br>GENTAMICIN<br>mezlocillin or piperacillin<br>ticarcillin<br>amoxicillin–clavulanic acid or ampicillin–sulbactam<br>ticarcillin–clavulanic acid<br>cefotetan or cefoxitin<br>cefamandole, cefonicid, cefuroxime<br>cefotaxime, ceftizoxime, ceftriaxone<br>imipenem<br>amikacin<br>ciprofloxacin<br>trimethoprim–sulfamethoxazole |
| From urine | Same as above with: carbenicillin; cinoxacin; lomefloxacin, norfloxacin, ofloxacin; loracarbef; nitrofurantoin; sulfisoxazole; and trimethoprim–sulfamethoxazole |
| *Staphylococcus* sp. | |
| From blood and tissue | PENICILLIN<br>OXACILLIN or METHICILLIN<br>CEFAZOLIN or CEPHALOTHIN<br>amoxicillin–clavulanic acid or ampicillin–sulbactam<br>vancomycin<br>azithromycin, clarithromycin, erythromycin<br>trimethoprim–sulfamethoxazole |
| From urine | Same as above with: lomefloxacin or norfloxacin, nitrofurantoin, sulfisoxazole, and trimethoprim–sulfamethoxazole |
| *Pseudomonas* sp., *Acinetobacter* sp., *Xanthamonas maltophilia* | |
| From blood and tissue | MEZLOCILLIN or TICARCILLIN<br>PIPERACILLIN<br>GENTAMICIN<br>CEFTAZIDIME<br>ticarcillin–clavulanic acid<br>cefoperazone<br>aztreonam<br>imipenem<br>amikacin<br>tobramycin<br>ciprofloxacin<br>trimethoprim–sulfamethoxazole |
| From urine | Same as above with: carbenicillin; ceftizoxime; tetracycline; lomefloxacin, norfloxacin, ofloxacin; and sulfisoxazole |
| *Enterococcus* sp. | |
| From blood and urine | PENICILLIN or AMPICILLIN<br>vancomycin |
| From urine | Same as above with: ciprofloxacin, norfloxacin, nitrofurantoin, and tetracycline |

[a]*Adapted from Reference 4.*
[b]*Upper case—Antimicrobial agents recommended for routine testing and results reporting. Lower case—Antimicrobial agents recommended for routine testing but selective results reporting.*

multicenter trial in endocarditis patients found that peak titers greater than 1:64 were associated with bacteriologic cure. In this trial, the SBT was predictive of bacteriologic cure only—not of bacteriologic failure or clinical outcome.[17]

## TEST INTERPRETATION AND CLINICAL RELEVANCE

Susceptibility tests can predict bacteriological but not clinical outcome.[18] Numerous factors can affect the in-

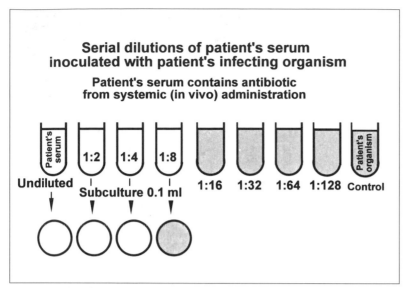

## Serial dilutions of patient's serum inoculated with patient's infecting organism

### Patient's serum contains antibiotic from systemic (in vivo) administration

**FIGURE 6.** This figure demonstrates the steps used in the serum bactericidal test (SBT). In this example, the serum inhibitory titer is 1:8 dilution and the serum bactericidal titer is 1:4.

terpretation of susceptibility testing results. Therefore, susceptibility tests are limited in predicting the success of antimicrobial therapy.

## Limitations

Antimicrobial therapy involves interactions among the host, the infecting bacteria, and the drug. Ideally, the drug will effectively eliminate the infecting organism and not cause toxicity to the host. These relationships are illustrated in Figure 7.

Interaction between the drug and host is determined by the pharmacokinetics of the drug—its absorption, distribution, metabolism, and excretion. Antibiotic serum

concentrations can be used to evaluate this interaction. Interaction between the host and infecting organism is represented by the serum bactericidal titer, a test that evaluates the host's immune system as it interacts with the infecting bacteria. The interaction between the infecting organism and the drug can be studied by several laboratory tests, including the antimicrobial susceptibility test, the MIC, and the MBC.

Susceptibility testing cannot adequately test all three of these associations simultaneously. As illustrated in Figure 7, susceptibility testing examines only one side of this triangle. This testing cannot reproduce in vivo conditions because host defense mechanisms, such as phagocytosis, are absent. No white cells (PMN leukocytes) are incorporated into these tests. Furthermore, the drug concentration is static during susceptibility testing, while in vivo the microorganism is exposed to varying drug concentrations over time. Finally, the number of bacteria used for susceptibility tests (inoculum size) is not always the same as in actual clinical infections.[18]

## Antimicrobial Dosage and Achievable Serum Concentration

As stated previously, bacteria are classified as S, I, or R based on zone size or MIC in relation to readily achievable serum concentrations of the agent tested following usual doses.[19] An organism is considered "susceptible" (S)

---

### ✎ Minicase 1

An intravenous (IV) drug user, Martin B., was admitted to the hospital with fevers as high as 103 °F (39.4 °C); a WBC count of 18,200 cells/mm³ (4800–10,800 cells/mm³) with 85% polymorphonuclear (PMN) leukocytes (45–73%), 10% bands (3–5%), and 5% lymphs (20–40%); and a faint heart murmur. Blood, urine, and sputum cultures were obtained. Two blood cultures grew *S. aureus* that was susceptible to nafcillin, cefazolin, vancomycin, clindamycin, and trimethoprim–sulfamethoxazole and resistant to penicillin. Urine and sputum cultures were negative.

Martin B. was being treated for presumptive endocarditis due to *S. aureus* with nafcillin 2 g IV every 6 hr. Each dose of nafcillin was infused over 30–45 min (via gravity); doses were administered at 6 a.m., noon, 6 p.m., and midnight.

After 6 days, Martin B. felt well, his temperature was 98.8 °F (37.1 °C), and his WBC count was 8000. The physician ordered a serum bactericidal titer. The sample, obtained at 10 a.m., had a titer of 1:4. The physician wanted to increase the nafcillin to 3 g IV every 4 hr to achieve a peak titer of at least 1:8.

*What is an appropriate response to this proposed change?*

**Discussion:** The serum sample for the titer was obtained at an inappropriate time, leading to a falsely low result. Serum samples should be obtained at the time of peak serum concentration of the antimicrobial agent. In this case, the SBT should be obtained shortly after the nafcillin infusion is complete (approximately 7 a.m.), but it was obtained 3 hr later. This minicase illustrates the need to understand the conditions under which laboratory tests are obtained so that results can be properly interpreted.

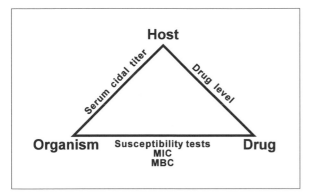

**FIGURE 7.** The triad of host, drug, and organism depicting the tests that can be applied to evaluate interacting components. Susceptibility tests alone, however, do not adequately describe these interactions. (Adapted, with permission, from Reference 18.)

if it is inhibited by serum drug concentrations that can be achieved using usual doses of the drug. This definition implies that an infection caused by the tested bacteria may be appropriately treated with the dosage of antimicrobial agent recommended for that type of infection and bacteria, unless otherwise contraindicated.[4]

An organism is considered "intermediate" (I) if it is inhibited by the maximal attainable concentration of the drug, such as the serum concentrations achieved with high doses of penicillins or cephalosporins or the urine concentration of drugs excreted unchanged by that route (e.g., quinolones and beta-lactams). The intermediate category includes isolates with antimicrobial agent MICs that approach usually attainable blood and tissue concentrations. Response rates for these bacteria may be lower than for susceptible strains.[4]

An organism is considered "resistant" (R) if it is not inhibited by the drug concentrations achieved in blood when usual doses are administered.

Many antimicrobial agents are effective in treating systemic infections if given orally, because achievable serum concentrations following oral administration are adequate to inhibit bacteria. Some agents are ineffective orally due to poor absorption, such as vancomycin and carbenicillin (oral carbenicillin is effective only for urinary tract infections). Organisms may be reported as "susceptible" to these antimicrobial agents, but that interpretation is based on serum concentrations following parenteral administration (Minicase 2).

As alluded to previously, both the site of infection and the ability of the antimicrobial agent to reach that site influence the interpretation of susceptibility results. For infections of the central nervous system (CNS), the ability of the antimicrobial agent to achieve adequate concentrations in CSF is crucial to the success of therapy. For example, a soft tissue infection caused by a cefazolin-susceptible *S. aureus* could be treated with cefazolin. However, cefazolin would be ineffective for treating this

## Minicase 2

A pediatrician called the pharmacist regarding a 6-year-old boy, Matthew P., with an infected puncture wound of the foot. Matthew P. stepped on a nail 5 days ago; the sole of his foot now showed an obvious puncture wound. The surrounding tissue was red and swollen. The wound itself was draining purulent material. Matthew P. had a low-grade fever of 100.5 °F (38 °C) and an elevated white count (15,000 WBC count with 80% PMN leukocytes and 10% bands).

A Gram stain of the foot drainage revealed numerous WBCs with many Gram-negative rods. When a sample of the drainage was cultured, it yielded heavy growth of *P. aeruginosa* (susceptible to carbenicillin, ticarcillin, gentamicin, ceftazidime, ciprofloxacin, and imipenem). A bone scan of the foot was negative for osteomyelitis, and surgical debridement was performed. Surgical cultures also grew *P. aeruginosa*. The pediatrician wanted to treat Matthew P. with oral antibiotics.

*What is an appropriate recommendation?*

**Discussion:** Only two of the listed antimicrobial agents are available in oral form: carbenicillin (useful only for urinary tract infections) and ciprofloxacin (not recommended for young children). Unfortunately, Matthew P. needs to be treated with a parenteral drug. Of the available products, ceftazidime is probably the most cost effective and convenient for administration in the home setting by a home IV therapy provider. Gentamicin and tobramycin, while inexpensive, require frequent renal function and drug serum concentration monitoring because of the potential for nephrotoxicity.

Imipenem is the most costly choice and offers an extended spectrum of antimicrobial activity that is not necessary for Matthew P. Ceftazidime is more costly than oral therapy but is well tolerated, does not require serum drug concentration monitoring, can be safely administered in the home environment in three daily doses, and is highly effective against pseudomonal infections.

This child should be treated until the infection and surrounding cellulitis have healed; he may require 7–10 days of therapy.

This case illustrates that a practitioner cannot solely depend on culture and susceptibility results for therapy decisions. Patient factors (in this case, age and severity of infection) and drug pharmacokinetics and toxicities must also be considered.

same organism if it had come from the CSF, because so little cefazolin enters the CSF.

Likewise, for urinary tract infections, the urinary concentration of the agent rather than its serum concentration is important. Sometimes, uncomplicated urinary tract infections with reportedly resistant bacteria can be treated with antimicrobial agents, to which they are normally resistant, because many drugs (e.g., penicillins, cephalosporins, and aminoglycosides) are concentrated in the urine.

## Factors to Consider

The affinity of a drug for binding to proteins is one characteristic that affects its distribution. The extent of protein binding of an antimicrobial agent may adversely affect the drug's ability to exert its antimicrobial effect. Clinical failures experienced while treating patients with highly protein-bound drugs such as cefonicid (>90% protein bound) may have resulted from low serum concentrations of unbound (microbiologically active) drug. Serum concentrations of antimicrobial agents include both bound and unbound drug. In contrast, MIC determinations and disk susceptibility testing procedures do not consider protein binding.

The underlying condition of host defenses must also be considered (Minicase 3). For example, a neutropenic cancer patient may not respond adequately to an appropriate antimicrobial regimen because of a lack of WBCs. Due to their immunosuppressive effects, corticosteroids may also interfere with drug therapy. In such cases, the clinician should choose a highly bactericidal antibiotic so that dependence on host factors for killing bacteria is minimal. Patients with severe underlying diseases also respond more poorly to antibiotic therapy due to relative immuno-incompetence.

Several other factors are useful when applying susceptibility results to patient care. Antimicrobial therapy alone is frequently ineffective when treating undrained abscesses. Likewise, infection in the presence of a foreign body (e.g., central venous catheter, heart valve, or hip prosthesis) is difficult or impossible to cure. Appropriate surgical intervention (e.g., drainage of abscess or removal of prosthetic device), in conjunction with antimicrobial therapy, is often necessary.

## Antimicrobial Agent Combinations

As discussed in Minicase 4, combinations of antimicrobial agents can be prescribed for a patient to

➢ Expand the spectrum of antimicrobial activity.
➢ Minimize the development of resistant strains of microorganisms.
➢ Produce a synergistic effect (greater than the sum of the effects of the individual agents).

Methods used to test antimicrobial combinations are not available in many hospital laboratories. Discussion of the various methods used to test antimicrobial combinations can be found in References 20 and 21.

---

### ✎ Minicase 3

A 16-year-old, 6-ft-tall male with Hodgkin's disease, Randy M., developed a fever and shaking chills at home 10 days after his first chemotherapy treatment. His family took him to the emergency room. He had a temperature of 104 °F (40 °C) and a WBC count of 200 cells/mm³ (4800–10,800 cells/mm³) with 20% PMN leukocytes (45–73%), 0% bands (3–5%), and 80% lymphs (20–40%). His physical exam showed no obvious site of infection.

The two blood cultures that were obtained both grew *Serratia marcescens*, which is susceptible to piperacillin, ceftriaxone, gentamicin, trimethoprim–sulfamethoxazole, imipenem, and ticarcillin–clavulanate. Randy M.'s renal function was good—his serum creatinine was stable at 0.8 mg/dL (0.7–1.5 mg/dL).

The physician prescribed trimethoprim–sulfamethoxazole 10 mL IV every 12 hr. After 4 days, Randy M. was still spiking fevers to 103 °F (39.4 °C). His WBC count was only 1000 cells with 50% PMN leukocytes, 30% bands, and 20% lymphs.

*Why is this patient responding so poorly to the trimethoprim–sulfamethoxazole when the drug was shown to be active against the pathogen on susceptibility testing?*

**Discussion:** Again, this case illustrates that culture and susceptibility results cannot be interpreted in isolation. Randy M. is seriously ill with Gram-negative bacillary bacteremia. Several theories may explain his lack of response:

1. The dose of antimicrobial agent is inadequate. The dosage prescribed, given this patient's body size,

type of infection, organism, and renal function, is low and could be increased substantially.
2. The patient's immune system is depressed. The fact that *S. marcescens* was isolated (an opportunist) is evidence of a depressed immune system. Combination therapy with the addition of another antibiotic may help to compensate for his severely depressed immune system. Optimally dosed aminoglycosides plus aggressive doses of trimethoprim–sulfamethoxazole could be considered.
3. Resistant organisms may have emerged or superinfection may have developed. Repeat blood, urine, and sputum cultures should be obtained in a search for new causes of fever (e.g., nosocomial pneumonia and IV site infection). Strong consideration should be given to broadening the spectrum of therapy to include *Pseudomonas* sp. and anaerobes, as neither is covered by trimethoprim–sulfamethoxazole. Empiric antifungal therapy can also be considered.
4. A pocket of infection, such as an undrained abscess, may exist. Although Randy M. did not have obvious signs of this infection, examination of his abdomen with appropriate physical and radiological tests (if necessary) should be done.
5. The continuance of neutropenia is a problem. Evidence suggests that the patient's bone marrow is recovering from chemotherapy (second WBC is improved). He may respond better as his WBC count continues to improve.

A hospital was under increasing pressure to cut costs. Since antimicrobial agents were a significant portion of annual hospital drug costs, the administrator was looking closely at this area. He asked why less costly agents were not recommended in the following two cases.

Case 1. A 29-year-old woman with appendicitis and perforation was growing an *E. coli* susceptible to cefazolin from her intraoperative cultures. The surgeon prescribed cefotetan 1 g IV every 12 hr, which was more costly than cefazolin.

*Why not switch to cefazolin since it is less expensive and the culture report showed that the drug would be effective?*

Case 2. A 17-year-old patient, admitted with pneumococcal meningitis, was being treated with ceftriaxone.

*Why not use cefazolin since the organism was reported to be susceptible to penicillin, cefuroxime, and cefazolin?*

**Discussion:** In the first case, cefazolin, while adequate for the *E. coli*, will not provide proper coverage for intra-abdominal anaerobic organisms. No anaerobes grew on culture, but that result may be because of technical errors in obtaining the culture or performing the tests in the laboratory. Since normal bowel flora contains a high concentration of anaerobic organisms (including *B. fragilis*) and since the patient had perforated appendicitis, a drug with good activity against intra-abdominal anaerobes should be part of the regimen. A combination, such as cefazolin (to cover the *E. coli*) and metronidazole (to cover anaerobic organisms), could be considered as an alternative. However, cefazolin alone is inadequate. This case demonstrates the importance of knowing the most likely organisms that can infect a specific site.

In the second case, antibiotic choices are restricted because of the site of infection. Not all antimicrobial agents attain CSF concentrations adequate for the treatment of meningitis. Cefazolin does not penetrate into the CSF to any appreciable extent. In high doses, penicillin or cefuroxime could be considered as ceftriaxone alternatives. This case illustrates the importance of knowing the site of infection and basic pharmacokinetic characteristics of antimicrobial agents.

## TESTS TO DIAGNOSE SPECIFIC INFECTIOUS DISEASES

### Mycobacteria

Numerous pathogenic mycobacteria exist. The most common are *Mycobacterium tuberculosis* and *Mycobacterium avium complex* (MAC), which includes *Mycobacterium avium* and *Mycobacterium intracellularae*.[22] In the past, there were hopes of eradicating TB in the United States. Unfortunately, there is a resurgence of TB in the United States and multidrug-resistant TB is also a growing problem. MAC commonly infects individuals with AIDS, leading to significant morbidity and mortality.

Mycobacteria grow slowly compared to conventional bacteria. They require specialized growth media, identification techniques, and susceptibility testing techniques unavailable in the average clinical laboratory.

Unlike conventional bacteria, mycobacteria are poorly visualized with a Gram's stain. Specialized stains, which can be performed by most clinical laboratories, improve visualization.[23] A relatively large concentration of organisms must be present in the specimen (usually sputum) to be seen with light microscopy. Concentrated sputum samples can increase the ability to detect mycobacteria, but they are unavailable in many laboratories.

Absence of bacteria on a smear (smear-negative specimen) does not rule out the presence of mycobacteria. Organisms may be present in concentrations too low to be reliably visualized by light microscopy. Staining techniques do not allow determinations of the (1) type of mycobacteria seen and (2) viability or nonviability of organisms.[23] These determinations require culturing of the specimen.

### *BACTEC System*

The conventional mycobacterial culturing technique takes 4 weeks, with several additional weeks for susceptibility testing.[24] Several newer systems speed up this process. With the BACTEC system, organisms growing in liquid media liberate $^{14}CO_2$ from a radiolabeled substrate.[22] The $^{14}CO_2$ is detected by the BACTEC instrument and translated into a "growth index." When the growth index is high enough, samples are examined for mycobacteria.[22] If the stain is positive (mycobacteria are present), the medium can be subcultured and/or concentrated for susceptibility testing and other studies. Compared to conventional techniques, the BACTEC system has reduced culturing time by 2 weeks.

### *Septi-Check AFB System*

The Septi-Check AFB system is a different, newly developed culture system.[22] A bottle of liquid culture medium is attached to a paddle containing three types of solid media. The apparatus is regularly tipped so the media is repeatedly inoculated. When growth is detected, samples are removed for further testing. While more rapid than conventional techniques, Septi-Check AFB is not as rapid as the BACTEC system.

### *Susceptibility Testing*

The conventional susceptibility testing method for *M. tuberculosis* is known as the proportion method. Testing can be performed using (1) a clinical specimen containing mycobacteria ("direct" susceptibility testing) or (2) mycobacteria grown in culture media (e.g., BACTEC, Septi-Check AFB, and conventional cultures).[22] Once the proportion method is set up, it requires 2–3 weeks.

Susceptibility testing using the radiometric BACTEC system has several advantages compared to the proportion method. The BACTEC system requires 1 week compared to 2 or 3 weeks for the proportion method. Additionally, the BACTEC system can generate an actual MIC while the proportion method cannot.[23] MIC information can (1) be linked with patient serum concentration data to determine the potency of an agent in the patient's drug regimen and (2) be useful for adjusting dosages to maximize the therapeutic response.

Susceptibility testing methods for MAC have been adapted directly from TB testing methods. However, these methods have not been validated for MAC, so no correlation exists between in vitro susceptibility results and clinical efficacy.[25,26] Rapid identification and susceptibility testing are areas of active investigation; numerous new techniques are being studied.[22,26–28]

## Meningitis

When a patient is suspected of having an infectious disease involving the CNS, CSF is frequently obtained to aid the diagnosis. Several tests are routinely ordered on CSF including Gram stain and bacterial culture, WBC count and differential, and glucose and protein measurements.[29] Table 5 includes the usual results of these tests for several types of meningitis.

### Gram's Stain

The stain is usually positive (bacteria are detected) in bacterial meningitis. However, the stain is often negative in cases of partially treated meningitis. In this situation, the patient has already received some antibiotics that have killed enough of the organisms to render the Gram's stain negative but not enough to treat the infection fully. A Gram's stain is also negative in nonbacterial (e.g., viral) meningitis. A positive Gram's stain is helpful with regard to selecting empiric therapy.

### Latex Agglutination (LA)

Special studies can be performed on the CSF to detect bacterial antigens. These studies include[30]

➤ Counterimmunoelectrophoresis.
➤ Coagglutination.
➤ Latex agglutination.

LA tests are among the most useful, especially when previous antimicrobial therapy has been given. They can detect various infectious diseases more rapidly than routine culturing of the sample.

To perform the test, latex particles coated with antibody (or antigen) are mixed with the specimen to be tested (Chapter 2). The specimen in this case is CSF, but it could also be serum or urine. If the clinical sample contains antigens that react with the antibody, cross-linkages between antigen and antibody form, causing a visible clumping (agglutination) of the latex particles.[31] If visible agglutination does not occur, either the antigen tested for is not present or it is present in amounts too small to cause agglutination.

LA tests are generally specific for the antigens of *S. pneumoniae* and many types of *Neisseria meningitidis*, the two most frequent causes of bacterial meningitis in adults. The LA test can also detect the antigens of *H. influenzae* (a common cause of meningitis in young children) and Group B streptococci (a common cause of meningitis in children less than 1 month old). Moreover, the LA test can detect antigens of *Cryptococcus neoformans*, a fungus that frequently causes meningitis in AIDS patients and other immunosuppressed individuals.[29]

If the Gram's stain is negative but the LA test for a specific bacterial or fungal antigen is positive, the clinician has some immediate information about the probable pathogen and the type of antimicrobial coverage to give the patient pending final CSF culture and susceptibility results. Because morbidity and mortality can occur quickly in acute CNS infections, it is important to make a diagnosis and to institute appropriate antibiotic therapy rapidly. Presumptive therapy must be started. Gram's stains and antigen detection tests are valuable because they yield results quickly.

## Viruses

Diagnostic techniques for viral infections are becoming increasingly important. Patients immunosuppressed due

**TABLE 5.** Composition of CSF[a]

| Source (Adults) | CSF Laboratory Value | | |
| --- | --- | --- | --- |
| | Protein (mg/dL) | Glucose (mg/dL) | WBC (per mm³) |
| Healthy | 15–50 | 40–80 | 0–10 |
| Bacterial meningitis | >100 | <40[b] | >1000 (mostly PMN leukocytes) |
| Fungal meningitis | Increased | <30 | Increased (mostly lymphocytes) |
| Viral meningitis | <100 | Normal | <500 (PMN leukocytes early in course and lymphocytes late) |

[a]Adapted from Reference 30.
[b]Less than 50% of a simultaneous serum sample.

to organ transplantation, cancer chemotherapy, or HIV are at increased risk of infection from numerous viruses. These viruses can lead to significant morbidity and/or mortality.

Viral detection can be useful in patient management, epidemiologic monitoring, and education of clinicians and patients. Viral detection can also better define the disease process and patient prognosis.[32]

Three techniques are useful in the diagnosis of viral infections. However, they are sometimes unavailable in the hospital laboratory and must be obtained from reference laboratories. The techniques include

> ➤ Viral culture.
> ➤ Antigen detection.
> ➤ Serologic testing.

### Viral Culture

Because viruses require living cells to support their replication, cell cultures are necessary for viral culture. Clinical specimens are inoculated on to a bed of living cells. The cell culture is examined for cytopathic effect (an observable change that occurs in cells as a result of viral replication). The nature of this effect helps the virologist to identify the suspected virus.

Different cell types can be used to culture different viruses, just as different types of media can be used for the growth of different types of bacteria. Traditional cell culturing techniques require a week or more to yield a result. A rapid cell culture technique, known as the shell vial assay, can yield results in only 24–48 hr.

Shell vial assays are useful in the identification of viruses such as cytomegalovirus (CMV), herpes simplex virus (HSV), and varicella zoster.[33] These viruses grow well in cell cultures.

### Antigen Detection

When clinical specimens contain high concentrations of viruses, antigen detection methods may be useful. Additionally, for viruses that do not grow well in cell cultures, other diagnostic techniques must be used.[33] Fluorescence or enzyme immunoassays are useful for the detection of viral antigens of respiratory syncytial virus, a virus that may not replicate in usual cell cultures. HSV can also be detected by these methods. In just a few hours, results from immunoassays can be obtained.

### Serologic Testing

Serologic tests are useful for the diagnosis of infections from viruses that do not replicate well in cell culture. These tests are also useful for viruses for which no reagents or techniques have been developed to identify them directly from a clinical specimen (antigen detection).[33] Examples of these viruses include Epstein–Barr, rubella, measles, hepatitis, and HIV.

Traditional serologic tests allow for detection of disease by collecting serum during the illness (acute) and after the illness (convalescent) and by comparing the antibody titers to the suspected virus in each sample. A rise in immunoglobulin G (IgG) antibody titer to the suspected virus—from the acute to the convalescent samples—suggests that the patient was infected with that virus. Traditional viral serology, by its nature, gives the diagnosis in retrospect. Acute and convalescent serum samples are generally separated by 2–3 weeks. By the time the results are obtained, the patient has usually recovered from the illness.

Currently, only a single (acute) serum sample is usually collected and examined for an increase in immunoglobulin M (IgM) antibody to the suspected virus. IgM antibody titers increase sooner than IgG antibody titers, so an increase in IgM indicates recent viral infection.[33] Use of a single serum specimen, rather than paired acute and convalescent specimens, increases the speed with which viral infections can be detected. This increase in speed makes serology more useful in patient management.

## Human Immunodeficiency Virus

In the past, HIV was referred to as the human T-cell lymphotropic virus type III (HTLV-III) or the lymphadenopathy-associated virus (LAV). HIV is the causal agent of AIDS. This disease can be transmitted[34]

> ➤ By sexual contact.
> ➤ By use of contaminated needles.
> ➤ By injection of infected blood or blood products.
> ➤ Through the placenta linking mother to fetus.

These routes of transmission seem to explain why the groups at greatest risk for contracting the disease in the United States are homosexual and bisexual men, IV drug abusers, hemophiliacs, and infants of infected mothers.[35] However, heterosexual transmission is now becoming a more commonly reported mode of infection.

A period of viremia, without detectable antibodies, occurs within 4–6 weeks after infection with HIV.[36] During this initial period, HIV can be cultured from plasma, and antigen corresponding to viral core protein (p24 antigen) can also be detected in plasma. Seroconversion, the production of antibodies to HIV in quantities sufficient for detection, occurs usually within 2–12 months (Minicase 5, next page). Within 6 months, most patients seroconvert[36] (Figure 8, next page).

### Enzyme-Linked Immunosorbent Assay (ELISA)

Antibody to HIV can be detected by an ELISA assay that is quite sensitive. In 1985, this assay was developed to screen donated blood and blood products. ELISA is the most common screening test used for HIV because it is inexpensive, reliable, standardized, and quick.[36]

If the HIV ELISA is negative, the result is reported as "nonreactive." If the result is "reactive," the test is repeated. If the result is still reactive, a more specific test is required to verify the result. This test can be either the Western blot or an indirect immunofluorescence assay.[37]

Although the ELISA is highly sensitive and specific, false-positive and false-negative results can occur. In a population at low risk for HIV, where the prevalence of HIV is 0.01% or less, a reactive test is more likely to be a false positive than a true positive. Conversely, in high-risk groups where the prevalence of HIV is high, a reactive test is more likely to be a true positive.[37]

False-positive ELISAs have been detected in patients with hematologic malignancies, autoimmune diseases [systemic lupus erythematosus (SLE)], multiple myeloma, alcoholic hepatitis, or positive rapid plasma reagin (RPR).[36–38] Human or technical errors in performing the test can also result in false-positive results. Antibodies to proteins of other viruses can cross-react with the ELISA, resulting in false positives in some patients administered influenza and hepatitis B vaccine.

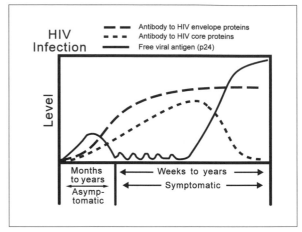

**FIGURE 8.** Basic time frame of antigen detection and antibody production following HIV infection. (Adapted, with permission, from Pizzo PA, Wilfert CM. Pediatric AIDS. Baltimore, MD: Williams & Wilkins; 1991:161.)

Babies of HIV-positive mothers receive maternal IgG antibodies to HIV through placenta transfer. These antibodies last for many months, making ELISAs unreliable for testing infants less than 15 months of age. Therefore, other diagnostic methods are being investigated to identify HIV-infected infants at a younger age.[39]

False-negative ELISAs can occur in truly infected patients early in the course of their disease, prior to seroconversion. Immunosuppressed patients, even in the late stages of AIDS, can also have false-negative ELISAs.[36]

### Western Blot

The Western blot for HIV detects antibodies to individual HIV proteins and glycoproteins that have been electrophoretically separated, according to their molecular weights, and transferred to strips of nitrocellulose paper.[37] These strips are incubated with the patient's serum. If antibodies to the HIV proteins are present, they bind to the paper and can be seen as colored bands. The spectrum of bands is used to interpret the test result; however, there is no agreement on a standardized interpretation of the bands. Interpretation guidelines within package inserts and labeling of the licensed tests are not uniform.

False-negative Western blots or indeterminate results can occur if the serum sample is collected prior to complete seroconversion. Western blots should not be used as screening tests but should be reserved to confirm repeatedly reactive ELISAs. Studies of blood donors with no HIV risk factors and nonreactive ELISAs showed that 20–40% may have an indeterminate Western blot.[37]

Detection of anti-HIV antibodies by ELISA and Western blot techniques cannot be interpreted as "positive AIDS" tests. AIDS is a diagnosis based on clinical and laboratory data in addition to positive serologic tests. HIV antibody tests are also useful in detecting and removing potentially infectious blood from the blood supply.

### Minicase 5

Renee N., a recent graduate from nursing school, was working in a university teaching hospital in New York City. Last week, while she performed an arterial puncture to obtain an arterial blood gas, the patient moved and Renee N. was scratched with the bloody needle used to obtain the specimen. The patient had AIDS and was admitted with recurrent pneumonia. Therefore, the employee health clinic advised Renee N. to submit a blood sample immediately and to return at regular intervals during the next 6 months for additional samples. These samples would be checked for HIV.

Renee N. was relieved because the blood sample she submitted on the day of exposure was negative. She felt that she did not get "AIDS" from the patient and did not understand why further testing was recommended.

*What is an appropriate answer?*

**Discussion:** The laboratory is performing an ELISA to detect the presence of anti-HIV antibodies in Renee N.'s blood. A negative test on the first sample serves as a baseline only. If Renee N. does not engage in behavior that puts her at risk for HIV (other than the risks entailed in her job performance), any change in the test results over the next 6 months will be attributed to her hospital exposure. Subsequent tests are required because, if Renee N. was infected with HIV at the time of the exposure, it would take several weeks to months for her immune system to produce anti-HIV antibody detectable by the ELISA.

If Renee N. seroconverts, she will have HIV but not "AIDS." The diagnosis of AIDS is a clinical one. Renee N. should be encouraged to return to the employee health clinic for an explanation of these matters and related issues.

## Mycoplasma

Mycoplasmas are the smallest, free living organisms. They lack a cell wall, so they are not true bacteria; they can grow on cell-free media, so they are not true viruses.[40] *Mycoplasma pneumoniae* is clinically the most important mycoplasma causing human infections. Techniques for culturing this organism are not widely available. Additionally, these organisms grow so slowly that often 10–14 days are required for culture results—approximately the length of time required for serologic testing.[41] Therefore, serologic tests are the most widely used methods for diagnosis. Detection of cold hemagglutinin, a common serologic test, is useful in diagnosing this infection.[41]

### Cold Hemagglutinin

Cold hemagglutinin is an antibody that reacts to an antigen on red blood cells. The antibody is best detected at 39.2 °F (4 °C). It usually develops by the second week of the illness and is positive in as many as 50% of patients with *Mycoplasma* infection.[41] Hemagglutinin is more commonly detected in seriously ill patients; they are more likely to be hospitalized and require a specific diagnosis.

The cold hemagglutinin test can be performed at the patient's bedside. A blood sample is mixed with an anticoagulant and immersed in ice for several minutes. If cold hemagglutinin is present, it usually is visible both macroscopically and microscopically. Warming the blood to 98.6 °F (37 °C) results in disappearance of hemagglutination.[41] Unfortunately, many other respiratory infections may cause a positive cold hemagglutination reaction. However, most cases with titers greater than or equal to 1:128 are caused by *M. pneumoniae*.[41]

### Complement Fixation

Another serologic test is complement fixation. This test measures antibody titers to *M. pneumoniae*. A fourfold rise in titer between acute and convalescent sera is diagnostic of a recent infection.

## Lyme Disease

Lyme disease is due to infection from the spirochete *Borrelia burgdorferi*, leading to numerous signs and symptoms. Diagnosis of this disease is based on the clinical profile as well as evidence of an antibody response to the spirochete.[42] Infection can rarely be proven because the affected tissues contain so few spirochetes that their identification with histologic staining is difficult. Moreover, the organism is not easily grown in the laboratory (unlike many other bacteria).[43]

After infection, the patient typically mounts an antibody response in which IgM can be detected 2–4 weeks after the onset of skin rash (known as erythema migrans), peaks at 6–8 weeks, and declines to the normal range over 4–6 months. IgG antibody becomes elevated by 6–8 weeks, peaks at 4–6 months, and often remains elevated for many months.[43,44]

### Enzyme-Linked Immunosorbent Assay

The most common method used to detect both IgM and IgG antibodies is the ELISA. Unfortunately, the exact ELISA methods for Lyme disease have not been standardized, so wide interlaboratory variations can exist on identical serum samples. Since IgM antibodies cannot be detected until 2–4 weeks after the onset of the illness and IgG antibodies cannot be detected until 6–8 weeks, testing serum too soon in the patient's clinical course leads to false-negative results. False-positive results can be detected in patients with illnesses, such as infectious mononucleosis, rheumatoid arthritis, SLE, bacterial endocarditis, and other spirochetal infections (e.g., periodontal disease).[43,44]

### Western Blot

Western blot testing may be useful in separating false- from true-positive ELISA results.[43] The test can detect antibodies in the patient's serum that are specifically reactive to proteins found in the *B. burgdorferi* spirochete. However, the Western blot test may not be positive until several months after illness.[43]

Even if the patient has serologic evidence (a positive ELISA for IgM or IgG antibodies or a positive Western blot), it indicates only that the patient was previously exposed to the spirochete, not that the patient is currently suffering from Lyme disease. Serologic tests should only be ordered when the patient's signs and symptoms suggest Lyme disease. In this situation, a positive test result can be used to confirm the diagnosis.[43]

Despite the use of these criteria, numerous patients can still be misdiagnosed.[42] In a recent review of patients referred to a clinic, only 23% had active Lyme disease. Twenty percent had previous Lyme disease (positive serologic tests) with another current illness, and the remaining 57% did not have Lyme disease. Of the patients who did not have the disease, 45% presented to the clinic with at least one positive serologic test. None of these patients was seropositive when tested by the clinic laboratory.

The clinician should be cautious in interpreting the results of serologic tests and should always correlate test results with the patient's clinical profile.

## Fungal Infections

Patients who are immunosuppressed, receive broad-spectrum antibiotics, or have intravascular catheters in place are at risk for invasive fungal infections.[45] In these patients, fungal infections can lead to devastating complications and increased mortality. Use of blood culturing techniques is the primary method of diagnosing invasive fungal infections. Commercially available systems can be used to culture fungus. However, positive culture results often take longer to develop for fungal isolates (2–10 days, depending on the specific fungus) than for bacteria (1–2 days). Common fungi include *Candida albicans* and other *Candida* sp., *Aspergillus* sp., *Torulopsis* sp., and *Histoplasma* sp.

## Sexually Transmitted Diseases (STDs)

More than a dozen diseases can be transmitted sexually. However, only gonorrhea, syphilis, and chlamydial infections are discussed in this section. Hepatitis B, which can be transmitted sexually, is discussed in Chapter 11.

### Gonorrhea

*N. gonorrhoeae* can cause various infections,[46] including localized, uncomplicated genital infections and pharyngeal and anorectal infections in both men and women. Approximately 10–20% of women with untreated genital gonococcal infection develop ascending infection leading to pelvic inflammatory disease. Occasionally, disseminated gonococcal infection occurs with bacteremia, fever, septic arthritis, and rash (gonococcal–dermatitis–arthritis syndrome). Coinfection with other STDs, such as syphilis and *Chlamydia trachomatis*, is not uncommon. Diagnosis and treatment of coinfection with chlamydia and treatment of sexual partners are important considerations in the control of STDs.

The diagnosis of uncomplicated genital infections is usually made by culture of urethral or cervical discharge with subsequent isolation of *N. gonorrhoeae*. Gram's staining of clinical specimens, if positive for Gram-negative cocci in association with neutrophils, can be helpful; if negative, infection is not ruled out.

Cultures should be performed on all patients with suspected gonococcal infections and their sexual partners. Susceptibility testing of gonococci should be performed for epidemiological purposes. Patients are treated prior to the availability of susceptibility results. In the past, gonococci were almost universally susceptible to penicillin, and procaine penicillin was the preferred treatment. Currently, the incidence of beta-lactamase-producing, penicillin-resistant gonococci is such that treatment regimens consist of drugs active against these isolates. These drugs include ceftriaxone, oral ciprofloxacin, ofloxacin, and cefixime.[47]

### Syphilis

The STD commonly known as syphilis is caused by the spirochete *Treponema pallidum*. Syphilis is a complex disease, with its natural course arbitrarily categorized as follows:[48]

1. Incubation.
2. Primary stage (characterized by a nonpainful skin lesion also known as a chancre).
3. Secondary stage (with generalized mucocutaneous lesions often involving palms or soles of feet).
4. Latent stage (subclinical infection detected only

by serologic tests).
5. Late/tertiary stage (occurs in a few untreated patients as a progressive disease usually involving the ascending aorta and/or CNS).

Unlike bacteria, the spirochete cannot be grown in the laboratory. Therefore, the diagnosis of syphilis depends on direct identification of the spirochete in specimens obtained from lesions, or serologic studies. Darkfield inspection of fluid from skin lesions enables the examiner to see the spirochetes under the microscope. Exudate from suspected syphilitic lesions is examined under a microscope with a darkfield condenser.[49] *T. pallidum* can be visualized as corkscrew-shaped organisms.

To perform the direct fluorescent antibody test, the specimen is incubated with fluorescein-labeled anti-*T. pallidum* antibody. Then the stained smear is examined by fluorescence microscopy.[49] Darkfield examinations and direct fluorescent antibody tests of lesion exudate or tissue are definitive methods for diagnosing early syphilis.[47]

Serologic tests can be helpful in screening blood for syphilis, diagnosing the disease, and monitoring therapy.[48] Two types of serologic tests are useful for these purposes:

➤ Tests that detect nonspecific nontreponemal reaginic antibody.
➤ Tests specific for detecting treponemal antibody.

*Nonspecific nontreponemal reaginic antibody tests.* One of the first serologic tests for syphilis was developed by A. P. Wassermann, using an extract from syphilitic liver. Later discoveries revealed that the main component of the extract had nothing to do with infections from *T. pallidum* and that the substance was present in other tissues besides the liver.[50] The extract was actually a phospholipid called cardiolipin; it is now commercially prepared from beef heart.

In patients with syphilis, an antibody (reagin) is produced that reacts with a cardiolipin–lipoprotein complex. It is not understood why reagin is produced, since it is not an antibody specific to *T. pallidum*. Today, two nonspecific serologic tests that utilize the reaction between reaginic antibody and cardiolipin are commonly used: the Venereal Disease Research Laboratories (VDRL) test and the RPR card test.

The VDRL test is performed by mixing patient serum with the antigen cardiolipin on a glass slide. Flocculation is read microscopically, and the result is reported as reactive (medium and large clumps), nonreactive (small clumps), or weakly reactive (very small clumps).[49] The test can be performed in a quantitative manner by preparing and testing several dilutions of the patient's serum. The greatest serum dilution that produces a fully reactive result is the reported titer (e.g., 1:8 or 1:32).

Because the VDRL test is nonspecific, false-positive results can occur in numerous situations (Table 6). In the general population, the false-positive rate is 1–2%. The

**TABLE 6.** Causes of False-Positive Serologic Tests for Syphilis[a]

| Nontreponemal Tests | Bacterial | Viral | Noninfectious |
|---|---|---|---|
| RPR | Pneumococcal pneumonia | Vaccinations | Pregnancy |
| VDRL | Leprosy | Chickenpox | IV drug abuse |
| | Endocarditis | HIV | Multiple myeloma |
| | TB | Measles | SLE |
| | *M. pneumoniae* | Mumps | Arthritis |
| | | Infectious mononucleosis | Multiple blood transfusions |
| | | Hepatitis | |

| Treponemal Tests | Infectious | Noninfectious |
|---|---|---|
| Fluorescent treponemal antibody absorption test | Lyme disease | SLE |
| Microhemagglutination assay for *T. pallidum* | Leprosy | |
| | Malaria | |
| | Infectious mononucleosis | |

[a]Adapted from Reference 51.

titers of these reactions are generally less than 1:8, while titers of active infection are usually greater than 1:32.[52]

Following infection with *T. pallidum*, several weeks are required to develop a positive VDRL test. False-negative results can occur in the early stages of the disease. Up to 25% of cases of primary syphilis may have nonreactive (negative), nonspecific serologic tests.[52] Therefore, the clinician must correlate the patient's signs, symptoms, and disease history with the test results.

The VDRL test is commonly used to monitor a patient's response to therapy. The high titers present in untreated disease (e.g., 1:32) traditionally decrease four fold by 6–12 months and are undetectable in 1–2 years. Clinicians should follow patients until they are clinically disease free and have become seronegative or have reached a very low, stable titer.[51]

The RPR card test, a modification of the VDRL test, is used by many laboratories and blood banks for routine syphilis screening.[48] It has the same limitations (false-positive and false-negative reactions) as the VDRL test. Results are also reported the same way as for the VDRL test.

*Specific treponemal tests.* While nontreponemal tests are useful for screening and monitoring therapeutic response, a positive result must be confirmed with a more specific test. Two specific treponemal tests are[51]

> ➤ Fluorescent treponemal antibody absorption (FTA-abs) test.
> ➤ Microhemagglutination assay for *T. pallidum* (MHA-TP).

The FTA-abs test is used to assay the patient's serum for antibodies specific to *T. pallidum*.[48] Patient serum is mixed with *T. pallidum* antigen and then mixed with fluorescein-labeled antihuman globulin. Fluorescence is detected and reported as reactive, nonreactive, or reactive minimal.[49] Because the technician must subjectively grade the amount of fluorescence in the specimen, the test is difficult to standardize among laboratories. It is also fairly expensive. For these reasons, the FTA-abs test is not used for screening. Its principal use is to verify the diagnosis of syphilis in patients with positive nontreponemal test results.

The FTA-abs test can detect antibodies earlier in the course of syphilis than nontreponemal tests. Once positive, the test remains positive for the life of the patient, unlike the nontreponemal tests.

The MHA-TP is performed using sheep erythrocytes that have been coated with lyzed *T. pallidum*.[49] The erythrocytes are mixed with patient serum. If the patient serum contains antibodies to *T. pallidum*, agglutination of the sheep erythrocytes occurs. The result is reported as reactive (positive) or nonreactive (negative).

### *Chlamydia trachomatis*

*C. trachomatis* infections are the most common STDs in the United States. An estimated $1 billion or more is spent annually on the direct and indirect costs of these infections.[53] In men, chlamydial infections can cause urethritis (now 2.5 times more common than gonococcal urethritis) and epididymitis (currently about 500,000 cases per year).[54]

Many chlamydial infections are asymptomatic, but some—especially in women—have serious sequelae. Chlamydial infections are a common cause of mucopurulent cervicitis and the urethral syndrome, the female equivalent of chlamydial urethritis. *C. trachomatis* causes approximately 50% of the 1 million cases of pelvic inflammatory disease that occur annually. This disease also contributes to female infertility and ectopic pregnancies.[54]

The laboratory diagnosis of chlamydial infections is based on tests that detect chlamydial antigens by a special staining technique or an enzyme assay. Isolation of the organism is the more logical way to diagnose the disease, but it is costly and technically difficult and requires 48 hr to yield results.[53] Therefore, other approaches to the laboratory diagnosis have been developed, including the direct fluorescent antibody (DFA) test.

The chlamydia spends a portion of its life cycle as an extracellular, infectious form (the elementary body). The rest of its life cycle is spent as a reproducing, intracellular form. The DFA test involves staining smears of secretions from patients with fluorescein-labeled monoclonal antibodies.[54] If the patient is infected, these antibodies react with the elementary bodies of the chlamydia in the secretions. Under appropriate conditions, the antigen–antibody complex undergoes fluorescence. The DFA test is highly specific and takes less than 1 hr to perform.

## SUMMARY

Although infectious disease is a rapidly changing field because of new challenges and technological advances, the diagnosis of many infectious illnesses depends on proper performance and interpretation of numerous basic laboratory tests. For example, the Gram's stain is a readily available, invaluable tool for examining clinical specimens for the presence of bacteria. Culture of clinical specimens using agar plates allows growth of many of the usual infecting bacteria in the clinical laboratory. Subjecting the cultured bacteria to a Gram's stain and further tests will result in exact identification of the organism. Because empiric antimicrobial therapy is based on the patient's history and clinical condition, information from a Gram's stain or identification of the organism is useful in tailoring therapy.

Susceptibility tests for rapidly growing aerobic bacteria are commonly performed using an automated microdilution or a manual disk diffusion method. Bacterial susceptibilities to various antimicrobial agents are reported as susceptible, intermediate, or resistant. National standards for the performance of the test, choice of antimicrobial agents, and susceptibility reporting procedures should be followed by the clinical laboratory. Moreover, susceptibility information should be considered in conjunction with patient-specific data (e.g., clinical condition, sites of infection, drug allergies, and renal function) to design an appropriate antimicrobial drug regimen for a patient.

The SBT is intriguing because it combines the pharmacokinetics and the pharmacodynamics of a given antimicrobial agent against the patient's infecting organism. Unfortunately, the SBT is more cumbersome to perform than traditional susceptibility testing, and interpretation of its results is controversial.

A selected group of infectious diseases has been considered in more detail. Mycobacterial diseases challenge the clinical laboratory due to their requirements for specialized staining, culturing, and susceptibility testing procedures.

Meningitis is a serious, rapidly progressive, and potentially fatal disease that requires antigen detection techniques (e.g., latex agglutination) to aid in rapid identification of infecting organisms.

Viruses cannot be visualized on a Gram's stain or grown on agar plates. Diagnostic techniques include use of cell culture, immunoassays for viral antigen detection, and serologic tests for antibodies directed against viral components. HIV is detected primarily by serologic tests. These tests are also useful in the diagnosis of infections due to *M. pneumoniae* (complement fixation), *B. burgdorferi* (immunosorbent assay), and *T. pallidum* (VDRL, RPR, FTA-abs, and MHA-TP).

Fungal infections are becoming more common as patients become increasingly immunosuppressed, subjected to IV access devices, or treated with antibiotics that disrupt normal bacterial flora. Many types of fungi can be cultured using media available in most clinical laboratories, although their growth characteristics are slower than most bacteria.

## REFERENCES

1. Washington JE. Bacteria, fungi, and parasites. In: Mandell GL, Douglas RG, Bennett JE, eds. Principles and practice of infectious diseases. New York: Churchill Livingstone; 1990:160–93.
2. Isenberg HD, Schoenknecht FD, von Graevenitz A. Cumitech 9-collection and processing of bacteriological specimens. Washington, DC: American Society for Microbiology; 1979:1–22.
3. Methods for testing antimicrobial effectiveness. In: Finegold SM, Baron EJ, eds. Bailey and Scott's diagnostic microbiology. St. Louis, MO: C.V. Mosby; 1990:171–94.
4. National Committee for Clinical Laboratory Standards. Methods for dilution antimicrobial susceptibility tests for bacteria that grow aerobically. Approved standard M7-A3. Villanova, PA: National Committee for Clinical Laboratory Standards; 1993.
5. National Committee for Clinical Laboratory Standards. Performance standards for antimicrobial disk susceptibility tests, 5th ed. Approved standard M2-A5. Villanova, PA; National Committee for Clinical Laboratory Standards; 1993.
6. Rosenblatt JE, Brook I. Clinical relevance of susceptibility testing of anaerobic bacteria. *Clin Infect Dis.* 1993; 16(Suppl 4):S446–8.
7. National Committee for Clinical Laboratory Standards. Methods for antimicrobial susceptibility testing of anaerobic bacteria, 3rd ed. Approved standard Mll-A3. Villanova, PA: National Committee for Clinical Laboratory Standards; 1993.
8. Sutter VL, Citron DM, Edelstein MAC, et al. Susceptibility testing of anaerobes. In: Wadsworth anaerobic bacteriology manual. Belmont, CA: Star Publishing; 1985:79–90.

9. Olsson-Liljequist B, Nord CE. Methods for susceptibility testing of anaerobic bacteria. *Clin Infect Dis.* 1994; 18(Suppl 4):S293–6.

10. Sanchez ML, Jones RN. E test, an antimicrobial susceptibility testing method with broad clinical and epidemiologic application. *Antimicrob Newsl.* 1993; 8:1–7.

11. Jorgenson JH. Antimicrobial susceptibility testing of bacteria that grow aerobically. *Infect Dis Clin North Am.* 1993; 7:393–409.

12. Citron DM. Susceptibility testing of anaerobic bacteria: a review of current methods and future prospects. *Antimicrob Newsl.* 1992; 8:53–8.

13. Jorgenson JH. Detection of antimicrobial resistance in Streptococcus pneumoniae by use of standardized susceptibility testing methods and recently developed interpretive criteria. *Clin Microbiol Newsl.* 1994; 16:97–101.

14. Reller LB. The serum bactericidal test. *Rev Infect Dis.* 1986; 8:803–8.

15. Stratton CW. Serum bactericidal test. *Clin Microbiol Rev.* 1988; 1:19–26.

16. Wolfson JS, Swartz MN. Serum bactericidal activity as a monitor of antibiotic therapy. *N Engl J Med.* 1985; 312:968–75.

17. Weinstein MP, Stratton CW, Ackley A, et al. Multicenter collaborative evaluation of a standardized serum bactericidal test as a prognostic indicator in infective endocarditis. *Am J Med.* 1984; 78:262–9.

18. Amsterdam D. The MIC: myth and reality. *Antimicrob Newsl.* 1992; 8:9–12.

19. Tilton RC. Interpreting MICs and MBCs. *Infect Med.* 1986; May/June:218–25.

20. Eliopoulos GM, Eliopoulos CT. Antibiotic combinations: should they be tested? *Clin Microbiol Rev.* 1988; 1:139–56.

21. Rahal JJ. Antibiotic combinations: the relevance of synergy and antagonism. *Medicine (Balt).* 1978; 57:179–95.

22. Witebsky FG, Conville PS. The laboratory diagnosis of mycobacterial diseases. *Infect Dis Clin North Am.* 1993; 7:359–76.

23. Peloquin CA, Berning SE. Infection caused by mycobacterium tuberculosis. *Ann Pharmacother.* 1994; 28:72–84.

24. Wolinsky E. Conventional diagnostic methods for tuberculosis. *Clin Infect Dis.* 1994; 19:396–401.

25. Woods GL. Disease due to the mycobacterium avium complex in patients infected with human immunodeficiency virus: diagnosis and susceptibility testing. *Clin Infect Dis.* 1994; 18(Suppl 3):S227–32.

26. Inderlied CB, Kemper CA, Bermudez LEM. The mycobacterium avium complex. *Clin Microbiol Rev.* 1993; 6:266–310.

27. Jacobs WR Jr, Barletta RG, Udani R, et al. Rapid assessment of drug susceptibilities of mycobacterium tuberculosis by means of luciferase reporter phages. *Science.* 1993; 260:819–22.

28. Jacobs RF. Multiple-drug-resistant tuberculosis. *Clin Infect Dis.* 1994; 19:1–10.

29. McGee ZA, Baringer JR. Acute meningitis. In: Mandell GL, Douglas RG, Bennett JE, eds. Principles and practice of infectious diseases. New York: Churchill Livingstone; 1990:741–55.

30. Gray LD, Fedorko DP. Laboratory diagnosis of bacterial meningitis. *Clin Microbiol Rev.* 1992; 5:130–45.

31. Power DA, McCuen PJ, eds. Manual of BBL products and laboratory procedures. Cockeysville, MD: Becton Dickinson Microbiology Systems; 1988:77.

32. Drew WL. Controversies in viral diagnosis. *Rev Infect Dis.* 1986; 8:814–24.

33. Smith TF, Wold AD, Espy MJ, et al. New developments in the diagnosis of viral diseases. *Infect Dis Clin North Am.* 1993; 7:183–201.

34. Health and Public Policy Committee, American College of Physicians and the Infectious Diseases Society of America. Acquired immunodeficiency syndrome. *Ann Intern Med.* 1986; 104:575–81.

35. Brettman LR. Serologic and epidemiologic assessment of AIDS risk. *Infect Med.* 1986; 3:18–33.

36. Bylund DJ, Ziegner UHM, Hooper DG. Review of testing for human immunodeficiency virus. *Clin Lab Med.* 1992; 12:305–33.

37. Proffitt MR, Yen-Lieberman B. Laboratory diagnosis of human immunodeficiency virus infection. *Infect Dis Clin North Am.* 1993; 7:203–19.

38. Barthel HR, Wallace DJ. False-positive human immunodeficiency virus testing in patients with lupus erythematosis. *Semin Arthritis Rheum.* 1993; 23:1–7.

39. Sison AV, Campos JM. Laboratory methods for early detection of human immunodeficiency virus type I in newborns and infants. *Clin Microbiol Rev.* 1992; 5:238–47.

40. Couch RB. Mycoplasma diseases: introduction. In: Mandell GL, Douglas RG, Bennett JE, eds. Principles and practice of infectious diseases. New York: Churchill Livingstone; 1990:1445–6.

41. Couch RB. Mycoplasma pncumoniae (primary atypical pneumonia). In: Mandell GL, Douglas RG, Bennett JE, eds. Principles and practice of infectious diseases. New York: Churchill Livingstone; 1990:1446–58.

42. Steere AC, Taylor E, McHugh GL, et al. The overdiagnosis of Lyme disease. *JAMA.* 1993; 269:1812–6.

43. Rahn DW, Malawista SE. Lyme disease: recommendations for diagnosis and treatment. *Ann Intern Med.* 1991; 114:472–81.

44. Berger BW. Laboratory tests for Lyme disease. *Dermatol Clin.* 1994; 12:19–24.

45. Geha DJ, Roberts GD. Laboratory detection of fungemia. *Clin Lab Med.* 1994; 14:83–97.

46. Handsfield HH. Neisseria gonorrhoeae. In: Mandell GL, Douglas RG, Bennett JE, eds. Principles and practice of infectious diseases. New York: Churchill Livingstone; 1990:1613–31.

47. Centers for Disease Control and Prevention. 1993 sexually transmitted diseases treatment guidelines. *MMWR.* 1993; 42(RR-14).

48. Tramont EC. Treponema pallidum (syphilis). In: Mandell GL, Douglas RG, Bennett JE, eds. Principles and practice of infectious diseases. New York: Churchill Livingstone; 1990:1794–1808.

49. Hart G. Syphilis tests in diagnostic and therapeutic decision making. *Ann Intern Med.* 1986; 104:368–76.

50. Ravel R. Tests for syphilis. In: Ravel R. Clinical laboratory medicine. Clinical application of laboratory data. Chicago, IL: Year Book Publishers; 1978:384–6.

51. Thomas DL, Quinn TC. Serologic testing for sexually transmitted diseases. *Infect Dis Clin North Am.* 1993; 7:793–824.

52. Larsen SA, Bradford LL. Serodiagnosis of syphilis. In: Rose NR, Friedman H, Fahey JL, eds. Manual of clinical laboratory immunology. Washington, DC: American Society for Microbiology; 1986:425–34.

53. Chlamydia trachomatis infections. Policy guidelines for prevention and control. *MMWR.* 1985; 34:53S–74S.

54. Bell TA, Grayston JT. Centers for Disease Control guidelines for prevention and control of Chlamydia trachomatis infections: summary and commentary. *Ann Intern Med.* 1986; 104:524–6.

## QuickView—HIV Antibody Test (ELISA)

| Parameter | Description | Comments |
|---|---|---|
| **Common reference ranges**<br>    **Adults and pediatrics** | Negative<br>Also called "nonreactive" | Sensitivity >99%<br>Specificity >99% |
| **Critical value** | Positive | Confirmed with Western blot test |
| **Natural substance?** | Yes | But antibody not normally found in serum |
| **Inherent activity?** | Yes | Immunologic antagonist to AIDS virus (HIV) |
| **Major causes of . . .**<br>    **Positive results** | Presence of antibodies to HIV | Recent infection by AIDS virus (HIV) |
|       **Associated signs and symptoms** | Mononucleosis-like syndrome<br>Lymphadenopathy<br>Lymphopenia<br>Kaposi's sarcoma<br>*Candida* and other opportunistic infections<br>Encephalopathy | Months to years after infection<br>Opportunistic infections associated with low $CD_4$ counts |
| **After insult, time to . . .**<br>    **Positive results** | Usually 2 weeks to 3 months | Rarely >6 months |
|     **Peak values** | Months to years | Quantitative results not reported |
|     **Antibody not detectable** | Late in disease | In patients with severe immunosuppression |
| **Causes of spurious results** | **False Positive**<br>Hematologic malignancies<br>SLE or multiple myeloma<br>Positive RPR<br>Alcoholic hepatitis<br>Viral vaccinations<br>Presence of maternal antibody<br>Unreliable in infants <15 months—maternal antibody persists | **False Negative**<br>Testing too early after infection<br>Human error<br>Severely immunosuppressed patients |

## QuickView—Lyme Disease Antibody Test (ELISA)

| Parameter | Description | Comments |
|---|---|---|
| **Common reference ranges**<br>    **Adults and pediatrics** | Negative | |
| **Critical value** | Positive | Treatment required |
| **Natural substance?** | Yes | But antibody not normally found in serum |
| **Inherent activity?** | Yes | Immunologic antagonist to *B. burgdorferi* |
| **Major causes of . . .**<br>    **Positive results** | Presence of antibodies to *B. burgdorferi* | Recent bite of tick carrying organism |
|       **Associated signs and symptoms** | Rash (erythema migrans), flu-like illness, headache, stiff neck, meningitis, heart block, congestive heart failure, asymmetric arthritis | Rash: 1–4 weeks<br>CNS/heart disease: days–months<br>Arthritis: months–years |

## QuickView—Lyme Disease Antibody Test (ELISA) *continued*

| Parameter | Description | Comments |
|---|---|---|
| **After infection, time to . . .** | | |
| **Initial elevation or positive result** | IgM: 2–4 weeks<br>IgG: 6–8 weeks | If untreated |
| **Peak values** | IgM: 6–8 weeks<br>IgG: 4–6 months | |
| **Antibody not detectable** | IgM: 4–6 months<br>IgG: many months | Assumes adequate treatment |
| **Causes of spurious results** | Mononucleosis (positive)<br>Syphilis (positive)<br>Rheumatoid arthritis (positive)<br>Endocarditis (positive)<br>SLE or endocarditis (positive)<br>Periodontal disease (positive) | Testing too early after infection may yield false negative |

## QuickView—Syphilis, VDRL Test

| Parameter | Description | Comments |
|---|---|---|
| **Common reference ranges**<br>**Adults and pediatrics** | Negative | |
| **Critical value** | Positive | Syphilis |
| **Natural substance?** | No | |
| **Inherent activity?** | No | |
| **Major causes of . . .** | | |
| **Positive results** | Syphilis | |
| **Associated signs and symptoms** | Signs and symptoms of above | |
| **After infection, time to . . .** | | |
| **Positive results** | Several weeks | |
| **Peak values** | Not applicable | |
| **Antibody not detectable** | 1–2 years after therapy | May take longer |
| **Causes of spurious results** | False positives (Table 6)<br>Early or treated syphilis (negative) | |

# Chapter 17

# Rheumatic Diseases

*Dwight A. Marble*

Laboratory tests in the medical specialty of rheumatology can vary from the general and nonspecific to the specific for a particular disease. Diagnosis and management of most rheumatic diseases depend primarily on clinical manifestations. However, the results of specific laboratory tests may be essential when establishing the diagnosis of a disease such as crystal-deposition arthritis. In conjunction with signs and symptoms, certain laboratory tests are important diagnostic tools. Some test results also may be used to assess current disease severity and to monitor therapy.

The diagnostic utility of a laboratory test depends on its sensitivity, specificity, and predictive value (Chapter 1). Laboratory tests that are highly sensitive and specific for certain rheumatic diseases often have low predictive values because the prevalence of the suspected rheumatic disease is low. The pretest probability of disease, or a clinician's estimated likelihood that a certain disease is present, is the most important determinant of a laboratory test's diagnostic utility. As the number of disease-specific signs and symptoms increases and approaches diagnostic confirmation, the pretest probability also increases.

After describing pertinent physiology, this chapter discusses the interpretation of test results relating to rheumatoid arthritis, systemic lupus erythematosus (SLE), other rheumatic diseases, and gout. Tests used to monitor antirheumatic drug therapy also are described.

## OBJECTIVES

Upon completion of this chapter, the reader should be able to

1. Recognize appropriate clinical applications for laboratory tests commonly used to diagnose or determine the activity of rheumatic diseases.
2. Given a clinical situation, interpret the results of a laboratory test associated with rheumatic diseases.
3. Recognize and interpret the results of rheu-

matologic laboratory tests used to monitor therapeutic response.
4. Identify adverse reactions to drugs used to treat rheumatic diseases by monitoring appropriate tests.
5. Describe the clinical use and interpretation of laboratory test results unique to the management of hyperuricemia.

## STRUCTURE AND PHYSIOLOGY OF IMMUNOGLOBULINS

Many rheumatologic laboratory tests involve detection of antibodies directed against normal cellular components. Therefore, to facilitate comprehension, the basic anatomy and physiology of immunoglobulins (i.e., antibodies) are presented first.

When the immune system is challenged by a foreign substance (antigen), activated B lymphocytes (Chapter 14) differentiate into immunoglobulin-producing plasma cells. All immunoglobulins are Y shaped (Figure 1, next page). Each immunoglobulin has two identical antigen-binding sites (labeled Fab or fraction antigen binding). One site is located on each "arm," and each arm is composed of a light amino acid chain and a heavy amino acid chain. *Light* and *heavy* refer to the number of amino acids in each chain. Since the heavy chain has more amino acids than the light chain, it is longer and has a higher molecular weight.

Chains contain both a variable region and a constant region. The *variable* regions of both chains make up the antigen-binding sites and vary in amino acid sequence. The sequences vary to allow immunoglobulins to recognize and specifically bind thousands of different antigens. The *constant* region of the light chain ($C_L$) is a single section. Immunoglobulins that have identical constant regions in their heavy chains (e.g., $C_H1$, $C_H2$, and $C_H3$) are of the same class.

The five classes of immunoglobulins are IgA, IgD, IgE, IgG, and IgM. Depending on the immunoglobulin,

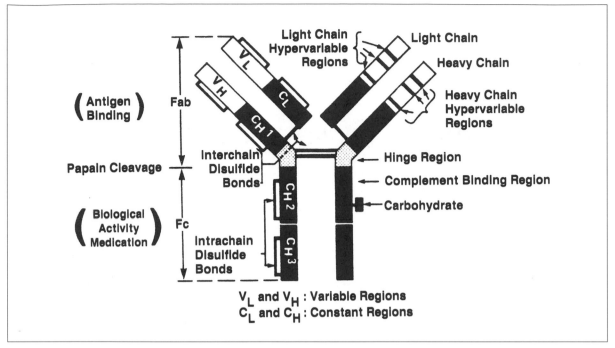

**FIGURE 1.** Prototypic IgG immunoglobulin. (Adapted from Wasserman RL, Capra JD. Immunoglobulins. In: Horowitz MI, Pigman W, eds. The glycoconjugates. New York: Academic Press; 1977. Reproduced, with permission, from Koopman WJ, Griffin JA. B-lymphocytes. In: Kelley WN, Harris ED Jr, Ruddy S, et al., eds. Textbook of rheumatology, 3rd ed. Philadelphia, PA: W. B. Saunders; 1989.)

the constant region of the heavy chain has either three domains and a hinge region (IgA, IgD, and IgG) or four domains without a hinge region (IgE and IgM). Thus, the immunoglobulin's heavy chain determines its class (α heavy chains, IgA; δ heavy chains, IgD; ε heavy chains, IgE; γ heavy chains, IgG; and μ heavy chains, IgM).

In Figure 1, the second and third domains ($C_H 2$ and $C_H 3$) of the heavy chain are part of the Fc (fraction crystallizable) portion of the immunoglobulin. This portion has two important functions:

> ➤ Binding of complement (discussed later).
> ➤ Binding of immunoglobulins (which react with and bind antigen) to cell surface receptors of polymorphonuclear leukocytes, monocytes, macrophages, and platelets.

Except when bound to platelets, the cell-surface-bound antigen–antibody complex is engulfed and destroyed.[1,2]

## TESTS TO DIAGNOSE OR ASSESS RHEUMATIC DISEASES

Blood tests used to diagnose or assess rheumatoid arthritis, SLE, and other rheumatic diseases include relatively specific tests such as rheumatoid factor, antinuclear antibodies (ANAs), antineutrophil cytoplasmic antibodies (ANCAs), and complement, as well as nonspecific tests such as erythrocyte sedimentation rate (ESR), C-reactive protein, and analysis of synovial fluid.

## Rheumatoid Factor

Rheumatoid factors are immunoglobulins that are abnormally directed against the Fc portion of IgG. These immunoglobulins do not recognize the IgG as being "self." Therefore, the presence of rheumatoid factor in the blood indicates an autoimmune process. The only rheumatoid factor measured in most laboratories is *IgM-anti-IgG* (an IgM antibody that specifically binds IgG antibody). Like all IgM antibodies, IgM rheumatoid factor is composed of five subunits whose Fc portions are attached to the same base (Figure 2). The variable regions of each IgM antibody can bind up to five IgG molecules at its multiple binding sites, making IgM rheumatoid factor the most stable as well as the easiest rheumatoid factor to quantify.

As depicted in Figure 3, each IgM rheumatoid factor reacts maximally with five IgG molecules. The complexes that exist in serum, however, most likely contain fewer than five IgG molecules. The positions of the IgG molecules shown in Figure 3 do not imply an antigenic determinant at the end of the Fc fragments.

Although rheumatoid factors are most commonly identified and quantified in serum, they also are found in synovial fluid (IgG, discussed later) and saliva. IgA rheumatoid factor can be produced locally in saliva, and IgE rheumatoid factor is found in patients with bronchial asthma. IgD rheumatoid factors have not been identified. Non-IgM rheumatoid factors remain laboratory research tools because their clinical relevance is still being

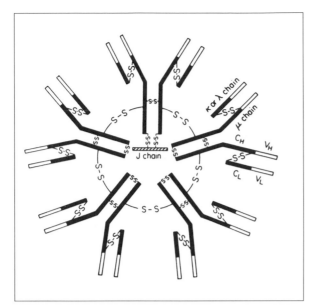

**FIGURE 2.** Polypeptide structure of a 19S IgM pentamer. (Reproduced, with permission, from Koopman WJ, Schrohenloher RE. Rheumatoid factor. In: Utsinger PO, Zvaifler NJ, Ehrlich GE, eds. Rheumatoid arthritis: etiology, diagnosis, management. Philadelphia, PA: J. B. Lippincott; 1985.)

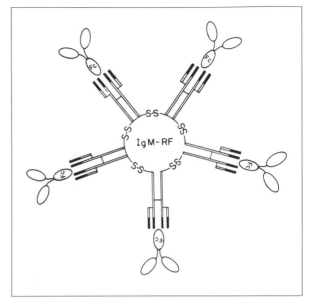

**FIGURE 3.** Schematic representation of the 22S immune complex between an IgM rheumatoid factor (IgM-RF) molecule and IgG molecules. (Reproduced, with permission, from Mannik M. Rheumatoid factors. In: McCarty DJ, ed. Arthritis and allied conditions: a textbook of rheumatology. Philadelphia, PA: Lea & Febiger; 1989.)

determined.[3]

Rheumatoid factor and antinuclear antibodies are the specific rheumatologic tests that are most frequently ordered. The following sections for each of these tests discuss quantitative assay results (antibody concentrations considered positive or negative), qualitative assay results (significance of positive or negative assay results as they relate to diagnosing and monitoring various rheumatic diseases), and their use in the most frequently diagnosed rheumatic diseases, other rheumatic diseases, and nonrheumatic diseases. ANCAs, though still incompletely understood, now have limited but important clinical significance. Their clinical significance will be discussed in terms of quantitative as well as qualitative assay results.

### Quantitative Assay Results
*Normal values: <1:160 and ≤40 IU/mL*

When a quantitative rheumatoid factor test is performed, results are reported as either a titer or a concentration in international units per milliliter. A rheumatoid factor titer of 1:160 or greater or a rheumatoid factor concentration greater than 40 IU/mL is considered positive. In general, rheumatoid factor titers of at least 1:320 are seen in rheumatoid arthritis patients. Even though a positive rheumatoid factor fulfills one of the American College of Rheumatology's criteria for the diagnosis of rheumatoid arthritis[4] (Table 1, next page), results of the rheumatoid factor test are always interpreted in conjunction with the patient's clinical signs and symptoms.

### Qualitative Assay Results

The titer chosen to indicate positivity for IgM rheumatoid factor routinely excludes 95% of the normal population. However, approximately 70–90% of rheumatoid arthritis patients diagnosed by other criteria have a positive latex agglutination test, indicating the presence of IgM rheumatoid factor.[3,5] Even though the remaining 10–30% of patients are often described as seronegative, approximately two-thirds of them (7–20% of all rheumatoid arthritis patients) probably have non-IgM rheumatoid factor circulating, predominantly IgG rheumatoid factor. The remaining 3–10% of these patients are considered to be truly seronegative.

In comparison with rheumatoid factor positive patients, seronegative patients are more likely to have milder arthritis and less likely to develop nonjoint manifestations of rheumatoid arthritis (e.g., rheumatoid nodules, lung disease, and vasculitis). In fact, the possibility that true seronegative patients may not have rheumatoid arthritis, but a clinically distinct rheumatic disease, has been debated. Thus, rheumatoid arthritis patients may or may not have a positive IgM rheumatoid factor or IgG rheumatoid factor; conversely, the presence of rheumatoid factor is not, by itself, diagnostic for rheumatoid arthritis.[3,5,6]

As support grows for early treatment of rheumatoid arthritis—before end-organ damage—all clinicians need to be aware of the relationship between disease onset and rheumatoid factor development. The rheumatoid factor test is least likely to be positive at the onset of rheumatoid arthritis, when it might be of the most help. Of all pa-

**TABLE 1.** American Rheumatism Association 1987 Revised Criteria for Classification of Rheumatoid Arthritis[a]

| Criterion | Definition |
|-----------|------------|
| 1. Morning stiffness | Morning stiffness in and around joints that lasts ≥1 hr before maximal improvement |
| 2. Arthritis of three or more joint areas | At least three joint areas simultaneously have had soft tissue swelling or fluid (not bony overgrowth alone) observed by physician[b] |
| 3. Arthritis of hand joints | At least one area swollen (as defined in 2) in wrist, MCP, or PIP joint |
| 4. Symmetric arthritis | Simultaneous involvement of same joint areas (as defined in 2) on both sides of body (bilateral involvement of PIPs, MCPs, or MTPs acceptable without absolute symmetry) |
| 5. Rheumatoid nodules | Subcutaneous nodules over bony prominences or extensor surfaces or in juxta-articular regions observed by physician |
| 6. Serum rheumatoid factor | Demonstration of abnormal amounts of serum rheumatoid factor by any method for which the result has been positive in <5% of normal control subjects |
| 7. Radiographic changes | Radiographic changes typical of rheumatoid arthritis on posteroanterior hand and wrist radiographs; must include erosions or unequivocal bony decalcification localized in or most marked adjacent to involved joints (not osteoarthritis changes alone) |

[a]*Adapted from Reference 4. Patients with four or more of the above criteria are considered to have rheumatoid arthritis. In addition, the first four criteria must be present for at least 6 weeks. However, patients with only two of the above criteria may not be excluded from having the disease.*
[b]*The 14 possible areas are right or left proximal interphalangeal (PIP), metacarpophalangeal (MCP), wrist, elbow, knee, ankle, and metatarsophalangeal (MTP) joints.*

tients who develop rheumatoid factor, only 33 and 60% are seropositive during the first 3 and 6 months, respectively.[5]

### Rheumatoid Arthritis

Rheumatoid factors are most commonly associated with, but are not specific for, rheumatoid arthritis. Although rheumatoid factors are predominantly obtained from the general circulation and rheumatoid arthritis is a systemic disease, pathophysiologically rheumatoid arthritis is an extravascular autoimmune disease affecting the synovium. Affected diarthrodial joints have an inflamed and proliferating synovium infiltrated with T lymphocytes and plasma cells. Plasma cells in the synovial fluid generate large amounts of IgG rheumatoid factor and abnormally low amounts of normal IgG. However, plasma cells in the bloodstream of a rheumatoid arthritis patient produce IgM rheumatoid factor predominantly.[3]

In contrast, degenerative joint disease (osteoarthritis) is not an autoimmune disease. The synovium is normal, and the synovial fluid usually lacks inflammatory cells. While affected joints are painful, they are not swollen or inflamed. Moreover, rheumatoid factors are usually absent.

For classification purposes, a patient is said to have rheumatoid arthritis if he or she satisfies at least four of the seven criteria outlined in Table 1. In addition, the first four criteria must be present for at least 6 weeks. However, patients with only two clinical criteria are not

excluded. Designation as classic, definite, or probable rheumatoid arthritis is no longer made.

For patients who already meet diagnostic criteria (Table 1) for rheumatoid arthritis, the rheumatoid factor test should not be performed; a negative rheumatoid factor may actually mislead clinicians, and a positive test contributes nothing. Likewise, rheumatoid factor tests should not be used to screen patients with minimal or no symptoms. These tests are useful when the pretest likelihood of rheumatoid arthritis is neither very low nor very high.[5]

After rheumatoid arthritis has been diagnosed, rheumatoid factor titers are not routinely used to assess or predict disease severity or treatment efficacy. A specific titer or a change in titers for an individual does not correlate reliably with disease activity. Statistically, when assessed retrospectively, the presence of rheumatoid factor increases the likelihood of severe disease[7] and patients with higher titer rheumatoid factor will have more severe disease.[8,9] Although often reported in therapeutic trials, neither rheumatoid factor nor rheumatoid factor titers are used to assess a patient's current clinical status, to modify a therapeutic regimen, or to determine prognosis.

### Juvenile Rheumatoid Arthritis (JRA)

Rheumatoid factors also are associated with JRA, although much less frequently than with adult rheumatoid arthritis. IgM rheumatoid factor is detected by latex agglutination testing in only 7–10% of JRA patients. A positive rheumatoid factor is rarely seen before the age of 7 and is present in fewer than 4% of children at disease onset. It is most commonly seen when onset is late in childhood, predominantly in girls with late-onset polyarticular disease. Based on these observations, the rheumatoid factor is of little diagnostic value. In addition, seropositivity is frequently observed in other childhood connective-tissue diseases.

Like adult rheumatoid arthritis patients, most children who are seronegative for IgM rheumatoid factor (via latex agglutination testing) are actually positive via the enzyme-linked immunosorbent assay (ELISA) for IgM rheumatoid factor (22–35%), IgA rheumatoid factor (30–60%), or IgG rheumatoid factor (4–6%). In a significant percentage of seronegative JRA patients, "hidden" IgM rheumatoid factor has been detected. Detection of IgM rheumatoid factor via latex agglutination occurs when IgG, attached to latex particles, binds unbound serum IgM rheumatoid factor. However, circulating IgM rheumatoid factor is already bound to IgG in the serum in 65–75% of patients with seronegative JRA. Therefore, the bound IgM rheumatoid factor is undetected—"hidden"—when latex agglutination is used.

Hidden IgM rheumatoid factor can be detected in the IgM-containing fraction of serum by latex agglutination after dissociation from serum IgG by acid-gel filtration. Due to the technical difficulty of this laboratory procedure, hidden rheumatoid factors are not routinely detected and their clinical significance remains unknown.[10,11]

The diagnosis of JRA is based on clinical signs and symptoms during the first 6 months. Three distinct types of onset occur, as described here.[10–12]

*Polyarticular onset (polyarthritis).* This type occurs in 40% of JRA patients. JRA begins in five or more joints, usually in a symmetrical pattern involving the large and sometimes the small joints of the hands or feet. Asymmetric temporomandibular joint involvement, leading to bite limitation and micrognathia, is relatively common.[11]

Rheumatoid factor, rarely detected before the age of 8, is positive in 15–20% and hidden in about 85% of this group. Children who are consistently rheumatoid factor positive have more joint erosions and extra-articular manifestations (rheumatoid nodules and vasculitis) as well as a worse prognosis. Lawrence et al.[10] divided these patients into two subgroups:

> ➤ Younger children with serum negative IgM rheumatoid factor by latex agglutination.
> ➤ Older girls with serum positive for IgM rheumatoid factor by latex agglutination and disease clinically similar to adult rheumatoid arthritis.

*Pauciarticular onset (oligoarthritis).* This type occurs in half of JRA patients; they are predominantly rheumatoid factor negative. One to four joints are involved. In 33–50%

of these patients, the onset begins in a single joint, usually the knee. Lawrence et al.[10] divided these patients into two subgroups:

> ➤ Early onset—young girls with iridocyclitis and positive ANAs.
> ➤ Late onset—boys with human lymphocytic antigen (HLA) B27 and early onset of ankylosing spondylitis.

*Systemic onset.* This type occurs in 10–20% of JRA patients and is characterized by severe signs and symptoms including a high fever that spikes once or twice daily, accompanied by a brief, migratory, measles-like rash. These two signs are practically diagnostic of systemic onset. Hepatosplenomegaly, lymphadenopathy, and pleural or pericardial effusions are common. Arthritis can first present at symptom onset or weeks to months later. Although leukocytosis and anemia occur, rheumatoid factors and ANAs are usually negative. In fact, rheumatoid factor is hidden 60% of the time.

### Other Rheumatic Diseases

Other rheumatic diseases in which circulating rheumatoid factors have been identified include SLE, progressive systemic sclerosis (scleroderma), mixed connective-tissue disease, and Sjögren's syndrome.[3] The significance of rheumatoid factors in these diseases remains unknown.

### Nonrheumatic Diseases

The presence of rheumatoid factor does not necessarily imply that a rheumatic disease exists. Patients with various acute and chronic inflammatory diseases as well as normal individuals have been identified as rheumatoid factor positive. Nonrheumatic diseases associated with rheumatoid factors include mononucleosis, hepatitis, malaria, tuberculosis, syphilis, subacute bacterial endocarditis, cancers after chemotherapy or irradiation, chronic liver disease, hyperglobulinemia, and cryoglobulinemia.

With advancing age, the percentage of individuals with positive rheumatoid factor concentrations, as well as the mean rheumatoid factor concentration of a population as a whole, increases. Although rheumatoid factors are associated with several rheumatic and many nonrheumatic diseases, the concentrations of rheumatoid factors in these diseases are lower than those observed in patients with rheumatoid arthritis. As serum titers of rheumatoid factor increase, its specificity for rheumatoid arthritis also increases.[3]

## Antinuclear Antibodies

Although rheumatoid factor is the most commonly ordered immunologic test in rheumatology, another expanding collective group of autoantibodies directed against nucleic acids and nucleoproteins within the nucleus and

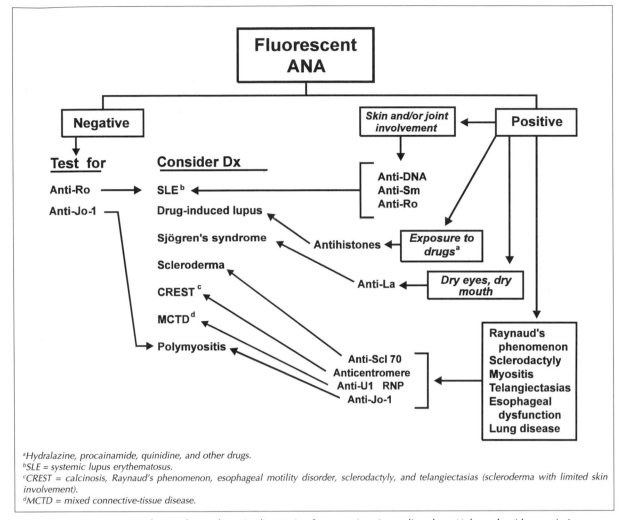

**FIGURE 4.** ANA test rationale, results, and use in diagnosis of connective-tissue disorders. (Adapted, with permission, from Reference 13.)

cytoplasm is expanding. Intracellular targets of these autoantibodies include deoxyribonucleic acid (DNA), ribonucleic acid (RNA), histones, acidic nuclear proteins, and complexes of these molecular elements.

This heterogeneous group of autoantibodies is collectively referred to as ANAs. ANAs most often are associated with SLE. On the average, an SLE patient has three different detectable autoantibodies circulating at one time.[13] However, most individuals with a positive ANA test do not have SLE or any other systemic inflammatory disease.

A positive ANA test occurs in 2–5% of healthy individuals, in females more than males. This false-positive rate increases with increasing age. As a result, the probability of diagnosing SLE in an ANA-positive patient may be as low as 1 in 100. However, in black females 15–40 years of age, the prevalence of SLE is 1 in 250 instead of 1 in 2000. The probability of diagnosing SLE in an ANA-positive patient may be as high as 1 in 10 in this specific patient population. In addition, positive ANAs frequently occur in other rheumatic and nonrheumatic diseases.[6]

Due to a significant lack of specificity, the ANA test should not be used to screen (asymptomatic patients) for SLE or any rheumatic or nonrheumatic disease. Figure 4 provides guidelines for the use of the ANA test in rheumatic disease diagnosis. The titer or quantitative value should be considered when evaluating the clinical significance of ANA test results.

### Quantitative Antinuclear Antibody Assay Results
*Normal: varies among laboratories*

The ANA titer, the highest serum dilution positive for ANAs, is usually reported by a laboratory. ANA titers less than two times the normal titer for a laboratory should be viewed with reservation because false-positive ANAs tend to be low titer (<1:40). High titers (>1:320) are most commonly seen in patients with SLE, drug-induced lupus, scleroderma, mixed connective-tissue disease, polymyositis/dermatomyositis, and Sjögren's syndrome. Unfortunately, there is no consistent correlation between disease activity and ANA titer.[13,14] When titers are high or considered positive, immunofluorescent staining patterns of the nucleus are assessed.

### Qualitative Antinuclear Antibody Assay Results

The pattern of nuclear fluorescence after staining provides limited—but sometimes clinically useful—information. Different patterns of fluorescence correspond with the component(s) of the nucleus against which the patient's ANAs are directed. The four common immunofluorescent patterns are

> *Homogeneous.* This pattern is seen most frequently in patients with SLE and can be observed in patients with drug-induced SLE, rheumatoid arthritis, vasculitis, and polymyositis.
> *Speckled.* This pattern also is seen most frequently in SLE patients but can appear in patients diagnosed with mixed connective-tissue disease, Sjögren's syndrome, progressive systemic sclerosis, polymyositis, and rheumatoid arthritis.
> *Nucleolar.* This pattern is infrequently observed in patients with SLE but is more frequently seen in patients with polymyositis, progressive systemic sclerosis, and vasculitis.
> *Nuclear rim.* This pattern is the only one highly specific for any rheumatic disease[13] and is observed predominantly (98%) in SLE patients.[15]

Patterns of immunofluorescence are less specific than the identification (or titer) of ANA to specific nuclear antigens. However, there are potential clinical applications for some ANAs associated with high disease specificity and low to moderate sensitivity. Table 2 (next page) summarizes the most frequently identified ANAs, their corresponding immunofluorescent staining patterns and targeted cellular material, and disease sensitivities and specificities.[13–17]

### Rheumatoid Arthritis

The frequency of positive ANAs in patients diagnosed with rheumatoid arthritis is highly variable. As determined by indirect immunofluorescence, this frequency varies from about 10 to 70%, depending on the substrate used and the titer considered positive. Regardless of frequency, however, a positive ANA test is generally low titer with a homogeneous pattern caused by antihistone antibodies.[17,18]

### Systemic Lupus Erythematosus

With current test methods, 95–98% of active, untreated patients with SLE have a positive ANA. For patients presenting with rheumatic signs and symptoms (e.g., joint pain, joint swelling, and morning stiffness) and SLE indicative signs (e.g., butterfly rash, photosensitivity, oral ulcers, and discoid rash), a positive ANA test can be con-

sidered one of the possible 11 SLE classification criteria established by the American College of Rheumatology (Table 3, page 379). As with the rheumatoid factor test, results of an ANA test are always interpreted in conjunction with a patient's clinical signs and symptoms.[19]

These diagnostic criteria were developed as a guide for selecting a more homogeneous patient population for research studies. The diagnosis of SLE could be made if any four of the 11 classification criteria are present, serially or simultaneously, during any observation period. Even if four criteria are fulfilled, however, a health care professional may elect not to diagnose SLE based on a history and physical examination. Likewise, patients with only three classification criteria may have their signs and symptoms diagnosed as SLE when strong clinical suspicion is present.[14]

Two other highly specific tests for SLE are anti-double-stranded DNA and anti-Sm. The anti-double-stranded DNA test is commonly used when the SLE diagnosis is questionable and the ANA titer is low or moderate with an immunofluorescent rim pattern. A positive anti-double-stranded DNA test is very specific for, and essentially diagnostic of SLE (Minicase 1, page 380). In contrast, testing for antibodies to single-stranded DNA has poor diagnostic specificity for SLE even though it is more sensitive (90%). Although this antibody appears to be important in the immunopathogenesis of SLE, the test has no clinical application because of poor specificity.

There is considerable evidence that antibodies to both double-stranded DNA and single-stranded DNA are important in the pathogenesis of lupus nephritis; they seem to correlate with its presence and severity. Titers of these antibodies tend to fall with successful treatment, frequently becoming undetectable during sustained remission.[13] If the ANA test is positive with a speckled pattern, an anti-Sm test may be done instead of an anti-double-stranded DNA test. Again, a positive anti-Sm is very specific for the diagnosis of SLE. Anti-Sm antibodies are detected in 30–40% of Asian or African SLE patients whereas only 10–20% of Caucasian SLE patients are positive (Table 2).

### Pediatric Rheumatic Diseases

Although a positive ANA is not part of official JRA diagnostic criteria, ANA testing may be useful clinically. JRA accounts for approximately 75% of all pediatric connective-tissue diseases. Approximately 50–70% of children specifically diagnosed with poly- or oligoarticular onset JRA demonstrate a positive ANA, making it a more useful test than rheumatoid factor. The staining pattern is usually homogeneous or speckled and diffuse, and the titer is usually low to moderate (≤1:256). The highest prevalence of ANA seropositivity (65–100%) is seen in young girls with oligoarticular onset JRA and uveitis. Chronic uveitis occurs in over one-third of JRA patients with oligoarticular onset.[10,11]

**TABLE 2.** Laboratory and Clinical Characteristics of Antibodies to Nuclear/Cytoplasmic Antigens[a]

| ANA | Immunofluorescent Staining Pattern | Targeted Cellular Material | Sensitivity | Specificity |
|---|---|---|---|---|
| Anti-dsDNA[b] | Rim | dsDNA | SLE[b] 60–70% | High: SLE >90% if present in high titer |
| Anti-Sm[c] (rarely occurs by itself) | Fine speckled | Nuclear ribonucleoproteins | SLE 25% (Asian/African 30–40%; Caucasian 10–20%) | High: SLE 98% |
| Anti-ssDNA[b] | Rim | ssDNA | SLE 90%; RA[b] 60%; drug-induced SLE 55% | |
| Antihistone | Homogeneous | Chromatin and DNA-packing protein | Drug-induced SLE 100%; SLE 30%; RA 15–20% | |
| Anti-$U_1$RNP[b] | Fine speckled | Nuclear ribonucleoproteins | MCTD[b] 100%; SLE 30%; scleroderma 20–30%; discoid lupus 20–30%; RA 10%; polymyositis 10% | |
| Anti-Ro[c]/SSA[d] | Fine speckled | Nuclear ribonucleoproteins | Sjögren's syndrome 90%; SLE 25–50%; polymyositis 18%; RA 5%; scleroderma 5% | |
| Anti-La[c]/SSB[d]/Ha[c] (rarely occurs by itself) | Fine speckled | Nuclear ribonucleoproteins | Sjögren's syndrome 85%; SLE 10–15% | |
| Anticentromere | Discrete large speckled | Chromatin and centromere | Scleroderma 10–15%; CREST[b] 50–90%; Raynaud's phenomenon 15–30% | High: scleroderma, CREST, or Raynaud's phenomenon >95% |
| Antitopoisomerase I (anti-Scl$_{70}$) | Grainy speckled | Chromatin and DNA-catalyzing protein | Scleroderma 15–20% | High: scleroderma >95% |
| Anti-Jo-1 | Cytoplasmic | Cytoplasm and histidyl t-RNA synthetase | Polymyositis 20–30%; Jo-1 syndrome 50% | High: polymyositis with interstitial lung disease or Jo-1 syndrome |

[a]Adapted from References 13–17.
[b]Anti-dsDNA = anti-double-stranded DNA; anti-ssDNA = anti-single-stranded DNA; anti-$U_1$RNP = anti-uridine-rich ribonuclear protein; SLE = systemic lupus erythematosus; RA = rheumatoid arthritis; MCTD = mixed connective-tissue disease; CREST = calcinosis, Raynaud's phenomenon, esophageal motility disorder, sclerodactyly, and telangiectasias.
[c]Represents the first two letters of the patient's name whose serum was used to identify the reaction in agar diffusion.
[d]Sjögren's syndrome A and B.

**TABLE 3.** 1982 Revised Criteria for Classification of SLE[a]

| Criterion | Definition |
|---|---|
| 1. Malar rash | Fixed erythema, flat or raised, over malar eminences, tending to spare nasolabial folds |
| 2. Discoid rash | Erythematous raised patches with adherent keratotic scaling and follicular plugging; atrophic scarring may occur in older lesions |
| 3. Photosensitivity | Skin rash as result of unusual reaction to sunlight, observed by physician or in patient history |
| 4. Oral ulcers | Oral or nasopharyngeal ulceration, usually painless, observed by physician |
| 5. Arthritis | Nonerosive arthritis involving two or more peripheral joints and characterized by tenderness, swelling, or effusion |
| 6. Serositis | Pleuritis—convincing history of pleuritic pain or rub, heard by physician or with evidence of pleural effusion<br>*or*<br>Pericarditis—documented by electrocardiogram or rub or with evidence of pericardial effusion |
| 7. Renal disorder | Persistent proteinuria >0.5 g/day or >3+ if quantitation not performed<br>*or*<br>Cellular casts—red cell, hemoglobin, granular, tubular, or mixed |
| 8. Neurologic disorder | Seizures or psychosis—in absence of offending drugs or known metabolic derangements (e.g., uremia, ketoacidosis, and electrolyte imbalance) |
| 9. Hematologic disorder | Hemolytic anemia—with reticulocytosis<br>*or*<br>Leukopenia—<4000/mm³ total on two or more occasions<br>*or*<br>Lymphopenia—<1500/mm³ on two or more occasions<br>*or*<br>Thrombocytopenia—<100,000/mm³ in absence of offending drugs |
| 10. Immunologic disorder | Positive lupus erythematosus cell preparation<br>*or*<br>Anti-DNA: antibody to native DNA in abnormal titer<br>*or*<br>Anti-Sm: presence of antibody to Sm nuclear antigen<br>*or*<br>False-positive serologic test for syphilis known to be positive for at least 6 months and confirmed by *Treponema pallidum* immobilization or fluorescent treponemal antibody absorption test |
| 11. ANA | Abnormal titer of ANA by immunofluorescence or equivalent assay at any time and in absence of drugs known to be associated with drug-induced lupus syndrome |

[a]*Adapted from Reference 19.*

Although the sensitivity of the ANA test in JRA patients is not high, its specificity is moderate; children diagnosed with SLE or scleroderma (either linear or systemic) can also have a positive ANA.[12] Clinically, the acute onset of SLE in children, which represents 10% of all pediatric connective-tissue diseases, can initially resemble systemic onset of JRA. The SLE diagnosis is likely to be made if the ANA test is positive, because the test is rarely positive in a child with systemic onset JRA (≤10%).

Polyarticular and oligoarticular onset JRA, however, cannot be easily differentiated from SLE. Usually, additional characteristic signs or symptoms of SLE must develop before a diagnosis is possible. All children diagnosed with SLE are ANA positive.[11]

Although scleroderma in children is associated with a positive ANA test in more than 50% of the cases, disease onset is usually within ages 3–14 years as compared to an onset of JRA in ages 1–3 years. Furthermore, skin conditions characteristic of scleroderma (e.g., skin tightening, thinning, and atrophy on hands and face) usually exist at presentation.[20]

## Other Rheumatic Diseases

Two other rheumatic diseases include a positive ANA test

---

### Minicase 1

A 50-year-old white male, Joe A., went to his family physician complaining of fever and sore throat and being run down for 5 days. Even though he had stayed home from work for the past 5 days, Joe A.'s skin appeared to be slightly sunburned in areas exposed to the sun.

Joe A.'s medical history was significant for a 20-year smoking habit (one pack a day), hypertension, and a myocardial infarction 6 months ago complicated by arrhythmias afterward. The physician had referred him to a rheumatologist approximately 11 months ago because of intermittent joint pain that was not characteristic of osteoarthritis. No diagnosis was made at that visit. The results of laboratory tests done at that time, however, were significant for a low-titer rheumatoid factor (1:80) and a positive ANA rim pattern at a titer of 1:160.

Joe A.'s current medications, unchanged for 6 months, included enalapril, ibuprofen, procainamide, and one aspirin a day. He was allergic to penicillin and intolerant to erythromycin.

After her examination, the physician performed a rapid strep test (negative), set up a throat culture, and prescribed tetracycline. The patient continued to take tetracycline after his physician's office notified him of the positive throat culture for *Streptococcus pyogenes*.

Five days after starting tetracycline, Joe A. returned to his physician's office because of continued fever and malaise. His sore throat had resolved. Upon examination, the physician noticed a continued fever; slightly labored breathing without productive cough, signs of pneumonia, bronchitis, or congestive heart failure; and with sunburned arms and neck. Joe A. mentioned that he had done light yard work, having forgotten that his antibiotic could make his skin sensitive to the sun.

When asked about his breathing, Joe A. indicated that he could not breathe deeply when he exerted himself because it was beginning to hurt more. However, the pain was not like what he had during his heart attack. Joe A. also mentioned that he had started taking more ibuprofen because his fingers and knees hurt.

Reluctant to put this patient on steroids, the physician asked him to stop taking tetracycline. She gave him a prescription for enough trimethoprim–sulfamethoxazole to complete 7 days of antibiotic therapy. Furthermore, she had blood drawn for a complete blood count (CBC) with differential, chemistry panel, rheumatoid factor, and ANAs. In addition, Joe A. was given an appointment to see the rheumatologist.

When Joe A. went to the rheumatology office, he had completed his antibiotic. His fever was still present, and all other signs and symptoms were unchanged except that his breathing was slightly more painful and labored and his sunburn was better.

The rheumatologist looked at Joe A.'s new laboratory results:

- A low white blood cell (WBC) count of 2000 cells/mm³ (4800–10,800 cells/mm³) without a left shift: bands 3% (3–6%) and no metamyelocytes.
- A normal percentage of 20% lymphocytes (20–40%).
- An unchanged rheumatoid factor titer (1:80).
- A high-titer (1:320) ANA rim pattern.

After getting a urine sample from the patient, the rheumatologist found that a dipstick test for protein was significantly positive. Blood was drawn to identify the specific ANAs present. When the lab results became available, anti-double-stranded DNA antibodies were identified.

*What diagnosis and treatment should the rheumatologist recommend?*

**Discussion:** This case demonstrates how difficult it is to diagnose SLE. Joe A.'s initial presentation was typical of an ongoing viral or bacterial infection. As a result of documented drug allergies and intolerances, tetracycline was a rational choice for the patient's bacterial infection. Moreover, his reaction to sunlight was not unexpected. However, both fever and photosensitivity are potential presenting symptoms for SLE or drug-induced SLE, often recognized weeks to months after nonacute presentations.

Joe A.'s previous arthritic symptoms occurred before procainamide was started, making drug-induced SLE less likely. Even though the first rheumatoid factor and ANA (rim pattern) tests were positive, the patient was febrile, and photosensitivity was present prior to tetracycline ingestion, SLE was not diagnosed at that time. However, after completion of antibacterial therapy, Joe A.'s symptoms continued and evidence of mild pleuritis occurred. Therefore, the family physician referred him to a rheumatologist.

With additional evidence of a lupus-like syndrome (leukopenia and proteinuria), a specific ANA test was ordered and anti-double-stranded DNA antibodies were detected. Based on the patient's symptoms, their time of presentation, and highly specific anti-double-stranded DNA antibodies, the diagnosis of SLE was made. Treatment with prednisone should resolve or improve all signs and symptoms in this patient.

---

in their diagnostic criteria. Virtually all patients diagnosed with mixed connective-tissue disease and drug-induced SLE have a positive ANA test. Other rheumatic diseases for which at least 75% of patients have positive ANAs include scleroderma, polymyositis/dermatomyositis, and Sjögren's syndrome.[13]

Three specific ANAs have high disease specificities. The anticentromere and antitopoisomerase I (Scl₇₀) antibodies are highly specific for scleroderma and related diseases such as CREST and Raynaud's disease. Anti-Jo-1 is highly specific for polymyositis with interstitial lung disease, Raynaud's phenomenon, and destructive polyarthritis (Jo-1 syndrome). However, these tests have little clinical utility because of their low sensitivity[15,16] (Table 2).

Four other specific ANAs have potential clinical importance. In women of childbearing age who have a known connective-tissue disease (e.g., SLE, mixed connective-tissue disease, or early undifferentiated connective-tissue disease), a positive anti-Ro/Sjögren's syndrome A (SSA) is associated with an infrequent but definite risk of bearing a child with neonatal SLE and congenital heart block.[15] In patients who are ANA negative but have clinical signs of SLE, a positive anti-Ro/SSA increases the probability of diagnosing SLE. Anti-Ro/SSA occurs in 62% of ANA-negative SLE patients. In some patients, anti-La/Sjögren's syndrome B (SSB)/Ha is a useful marker in the diagnosis of Sjögren's syndrome.[13]

In a patient with possible mixed connective-tissue disease, a negative anti-uridine-rich ribonuclear protein (anti-U$_1$RNP) virtually excludes this diagnosis. However, a positive test in the same patient increases the probability of mixed connective-tissue disease, even though the test is nonspecific.[15] A similar situation applies to antihistone testing in patients with suspected drug-induced SLE. Most of these cases are readily diagnosed because a commonly implicated drug (e.g., chlorpromazine, hydralazine, isoniazid, or procainamide) is being taken or a strong temporal relationship exists between drug initiation and the onset of SLE signs and symptoms. However, in some cases of potential drug-induced SLE, testing for histone autoantibodies can be helpful. The same logic applies to interpretation of anti-U$_1$RNP results and the association with mixed connective-tissue disease.[13,15]

*To be useful in patient management, specific ANAs need to correlate consistently with disease activity.* The only test that may consistently fluctuate with disease activity is anti-double-stranded DNA in a patient diagnosed with SLE. Even here, however, clinical and other laboratory findings are usually more consistent and more helpful than the anti-double-stranded DNA test for patient management decisions.[14]

### Nonrheumatic Diseases

ANAs are associated with various genetic and environmental factors (e.g., intravenous drug abuse) as well as hormonal factors and age. They also are associated with nonrheumatic diseases, both immunologically mediated (e.g., Hashimoto's thyroiditis, idiopathic pulmonary fibrosis, primary pulmonary hypertension, idiopathic thrombocytopenic purpura, and hemolytic anemia) and not immunologically mediated (e.g., infections—viral, parasitic, or bacterial; chronic or acute; neoplasm). Most laboratories use indirect immunofluorescence in initial ANA testing.[13]

## Antineutrophil Cytoplasmic Antibodies

In 1982, Davies et al. reported the presence of autoantibodies to cytoplasmic components of granulocytes in some patients with segmental necrotizing glomerulonephritis.[21] Four patients with systemic vasculitis (three patients had necrotizing glomerulonephritis) were reported to have the same autoantibodies.[22]

In 1985, Van der Woude et al. described a sensitive and specific marker for active Wegener's granulomatosis.[23] After ethanol fixation, indirect immunofluorescence pro-

duced a characteristic cytoplasmic pattern. These autoantibodies are now designated as cytoplasmic ANCAs (c-ANCAs). Other authors also noted that the c-ANCA titer correlated with Wegener's granulomatosis disease activity.[24] Furthermore, c-ANCAs were subsequently found in patients with polyarteritis nodosa, Churg-Strauss syndrome, and idiopathic crescentic glomerulonephritis. In 1988, c-ANCA was reported to be positive over a broad clinical spectrum, ranging from disease limited to necrotizing, crescentic glomerulonephritis without immune complex deposition to systemic polyarteritis nodosa and Wegener's granulomatosis.[24]

Antibodies producing a perinuclear pattern on ethanol-fixed neutrophils were first detected in patients with rheumatoid arthritis, ulcerative colitis, and chronic hepatitis, as described in 1959.[25] Unlike antibodies in SLE, these antibodies have affinity for nucleoproteins of neutrophils only and are now known as granulocyte-specific ANAs (GS-ANAs).[26]

ANCAs producing a perinuclear immunofluorescent pattern are now designated as perinuclear ANCAs (p-ANCAs). Numerous later reports determined that GS-ANAs and p-ANCAs were the same autoantibodies.[24] Originally, myeloperoxidase (MPO), a serine protease in the cytoplasmic granules of neutrophils and monocytes, was considered the specific antigenic target of p-ANCAs. However, when the MPO-specific ELISA is used (Chapter 2), anti-MPO antibodies are rarely detected in p-ANCA-positive sera from patients with various diseases.[27]

The detection and identification of ANCAs is probably most useful in diagnosing noninfectious systemic vasculitis, an often diagnostically confusing disease in which blood vessel walls are infiltrated by inflammatory cells. Most patients with this disease do not present with a classic clinical picture. Initial presentation is usually comprised of random flu-like symptoms (e.g., arthralgias, myalgias, anorexia, fever, and/or weight loss). Clinically, signs and symptoms may be consistent with many different diseases but still be diagnostically inconsistent with any particular disease. Serologic tests for SLE are negative (e.g., ANA, anti-Sm, and anti-double-stranded DNA) and complement concentrations are within normal limits, but ESR or C-reactive protein is elevated. Many times, pathologic confirmation of vasculitis is usually not available or is missed at biopsy. Vasculitic involvement of organs occurs sequentially, and the disease becomes obvious only retrospectively.

### Quantitative Assay Results

Disease activity of Wegener's granulomatosis and related disorders has been followed using c-ANCA. In a prospective study, Cohen Tervaert et al. demonstrated that c-ANCA titer elevations predicted, with high sensitivity and specificity, rises in disease activity. Relapses of Wegener's granulomatosis were preceded by c-ANCA titer increases by a median of 49 days.[28] Egner and Chapel confirmed these findings.[29]

In another prospective study, Wegener's granulomatosis patients were randomized to either immunosuppressive treatment or no treatment when c-ANCA titers increased and signs and symptoms of disease had not yet recurred. During a 2-year observation period, c-ANCA titers rose in 20 of 58 patients. Nine of these patients received immunosuppressive treatment, and no relapses occurred. Of the 11 patients who were not treated when c-ANCA titers rose, nine relapsed. The total amount of immunosuppression administered was lower in the prospectively treated group.[30] Serial quantitative titers of c-ANCAs may be useful for monitoring and predicting Wegener's granulomatosis disease activity as well as guiding "prophylactic" treatment.[27]

p-ANCAs have been detected in the sera of patients with various diseases, both rheumatic and nonrheumatic. Antigen-specific and nonspecific p-ANCAs range widely in sensitivity and specificity. Variable correlations exist between p-ANCA titer and disease activity. To date, a positive p-ANCA test and corresponding titers have limited diagnostic and therapeutic significance.[27]

Anti-MPO antibodies occur in patients with different forms of vasculitis and/or crescentic glomerulonephritis. In comparison to titers in sera obtained during remission, higher titers are associated with active disease. Although observed titers have increased prior to disease relapses, no prospective study has demonstrated the use of serial titer monitoring for predicting disease activity or initiating prophylactic treatment.

### Qualitative Assay Results

The antigenic target for c-ANCAs is proteinase 3 (a glycoprotein with serine protease, antibiotic, and growth-promoting activity) contained within azurophilic granules in the cytoplasm of neutrophils and monocytes. Originally, p-ANCAs were thought to react with MPO present in the same granules of the same cells. However, the perinuclear immunofluorescent pattern of p-ANCAs was an artifact of ethanol fixation. Ethanol fixation disrupts the membrane of the azurophilic granules; then MPO, a highly cationic protein, and other substances move from the disrupted granules and bind to the negatively charged outer surface of the nuclear membrane. Cross-linking fixatives, such as formalin, prevent granular leakage; a diffuse, granular cytoplasmic fluorescent pattern is produced. Although most p-ANCAs are no longer anti-MPO specific, the still unspecified antigenic targets are within the same cytoplasmic granules as MPO.[27]

For active Wegener's granulomatosis, the c-ANCA test (anti-Pr3) is highly sensitive. In classic (extended, restrictive) Wegener's granulomatosis (characterized by granulomatous inflammation of the respiratory tract, systemic vasculitis, and necrotizing crescentic glomerulo-

nephritis), c-ANCAs are present in more than 90% of patients. The c-ANCA test is 67–86% sensitive in patients with "limited" (no renal involvement) Wegener's granulomatosis.[28,31,32] When these two patient groups are combined, the sensitivity drops to 80%.

The sensitivity of the c-ANCA test for different vasculitic diseases is listed in Table 4. The presence of c-ANCAs denotes a spectrum of diseases, ranging from idiopathic pauci-immune, necrotizing glomerulonephritis to extended Wegener's granulomatosis. In most cases of vasculitis, renal disorder, and granulomatous disease, patient sera are invariably negative for c-ANCAs. The specificity of c-ANCAs for the spectrum of Wegener's granulomatosis disease is high (98%).[27]

The p-ANCA test has limited diagnostic value. A positive p-ANCA test should be followed by antigen-specific assays such as anti-MPO. The prevalence of p-ANCAs in various diseases also is listed in Table 4. In ulcerative colitis, the p-ANCA test has been reported to be as high as 94% specific. However, with only moderate sensitivity and inconsistent correlation between titers and disease activity, p-ANCA screening may be of little value. Although sensitivity can reach 85% in primary sclerosing cholangitis, the p-ANCA test lacks specificity in the differential diagnosis of autoimmune hepatic diseases. In rheumatoid arthritis, p-ANCAs may be related to aggressive, erosive disease. Test sensitivity increases in rheumatoid arthritis complicated by vasculitis, but specificity remains low.

In groups of patients with renal disorders and vasculitic diseases, anti-MPO antibodies are highly specific for systemic vasculitis and/or idiopathic crescentic glomerulonephritis. Disease-specific sensitivities and specificities are listed in Table 4.

## Complement

Complement is a well-defined system of 14 different plasma proteins that routinely circulate in precursor (inactive) form. Six plasma control proteins and five integral membrane control proteins regulate this cascade. Activation of this system can occur through either the classic or alternative pathway. When the initial protein of either pathway is activated, it then activates the next protein in a cascading fashion, similar to that seen with clotting factors (Chapter 15). Both activation pathways can activate the same final common cascade of proteins, known as the terminal sequence.

Each activated protein of the complement system has unique effects on the immune and inflammatory systems. At the same time, through the terminal sequence, activation of cascading proteins leads to the complement system's end-product. This end-product is a complex of the proteins C5–C6–C7–C8–C9, known as the *membrane attack complex*. This complex functions to lyse and destroy a targeted cell.[33]

**TABLE 4.** Disease Associations of ANCAs[a]

| ANCA | Targeted Cellular Material | Sensitivity | Specificity |
|---|---|---|---|
| c-ANCA (antiproteinase 3; anti-Pr3) | Proteinase 3, serine protease in azurophilic cytoplasmic myeloid granules | Extended Wegener's granulomatosis >90%; limited Wegener's granulomatosis 70–85%; microscopic polyarteritis 50%; polyangiitis overlap syndrome 40%; idiopathic crescentic glomerulonephritis 30%; Churg-Strauss syndrome 10%; classic polyarteritis nodosa 10% | Wegener's granulomatosis disease spectrum 98% (extended Wegener's granulomatosis; limited Wegener's granulomatosis-microscopic polyarteritis; polyangiitis overlap syndrome; and idiopathic crescentic glomerulonephritis) |
| p-ANCA | Unknown | Ulcerative colitis 60–75%; Crohn's disease 10–20%; autoimmune chronic active hepatitis 60–70%; primary biliary cirrhosis 30–40%; primary sclerosing cholangitis 60–85%; RA[b] with Felty's syndrome 90–100%; RA with vasculitis 50–75%; RA 20–40% | Ulcerative colitis >90%; all others low |
| anti-MPO | MPO, in azurophilic cytoplasmic myeloid granules | Idiopathic crescentic glomerulonephritis 70%; Churg-Strauss syndrome 70%; microscopic polyarteritis 50%; Wegener's granulomatosis 20%; classic polyarteritis nodosa 20%; polyangiitis overlap syndrome 20% | Systemic vasculitis and/or idiopathic crescentic glomerulonephritis 94–99% |

[a]Adapted from Reference 27.
[b]RA = rheumatoid arthritis.

Although existing immunoassays can identify each individual protein, test results are highly variable. Specific tests can measure the hemolytic capabilities of each activation pathway and the terminal sequence, but they are difficult to perform and often are used inappropriately in the diagnosis of rheumatic diseases.[34] To assess the complement system, a complement screen should include measurements of C3, C4, and total hemolytic activity by the complement hemolytic 50% ($CH_{50}$) test.[33]

Three important aspects need to be considered when interpreting complement test results:[33]

1. Normal ranges are relatively wide. Therefore, new test results should be compared with previous test results rather than with a normal range. It is most useful to examine serial test results and correlate changes with a patient's clinical picture.
2. Normal results should be compared with previous results, if available. For example, some SLE patients have concentrations of specific complement components two to three times the upper limit of normal when their disease is clinically inactive. As SLE disease activity increases, the concentrations drop into the normal range. If misinterpreted, normal concentrations would indicate an inactive complement system.
3. Complement responses do not consistently correlate with disease activity. In some patients, the

increase and decrease of the complement should not be used to assess disease activity.

### Complement Hemolytic 50%
*Normal range: 100–250 IU/mL*

One test still used in the clinical setting is the $CH_{50}$. It measures the ability of a patient's serum to lyse 50% of a standard suspension of sheep erythrocytes coated with rabbit antibody; the reaction includes the entire classic complement pathway. The $CH_{50}$ screening test may be useful when a complement deficiency is suspected or a body fluid other than serum is involved. For patients with SLE and lupus nephritis, serial monitoring of $CH_{50}$ may be recommended for guiding drug therapy.[6,35]

### C3 and C4
*Normal ranges: C3, 72–156 mg/dL or 0.72–1.56 g/L; C4, 20–50 mg/dL or 0.2–0.5 g/L*

Two other tests, for complement components C3 and C4, are routinely available. Since it is the most abundant complement protein, C3 was the first to be purified and measured by immunoassay. However, C4 concentrations appear to be more sensitive to smaller changes in complement activation and to be specific for identifying complement activation by the classic pathway.[33]

### Use of Complement Tests in Rheumatic Diseases
Hypocomplementemia occurs when the C3 or C4 con-

centration falls below its reference range. Most cases of hypocomplementemia are associated with hypercatabolism due to activation of the immune system and are not associated with decreased production of complement components (hyposynthesis). However, any disease that is associated with IgG- or IgM-containing circulating immune complexes can cause hypocomplementemia. Rheumatic diseases included in this category are SLE, rheumatoid arthritis with extra-articular disease, and systemic vasculitis. Synovial fluid of rheumatoid arthritis patients is often markedly low in complement concentrations.[33]

In SLE patients, decreases in complement concentrations have been associated with increased disease activity, specifically renal involvement. Decreases in complement have occurred prior to clinical exacerbations when followed serially.[33] The results of regularly scheduled complement tests have been used to guide decisions regarding immunosuppressive therapy of lupus nephritis. From a 10-year prospective study, findings in three consecutive reports (at 2, 5, and 10 years) positively correlated normalization of $CH_{50}$ with histologic stabilization and improvement of lupus nephritis. No correlation was found between concentrations of anti-double-stranded DNA and disease course.[36-38] Another study demonstrated improvement in renal function.[35]

## Related Nonspecific Tests

A heterogeneous group of plasma proteins, *acute-phase proteins* or *acute-phase reactants*, increases in concentration in response to inflammatory stimuli such as tissue injury and infection. Concentrations of C-reactive protein, serum amyloid A protein, $\alpha_1$-acid glycoprotein, fibrinogen, haptoglobin, prealbumin, and complement characteristically increase while transferrin and albumin concentrations decrease. Prealbumin and fibrinogen are described in Chapters 11 and 15, respectively. Their collective change is referred to as the *acute-phase response*.

In general, if the inflammatory stimulus is acute and of short duration, these proteins return to normal within days to weeks. If tissue injury or infection is persistent, however, acute-phase changes also may persist. Additionally, WBC and platelet counts may be elevated significantly.

Rheumatic diseases are chronic and are associated with varying severities of inflammation. Two acute-phase proteins are frequently measured, and the results are used in both research and general patient care settings. Fibrinogen is measured indirectly by the ESR, and C-reactive protein is measured directly.[39]

### Erythrocyte Sedimentation Rate
*Normal range: 0–10 mm/hr for males or*
*0–20 mm/hr for females*

The ESR is a nonspecific test that has been used widely in clinical medicine for over 60 years. It is simple to perform and commonly recognized. Moreover, a tremendous amount of data is available concerning its clinical significance in numerous diseases. The ESR is an important outcome variable when used in multicenter clinical trials assessing drug efficacy in the treatment of rheumatoid arthritis.[39]

Relative to rheumatic diseases, an increase in the ESR is related to an increased concentration of fibrinogen, the major component of the acute-phase response. The ESR is not, however, a direct reflection of fibrinogen concentrations. The Westergren method of performing an ESR test is still used routinely because of its relative ease in any clinical or laboratory setting; it is procedurally better than the Wintrobe ESR.

As mentioned in Chapter 14, the zeta-sedimentation ratio is the only procedure that corrects for anemia and gives a technically accurate measurement of the effect of altered plasma protein concentrations on erythrocyte aggregation. However, even this ratio is nonspecific. In addition, a special centrifuge is required, making it very unlikely that the zeta-sedimentation method will be used often.[39]

Despite its technical problems, the Westergren ESR is often used clinically. Evaluating serial Westergren ESR results and correlating them with patient data may influence therapeutic decisions. Two rheumatic diseases, polymyalgia rheumatica and temporal arteritis (giant cell arteritis), are almost always associated with an elevated Westergren ESR. The ESR is usually above 60 mm/hr and frequently is above 100 mm/hr. During initial therapy or therapy instituted after a flare, a significant decrease or a return to a normal ESR probably indicates that systemic inflammation has significantly decreased. In the absence of clinical symptoms, an increased ESR may indicate that more aggressive therapy is needed. Disease activity then could be monitored by ESR results. Of course, if symptoms are present, they should not be ignored.[39]

### C-Reactive Protein
*Normal range: 0–0.5 mg/dL or 0–0.005 g/L*

C-reactive protein is a plasma protein of the acute-phase response. In response to a stimulus, C-reactive protein can increase up to 1000 times its baseline concentration. Although C-reactive protein concentrations increase in response to tissue injury and infection, no specific C-reactive protein function has been identified. One suggested role is it binds with necrotic cell membranes at inflammation sites, allowing phagocytes to adhere and activate the complement system. Because it more accurately reflects immune system activity, C-reactive protein may be a better test than the Westergren ESR.

With the advancement of technology, C-reactive protein is no longer reported as simply "present" or "absent." Most patients and normal individuals have concentrations of 1 mg/dL or less. Moderate increases range from 1 to 10 mg/dL, and marked increases are greater than 10 mg/dL. Bacterial infections are often associated with values above 10 mg/dL. As with the Westergren ESR, serial measurements of C-reactive protein are the most valuable, especially in chronic inflammatory diseases.

Currently, the routine use of C-reactive protein is limited. As with the ESR test, C-reactive protein concentrations generally increase and decrease with worsening or improving signs and symptoms, respectively. Nevertheless, C-reactive protein concentrations are not disease specific, nor are they part of the diagnostic criteria for any rheumatic disease. Unlike the ESR test, the C-reactive protein test is difficult to perform without expensive equipment. However, concentrations are not affected by age, anemia, pregnancy, and hyperglobulinemia.

Most published studies were conducted before quantitative technology became available. One potential clinical application of C-reactive protein is in patients with SLE. If the C-reactive protein concentration reaches 6–8 mg/dL in an SLE patient, the possibility of infection should be ruled out as the signs and symptoms of SLE are assessed.[39]

## Synovial Fluid Analysis

Synovial fluid is essentially a dialysate of plasma to which synovial cells add hyaluronate. This fluid lubricates and nourishes the avascular articular cartilage. Normally, synovial fluid is present in small amounts and is clear and acellular (<200 cells/mm$^3$) with a high viscosity because of the hyaluronic acid concentration. The fluid does not clot because fibrinogen and clotting factors do not enter the joint space from the vascular space.

For arthrocentesis, or joint aspiration, a needle is introduced into the joint space of a diarthrodial joint. With a syringe, all easily removed synovial fluid is drained from the joint space. Arthrocentesis is indicated as a diagnostic procedure when septic arthritis, hemarthrosis (blood within a joint), or crystal-induced arthritis is suspected. Furthermore, arthrocentesis may be indicated in any clinical situation, rheumatic or nonrheumatic, if the cause of new or increased joint inflammation is unknown. Arthro-

centesis also is performed to administer intra-articular corticosteroids.

When arthrocentesis is done, the synovium may be inflamed, allowing fibrinogen, clotting factors, and other proteins to diffuse into the joint. Therefore, the collected synovial fluid should be placed in heparinized tubes to prevent clotting and to allow determination of cell type and cell number.

Synovial fluid is usually classified as inflammatory or noninflammatory. Table 5 presents the characteristics of four pathological types. In addition to sending heparinized fluid for Gram's staining and culture, synovial fluid should be examined for crystals. The presence of crystals, identified by polarized light microscopy with red compensation, can be diagnostic (Table 6, next page). Monosodium urate crystals are associated with gout, and calcium pyrophosphate dihydrate crystals are associated with calcium pyrophosphate deposition disease (pseudogout).[40] (Minicase 2, next page.)

## Miscellaneous Tests

The three most commonly performed "nonrheumatic" tests in rheumatology are

➤ CBC with a WBC differential and platelet count.
➤ Chemistry panel, including electrolytes and tests of hepatic, renal, and pancreatic functions.
➤ Urinalysis with microscopic analysis.

Tables 7 and 8 (page 387) contain information on interpreting results of these tests for common rheumatic disorders. These tests are discussed from a more general perspective in other chapters.

# TESTS TO MONITOR ANTIRHEUMATIC DRUG THERAPY

Antirheumatic therapies can cause significant adverse reactions that are reflected in laboratory test results. Abnormal test results may necessitate dose reduction, temporary discontinuation, or permanent withdrawal of the

**TABLE 5.** Synovial Fluid Classification[a]

| Synovial Fluid Type | Color | Clarity | WBC (/mm$^3$) | PMN[b] | Culture | Protein (g/dL) |
|---|---|---|---|---|---|---|
| Normal | Colorless | Clear | <200 | <25 | Negative | <2.0 |
| Noninflammatory | Straw | Transparent | <2000 | <25 | Negative | >3.5 |
| Inflammatory | Yellow | Translucent | 2000–80,000 | Variable | Negative | >3.5 |
| Septic | Variable | Opaque | 2000–100,000 | Usually present | Usually positive | >3.5 |

[a]Adapted from Reference 40.
[b]PMN = polymorphonuclear leukocyte.

**TABLE 6.** Synovial Fluid Crystal Morphology[a]

| Crystal | Birefringence | Shape | Size (microns) |
|---|---|---|---|
| Monosodium urate | Negative | Needle | 1–20 |
| Calcium pyrophosphate dihydrate | Positive (weak) | Rod | 5–100 |
| Dicalcium phosphate dihydrate | Positive (strong) | Variable | Variable |
| Hydroxyapatite | – | Needle | 0.1–1 |
| Cholesterol | Negative | Flat rhomboid plates with notched corners or needle | >100 |
| Calcium oxalate | Positive | Cuboidal | 2–10 |
| Corticosteroid | Positive and negative | Variable | 1–20 |
| Others [cartilage fragments, metal fragments (joint prosthesis), and amyloid fragments] | Usually present | Variable | Variable |

[a]Adapted from Reference 40.

offending drug. The laboratory tests most commonly affected are the WBC count, platelet count, hepatic transaminases, and urinalysis (Table 9, pages 388 and 389).

Decreases in WBCs are considered to be clinically significant when the total count is 3000–3500/mm³ or lower, because immune defenses are compromised. The various types of WBCs are discussed in Chapter 14. The low WBC counts are primarily due to a relative and absolute decrease of neutrophils. Pancytopenia indicates a suppression of all cell lines, including red blood cells and platelets; aplastic anemia indicates a complete arrest of blood cell production in the bone marrow.

---

### ✎ Minicase 2

Nathan S., an 85-year-old male, came to the emergency department unable to bear weight on his right leg. His right knee was swollen, inflamed, and painful. He had no signs or symptoms of infection and otherwise was in good health, except for several gout attacks over the past 10 years.

Nathan S.'s knee was aspirated and drained with a needle and syringe. Several drops of slightly cloudy, light yellow aspirate were placed on a slide, and the slide was sent to pathology. The remaining knee aspirate in the syringe was sent, in heparinized tubes, to the laboratory for Gram's stain, bacterial culture, cell count, and chemistry panel.

Examination of the slide showed a mixture of needle, rhomboid or rod, and variably shaped crystals. The slide was then viewed under a polarizing light microscope with a first-order red plate compensator. Although some crystals demonstrated either strongly positive or strongly negative birefringence, most were not birefringent (splitting a ray of light in two).

Upon receiving the pathology report, the emergency department physician looked at the preliminary laboratory results of the knee aspirate:

♦ 55,000 WBCs/mm³.
♦ 10% polymorphonuclear leukocytes.
♦ 5 g/dL protein.

No bacteria or other organisms were seen on the Gram's stain. (Tables 5 and 6 provide reference values.)

*What is Nathan S.'s diagnosis? What should be the plan for his treatment?*

**Discussion:** When Nathan S. presented initially, the worst was expected: septic arthritis. It was not ruled out by the absence of systemic signs and symptoms of infection. However, needle aspiration and drainage are diagnostic for calcium pyrophosphate dihydrate disease. Aspirating cloudy, yellow fluid from a red, swollen, and painful knee is consistent with infection and inflammation. Therefore, appropriate diagnostic tests were performed.

The patient's history of gout might have indicated a recurrent acute gouty attack as the most likely diagnosis. However, when microscopic examination found a mixture of crystal shapes, the slide was then examined under a polarizing light microscope to distinguish their most likely chemical composition. Based on birefringence findings and the differing shapes, most crystals were composed of calcium pyrophosphate dihydrate. The other two types of crystals were likely dicalcium phosphate dihydrate and uric acid.

Even though the synovial fluid findings, clinical presentation, and patient's age were consistent with the diagnosis of calcium pyrophosphate deposition disease (pseudogout), the presence of other crystal types is common. Nathan S. should take ibuprofen 600–800 mg four times a day for 4–5 days at home. After approximately 48 hr, as should be done whenever there is laboratory and clinical evidence of intra-articular inflammation, the physician should call the microbiology laboratory for the synovial fluid culture results. If no growth of bacteria happens, the patient can stay at home and continue his current therapy.

**TABLE 7.** Miscellaneous Abnormal Test Results in Rheumatoid Arthritis[a]

| Laboratory Test | Significant Result | Interpretation | Comments |
|---|---|---|---|
| CBC | Low hemoglobin; low hematocrit | Normochromic, normocytic anemia of chronic disease | Not erythropoietin deficiency |
| | MCV[b] <80 | Microcytic, hypochromic anemia—iron deficiency | Administration of iron to correct anemia in proportion to degree of iron deficiency |
| | | GI[b] blood loss (steroid or NSAID[b] associated?) | Identify source—guaiac testing, endoscopy; change drug regimen? |
| Platelet count | Thrombocytosis | Clinically active rheumatoid arthritis | Part of acute-phase response; as disease improves spontaneously or as result of drug therapy, platelet count returns toward normal |
| WBC and differential | Eosinophilia (>5% of WBC differential) | Associated with rheumatoid factor-positive severe disease | |
| | Granulocytopenia<br>• relative<br>• absolute (<2000 cells/mm³) | Felty's syndrome | |
| Chemistry panel (SMA 20, Chem 20) | Low albumin; low total protein | Poor nutrition; loss of nutrients | Loss of appetite |

[a]Adapted from Reference 41.
[b]MCV = mean corpuscular volume; GI = gastrointestinal; NSAID = nonsteroidal anti-inflammatory drug.

**TABLE 8.** Miscellaneous Abnormal Test Results in SLE[a]

| Laboratory Test | Significant Result | Interpretation | Comments |
|---|---|---|---|
| CBC | Low hemoglobin; low hematocrit | Normocytic, normochromic anemia | Not erythropoietin deficiency |
| | | Hemolytic anemia due to antierythrocyte antibodies with reticulocytosis | One of 11 diagnostic criteria; 10% patients; majority have positive Coomb's test |
| | MCV[b] <80 | Microcytic, hypochromic anemia—iron deficiency | Administration of iron to correct anemia in proportion to degree of iron deficiency |
| | MCV >80 | Macrocytic, normochromic anemia—hemolytic | |
| WBC and differential | Leukopenia; absolute lymphopenia | Clinically active SLE—antilymphocyte antibodies | One of 11 diagnostic criteria |
| Platelet count | Thrombocytopenia | Clinically active SLE—antiplatelet antibodies | Usually mild, between 100,000 and 150,000/mm³ |
| Chemistry panel | "Transaminitis"—increased ALP[b], ALT[b], and AST[b] | Possible chronic active hepatitis, granulomatous hepatitis, cirrhosis, acute hepatitis, fatty change, or cholestasis | Usually present only at onset of disease; decreases as disease improves |
| Urinalysis with microscopic analysis | Proteinuria >500 mg in 24 hr | | ~50% of patients; renal disease may still be present if urinalysis is normal |
| | Hematuria >2 RBC/hpf[b] in spun sediment | | ~35% of patients |
| | Pyuria >5 WBC/hpf in spun sediment | | ~30% of patients |

[a]Adapted from Reference 42.
[b]MCV = mean corpuscular volume; ALP = alkaline phosphatase; RBC = red blood cells; ALT = alanine aminotransferase; AST = aspartate aminotransferase; hpf = high-power field.

**TABLE 9.** Routine Laboratory Tests to Monitor Patients Receiving Selected Drugs for Treatment of Rheumatoid Arthritis or SLE

| Drug | Disease | Laboratory Test | Adverse Drug Reaction | Incidence (%) | References |
|---|---|---|---|---|---|
| Injectable gold (gold sodium thio-malate and sodium aurothioglucose) | RA[a] | CBC with differential and platelet count | Thrombocytopenia<br>Leukopenia<br>Pancytopenia | 1–3<br><1<br><0.5 | 43, 44<br>45, 46<br>45, 46 |
| | | Hepatic profile | Transaminitis | 4 | 45 |
| | | Urinalysis | Proteinuria | 1.3 | 45 |
| Oral gold (auranofin) | RA | CBC with differential and platelet count | Thrombocytopenia<br>Leukopenia | 0–1.3<br>0.5–1.3 | 45–48<br>45–48 |
| | | Hepatic profile | Transaminitis | 0–3.8 | 45–48 |
| | | Urinalysis | Proteinuria | 0–2.6 | 45–48 |
| Methotrexate | RA | CBC with differential and platelet count | Leukopenia<br>Pancytopenia | 0–2.6<br>0–2.1 | 48–51<br>48–51 |
| | | Hepatic profile, albumin | Transaminitis | 4.3–21 | 48–51 |
| D-Penicillamine | RA | CBC with differential and platelet count | Thrombocytopenia<br>Leukopenia | 0.1<br>0.9–5.3 | 52–58<br>52–58 |
| | | Hepatic profile | Transaminitis | 0.9 | 56 |
| | | Urinalysis | Proteinuria<br>Hematuria | 0–10.5<br>1.1 | 52–58<br>52 |
| Azathioprine | RA | CBC with differential and platelet count | Leukopenia | 0–31.6 | 54, 56, 59–64 |
| | | Hepatic profile | Transaminitis | 0–4.8 | 54, 56, 59–64 |
| | | Urinalysis | Proteinuria | 2.3 | 63 |
| Hydroxychloroquine | RA | CBC with differential and platelet count | Thrombocytopenia | 0–5.6 | 65–67 |
| | | Urinalysis | Proteinuria | 0–5.6 | 65–67 |
| Sulfasalazine | RA | CBC with differential and platelet count | Leukopenia | 0–3.3 | 68–76 |
| | | Hepatic profile | Transaminitis | 1.4 and 5.5 | 73, 74 |
| Chlorambucil | RA | CBC with differential and platelet count | Leukopenia<br>Thrombocytopenia<br>Acute myelogenous leukemia<br>Malignant histocytosis | 50<br>32.1<br>3.6 (one case)<br>3.6 (one case) | 77<br>77<br>77<br>77 |
| Cyclophosphamide | RA | CBC with differential and platelet count | Leukopenia | 40 and 0<br>0<br>31.6 and 5.6 | b, c<br>d<br>e, f |
| | | Urinalysis | Proteinuria<br>Hematuria | 7.9 and 8.3<br>26.1<br>19.4 and 15.8 | e, f<br>d<br>e, f |
| NSAID,[a] including aspirin | RA, SLE | CBC with differential and platelet count | Low hemoglobin; low hematocrit due to NSAID gastropathy or ulceration leading to blood loss | Unknown[g] | 81 |

**TABLE 9** *(continued)*

| Drug | Disease | Laboratory Test | Adverse Drug Reaction | Incidence (%) | References |
|---|---|---|---|---|---|
| | | Hepatic profile | Transaminitis with salicylates | Very rare | 82 |
| | | | Increased serum creatinine, blood urea nitrogen, and potassium;[h] increased or decreased sodium; decreased uric acid from anti-inflammatory doses of aspirin | Very rare | 83 |
| | | Urinalysis | Proteinuria; hematuria; pyuria | Very rare | 83 |
| Corticosteroids (most commonly prednisone) | RA, SLE | CBC with differential and platelet count | Peptic ulceration blood loss leading to low hemoglobin and hematocrit | Unknown | 84 |
| | | Hepatic profile | Low potassium; increased bicarbonate and creatine kinase (steroid myopathy) | Unknown | 84 |
| | | Urinalysis | Glycosuria | Unknown | 84 |

[a]RA = rheumatoid arthritis; NSAID = nonsteroidal anti-inflammatory drug.
[b]High dose, 150 mg/day maximum (78).
[c]Low dose, 15 mg/day maximum (78).
[d]Only dose, 1.8 mg/kg/day (79).
[e]High dose, 150 mg/day maximum (80).
[f]Low dose, 75 mg/day maximum (80).
[g]Incidence unknown due to lack of correlation of GI damage and symptoms.
[h]Due to worsening of preexisting mild to moderate renal dysfunction.

Thrombocytopenia (a decrease in platelet count) is discussed in Chapter 15. Increases in hepatic transaminases of two to three times baseline may be important (Chapter 11). The most common abnormalities identified by urinalysis are proteinuria, hematuria, pyuria, and casts (Chapter 7).

In Table 9, incidences are listed only if the adverse reaction led to temporary discontinuation or withdrawal of the implicated drug therapy. "Abnormal" test results that were transient or persistent but clinically not serious enough to warrant temporary discontinuation or withdrawal of drug therapy are not included; changes in dose either resolved or stabilized the affected laboratory parameters.

## TESTS TO GUIDE MANAGEMENT OF HYPERURICEMIA

The two most common tests used to diagnose or assess treatment of gout are serum uric acid and urine uric acid.

### Serum Uric Acid
*Normal range: 3.4–7 mg/dL or 202–416 μmol/L for males >17 years old or 2.4–6 mg/dL or 143–357 μmol/L for females >17 years old*[85]

Uric acid is the metabolic end-product of the purine bases of DNA. In humans, uric acid is not metabolized further and is eliminated unchanged by renal excretion. It is completely filterable at the renal glomerulus and is almost completely reabsorbed. Most excreted uric acid (80–86%) is the result of active tubular secretion at the distal end of the proximal convoluted tubule.[86]

As urine becomes more alkaline, more uric acid is excreted because the percentage of ionized uric acid molecules increases. Conversely, reabsorption of uric acid within the proximal tubule is enhanced and uric acid excretion is suppressed as urine becomes more acidic.

In plasma at normal body temperature, the physicochemical saturation concentration for urate is 7 mg/dL. However, plasma can become supersaturated, with the concentration exceeding 12 mg/dL. In nongouty subjects with normal renal function, urine uric acid excretion abruptly increases when the serum uric acid concentration approaches or exceeds 11 mg/dL. At this concentration, urine uric acid excretion usually exceeds 1000 mg/24 hr.

### Hyperuricemia

When serum uric acid exceeds the upper limit of normal, the biochemical diagnosis of hyperuricemia can be made. Hyperuricemia can result from an overproduction of purines and/or reduced renal clearance of uric acid. When specific factors affecting the normal disposition of uric acid cannot be identified, the problem is diagnosed as primary hyperuricemia. When the specific factors can be identified (e.g., another disease or drug therapy), the problem is diagnosed as secondary hyperuricemia.

Severe hyperuricemia is defined as a uric acid concentration greater than 12 mg/dL.[85] As the serum urate concentration increases above the upper limit of normal, the risk of a patient developing clinical signs and symptoms of gouty arthritis, renal stones, urate nephropathy, uric acid nephropathy, and subcutaneous tophaceous deposits increases. However, many patients who are labeled hyperuricemic are clinically asymptomatic. If a patient is hyperuricemic, it is important to look initially for potential causes of false laboratory test elevation and contributing extrinsic factors.

In general:[87]

> Renal function is not adversely affected by chronic hyperuricemia.
> Renal disease accompanying hyperuricemia often is related to uncontrolled hypertension.
> Correction of hyperuricemia has no measurable effect on renal function.

Hypouricemia, although associated with low-protein diets, renal tubular defects, xanthine oxidase deficiency, and drugs (e.g., high-dose aspirin, allopurinol, probenecid, and megadose vitamin C), is not important pathophysiologically.

*Extrinsic causes.* The most common extrinsic causes of hyperuricemia are medications. The therapeutic action of cancer chemotherapeutic agents (e.g., methotrexate, nitrogen mustards, vincristine, 6-mercaptopurine, and azathioprine) may increase the turnover rate of nucleic acids and the production of uric acid. Medications that interfere with renal clearance of uric acid include acetazolamide, hydralazine, ethacrynic acid, furosemide, and thiazide diuretics. Nephrotoxic drugs, such as mitomycin C, also can alter uric acid renal clearance.[88]

Salicylates, including aspirin, taken in low doses (1–2 g/day) may decrease urate renal excretion. Moderate doses (2–3 g/day), however, usually do not alter urate excretion. Large doses (>3 g/day) generally increase urate renal excretion, thus lowering serum urate concentrations.[82]

Drug-induced hyperuricemia following cancer chemotherapy, especially high-dose regimens, can lead to acute renal failure. Allopurinol is routinely administered prophylactically to decrease uric acid formation. In other clinical situations, drug-induced hyperuricemia may not be clinically significant.

The decision to continue or discontinue a drug that may be causing hyperuricemia is dependent on several factors:

> Risk of precipitating gouty symptoms, based on the patient's past history and current clinical status.

> Feasibility of substituting another drug that is less likely to affect uric acid disposition.
> Plausibility of temporarily or permanently discontinuing the drug.

If the regimen of the causative drug must remain unchanged, pharmacological treatment of hyperuricemia may be instituted.

Diet is another extrinsic cause of hyperuricemia. High-protein weight-reduction programs can greatly increase the amount of ingested purines and subsequent uric acid production. If the average daily diet contains a high proportion of meats, the excess nucleoprotein intake can lead to increased uric acid production. Fasting or starvation also can cause hyperuricemia because of increased muscle catabolism. Furthermore, lead poisoning from paint, batteries, or moonshine, in addition to recent alcohol ingestion, obesity, diabetes mellitus, and hypertriglyceridemia, is associated with increases in serum uric acid concentration[85,88] (Minicase 3).

*Intrinsic causes.* Intrinsic causes of hyperuricemia include diseases, abnormal physiological conditions that may or may not be disease related, and genetic abnormalities. Diseases include

> Renal diseases (e.g., renal failure).
> Those associated with increased destruction of nucleoproteins (e.g., leukemia, lymphoma, polycythemia, hemolytic anemia, sickle cell anemia, toxemia of pregnancy, and psoriasis).
> Endocrine abnormalities (e.g., hypothyroidism, hypoparathyroidism, pseudohypoparathyroidism, nephrogenic diabetes insipidus, and Addison's disease).

Predisposing abnormal physiological conditions include shock, hypoxia, lactic acidosis, diabetic ketoacidosis, alcoholic ketosis, and violent muscular exercise. In addition, males and females are at risk of developing asymptomatic hyperuricemia at puberty and menopause, respectively.

Genetic abnormalities include Lesch-Nyhan syndrome, gout with partial absence of the enzyme hypoxanthine guanine phosphoribosyltransferase, increased phosphoribosyl pyrophosphate P-ribose-pp synthetase, and glycogen storage disease type I.[85]

### Assays and Interferences

In the laboratory, the concentration of uric acid is measured by either the phosphotungstate colorimetric method or the more specific uricase method. With the colorimetric method, ascorbic acid, caffeine, theophylline, levodopa, propylthiouracil, and methyldopa can all cause falsely elevated uric acid concentrations. With the uricase method, dipyrone, calcium dobesilate, purines, and total bilirubin greater than 10 mg/dL can cause a false depression of

---

A 45-year-old, obese, male, Marvin B., recently began a daily exercise program to lose 50 lb. In addition, he began a new high-protein liquid diet because he knew how bad fatty foods were for him.

Two weeks after his new commitment, Marvin B. went to his family physician for his first complete physical examination in approximately 7 years. He told his physician not to tell him that he had to lose weight because he was already walking briskly for 1 hr three times a week and was carefully watching his diet. During the examination, the only abnormal finding was a high blood pressure (BP) of 150/95. After drawing blood for a CBC with differential and a full chemistry panel and obtaining a urine sample for urinalysis, his physician prescribed hydrochlorothiazide 25 mg once a day for hypertension. Three days later, Marvin B. was notified that his laboratory results, including uric acid, were normal.

Two weeks later, Marvin B. returned on crutches to see his physician. He explained that he had injured his right foot 3 days ago; when walking before sunrise, he had accidentally stubbed his right toes on a rock. Two nights ago, he had awakened with a fever and felt as if his right big toe was in a vise while an ice-cold knife was being pushed into the joint.

Upon examination of Marvin B.'s right foot, the physician noted abrasions on all five toes. The skin of the big toe looked shiny, and the toe was swollen and warm to the touch. Marvin B. was in obvious pain. Whitish fluid was oozing from a small wound on the dorsal aspect of the big toe. After anesthetizing it, the physician aspirated several drops of whitish fluid. He then performed a Gram stain and examined the fluid on a slide, finding needle-shaped crystals but no bacteria. Then he ordered a chemistry profile.

*What is this patient's diagnosis? What is an appropriate therapy?*

**Discussion:** Marvin B. had his first gout attack. Although his previous serum uric acid concentration was unknown, one intrinsic and two extrinsic factors were etiologic in the attack. In addition to hypertension, the sudden change to a high-protein diet greatly increased the amount of purines he was ingesting. In conjunction with this change, hydrochlorothiazide, an inhibitor of uric acid renal clearance, was started. His abrupt change in physical exertion probably did not contribute to the attack since it was low

in intensity.

Although Marvin B. attributed his condition to his traumatic toe-stubbing event, his physician noted that none of his other abraded toes appeared to be "infected." Having confidence and using a polarizing-light microscope, he was able to identify monosodium urate crystals while noting the significant absence of bacteria and daily febrile episodes (Table 6).

An appropriate therapy would be indomethacin 50 mg three times a day for 5 days. Marvin B. also should stop taking hydrochlorothiazide for 2 weeks.

**Minicase 3 (continued):** After explaining the health risks of a high-protein diet, the physician convinced Marvin B. to find a better balanced diet. He told Marvin B. that he would feel much better in 24 48 hr. Furthermore, if Marvin B.'s uric acid concentration was highly elevated the following week, he probably would add a drug called allopurinol.

Four days later, Marvin B. received a call from his physician and was told that his serum uric acid concentration was high at 9.8 mg/dL. His physician mentioned that he would not prescribe allopurinol at this time but asked Marvin B. to return in 2 weeks for a repeat blood test and reevaluation of his BP.

*Why did the physician decide to take this action? Why did he delay allopurinol therapy?*

**Discussion (continued):** After discontinuing Marvin B.'s hydrochlorothiazide and recommending a balanced low-fat diet plan, the physician decided to wait and see if the elevated serum uric acid concentration would decline without allopurinol. In 2 weeks, he would consider starting allopurinol if the repeat serum uric acid concentration was not near normal. He also should consider starting an angiotensin-converting enzyme inhibitor, such as enalapril, for Marvin B.'s hypertension.

Some clinicians recommend only observation after just one gout attack. However, if material aspirated from a joint is tophaceous (sheets of crystals in large numbers), allopurinol should be started immediately, regardless of the serum uric acid concentration or amount of uric acid in the urine. In this case, the physician decided to observe results before adding allopurinol to the patient's regimen.

---

uric acid concentrations. False elevations may occur if ascorbic acid concentrations exceed 5 mg/dL or if hemoglobin exceeds 300 mg/dL (in hemolysis).

## Urine Uric Acid

*Normal range: 250–750 mg/24 hr or 1.48–4.46 mol/24 hr*

In hyperuricemic patients who excrete an abnormal amount of uric acid in the urine (hyperuricaciduria), the risk of uric acid and calcium oxalate nephrolithiasis must be considered. The prevalence of stone formation is only twice that observed in the normouricemic population. When a stone does form, it rarely produces serious com-

plications. Furthermore, treatment can reverse stone disease related to hyperuricemia and hyperuricaciduria.[87]

Pathologically, uric acid nephropathy—a form of acute renal failure—is a direct result of uric acid precipitation in the lumen of collecting ducts and ureters. Uric acid nephropathy most commonly occurs in two clinical situations:

1. Patients with marked overproduction of uric acid secondary to chemotherapy-induced tumor lysis (leukemia or lymphoma).
2. Patients with gout and profound hyperuricaciduria.

Uric acid nephropathy also has developed after strenuous exercise or convulsions.[87]

In hyperuricemia unrelated to increased uric acid production, quantification of urine uric acid excreted in 24 hr can help to direct prophylaxis or treatment. Patients at higher risk of developing renal calculi or uric acid nephropathy (patients with gout or malignancies) excrete 1100 mg or more of uric acid per 24 hr. Prophylaxis of these patients may be recommended. To minimize the risk of nephrolithiasis, allopurinol should be used for prophylaxis instead of uricosuric agents. Furthermore, therapy could be started at the onset of gouty symptoms.[87]

## SUMMARY

Most specific rheumatologic laboratory tests are used in the management or diagnosis of patients with rheumatoid arthritis or SLE. By itself, none of these tests is diagnostic for any particular disease. Positive results of rheumatoid factor testing are most commonly seen in rheumatoid arthritis patients. Although higher concentrations of rheumatoid factor are associated with more severe cases of rheumatoid arthritis, rheumatoid factor titers or concentrations are not currently used to assess disease severity or clinical response to treatment.

ANA testing is most commonly used in SLE diagnosis. A positive ANA occurs in almost 100% of patients diagnosed with drug-induced SLE or mixed connective-tissue disease. Anti-double-stranded DNA and anti-Sm are disease specific for SLE.

c-ANCA is highly specific for the disease spectrum of Wegener's granulomatosis, and anti-MPO antibodies are highly specific for systemic vasculitis and/or idiopathic crescentic glomerulonephritis.

The most complete screen of complement activation includes measurements of C3, C4, and $CH_{50}$. Patients diagnosed with SLE and lupus nephritis may benefit from normalization of complement activity through the use of prednisone and/or azathioprine.

The degree of general systemic inflammation can be estimated with the Westergren ESR and C-reactive protein. In rheumatoid arthritis, polymyalgia rheumatica, and temporal arteritis (giant cell arteritis), elevated ESRs may indicate the need for more aggressive drug therapy. Unlike the ESR, C-reactive protein does not appear to increase with age and may be useful in assessing potential infection in SLE patients.

Patients diagnosed with rheumatoid arthritis or SLE commonly have routine laboratory work. Rheumatoid arthritis is usually associated with anemia of chronic disease and thrombocytosis. SLE is normally associated with anemia of chronic disease and thrombocytopenia and occasionally with hemolytic anemia. Proteinuria, hematuria, and pyuria are often seen in patients with active disease when a urinalysis is done. When rheumatoid arthritis or SLE patients begin antirheumatic drug therapy, labora-tory tests must be performed regularly to monitor for adverse drug reactions.

Patients with hyperuricemia are usually asymptomatic. Prophylaxis or treatment of gout, if initiated, is begun after the first attack. The severity and frequency of the attacks guide the decision. Allopurinol prophylaxis is recommended for patients who are known to form renal calculi.

## REFERENCES

1. Frangione B, Buxbaum JN. Immunoglobulins and their genes. In: Kelley WN, Harris ED Jr, Ruddy S, et al., eds. Textbook of rheumatology, 2nd ed. Philadelphia, PA: W. B. Saunders; 1985:5–21.
2. Lipsky PE, Davis LS, Meek K, et al. T cells and B cells. In: Kelley WN, Harris ED Jr, Ruddy S, et al., eds. Textbook of rheumatology, 4th ed. Philadelphia, PA: W. B. Saunders; 1993:108–54.
3. Carson DA. Rheumatoid factor. In: Kelley WN, Harris ED Jr, Ruddy S, et al., eds. Textbook of rheumatology, 4th ed. Philadelphia, PA: W. B. Saunders; 1993:155–63.
4. Arnett FC. Revised criteria for the classification of rheumatoid arthritis. *Bull Rheum Dis.* 1989; 38:1–6.
5. Shmerling RH, Delbanco T. The rheumatoid factor: an analysis of clinical utility. *Am J Med.* 1991; 91:528–34.
6. Pincus T. A pragmatic approach to cost-effective use of laboratory tests and imaging procedures in patients with musculoskeletal symptoms. *Prim Care.* 1993; 20:795–815.
7. Alarcon GS, Koopman WJ, Acton RT, et al. Seronegative rheumatoid arthritis. A distinct immunogenetic disease? *Arthritis Rheum.* 1982; 25:502–7.
8. Cats A, Hazevoet HM. Significance of positive tests for rheumatoid factor in the prognosis of rheumatoid arthritis: a follow-up study. *Ann Rheum Dis.* 1970; 29:254–9.
9. Feigenbaum SL, Masi AT, Kaplan SB. Prognosis in rheumatoid arthritis—a longitudinal study of newly diagnosed younger patients. *Am J Med.* 1979; 66:377–84.
10. Lawrence JM III, Moore TL, Osborn TG, et al. Autoantibody studies in juvenile rheumatoid arthritis. *Semin Arthritis Rheum.* 1993; 22:265–74.
11. Cassidy JT. Juvenile rheumatoid arthritis. In: Kelley WN, Harris ED Jr, Ruddy S, et al., eds. Textbook of rheumatology, 4th ed. Philadelphia, PA: W. B. Saunders; 1993:1189–208.
12. Singsen BH. Pediatric rheumatoid diseases: nonarticular rheumatism, juvenile rheumatoid arthritis, juvenile spondyloarthropathies. In: Schumacher HR Jr, ed. Primer on the rheumatic diseases, 9th ed. Atlanta, GA: Arthritis Foundation; 1988:160–4.
13. Craft J, Hardin JA. Antinuclear antibodies. In: Kelley WN, Harris ED Jr, Ruddy S, et al., eds. Textbook of rheumatology, 4th ed. Philadelphia, PA: W. B. Saunders; 1993:164–87.
14. Mills JA. Systemic lupus erythematosus. *N Engl J Med.* 1994; 330:1871–9.
15. White RH, Robbins DL. Clinical significance and interpretation of antinuclear antibodies. *West J Med.* 1987; 147:210–3.
16. Reichlin M. Antibodies to defined antigens in the systemic rheumatic diseases. *Bull Rheum Dis.* 1993; 42:4–6.
17. Aitcheson CT, Peebles C, Joslin F, et al. Characteristics of antinuclear antibodies in rheumatoid arthritis. Reactivity of rheumatoid factor with a histone-dependent nuclear antigen. *Arthritis Rheum.* 1980; 23:528–38.
18. Fries JF, Holman HR. Systemic lupus erythematosus: a

clinical analysis. Philadelphia, PA: W. B. Saunders; 1975.

19. Tan EM, Cohen AS, Fries JF, et al. The 1982 revised criteria for the classification of systemic lupus erythematosus (SLE). *Arthritis Rheum.* 1982; 25:1271–7.

20. Cassidy JT. Systemic lupus erythematosus, juvenile dermatomyositis, scleroderma, and vasculitis. In: Kelley WN, Harris ED Jr, Ruddy S, et al., eds. Textbook of rheumatology, 4th ed. Philadelphia, PA: W. B. Saunders; 1993:1224–47.

21. Davies DJ, Moran JE, Niall JF, et al. Segmental necrotizing glomerulonephritis with antineutrophil antibody: possible arbovirus aetiology? *BMJ.* 1982; 285:606.

22. Hall JB, Wadham B McN, Wood CJ, et al. Vasculitis and glomerulonephritis: a subgroup with an antineutrophil antibody. *Aust N Z J Med.* 1984; 14:277–8.

23. Van der Woude FJ, Rasmussen N, Lobatto S, et al. Autoantibodies to neutrophils and monocytes: a new tool for diagnosis and a marker of disease activity in Wegener's granulomatosis. *Lancet.* 1985; 2:425–9.

24. Falk RJ. ANCA-associated renal disease. *Kidney Int.* 1990; 38:998–1010.

25. Calabresi P, Edwards EA, Schilling RF. Fluorescent antiglobulin studies in leukopenic and related disorders. *J Clin Invest.* 1959; 38:2091–100.

26. Wiik A. Granulocyte-specific antinuclear antibodies. *Allergy.* 1980; 35:263–89.

27. Kallenberg CGM, Mulder AHL, Cohen Tervaert JW. Antineutrophil cytoplasmic antibodies: a still growing class of autoantibodies in inflammatory disorders. *Am J Med.* 1992; 93:675–82.

28. Cohen Tervaert JW, Van der Woude FJ, Fauci AS, et al. Association between active Wegener's granulomatosis and anticytoplasmic antibodies. *Arch Intern Med.* 1989; 149: 2461–5.

29. Egner W, Chapel HM. Titration of antibodies against neutrophil cytoplasmic antigens is useful in monitoring disease activity in systemic vasculitides. *Clin Exp Immunol.* 1990; 82:244–9.

30. Cohen Tervaert JW, Huitema MG, Hené RJ, et al. Prevention of relapses in Wegener's granulomatosis by treatment based on antineutrophil cytoplasmic antibody titre. *Lancet.* 1990; 336:709–11.

31. Nölle B, Specks V, Lüdemann J, et al. Anticytoplasmic autoantibodies: their immunodiagnostic value in Wegener's granulomatosis. *Ann Intern Med.* 1989; 111:28–40.

32. Andrassy K, Koderisch J, Rufer M, et al. Detection of clinical implication of antineutrophil cytoplasm antibodies in Wegener's granulomatosis and rapidly progressive glomerulonephritis. *Clin Nephrol.* 1989; 32:159–67.

33. Moxley G, Ruddy S. Immune complexes and complement. In: Kelley WN, Harris ED Jr, Ruddy S, et al., eds. Textbook of rheumatology, 4th ed. Philadelphia, PA: W. B. Saunders; 1993:188–200.

34. Bush TM, Shlotzhauer TL, Grove W. Serum complements. Inappropriate use in patients with suspected rheumatic disease. *Arch Intern Med.* 1993; 153:2363–6.

35. Lange K, Ores R, Strauss W, et al. Steroid therapy of systemic lupus erythematosus based on immunologic considerations. *Arthritis Rheum.* 1965; 8:244–59.

36. Appel AE, Sablay LB, Golden RA, et al. The effect of normalization of serum complement and anti-DNA antibody on the course of lupus nephritis. *Am J Med.* 1978; 64:274–83.

37. Jarrett MP, Sablay LB, Walter L, et al. The effect of continuous normalization of serum hemolytic complement on the course of lupus nephritis. *Am J Med.* 1981; 70:1067–72.

38. Laitman RS, Glicklich D, Sablay LB, et al. Effect of long-term normalization of serum complement levels on the course of lupus nephritis. *Am J Med.* 1989; 87:132–8.

39. Ballou SP, Kushner I. Laboratory evaluation of inflammation. In: Kelley WN, Harris ED Jr, Ruddy S, et al., eds. Textbook of rheumatology, 4th ed. Philadelphia, PA: W. B. Saunders; 1993:671–9.

40. Samuelson CO Jr, Ward JR. Examination of the synovial fluid. *J Fam Pract.* 1982; 14:343–9.

41. Harris ED Jr. Rheumatoid arthritis: the clinical spectrum. In: Kelley WN, Harris ED Jr, Ruddy S, et al., eds. Textbook of rheumatology, 2nd ed. Philadelphia, PA: W. B. Saunders; 1985:915–50.

42. Rothfield N. Clinical features of systemic lupus erythematosus. In: Kelley WN, Harris ED Jr, Ruddy S, et al., eds. Textbook of rheumatology, 2nd ed. Philadelphia, PA: W. B. Saunders; 1985:1070–97.

43. Deren B, Masi R, Weksler M. Gold-associated thrombocytopenia. *Arch Intern Med.* 1974; 134:1012–5.

44. Stafford BT, Crosby WH. Late onset of gold-induced thrombocytopenia. *JAMA.* 1978; 239:50–1.

45. Ward JR, Williams HJ, Egger MJ, et al. Comparison of auranofin, gold sodium thiomalate, and placebo in the treatment of rheumatoid arthritis. *Arthritis Rheum.* 1983; 10:1303–15.

46. Bombardier C, Ware J, Russell IJ, et al. Auranofin therapy and quality of life in patients with rheumatoid arthritis: results of a multicenter trial. *Am J Med.* 1986; 81:565–78.

47. Williams HJ, Dahl SL, Ward JR, et al. One-year experience in patients treated with auranofin following completion of parallel, controlled trial comparing auranofin, gold sodium thiomalate, and placebo. *Arthritis Rheum.* 1988; 31:9–14.

48. Williams HJ, Ward JR, Reading JC, et al. Comparison of auranofin, methotrexate, and the combination of both in the treatment of rheumatoid arthritis. A controlled clinical trial. *Arthritis Rheum.* 1992; 35:259–69.

49. Williams HJ, Willkens RF, Samuelson CO, et al. Comparison of low-dose oral pulse methotrexate and placebo in the treatment of rheumatoid arthritis: a controlled clinical trial. *Arthritis Rheum.* 1985; 28:721–30.

50. Weinblatt ME, Coblyn JS, Fox DA, et al. Efficacy of low-dose methotrexate in rheumatoid arthritis. *N Engl J Med.* 1985; 312:818–22.

51. Weinblatt ME, Kaplan H, Germain BF, et al. Low-dose methotrexate compared with auranofin in adult rheumatoid arthritis. *Arthritis Rheum.* 1990; 33:330–8.

52. Williams HJ, Ward JR, Reading JC, et al. Low-dose D-penicillamine therapy in rheumatoid arthritis: a controlled, double-blind, clinical trial. *Arthritis Rheum.* 1983; 26:581–92.

53. Dixon ASJ, Davies J, Dormandy TL, et al. Synthetic D (-) penicillamine in rheumatoid arthritis: double-blind controlled study of a high and low dosage regimen. *Ann Rheum Dis.* 1975; 34:416–21.

54. Halberg P, Bentzon MW, Crohn D, et al. Double-blind trial of levamisole, penicillamine, and azathioprine in rheumatoid arthritis. *Dan Med Bull.* 1984; 31:403–9.

55. Berry H, Linanage SP, Durance RA, et al. Azathioprine and penicillamine in treatment of rheumatoid arthritis: a controlled trial. *Br Med J.* 1976; 1:1052–4.

56. Paulus HE, Williams HJ, Ward JR, et al. Azathioprine versus D-penicillamine in rheumatoid arthritis patients who have been treated unsuccessfully with gold. *Arthritis Rheum.* 1984; 27:721–7.

57. Kean WF, Dwosh IL, Anastassiades TP, et al. The toxicity pattern of D-penicillamine therapy: a guide to its use in

rheumatoid arthritis. *Arthritis Rheum.* 1980; 23:158–64.

58. Shiokawa Y, Horiuchi Y, Honma M, et al. Clinical evaluation of D-penicillamine by multicenter double-blind comparative study in chronic rheumatoid arthritis. *Arthritis Rheum.* 1977; 20:1464–72.

59. Hamdy H, McKendry RJR, Mierins E, et al. Low-dose methotrexate compared with azathioprine in the treatment of rheumatoid arthritis: a twenty-four-week controlled clinical trial. *Arthritis Rheum.* 1987; 30:361–8.

60. Urowitz MB, Gordon DA, Smythe HA, et al. Azathioprine in rheumatoid arthritis: a double-blind, cross-over study. *Arthritis Rheum.* 1973; 16:411–8.

61. Urowitz MB, Hunter J, Bookman AAM, et al. Azathioprine in rheumatoid arthritis: a double-blind study comparing full dose to half dose. *J Rheumatol.* 1974; 1:274–81.

62. Dwosh IL, Stein HB, Urowitz MB, et al. Azathioprine in early rheumatoid arthritis: comparison with gold and chloroquine. *Arthritis Rheum.* 1977; 20:685–92.

63. Currey HLF, Harris J, Mason RM, et al. Comparison of azathioprine, cyclophosphamide, and gold in treatment of rheumatoid arthritis. *Br Med J.* 1974; 3:763–6.

64. Singh G, Fries JF, Spitz P, et al. Toxic effects of azathioprine in rheumatoid arthritis: a national post-marketing perspective. *Arthritis Rheum.* 1989; 32:837–43.

65. Husain Z, Runge LA. Treatment complications of rheumatoid arthritis with gold, hydroxychloroquine, D-penicillamine, and levamisole. *J Rheumatol.* 1980; 7:825–30.

66. Adams EM, Yocum DE, Bell CL. Hydroxychloroquine in the treatment of rheumatoid arthritis. *Am J Med.* 1983; 75:321–6.

67. Bunch TW, O'Duffy JD, Tompkins RB, et al. Controlled trial of hydroxychloroquine and D-penicillamine singly and in combination in the treatment of rheumatoid arthritis. *Arthritis Rheum.* 1984; 27:267–76.

68. McConkey B, Amos RS, Durham S, et al. Sulphasalazine in rheumatoid arthritis. *Br Med J.* 1980; 280:442–3.

69. Pullar R, Hunter JA, Capell HA. Sulphasalazine in rheumatoid arthritis: a double-blind comparison of sulphasalazine with placebo and sodium aurothiomalate. *Br Med J.* 1983; 287:1102–4.

70. Taggart AJ, Hill J, Astbury C, et al. Sulfasalazine alone or in combination with D-penicillamine in rheumatoid arthritis. *Br J Rheumatol.* 1987; 26:32–6.

71. Bax DE, Amos RS. Sulfasalazine: a safe, effective agent for prolonged control of rheumatoid arthritis: a comparison with sodium aurothiomalate. *Am Rheum.* 1985; 44:194–8.

72. Martin L, Sitar DS, Chalmers IM, et al. Sulfasalazine in severe rheumatoid arthritis: a study to assess potential correlates of efficacy and toxicity. *J Rheumatol.* 1985; 12:270–3.

73. Pinals RS, Caplan SB, Lawson JG, et al. Sulfasalazine in rheumatoid arthritis: a double-blind, placebo controlled trial. *Arthritis Rheum.* 1986; 29:1427–34.

74. Williams HJ, Ward JR, Dahl SL, et al. A controlled trial comparing sulfasalazine, gold sodium thiomalate, and placebo in rheumatoid arthritis. *Arthritis Rheum.* 1988; 31:702–13.

75. Farr M, Tunn EJ, Symmons DPM, et al. Sulphasalazine in rheumatoid arthritis: haematological problems and change in haematological indices associated with therapy. *Br J Rheumatol.* 1989; 28:134–8.

76. Amos RS, Pullar T, Bax DE, et al. Sulphasalazine for rheumatoid arthritis: toxicity in 774 patients monitored for one to 11 years. *Br Med J.* 1986; 293:420–3.

77. Cannon GW, Jackson CG, Samuelson CO Jr, et al. Chlorambucil therapy in rheumatoid arthritis: clinical experience in 28 patients and literature review. *Semin Arthritis Rheum.* 1985; 15:106–18.

78. Cooperating Clinics Committee of the American Rheumatism Association. A controlled trial of cyclophosphamide in rheumatoid arthritis. *N Engl J Med.* 1970; 283:883–9.

79. Townes AS, Sowa JM, Shulman LE. Controlled trial of cyclophosphamide in rheumatoid arthritis. *Arthritis Rheum.* 1976; 19:563–73.

80. Williams HJ, Reading JC, Ward JR, et al. Comparison of high and low dose cyclophosphamide therapy in rheumatoid arthritis. *Arthritis Rheum.* 1980; 23:521–7.

81. Marble DA, Ward JR. Managing NSAID-induced peptic ulcers. *Drug Ther.* 1989; 9:34–46.

82. Insel PA. Analgesic-antipyretics and antiinflammatory agents; drugs employed in the treatment of rheumatoid arthritis and gout. In: Gilman AG, Rall TW, Nies AS, et al., eds. Goodman and Gilman's the pharmacological basis of therapeutics. New York: Pergamon Press; 1990:647.

83. Clive DM, Stoff JS. Renal syndromes associated with nonsteroidal anti-inflammatory drugs. *N Engl J Med.* 1984; 310:563–72.

84. Haynes RC Jr. Adrenocorticotropic hormone; adrenocortical steroids and their synthetic analogs; inhibitors of the biosynthesis and actions of adrenocortical hormones. In: Gilman AG, Rall TW, Nies AS, et al., eds. Goodman and Gilman's the pharmacological basis of therapeutics. New York: Pergamon Press; 1990:48–52.

85. Jacobs DS, Kasten BL, DeMott WR, et al. Laboratory test handbook. St. Louis, MO: LexiComp/Mosby; 1988.

86. Hawkins DW. Gout and hyperuricemia. In: Dipiro JT, Talbert RL, Hayes PE, et al., eds. Pharmacotherapy: a pathophysiologic approach, 2nd ed. East Norwalk, CT: Appleton & Lange; 1992:1343–8.

87. Kelley WN. Approach to the patient with hyperuricemia. In: Kelley WN, Harris ED Jr, Ruddy S, et al., eds. Textbook of rheumatology, 4th ed. Philadelphia, PA: W. B. Saunders; 1993:498–506.

88. Wallach J. Interpretation of diagnostic tests: a synopsis of laboratory medicine. Boston, MA: Little, Brown; 1992.

# QuickView—Uric Acid

| Parameter | Description | Comments |
|---|---|---|
| **Common reference ranges** | | |
| Males | 3.6–8.5 mg/dL<br>214–506 µmol/L | *Prepuberty*: males and females have equal uric acid concentrations |
| | | *Postpuberty*: uric acid concentration stabilizes in early 20s; males have greater concentration than females |
| Females | 2.3–6.6 mg/dL<br>137–393 µmol/L | *Prepuberty*: females and males have equal uric acid concentrations |
| | | *Postpuberty*: uric acid concentration stabilizes in late teens to early 20s; females have lower concentration than males until menopause |
| | | *Postmenopausal*: females approach or equal males |
| **Critical value** | None | Concentrations greater than upper limit of normal: evaluation in conjunction with signs and symptoms |
| **Natural substance?** | Natural end-product of purine metabolism | Formed under normal circumstances |
| **Location** | | |
| Production | Throughout body | |
| Storage | None | |
| Secretion/excretion | Renal<br>Glomerular filtration 100%; proximal tubular reabsorption, 90%; net excretion, 10% | |
| **Major causes of . . .** | | |
| Hyperuricemia | Cancer chemotherapy, renal disease, malignancy, psoriasis, radiation therapy, hemolytic anemia, sickle cell anemia, polycythemia vera, starvation, fasting, high-protein weight reduction diets, obesity, ethanol, convulsions, severe exercise, tissue damage | Increased production or intake of purines |
| | Medication—acetazolamide, hydralazine, furosemide, thiazide diuretics, low-dose salicylates, mitomycin C<br>Renal—acidic urine, renal tubule disease, hypertension | Reduced renal clearance of uric acid |
| Associated signs and symptoms | Arthritis (gout), subcutaneous nodules, erosions/X-ray changes, nephrolithiasis (renal stones/calculi), urate nephropathy (renal insufficiency), uric acid nephropathy | |
| Normouricemia, hyperuricaciduria | Increased production or intake of purines<br>*and*<br>Normal or increased renal clearance of uric acid | |
| Associated signs and symptoms | Nephrolithiasis (renal stones/calculi) | |

  *continued*

## QuickView—Uric Acid *continued*

| Parameter | Description | Comments |
|---|---|---|
| **Hypouricemia** | Low protein diet and xanthine oxidase deficiency | Decreased production or normal intake of purines |
| | Medication—high-dose salicylates, allopurinol, probenecid<br>Renal—renal tubular defects and alkaline urine<br>Endocrine—hypothyroidism, hypoparathyroidism, nephrogenic diabetes insipidus, Addison's disease | Normal or increased renal clearance of uric acid |
| **Associated signs and symptoms** | None | |
| **After insult, time to . . .**<br>**Initial elevation or positive result** | Highly variable | Many patients do not have normal baseline uric acid concentrations recorded; first recorded results are often elevated, discovered incidentally in asymptomatic patient or as part of diagnostic workup for symptomatic patient |
| **Peak values** | Unknown | |
| **Normalization** | Hours, days | Assumes cause of hyperuricemia or hyperuricaciduria identified and treated |
| **Drugs often monitored with test** | Cancer chemotherapy | In hematologic malignancies |
| **Causes of spurious results** | Falsely low with uricase method (most specific) | Purines, total bilirubin (>10 mg/dL), calcium dobesilate, dipyrone |
| | Falsely high with phosphotungstate colorimetric method | Ascorbic acid, caffeine, theophylline, levodopa, propylthiouracil, methyldopa |
| | Falsely low with phosphotungstate colorimetric method | Ascorbic acid (>5 mg/dL) and hemoglobin (>300 mg/dL) |

# Appendix A
# Therapeutic Ranges of Drugs in Traditional and SI Units[a]

| Drug | Traditional Range | Conversion Factor[b] | SI Range |
|---|---|---|---|
| Acetaminophen | >5 mg/dL toxic | 66.16 | >330 µmol/L toxic |
| N-Acetylprocainamide | 4–10 mg/L | 3.606 | 14–36 µmol/L |
| Amitriptyline | 75–175 ng/mL | 3.605 | 180–720 nmol/L |
| Carbamazepine | 4–12 mg/L | 4.230 | 17–51 µmol/L |
| Chlordiazepoxide | 0.5–5.0 mg/L | 3.336 | 2–17 µmol/L |
| Chlorpromazine | 50–300 ng/mL | 3.136 | 150–950 nmol/L |
| Chlorpropamide | 75–250 µg/mL | 3.613 | 270–900 µmol/L |
| Clozapine | 450–? ng/mL | 0.003 | 1.38–? µmol/L |
| Cyclosporine | 100–200 ng/mL[c] | 0.832 | 80–160 nmol/L |
| Desipramine | 100–160 ng/mL | 3.754 | 170–700 nmol/L |
| Diazepam | 100–250 ng/mL | 3.512 | 350–900 nmol/L |
| Digoxin | 0.9–2.2 ng/mL | 1.281 | 1.2–2.8 nmol/L |
| Disopyramide | 2–6 mg/L | 2.946 | 6–18 µmol/L |
| Doxepin | 50–200 ng/mL | 3.579 | 180–720 nmol/L |
| Ethosuximide | 40–100 mg/L | 7.084 | 280–710 µmol/L |
| Fluphenazine | 0.5–2.5 ng/mL | 2.110 | 5.3–21 nmol/L |
| Glutethimide | >20 mg/L toxic | 4.603 | >92 µmol/L toxic |
| Gold | 300–800 mg/L | 0.051 | 15–40 µmol/L |
| Haloperidol | 5–15 ng/mL | 2.660 | 13–40 nmol/L |
| Imipramine | 200–250 ng/mL | 3.566 | 180–710 nmol/L |
| Isoniazid | >3 mg/L toxic | 7.291 | >22 µmol/L toxic |
| Lidocaine | 1–5 mg/L | 4.267 | 5–22 µmol/L |
| Lithium | 0.5–1.5 mEq/L | 1.000 | 0.5–1.5 µmol/L |
| Maprotiline | 50–200 ng/mL | 3.605 | 180–720 µmol/L |
| Meprobamate | >40 mg/L toxic | 4.582 | >180 µmol/L toxic |
| Methotrexate | >2.3 mg/L toxic | 2.200 | >5 µmol/L toxic |
| Nortriptyline | 50–150 ng/mL | 3.797 | 190–570 nmol/L |
| Pentobarbital | 20–40 mg/L | 4.419 | 90–170 µmol/L |
| Perphenazine | 0.8–2.4 ng/mL | 2.475 | 2–6 nmol/L |
| Phenobarbital | 15–40 mg/L | 4.306 | 65–172 µmol/L |
| Phenytoin | 10–20 mg/L | 3.964 | 40–80 µmol/L |
| Primidone | 4–12 mg/L | 4.582 | 18–55 µmol/L |
| Procainamide | 4–8 mg/L | 4.249 | 17–34 µmol/L |
| Propoxyphene | >2 mg/L toxic | 2.946 | >6 µmol/L toxic |
| Propranolol | 50–200 ng/mL | 3.856 | 190–770 nmol/L |
| Protriptyline | 100–300 ng/mL | 3.797 | 380–1140 nmol/L |
| Quinidine | 2–6 mg/L | 3.082 | 5–18 µmol/L |
| Salicylate (acid) | 15–25 mg/dL | 0.072 | 1.1–1.8 mmol/L |
| Theophylline | 10–20 mg/L | 5.550 | 55–110 µmol/L |
| Thiocyanate | >10 mg/dL toxic | 0.172 | >1.7 mmol/L toxic |
| Valproic acid | 50–100 mg/L | 6.934 | 350–700 µmol/L |
| Warfarin | 1–3 mg/L | 3.243 | 3.3–9.8 µmol/L |

[a]Also see Table 5 in Chapter 5.
[b]Traditional units are multiplied by conversion factor to get SI units.
[c]Whole blood assay.

# Appendix B
# Nondrug Reference Ranges for Common Laboratory Tests in Traditional and SI Units[a]

| Laboratory Test | Reference Range Traditional Units | Conversion Factor | Reference Range SI Units | Comment |
|---|---|---|---|---|
| Alanine aminotransferase (ALT) | 0–30 IU/L | 0.01667 | 0–0.50 µkat/L | SGPT |
| Albumin | 3.5–5 g/dL | 10.00 | 35–50 g/L | |
| Ammonia | 30–70 µg/dL | 0.587 | 17–41 µmol/L | |
| Aspartate aminotransferase (AST) | 8–42 IU/L | 0.01667 | 0.133–0.700 µkat/L | SGOT |
| Bilirubin (direct) | 0.1–0.3 mg/dL | 17.10 | 1.7–5 µmol/L | |
| Bilirubin (total) | 0.3–1.0 mg/dL | 17.10 | 5–17 µmol/L | |
| Calcium | 8.5–10.8 mg/dL | 0.25 | 2.1–2.7 mmol/L | |
| Carbon dioxide ($CO_2$) | 24–30 mEq/L | 1.000 | 24–30 mmol/L | Serum bicarbonate |
| Chloride | 96–106 mEq/L | 1.000 | 96–106 mmol/L | |
| Cholesterol (HDL) | >35 mg/dL | 0.026 | >0.91 mmol/L | desirable |
| Cholesterol (LDL) | <130 mg/dL | 0.026 | <3.36 mmol/L | desirable |
| Creatine kinase (CK) | 40–200 IU/L<br>35–150 IU/L | 0.01667 | 0.667–3.33 µkat/L<br>0.583–2.50 µkat/L | males<br>females |
| Serum creatinine (SCr) | 0.7–1.5 mg/dL | 88.40 | 62–133 µmol/L | |
| Creatinine clearance (CrCl) | 90–140 mL/min/1.73 m² | 0.017 | 1.53–2.38 mL/sec/1.73 m² | |
| Folic acid | ≥3.3 ng/dL | 2.212 | >7.3 nmol/L | |
| γ-glutamyl transpeptidase | 0–30 U/L (but varies) | 0.01667 | 0–0.50 µkat/L (but varies) | GGTP |
| Globulin | 2–3 g/dL | 10.00 | 20–30 g/L | |
| Glucose (fasting) | 70–110 mg/dL | 0.056 | 3.9–6.1 mmol/L | fasting |
| Hemoglobin (Hgb) | 14–18 g/dL<br>12–16 g/dL | 0.622 | 8.7–11.2 mmol/L<br>7.4–9.9 mmol/L | males<br>females |
| Iron | 50–150 µg/dL | 0.179 | 9–26.9 µmol/L | |
| Iron-binding capacity | 250–410 µg/dL | 0.179 | 45–73 µmol/L | TIBC |
| Lactate dehydrogenase | 100–210 IU/L | 0.01667 | 1.67–3.50 µkat/L | LDH |
| Serum lactate (venous) | 0.5–1.5 mEq/L | 1.000 | 0.5–1.5 mmol/L | Lactic acid |
| Serum lactate (arterial) | 0.5–2.0 mEq/L | 1.000 | 0.5–2.0 mmol/L | |
| Magnesium | 1.5–2.2 mEq/L | 0.500 | 0.75–1.1 mmol/L | |
| 5′ Nucleotidase | 1–11 U/L (but varies) | 0.01667 | 0.02–0.18 µkat/L (but varies) | |
| Phosphate | 2.6–4.5 mg/dL | 0.329 | 0.85–1.48 mmol/L | |
| Potassium | 3.5–5.0 mEq/L | 1.000 | 3.5–5.0 mmol/L | |
| Sodium | 136–145 mEq/L | 1.000 | 136–145 mmol/L | |
| Total serum thyroxine ($T_4$) | 4–12 µg/dL | 12.87 | 51–154 nmol/L | Total $T_4$ |
| Triglycerides | <200 mg/dL | 0.0113 | <2.26 mmol/L | |
| Total serum triiodothyronine ($T_3$) | 78–195 ng/dL | 0.0154 | 1.2–3.0 nmol/L | Total $T_3$ |
| Urea nitrogen, blood | 8–20 mg/dL | 0.357 | 2.9–7.1 mmol/L | BUN |
| Uric acid (serum) | 3.4–7 mg/dL | 59.48 | 202–416 µmol/L | |

[a]Some laboratories are maintaining traditional units for enzyme tests.

# Glossary of Medical Terms: Contextual Definitions

**Abscess**—Localized, walled-off collection of pus (white blood cells and cellular debris).

**Absorption, drug**—Extent of drug transfer from one body compartment (e.g., intestines) to another (bloodstream).

**Accuracy**—Degree of correlation of results between assay being investigated and alternative (usually standard) assay in analyzing patient samples.

**Acetylcholine**—Chemical released from nerve endings responsible for stimulating other nerves, muscles, and glands; neurotransmitter.

**Acidemia**—Abnormally acidic blood (pH < 7.35).

**Acidosis**—Process causing acidemia; pH is often less than 7.35 but may be higher if compensation mechanisms are effective.

**Actin**—Protein in muscle tissue that acts with myosin to allow muscle contraction and relaxation.

**Action potential**—Electrical activity developed in muscle or nerve cells responsible for propagating nerve signals or contraction.

**Addison's disease**—Adrenal gland dysfunction resulting in low or no output of hormones such as cortisone and aldosterone.

**Agglutination**—End-point of process used in certain assays. Clumping of cells (e.g., blood cells and bacteria) due to presence of antibodies. Use of known antigen (usually attached to latex particles) allows detection and identification of antibody in serum or other fluid (e.g., cerebrospinal fluid).

**Aggregation**—Clumping of cells due to electrostatic charges.

**Aldosteronism**—State of excessive aldosterone secretion by adrenal cortex.

**Alkalemia**—Abnormally alkaline blood (pH >7.45).

**Alkalosis**—Process causing alkalemia; pH is often greater than 7.45 but may be lower if compensation mechanisms are effective.

**Amyloidosis**—Generic term for group of clinically and biochemically diverse disease states characterized by deposition of insoluble fibrillar protein (including prealbumin or transthyretin) in extracellular space.

**Analyte**—Component intended to be measured in collected body fluid or tissue.

**Anemia**—Decrease in hemoglobin concentration or red blood cell count.

**Angiotensin**—Vasoconstrictor and stimulator of aldosterone secretion; formed from interaction of angiotensinogen (present in blood) and renin (released from kidneys); active form is angiotensin II.

**Antibody**—Protein produced by body in response to exposure to foreign proteins. As part of body's defense against invasion, antibodies help to increase efficiency of phagocytes and to activate complement.

**Antigen**—Foreign substance (e.g., bacteria, toxins, or proteins) that causes formation of antibodies.

**Antipyretic**—Having the ability to decrease elevated body temperatures. Examples are aspirin, ibuprofen, acetaminophen, and prednisone.

**Apparent distribution mass**—Mass or weight of body into which a drug apparently distributes; derivative of volume of distribution.

**Artifact**—False or spurious reading of laboratory test results caused by substance not usually present in specimen or assay equipment.

**Assay**—Test measuring concentration or activity of analyte.

**Asterixis**—Flapping tremor of fingers when arms and hands are outstretched; usually seen with hepatic encephalopathy and hypercapnia.

**Ataxia**—Incoordination of muscle action, usually without loss of muscle power; seen with excessive alcohol and phenytoin.

**Atherosclerosis**—Hardening of arteries with deposition of fat along inner arterial walls.

**Atrophy**—Reduction in size; can be normal physiological process (e.g., due to aging) or caused by disease.

**Autoimmune**—Specific humoral or cell-mediated immune response directed against constituents of body's own tissue.

**azo-**—Word root relating to nitrogen.

**Azotemia**—Excessive concentration of nitrogenous substances (e.g., blood urea nitrogen) in blood.

**Azoturia**—Excessive concentration of nitrogenous substances (e.g., blood urea nitrogen) in urine.

**Bacilli**—Rod-shaped bacteria (singular form: bacillus).

**Bacteremia**—Presence of bacteria in blood.

**Bacteria**—Single-celled procaryotic organisms that lack chlorophyll but have cell wall (unlike human cells).

**Basal**—Rate of process when body is at rest. For example, basal energy expenditure (also called basal metabolic rate) refers to amount of energy the body requires when at rest.

**Benign prostatic hypertrophy**—Noncancerous enlargement of prostate, usually seen in older men.

**Bioavailability**—Extent of drug absorption from gastrointestinal tract into bloodstream.

**B lymphocyte**—Thymus-independent, mononuclear white blood cell that is product of lymphoid tissue and participates in humoral immunity; also known as "B-cell."

**Canaliculi**—Very small ducts or channels; often refers to tiny bile ducts in liver between hepatocytes.

**Carpopedal**—Relating to both hands and feet.

**Catabolism**—Breakdown of tissue or protein in body; opposite of anabolism.

**Catalyst**—Substance that increases velocity of chemical reaction.

**Catecholamine**—Neurotransmitter that contains catechole ring and is produced by adrenal medulla or nerve cells. Examples are epinephrine, norepinephrine, and dopamine.

**Celiac disease**—Intestinal malabsorption, characterized by diarrhea, malnutrition, and predisposition to bleeding. Treatment is gluten-free diet.

**Cerebrospinal fluid**—Fluid occupying space between arachnoid membrane and pia matter; formed by choroid plexuses of cerebral ventricles and serves as fluid buffer for central nervous system, as reservoir for regulating contents of cranium, and as mechanism for exchange of nutrients and gases of nervous system. It may be a specimen in tests to assess integrity of central nervous system.

**Cheyne-Stokes respiration**—Rhythmical (periodic) rapid and shallow breathing occurring in grave conditions of central nervous system, heart, and lungs and during severe intoxication.

**Chief cell**—Cell in stomach lining; secretes pepsin and extrinsic factor aiding in digestion.

**Choreiform**—Usually relating to involuntary "spastic," purposeless movements that can be symptoms of chorea or side effects of central nervous system drugs.

**Chromatin**—Deoxyribonucleic acid attached to protein structure base.

**Chromogen**—Chemical substance that imparts color to specimen. This color may be made by substance intended for measurement in an assay or by unintended substance (interferent) such as noncreatinine chromogens (e.g., ketones and cefoxitin). A large number of interferents decreases an assay's specificity.

**Chromophore**—Chemical group that gives color to compound.

**Chronotropic**—Affecting rate; usually used in context of heart rate. See Inotropic.

**Chvostek's sign**— Spasm of facial muscles from tapping them or branches of facial nerves; associated with hypocalcemia.

**Circadian**—Relating to cycle of physiological events encompassed by a 24-hr day.

**Cirrhosis**—Disease characterized histologically by fibrosis and nodular formations in liver.

**Clinical**—Pertaining to patient. Throughout this book, clinical connotes information (symptoms and signs) that is readily obtainable from, or apparent in, patients (history and physical examination) in contrast to information obtained from tests or procedures.

**Cocci**—Sphere-shaped bacteria (singular form: coccus).

**Coefficient of variation**—In statistics, standard deviation of series expressed as percentage of arithmetic mean of series; used in measuring assay performance. The smaller the coefficient of variation, the more likely it is that the test result is accurate.

**Complement**— Group of nine proteins. When activated by antibody, they sequentially bind to cell membranes, causing cell lysis.

**Conjugation (metabolism)**—Combining of one compound with another to form third, often more water-soluble, compound which is more readily eliminated by body.

**Contagium**—Any microorganism, virus, or infectious matter producing or transmitting disease.

**CREST**—Indolent subgroup of systemic sclerosis historically referred to as acrosclerosis. CREST is acronym for calcinosis, Raynaud's phenomenon, esophageal hypomotility, sclerodactyly, and telangiectasia.

**Culture**—Quantity of microorganisms (e.g., bacteria and fungi) growing in artificial nutritive medium.

**Cushing's disease**—Disease characterized by adrenal gland hypersecretion of hormones such as cortisol (cortisone); manifests as truncal obesity, moonface, edema, hypertension, striae, and electrolyte imbalances.

**Cuvette**—Glass container having well-defined optical properties; used to hold solution being analyzed for color changes or light-scattering properties.

**Cyanosis**—Bluish coloration of skin and mucous membranes that results from excessive unoxygenated hemoglobin in blood; usually sign of respiratory disease.

**Cytosol**—Colloidal solution that comprises cellular fluid outside nucleus.

**Defervescence**—Lowering of elevated body temperature (fever); often seen when antibiotic therapy is effective in treating infection.

**Demographic**—Relating to statistical study of population's specific characteristics (e.g., age, weight, height, sex, and health).

**Depolarization**—Tendency of cell membranes to become more positive upon presentation of proper stimulus giving rise to action potentials.

**Diabetes mellitus**—Metabolic disorder characterized by hyperglycemia caused by absolute or relative lack of insulin.

**Diarthrodal**—Relating to joints that are normally freely movable.

**Disseminated**—Spread throughout entire body or particular organ.

**Disseminated intravascular coagulation**—Excessive activation of coagulation system resulting in clotting at multiple sites. Rapid consumption of clotting factors may then result in bleeding; also called consumptive coagulopathy.

**Duodenum**—First portion of small bowel beginning at pylorus and extending for about 12 in.

**Dyscrasia, blood**—Abnormal generation or production of one or more blood cell types; usually refers to inadequate formation of red blood cells, white blood cells, or platelets.

**Dysrhythmia**—Abnormal cardiac rhythm.

**Dysuria**—Discomfort or pain upon urination.

**Ecchymosis**—Appearance of bruises caused by blood leakage into skin.

**Eclampsia**—Toxic condition of late pregnancy characterized by increasing blood pressure, seizures, and ultimately coma.

**Ectopic**—In area other than its normal location. A heart beat originating from somewhere other than SA node is an example.

**Electrophoresis**—Separation of differently charged particles (often protein) by passing an electric current through mixture on support medium. Molecules move toward electrodes at different rates, depending on their charge and molecular configuration and on physical properties of support medium.

**Elution**—Separation of substance from adsorbent material (e.g., chromatography column) by extraction or washing with solvent.

**Embolism**—Blood clot that travels from one vascular location to distant site.

**-emia**—Suffix relating to blood.

**Endemic**—Any disease that is constantly prevalent in a particular area, sometimes in varying degrees.

**Endocarditis**—Condition characterized by inflammation of endocardium, particularly valves; usually due to bacterial infection.

**Endogenous**—Of or relating to substances normally found within body (e.g., urea, ammonia, or potassium).

**Enzyme-linked immunosorbent assay (ELISA)**—Procedures where enzyme activation indicates that immune reaction has occurred. Usually the enzyme is attached to an antibody. When it reacts with its antigen, the antibody undergoes changes that activate the enzyme. Indicator system employs enzyme substrate. Also available as enzyme-multiplied immunoassay technique (EMIT) and enzyme immunoassay (EIA).

**Enzyme-multiplied immunoassay (EMIT)**—See Enzyme-linked immunosorbent assay.

**Erythropoiesis**—Production of erythrocytes.

**Euthyroid**—Relating to normally functioning thyroid gland.

**Euthyroid sick state**—Decreased total serum thyroxine ($T_4$) level in seriously ill patient.

**Exogenous**—Of or relating to substances not normally found within body (e.g., drugs).

**Exophthalmos**—Abnormal protrusion of eyeball; seen in hyperthyroidism.

**Extracellular**—Outside of cells; includes interstitial and intravascular spaces.

**False negative**—Test result that is negative when it should be positive (i.e., disease tested for is actually present).

**False positive**—Test result that is positive when it should be negative (i.e., disease tested for is not present).

**Fibronectin**—Subendothelial structure that accompanies collagen. When these structures are exposed to circulation following injury, they cause a potent platelet adhesion reaction.

**Fluorophore**—Compound emitting wavelength of light longer than light it absorbs. This phenomenon results in fluorescence.

**Fulminant**—Coming on suddenly with great severity.

**Gestational diabetes**—Onset of glucose intolerance during pregnancy.

**Giant cell arteritis**—Vascular disease that typically manifests as headache and involves inflammation of carotid arteries; also known as temporal arteritis.

**Glanzmann's thrombasthenia**—Genetic (autosomal-recessive) disorder associated with normal clotting factors, normal platelet count, abnormal platelet function, and severe congenital bleeding.

**Glomerulus**—Filtering unit of nephrons of kidneys.

**Glucose intolerance**—Inability of body to process glucose properly; usually leads to hyperglycemia.

**-glyc-**—Word root relating to carbohydrates.

**Glycolysis**—Process of carbohydrate breakdown into smaller molecules.

**Glycosuria**—Presence of glucose in urine.

**Goiter**—Enlargement of thyroid gland.

**Gram negative**—Microorganisms that are decolorized by alcohol during Gram staining process. They appear pink under microscope. Examples are *Escherichia coli*, *Pseudomonas*, *Haemophilus*, *Klebsiella*, *Salmonella*, *Neisseria*, and *Bacteroides* species.

**Gram positive**—Microorganisms that retain stain during Gram staining process. They appear purple under microscope. Examples are *Streptococcus*, *Staphylococcus*, *Listeria*, *Clostridia*, and *Peptococcus* species.

**Granulocytopenia**—Decrease in number of granulocytes below normal range.

**Granulocytosis**—Increase in number of granulocytes above normal (reference) range.

**Half-life**—Time needed for original amount or concentration to be reduced to 50%. With drugs, half-life usually refers to time needed for serum concentration to fall from 20 to 10 µg/ml, for example.

**Hapten**—Part of antigen containing structure that determines its immunologic specificity.

**Haptoglobin**—Plasma protein that binds hemoglobin set free from erythrocytes to plasma.

**Hemagglutination**—Clumping of red blood cells.

**Hemarthrosis**—Hemorrhage into joint.

**Hematoma**—Collection of extravasated blood often caused by trauma or coagulopathy.

**Hematopoietic**—Pertaining to production of erythrocytes.

**Hemochromatosis**—Genetic disorder characterized by excessive deposition of hemosiderin and hemofuscin in some organs.

**Hemodynamics**—Study of blood movement and forces (pressures) concerned therein.

**Hemolysis**—Breakdown of red blood cells.

**Hemolytic**—Destructive of erythrocytes.

**Hemolytic uremic syndrome**—Disease characterized by acute microangiopathic hemolytic anemia, thrombocytopenia, and renal failure. It is most common in early childhood and in pregnant and postpartum women. See Uremic syndrome.

**Hemostasis**—Arrest of blood escaping from vessels.

**Hepatic**—Of or relating to liver.

**Homeostasis**—System of control mechanisms used by body to maintain normal balance of given substance or state.

**Human chorionic gonadotropin**—Gonad-stimulating hormone stimulated by anterior pituitary. Its secretion increases dramatically after pregnancy; elevated concentrations can be detected as early as 4 days after missed menses. It is, therefore, basis for most pregnancy tests.

**Humoral**—Pertaining to body fluids or substances contained in them.

**Hydrostatic pressure**—Pressure exerted by pumping of blood by heart. Hydrostatic pressure is roughly equivalent to arterial blood pressure but increases in standing person as one measures from the heart level to feet. It tends to push fluid out of vessels toward interstitial tissue.

**Hyper-**—Prefix meaning above normal or excessive.

**Hyperglycemia**—Abnormally high glucose concentration in blood.

**Hyperplasia**—Abnormal increase in number of cells in given tissue. For example, gingival hyperplasia involves gums.

**Hyperpyrexia**—Abnormally high fever (for given disease).

**Hypersegmented**—When referring to nucleus of granulocytes, nucleus has more lobes (segments) than usual; seen in some deficiency states.

**Hyperthyroid**—Condition that develops from excess of thyroid hormone activity.

**Hypo-**—Prefix meaning below normal or deficient.

**Hypochromic**—Referring to erythrocytes that appear more lightly colored than usual because of decreased amounts of hemoglobin.

**Hypoglycemia**—Abnormally low glucose concentration in blood.

**Hypophosphatasia**—Rare genetic disease of bone mineralization where serum alkaline phosphatase is about 25% (0–40%) of normal, serum phosphorus is normal, and serum and urine phosphoethanolamines are elevated.

**Hypothyroidism**—Condition that develops from deficiency of thyroid hormone activity.

**Hypovolemia**—Inadequate volume of blood in body.

**Iatrogenic**—Any disorder caused by clinician, practitioner, or drug.

**Ileum**—Terminal portion of small intestine.

**Immunofluorescence assay**—Any technique where a fluorescent marker is attached to one of the immune reactants. In *direct* testing, fluorescein or similar label is attached to a specific antibody that identifies the location of its specific antigen in tissue or in a specimen. In *indirect* testing, the label is attached to an antiglobulin serum which reacts with human antibody molecules. The fluorescent antiglobulin marker shows that an antigen-antibody reaction has occurred in the test system. The indirect method is used to reveal whether or not a fluid contains antibody.

**Immunoglobulin**—See Antibody.

**Inotropic**—Affecting force; usually used in context of heart contractions. See chronotropic.

**Insensible loss**—Small, gradual loss of body fluid that is not readily appreciated with naked eye. Examples include sweat and respiratory water vapor.

**Interferent**—Component of collected sample of body fluid or tissue, other than analyte, that falsely alters final results.

**Interstitial**—Fluid between cells or tissue; extracellular fluid excluding fluid in blood vessels.

**Intracellular**—Fluid within cells; opposite of extracellular.

**Intrinsic factor**—Protein produced in stomach that is necessary for intestinal absorption of vitamin $B_{12}$.

**Jodbasedow effect**—Development of hypothyroidism in previously euthyroid patient as result of exposure to increased quantities of iodine.

**-kal-**—Word root relating to potassium.

**Laboratorians**—Generic term denoting various workers within laboratories; may include technologists, technicians, phlebotomists, administrators, and pathologists.

**Leukocytosis**—Increased concentration of circulating white blood cells; often associated with infection or inflammation.

**Lipemia retinalis**—Whitish cast in vascular bed of retina due to light scattering by triglyceride particles in blood.

**Lumen**—Internal space of tube or tubule through which fluid flows; used commonly in reference to airways, kidney tubules, and blood or lymph vessels.

**Maceration**—Softening of tissue by action of liquid (e.g., effect on anal skin by persistent diarrhea).

**Macrocyte**—Erythrocyte that is larger than normal.

**Macrophage**—Phagocytic cell in organs such as spleen, liver, and lungs.

**Macroscopic**—Visible by naked eye without microscope.

**Mast cell**—Cell that has membrane binding sites for IgE and contains granules of histamine and other substances important in causing symptoms of immediate hypersensitivity reactions.

**Megakaryocyte**—Giant white blood cell in bone marrow that gives rise to platelets.

**Megaloblast**—Nucleated erythrocyte distinct from normal nucleated erythrocyte precursors; found in bone marrow and peripheral blood in vitamin $B_{12}$ and folic acid deficiencies.

**Mesenteric**—Relating to fold of peritoneum connecting small intestine with posterior abdominal wall.

**Microcytic**—Referring to erythrocytes that are smaller than normal.

**Microscopic**—Not visible by naked eye without microscope.

**Mineralocorticoids**—Corticosteroids (e.g., aldosterone) secreted by adrenal cortex. They cause sodium retention and potassium loss.

**Minimal bactericidal concentration**—See Chapter 16.

**Minimal inhibitory concentration**—See Chapter 16.

**Mixed connective-tissue disease**—Rheumatological diagnosis associated with symptoms commonly seen separately in systemic sclerosis, rheumatoid arthritis, polymyositis, and systemic lupus erythematosus. Symptoms are bonded together by presence of antiribonucleoprotein antibodies.

**Mononucleosis**—Disorder produced by infection by Epstein-Barr virus; characterized by fever, sore throat, malaise, swollen lymph glands, enlargement of liver and spleen, and typical rash.

**Morbidity**—Unhealthy state; untoward effects of disorder or drug.

**Morphologic**—Referring to form or appearance.

**Myeloproliferative**—Increase of cellular elements of bone marrow.

**Myoglobin**—Pigment in muscle that is similar to hemoglobin in action. It acts as oxygen reservoir within muscle fibers.

**Myosin**—Protein in muscle tissue that acts with actin to allow muscle contraction and relaxation.

**-natr-**—Word root pertaining to sodium.

**Nephelometry**—Determination of solute concentration by measurement of light-scattering properties of molecules in suspension. Degree of light scattering is proportional to molecule's concentration.

**Nephron**—Functional unit of kidneys.

**Nephrotic syndrome**—Disorder where glomerular lesions cause enhanced permeability to proteins; characterized by heavy loss of serum proteins to urine and low serum albumin.

**Neuroglycopenia**—Abnormally low glucose concentration in central nervous system; usually associated with hypoglycemia and manifests as confusion, seizures, and/or coma.

**Neurohypophysis**—Posterior lobe of pituitary gland; secretes antidiuretic hormone and oxytocin.

**Nucleic acid**—Either deoxyribonucleic acid (DNA) or ribonucleic acid (RNA).

**Nystagmus**—Involuntary rhythmic movement of eyeballs.

**Occult**—Hidden; referring to blood in specimen that can be discovered only by chemical tests or microscopy.

**Oliguria**—Diminution in urine production or excretion.

**Oncotic pressure**—Osmotic pressure developed at vascular capillary membrane by plasma proteins (e.g., albumin) that tends to hold fluid in bloodstream; also called colloid osmotic pressure.

**Osmolality**—Measure of pressure caused by solute concentration difference between opposite sides of semipermeable membrane.

**Osmolar gap**—Difference in osmolality between two compartments (e.g., intracellular and extracellular fluids).

**Osteoblast**—Bone cell responsible for bone production.

**Osteoclast**—Bone cell responsible for bone resorption and removal.

**Osteolytic**—Relating to promotion of bone dissolution.

**Osteomalacia**—Disease characterized by softening of bone, usually from vitamin D deficiency; seen in uremic syndrome.

**Ototoxicity**—Damage to function of ears.

**Parasite**—Organism that lives on surface of or within another organism and, by so doing, causes harm to that organism.

**Parietal cell**—Cell in stomach that produces gastric acid and intrinsic factor.

**Parotid gland**—Salivary gland, below and in front of the external ear. It produces amylase (ptyalin), which aids in initial breakdown of starches.

**Pathogenic**—Producing disease.

**Pathognomonic**—Information that definitively distinguishes one pathophysiological process, etiology, or diagnosis from another. For example, a theophylline concentration of 25 µg/mL without clinical signs of toxicity is not pathognomonic for theophylline toxicity.

**Peak (drug concentration)**—Highest drug concentration within dosing interval.

**Pelvic inflammatory disease**—Disease of female reproductive organs, commonly caused by infection due to gonococci or chlamydia.

**Performance, assay**—Tests used to determine overall usefulness of assay; may include testing for precision, accuracy, specificity, sensitivity, and substrate stability.

**Petechiae**—Small, pinpoint, purplish-red spots on skin caused by intradermal leakage of blood.

**Phagocyte**—Cell that ingests and digests microorganisms or other cells and foreign particles.

**Pheochromocytoma**—Tumor (usually benign) of adrenal medulla that secretes excessive catecholamines into blood; manifests primarily as hypertension.

**Pickwickian syndrome**—Disorder characterized by chronic alveolar hypoventilation, somnolence, polycythemia, hypoxemia, and hypercapnia; occurs in morbidly obese patients when excessive fat apparently limits movement of lungs.

**Plasma**—Aqueous component of blood consisting of 92% water and 8% solids (e.g., albumin, globulin, fibrinogen, clotting factors, minerals, nutrients, waste products, and enzymes).

**Plasma cell**—Terminally differentiated B lymphocytes that are devoted entirely to antibody production.

**Pluripotential**—Purported ability of certain stem cells to differentiate into numerous types of blood cell precursors.

**Polydipsia**—Excessive thirst; often associated with diabetes.

**Polymorphonuclear cell**—Cell containing nucleus with many lobes. Granulocytes are polymorphonuclear cells.

**Polymyalgia rheumatica**—Self-limited syndrome characterized by proximal joint and muscle pain, high erythrocyte sedimentation rate, malaise, low-grade fever, weight loss, and fatigue.

**Polymyositis**—Rheumatic disease characterized by interstitial inflammatory infiltrates of skeletal muscle, increased creatine phosphokinase, and symmetrical, proximal limb weakness.

**Polyphagia**—Excessive hunger; associated with diabetes.

**Porphyria**—Condition producing increased concentrations of any heme precursor.

**Postantibiotic effect**—Effect of some antibiotics (e.g., ciprofloxacin) against certain bacteria, characterized by inhibition of growth hours after antibiotic concentrations fall below minimal inhibitory concentration.

**Postprandial**—After a meal.

**Precision**—Degree of variation of assay results when known specimens are tested repeatedly in one run or over several days.

**Pre-eclampsia**—Syndrome of nausea, vomiting, headache, dypnea, and albuminuria; precedes onset of true eclampsia (hypertensive toxemia associated with seizures and coma).

**PR interval**—Part of electrocardiogram between onset of atrial activity (P wave) and ventricular activity (QRS complex); indicator of conduction between two chambers.

**Prodrome**—Advance clinical finding indicating approach of disease.

**Prostacyclin**—Prostaglandin metabolite in vascular tissue that is potent vasodilator and inhibitor of platelet aggregation.

**Pseudopod**—Temporary protrusion of outer membrane of ameba, platelet, etc.

**Purpura**—Confluent petechiae and/or ecchymoses.

**Pyelonephritis**—Inflammation of kidneys (usually caused by bacterial infection) that may be accompanied by flank pain and tenderness, bacteriuria (often bacteremia), pyuria, and fever.

**Pyuria**—White blood cells in urine.

**QRS complex**—Part of electrocardiogram representing ventricular activity.

**Radionuclide**—Atom or type of atom with unstable nucleus that spontaneously decays to more stable form while emitting radiation; also called radioisotope. Radionuclides used in scintigraphy are technetium-99m pyrophosphate and thallium-201.

**Raynaud's phenomenon**—Intermittent vasospasm in fingers or toes leading to blanching; brought on by cold and sometimes by emotion.

**Renal**—Pertaining to kidneys.

**Retention time**—Time between when compound is injected and its characteristic band emerges from chromatographic column.

**Rhabdomyolysis**—Disintegration or dissolution of muscle associated with elevated serum creatine phosphokinase and excretion of myoglobin in urine.

**Rheological**—Relating to study of (blood) flow.

**Scintigraphy**—Process of acquiring a scintigram—image of radioactivity distribution obtained with scintillation camera after internal administration of radionuclide; used in diagnosis of myocardial infarction.

**Scleroderma**—Multisystem disorder characterized by "hidebound" fibrotic skin, vascular lesions, and residual atrophy with fibrosis of multiple organs; now called progressive systemic sclerosis.

**Sensitivity**—Lowest quantity of substance that an assay can measure accurately. Also see Chapter 1 for meaning with qualitative tests.

**Serological**—Relating to (tests) detecting, identifying, and or quantifying antibodies (immunoglobulins) or antigens from serum; most useful in evaluating viral infections and (auto)immune diseases.

**Serum**—Aqueous portion of blood containing all plasma substances except fibrinogen and clotting factors. See plasma.

**$S_3$ heart sound**— Low-pitched extra heart sound that occurs during rapid ventricular filling; also referred to as $S_3$ gallop. It may occur normally in children and young adults. In older patients, however, it is usually produced by ventricular failure.

**$S_4$ heart sound**—Low-pitched extra heart sound that occurs when atria contracts against noncompliant ventricle; also referred to as $S_4$ gallop. Noncompliance is usually result of reduced ventricular wall distensibility or increased ventricular volumes.

**Sjögren's syndrome**—Diagnostic triad of dry eyes and dry mouth presence of rheumatic disease (usually rheumatoid arthritis). It is a chronic autoimmune disorder characterized by lymphocytic infiltration of lachrymal and salivary glands. Diagnosis of primary form is confirmed by minor salivary gland biopsy and presence of circulating autoantibodies.

**Solute**—Substance dissolved in solvent.

**Specificity**—Degree of assay cross-reactivity with unintended substances as opposed to substance being tested.

Also see Chapter 1 for meaning with qualitative tests.

**Specimen**—Sample of tissue or fluid (e.g., sputum, stool, or urine) to be tested.

**Spherocyte**—Red blood cell that is more spherical and fragile than normal. Spherocytosis is hereditary disease in which there is excessive hemolysis.

**Spirochete**—Spiral-shaped microorganism (e.g., Treponema).

**Steady state (drug concentration)**—See Chapter 5.

**Subluxation**—Sprain or incomplete dislocation.

**Supernatant**—Floating on surface of liquid.

**Susceptibility, bacterial**—Propensity of bacteria to be killed by antimicrobial agent.

**Synovium**—Tissue lining nonarticulating surfaces inside joint capsule of movable joint that maintains integrity of synovial fluid by supplying nutrients and clearing wastes.

**Systemic**—Referring to entire body (in contrast to "local").

**Tachypnea**—Abnormal breathing rate (respiratory rate) seen in patients with obstructive lung disorders, acidosis, etc.

**Tetany**—Syndrome manifested by muscle twitching, cramps, and convulsions; often due to hypocalcemia.

**Therapeutic range**—See Chapter 5.

**Third spacing**—Abnormal accumulation of fluid outside intravascular and intracellular spaces. Example is ascites.

**Thrombocythemia**—Increase in number of circulating blood platelets.

**Thrombocytopenia**—Decrease in number of platelets below normal (reference) range.

**Thrombocytosis**—Unusually large number of platelets in blood.

**Thromboplastin, tissue**—Complex mixture of substances in vascular intima that are released with vascular injury; initiating factor in extrinsic system for clotting.

**Thrombosis**—Development of blood clot.

**Tinnitus**—Ringing in ears.

**T lymphocyte**—Thymus-influenced leukocyte that helps B lymphocytes make antibodies, destroy cells infected with virus, activate phagocytes to destroy engulfed pathogens, and control level and quality of immune system.

**Trigeminal neuralgia**—Disease of trigeminal nerve typically characterized by sharp, shooting pains in jaw and face.

**Trousseau's sign**—Hand spasms and contortions after inflation of blood pressure cuff on arm; may indicate hypocalcemia.

**Turbidity**—Cloudiness; often refers to serum or urine.

**T wave**—Part of electrocardiogram representing ventricular repolarization.

**Urea**—Chief nitrogenous component of urine and principal end-product of protein metabolism; $NH_2$-CO-$NH_2$.

**Uremic syndrome**—Symptom complex associated with end-stage renal failure; characterized by headache, vertigo, vomiting, blindness, and, later, convulsions and coma; once believed to be due to excess urea in blood. Patients develop metabolic acidosis, electrolyte imbalances, hypertension, congestive heart disease, anemia, and osteomalacia.

**-uria**—Suffix relating to urine.

**Uricosuric**—Relating to ability to increase uric acid excretion in urine.

**Urticaria**—Allergic skin reaction also known as hives.

**Uveitis**—Iinflammation of iris, ciliary body, and choroid of eye.

**Vagus nerve**—Tenth cranial nerve; cholinergically innervates heart, lungs, esophagus, stomach, small intestine, liver, gallbladder, pancreas, and upper portions of colon and ureters.

**Valley (drug concentration)**—Lowest drug concentration within dosing interval.

**Volume of distribution, drug**—Volume of body tissue into which drug apparently distributes; not a real body space.

**Von Willebrand factor and disease**—Part of factor VIII molecule responsible for platelet adhesion and function; also called factor VIII/vWF. The disease is genetic (autosomal-dominant) deficiency of this factor, manifesting as bleeding.

**Wilson's disease**—Rare, hereditary liver disease where copper accumulates in liver and ultimately causes cirrhosis.

**Wolf-Chaikoff effect**—Iodide-induced hypothyroidism.

**Xanthoma**—Yellow skin plaque due to lipid deposition.

# Appendix D
# Blood Collection Tubes: Color Codes, Additives, and Appropriate Sample Volumes[a,b]

| Cap Color | Additive(s) | Number of Tube Inversions at Collection | Optimum Volume (mL) | Minimum Volume[c] (mL) | Laboratory Use and Comments[d] |
|---|---|---|---|---|---|
| Red | None | 0 | 10 | NA | For serum determinations in chemistry, serology, and blood banking. Serum should be separated from cells within 45 min |
| Lavender | Liquid potassium EDTA<br>Freeze-dried sodium EDTA | 8<br>8 | 7 | 2<br>2 | For whole-blood hematology determinations. Inversions prevent clotting |
| Light blue | 0.105 $M$ sodium citrate<br>0.129 $M$ sodium citrate | 8<br>8 | 4.5 | 4.5 | For coagulation determinations on plasma. Inversions prevent clotting. Some tests may require chilling |
| Royal blue | Heparin sodium<br>Sodium EDTA<br>None | 8<br>8<br>0 | 10<br>7<br>10 | 3.5<br>2.0<br>NA | For trace element, toxicology, and nutrient determinations |
| Green | Heparin sodium<br>Lithium heparin<br>Ammonium heparin | 8<br>8<br>8 | 10 | 3.5 | For plasma determinations in chemistry. Inversions prevent clotting. Used for arterial blood gases, ammonia (on ice), and electrolytes |
| Orange | Thrombin | 8 | 10 | NA | For stat serum determinations in chemistry. Inversions ensure clotting within 5 min |
| Gray | Potassium oxalate/sodium fluoride<br>Sodium fluoride<br>Lithium iodoacetate<br>Lithium iodoacetate/heparin | 8<br>8<br>8<br>8 | 10 | 10 | For glucose determinations. Glycolytic inhibitors stabilize glucose for ≤24 hr at room temperature (iodoacetate) and for ≤3 days with fluoride. Oxalate and heparin give plasma samples; without them, samples are serum. For lactate (on ice) |
| Light brown | Heparin sodium | 8 | 10 | 3.5 | For lead determinations. Inversions prevent clotting |
| Gold | Clot activator and gel for serum separation | 5 | 10 | NA | Serum separator tube for serum determinations in chemistry. Inversions ensure mixing of clot activator with blood and clotting within 30 min |
| Light green | Lithium heparin and gel for plasma separation | 8 | 10 | 3.5 | Plasma separation tube for plasma determinations in chemistry. Inversions prevent clotting |
| Yellow | Sodium polyanetholesulfonate (SPS) | 8 | | | For blood culture specimen collections in microbiology. Inversions prevent clotting |

[a]Compiled from (1) 1990 company literature (Becton Dickinson, Rutherford, NJ 07070) on Vacutainer collection systems; (2) Jacobs DS, Kasten BL Jr, Demott WR, et al., eds. Laboratory test handbook. St. Louis, MO: Lexi-Comp/Mosby; 1988; (3) National Committee for Clinical Laboratory Standards. Procedures for handling and processing of blood specimens, H18-A. Villanova, PA: 1989; and (4) editor's experience. NA = not applicable; EDTA = ethylenediaminetetraacetic acid.

[b]Colors and additives are specific only for Vacutainer tubes with Hemogard closure or stoppers from Becton Dickinson. Other types and brands may vary.

[c]If known, that volume of blood required to avoid spurious results due to inappropriate ratio of anticoagulant to specimen. In general, tubes with liquid additives should be filled.

[d]In general, specimens should not be chilled before delivery to the laboratory unless specified otherwise. Exceptions include lactic acid, blood gases, pyruvate, gastrin, ammonia, parathyroid hormone, catecholamines, and possibly activated partial thromboplastin time. Stoppers should not be removed outside the laboratory, because specimens may be oxidized, volatile, or contaminated by bacteria. Serum or plasma should be separated from contact with cells within 2 hr of collection unless specified otherwise.

# Index

The following symbols indicate whether the information is part of a table (t), figure (f), minicase (mc), or glossary (g). Material within QuickViews is not indexed.

results 265
cause of fasting hypoglycemia 267
cause of hyperlipidemia 283 (t)
cause of hypoglycemia 267
cause of hypomagnesemia 105
cause of hypophosphatemia 113
cause of hypozincemia 117 (t)
cause of iron deficiency anemia 305
cause of pancreatitis 214, 232
cause of porphyrias 291
interaction with warfarin 334 (t)
unsafe in hepatic porphyria 291 (t)
metabolism, factors affecting 52
nonlinear vs linear kinetics 67
signs and symptoms
at various blood levels 55
of chronic abuse 333 (mc)
withdrawal, cause of hypophosphatemia 113
Alcohol testing 43
confounded interpretation by glucosuria 53, 54 (mc)
confounded interpretation by microbes in urine 53, 54 (mc)
interference with assay 52–54
minicase 225
Aldesleukin, cause of thrombocytopenia 327 (t)
Aldosterone, effect on sodium and water balance 95 (f)
Aldosteronism
definition of 401 (g)
Alendronate, cause of hypocalcemia 110
Alkalemia
definition of 159, 401 (g)
Alkaline phosphatase (ALP) 218, 219
assay
interference by *N*-acetylcysteine 30, 38
interference by theophylline 30
serum
causes of nonhepatic elevation 219 (t)
circadian rhythm 6
decrease, causes of 219
effect of age on 4
elevation during growth spurts 218
elevation during late pregnancy 218
elevation in cholestasis 218, 219 (mc)
elevation in hyperthyroid 248 (t)
elevation, interpretation with other tests 218 (t)
false elevation after fatty meal 219
half-life 218
normal range 218
QuickView 240
tissues with high concentration of 218
Alkaline urine
cause of elevated urobilinogen 148
causes of 148 (t)

from *Proteus mirabilis* urinary infection 147
interference with proteinuria dipstick 146
Alkalosis
definition of 159, 401 (g)
metabolic 165–167
cause of elevated urine potassium 150
cause of hypokalemia 100, 102 (t)
causes of 166 (t)
decreased free serum calcium 108
definition of 159
minicase 166
test results in 164 (t)
urine chloride in 150 (t)
respiratory 167, 169
cause of hypophosphatemia 113
causes of 169 (t)
definition of 159
from salicylate toxicity 83
minicase 167
signs and symptoms 167
test results in 164 (t)
Allergic reactions
and basophil involvement 311
cause of eosinophilia 311, 312 (t)
Allopurinol
cause of elevated ALT, AST, and LDH 220 (t)
cause of thrombocytopenia 327 (t)
Alopecia from hypozincemia 118
ALP. *See* Alkaline phosphatase
$\alpha_1$-Acid glycoprotein, acute-phase reactant 384
$\alpha$-Adrenergic agonists
ADH stimulation by 269
cause of decreased insulin secretion 256 (t)
ALT. *See* Alanine aminotransferase, serum
Alteplase (t-PA). *See* Thrombolytics
Ameba, cause of infectious colitis 235
Amikacin
clinical pharmacokinetics 73, 74 (t)
Amiloride
cause of elevated SCr from tubular secretion inhibition 134
cause of hyperkalemia 102
treatment of nephrogenic diabetes insipidus 270
Amino acid intake
cause of insulin secretion 256 (t)
excessive, cause of azotemia 133 (t)
Aminocaproic acid
cause of elevated creatine kinase 190
inhibitor of fibrinolysis 325
Aminoglutethimide, cause of decreased thyroxine, serum 250 (t)
Aminoglycosides
assay interference
by heparin 87
by penicillins 31, 73
cause of elevated SCr 135 (t)
clinical pharmacokinetics 73

safe in hepatic porphyria 291 (t)
Aminosalicylic acid
cause of false elevation of AST 222
cause of vitamin $B_{12}$ malabsorption 302 (t)
Aminotransferases. *Also see* Alanine aminotransferase *and* Aspartate aminotransferase
algorithm for differential diagnosis of hepatitis 221 (f)
differential diagnosis with bilirubin 224 (t)
diurnal changes 220
elevation from HMG Co-A RI
elevation from niacin 286
elevation from salicylate toxicity 83
elevation from viral hepatitis 226, 230
false-positive screens 220
Amiodarone
cause of decreased thyroxine, serum 250 (t)
cause of elevated ALT, AST, and LDH 220 (t)
cause of elevated thyroxine, serum 250 (t)
cause of hyperglycemia 258 (t)
cause of hyperlipidemia 283 (t)
cause of hyperthyroidism 247 (t), 251
cause of primary hypothyroidism 247 (t), 251
cause of pseudoporphyria 291 (t)
free $T_4$ and TSH after 248 (t)
interaction with digoxin 78
interaction with phenytoin 82
interaction with quinidine 83
interaction with warfarin 334 (t)
iodine-containing product 251 (t)
Amitriptyline
cause of blue-green urine 143 (t)
protein binding and Vd 64 (t)
tissue-binding effect on Vd 64
therapeutic range 80 (t), 397
Ammonia
interference with cannabinoids assay 52 (t)
serum
causes of elevated 226
correlation with encephalopathy severity 226
minicase 225
normal range 225, 399
QuickView 243
Ammonium chloride
cause of acidic urine 148 (t)
cause of metabolic acidosis 165 (t)
Amoxicillin
cause of *C. difficile*-associated diarrhea 235 (t)
Amphetamines
cause of elevated thyroxine, serum 250 (t)
testing 44
cut-off for positive result 45 (t)
detection periods 46 (t)
interfering substances 45 (f), 53 (t)
QuickView 59

sensitivity of common assays 46 (t)
Amphotericin B
cause of elevated creatine kinase 190
cause of elevated SCr 135 (t)
cause of hypokalemia 102 (t)
cause of metabolic acidosis 165 (t)
cause of nephrogenic diabetes insipidus 98 (t)
cause of renal tubular acidosis 102
cause of thrombocytopenia 327 (t)
Ampicillin
cause of *C. difficile*-associated diarrhea 235 (t)
Amrinone, cause of thrombocytopenia 327 (t)
Amylase
fractionation 232, 233 (mc)
origin 214, 232
serum
causes of elevated 232, 233 (t)
circadian rhythm 6
effect of age on 4
elevation from hyperzincemia 118
elevation from salivary gland 266 (mc)
false depression of, by hypertriglyceridemia 233
half-life 232
normal range 232
urine
factitious elevation 233 (mc)
normal range 232
Amyloid A
acute-phase reactant 384
serum elevation after unstable angina 195
Amyloidosis
cause of azotemia 133 (t)
cause of elevated ALP 218
cause of hypophosphatemia 113
cause of proteinuria 146 (t)
definition of 401 (g)
from deposition of mutant prealbumin 215
ANA. *See* Antinuclear antibody test
Anabolic steroids, interaction with warfarin 334 (t)
Anaerobic bacteria. *See* Bacteria, anaerobic
Analgesics
chronic overuse, cause of azotemia 133 (t)
narcotic. *See* Opiates
Analyte
definition of 401 (g)
subforms and isoenzymes of 5
Analytical performance of assay 6
ANCA. *See* Antineutrophil cytoplasmic antibodies
Androgens
cause of decreased thyroxine-binding globulin 249 (t)
cause of hypercalcemia 111
Anemia
aplastic
cause of lymphopenia 312 (t)
cause of thrombocytopenia 326

GTT. *See* Glucose tolerance test
Guillain-Barré syndrome, cause of
    respiratory acidosis 166 (t)
GUSTO III heparin dosing
    nomogram 335 (f)

## H

H$_2$-antagonist drugs. *Also see*
    Cimetidine *and* Ranitidine
    cause of thrombocytopenia 327
    (t), 333 (mc)
*Haemophilus influenzae*
    beta-lactamase testing 353
    inability to test with automated
        microdilution method 351
    morphology and Gram-stain 348
        (t)
    usefulness of E test 353
    use of latex agglutination test for
        bacterial antigens 360
Hageman factor (XII), half-life
    324 (t)
Hair
    color change from hypomanga-
        nesemia 119
    dry coarse, from hypothyroidism
        247
Hair analysis for drugs of abuse 42,
    43
    effect of shampooing and
        bleaching on 42
Half-life (t½)
    definition of 404 (g)
    elimination 63 (f), 65 (f)
    relationship with Ke and Cl$_T$ 64
    selected drugs 74, 75 (t)
    with nonlinear and linear phar-
        macokinetics 67
Hallucinations
    from drugs of abuse 47
    from hypocalcemia 110
Haloperidol therapeutic range 85,
    397
Halothane
    cause of elevated ALT, AST, and
        LDH 220 (t)
    cause of elevated creatine kinase
        190
Hapten
    definition of 404 (g)
Haptoglobin
    acute-phase reactant 384
    causes of alteration 306
    decrease in hemolytic anemia
        blunted by steroids 306
    decreased in hemolytic anemia
        306
    definition of 404 (g)
    production by the liver 214
Hashimoto's thyroiditis. *See*
    Thyroiditis, Hashimoto's
HAV. *See* Hepatitis virus type A
HBcAg. *See* Hepatitis B virus core
    antigen
HBeAg. *See* Hepatitis B e antigen
HBsAg. *See* Hepatitis B virus
    surface antigen
HBV. *See* Hepatitis virus type B
HCP. *See* Porphyria, hereditary
    coproporphyria (HCP)
Hct. *See* Hematocrit
HCV. *See* Hepatitis virus type C
HDL. *See* High-density lipopro-

teins
HDV. *See* Hepatitis virus type D
Headache
    from folate deficiency anemia
        304
    from hypermanganesemia (body
        excess) 119
    from hypoglycemia 267
    from lithium 80
    from quinidine 75 (t), 83
    from theophylline 84
Heart. *Also see* Cardiac
    disease
        congenital, cause of cardiac
            dysfunction 188
        valvular, cause of cardiac dys-
            function 188
    murmur from endocarditis 356
        (mc)
    physiology 187, 188 (f)
    rate
        decrease by digoxin 77
        increase. *See* Tachycardia
        normal 188
Heat intolerance, from hyperthy-
    roidism 247
Heavy metal toxicity
    cause of epithelial cell casts in
        urine 145 (t)
    cause of hypophosphatemia 113
*Helicobacter pylori*
    assays and culture for 234
    cause of ulcer (peptic) disease
        234
Hemagglutination
    definition of 404 (g)
Hemangiomas, spider, from chro-
    nic alcohol abuse 333 (mc)
Hemarthrosis, from platelet
    dysfunction 328
    definition of 404 (g)
Hematin
    heme synthesis inhibition 289
Hematocrit (Hct)
    decreased in thyroid dysfunction
        248 (t)
    effect of age on 4
    evaluating hemostasis 325
    normal range 299 (t), 300
Hematomas, from platelet dys-
    function 328
    definition of 404 (g)
Hematopoiesis 297, 298 (f)
Hematopoietic
    definition of 404 (g)
Hematuria
    cause of red urine 144
    from platelet dysfunction 328
Heme
    synthesis 288, 289 (f)
Hemochromatosis
    algorithm for differential diag-
        nosis of hepatitis 221 (f)
    cause of elevated ALT, AST, and
        LDH 220 (t)
    definition of 405 (g)
Hemocult test
    positive in pseudomembranous
        colitis 235
Hemodynamics
    definition of 405 (g)
Hemoglobin
    normal range 399
Hemoglobin (Hgb), blood

blood pH buffer 160
    decreased in thyroid dysfunction
        248 (t)
    effect of age on 4
    effect of packed RBCs on hemo-
        globin 306
    evaluating hemostasis 325
    glycated. *See* Glycated hemo-
        globin
    glycosylated. *See* Glycated hemo-
        globin
    maximum daily regeneration 305
    metabolism to bilirubin 223
    normal range 299 (t), 300
    production from heme 288
Hemoglobin, serum
    cause of false fructosamine ele-
        vation 259
Hemoglobinuria. *Also see* Urine,
    hemoglobin
    cause of proteinuria 146 (t)
    cause of red-orange urine 143 (t)
    causes of 149
Hemolysis. *Also see* Anemia,
    hemolytic
    definition of 405 (g)
    in vivo
        cause of brown urine 143 (t)
        cause of elevated AST 222
        cause of elevated bilirubin 223,
            224
        cause of elevated LDH 222
        cause of elevated urobilinogen
            148
        cause of false elevation of gly-
            cated Hgb 259
        cause of hemoglobinuria 149
        cause of hyperkalemia 103 (t)
        cause of red-orange urine 143
            (t)
        cause of reticulocytosis 299 (t)
        from hypercupremia 116
        from hypophosphatemia 114
        from SLE 379
    specimen
        cause of elevated creatine
            kinase 190
        cause of elevated LDH 222
        cause of false elevations of ALT
            196
        cause of false elevations of LDH
            193
        cause of false hyperphospha-
            temia 114
        cause of false hyperzincemia
            118
        cause of hyperkalemia 104 (t)
        interference with AST assay
            222
Hemolytic uremic syndrome
    cause of thrombocytopenia 326
    definition of 405 (g)
    from anticancer drugs 326
Hemophilia A and B 331
Hemorrhage
    cause of azotemia 133 (t)
    cause of elevated urine bilirubin
        148
    cause of reticulocytosis 299 (t),
        300
    from liver disease 217
    from platelet dysfunction 328
    from thrombocythemia 326
    risk from heparin 337

variceal, from HDV infection
    231
Hemosiderin in iron metabolism
    305
Hemostasis
    definition of 405 (g)
    physiology 321–325, 322 (f), 324
        (f)
Henderson–Hasselbalch equation
    160
Heparin
    and antithrombin III inhibits
        coagulation 324
    assays 334, 335
    binding protein, cause of high-
        dose requirement 335
    bleeding risk from 337
    cause of elevated ALT 220
    cause of hyperkalemia 103 (t)
    cause of prolonged bleeding time
        329
    cause of prolonged prothrombin
        time 333, 336 (mc)
    cause of prolonged thrombin
        time 331
    cause of thrombocytopenia 326,
        327 (t)
    concentrations, plasma 334, 335
        QuickView 345
    dosing
        causes of high-dose require-
            ments 335
        general 334, 335
    effect on triglyceride levels 284
    effect on urine sodium 150
    in basophils 311
    interference with aminoglycoside
        assay 30, 87
    low molecular weight, and
        thrombocytopenia 327
    nomogram (GUSTO III) 335 (f)
    nonlinear vs linear kinetics
        67
    pseudoresistance 335, 336 (mc)
    therapeutic range (sec and U/
        mL) 334
    therapy, coagulation test results
        during 326 (t)
Hepatic
    definition of 405 (g)
Hepatitis
    alcoholic
        cause of false-positive ELISA
            HIV test 362
        cause of intrahepatic cholestasis
            217
    algorithm for differential diag-
        nosis 221 (f)
    autoimmune, cause of false-
        positive anti-HCV 230
    cause of elevated ALT 222
    cause of elevated AST 222
    cause of elevated LDH and LDH$_5$
        222
    cause of elevated lipid levels
        (plasma) 283 (t)
    cause of elevated serum globulin
        215
    cause of elevated thyroxine-
        binding globulin 249 (t)
    cause of hypermagnesemia 106
    chronic, antineutrophil cyto-
        plasmic antibodies in 381
    from cyclosporine 77